# Effects of Polyphenol-Rich Foods on Human Health

## Volume 1

# Effects of Polyphenol-Rich Foods on Human Health

## Volume 1

Special Issue Editor

**Giuseppe Grosso**

MDPI • Basel • Beijing • Wuhan • Barcelona • Belgrade

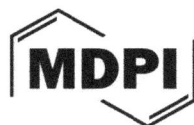

**MDPI**

*Special Issue Editor*
Giuseppe Grosso
Azienda Ospedaliera Universitaria Policlinico Vittorio Emanuele
Italy

*Editorial Office*
MDPI
St. Alban-Anlage 66
Basel, Switzerland

This is a reprint of articles from the Special Issue published online in the open access journal *Nutrients* (ISSN 2072-6643) from 2017 to 2018 (available at: http://www.mdpi.com/journal/nutrients/special_issues/polyphenol_rich_foods)

For citation purposes, cite each article independently as indicated on the article page online and as indicated below:

LastName, A.A.; LastName, B.B.; LastName, C.C. Article Title. *Journal Name* **Year**, *Article Number*, Page Range.

**Volume 1**
**ISBN 978-3-03897-135-1 (Pbk)**
**ISBN 978-3-03897-136-8 (PDF)**

**Volume 1–3**
**ISBN 978-3-03897-145-0 (Pbk)**
**ISBN 978-3-03897-146-7 (PDF)**

# Contents

# About the Special Issue Editor

**Giuseppe Grosso**'s research focuses on evidence-based nutrition, a recently emerged field as the bottom line of the Health Technology Assessment applied to food and nutrition. The main interests include the impact of dietary and lifestyle habits on common non-communicable diseases. In particular, he produced over 100 papers on the effects of dietary patterns (i.e., Mediterranean diet) and specific antioxidant-rich foods (i.e., coffee, tea), as well as individual antioxidants (i.e., polyphenols, n-3 PUFA) on cardiovascular and metabolic diseases, cancer, and depression. Dr. Grosso conducted his research on cohorts of individuals in both Mediterranean and non-Mediterranean countries collaborating with several research institutions. He is interested in evidence synthesis aimed to generate policy-oriented research in the area of public health nutrition. He is currently working as research fellow at Integrated Cancer Registry of Catania-Messina-Siracusa-Enna, southern Italy. He is a cum-laude graduated MD and PhD.

# Preface to "Effects of Polyphenol-Rich Foods on Human Health"

The global burden of non-communicable diseases (NCDs) has been rising over the last century, and among the main NCDs are cardiovascular diseases (CVDs), cancers and diabetes. Besides genetic, environmental, and social factors, exploring dietary factors influencing such conditions is of primary importance to better define effective strategies for reducing the burden of disease. In fact, higher adherence to healthy and equilibrated dietary patterns has been shown to be implicated in prevention of NCDs.

In recent years, polyphenols have received a great deal of attention due to their potential beneficial effects on human health. Contained in foods commonly consumed in all populations worldwide, polyphenols offer a range of beneficial effects and are contained not only in fruits and vegetables, characteristic components of healthy dietary patterns, but also in other plant-derived foods, such as tea, coffee, and cocoa, which only recently have been scientifically exploited as being beneficial for humans. In addition to the numerous biological properties, polyphenols have been indicated as being responsible for a decreased risk of several health outcomes. Numerous epidemiological studies have demonstrated the association between both polyphenols and polyphenol-rich foods intake and human health. For example, recent meta-analyses show that high consumption of polyphenols and polyphenol-rich foods decrease the risk of overall and CVD-related mortality, cancer, CVD, diabetes and neurodegenerative diseases. However, some studies reported null results, which could be at least partially explained by significant differences in dietary intake of polyphenols in different populations, differences in food processing (loss of phenolic content), absorption, bioavailability, and metabolism of polyphenols.

Several molecular mechanisms have been taken into account for the beneficial effects of polyphenols. The antioxidant effects of dietary polyphenols can be attributed to the regulation of redox enzymes through reducing reactive oxygen species (ROS) production and modulation of the II-phase enzymes responsible for the cellular oxidative response. Moreover, several studies have suggested that polyphenols may exert protective effects on cardio-metabolic health by reducing inflammatory response, lowering LDL oxidation and blood pressure, and by improving endothelial function. Finally, polyphenols may exert chemo-preventive effects through a variety of mechanisms, including elimination of carcinogenic agents, modulation of pathways responsible for cancer cell signaling and cell cycle progression, and by promotion of apoptosis.

Even though research is ongoing, further evidence is needed in order to better characterize dietary factors that may exert beneficial effects toward prevention of chronic diseases associated with oxidative stress and inflammation.

**Giuseppe Grosso**
*Special Issue Editor*

*nutrients*

MDPI

*Article*

# Absorption Profile of (Poly)Phenolic Compounds after Consumption of Three Food Supplements Containing 36 Different Fruits, Vegetables, and Berries

**Letizia Bresciani [1], Daniela Martini [1], Pedro Mena [1], Michele Tassotti [1], Luca Calani [2], Giacomo Brigati [1], Furio Brighenti [1], Sandra Holasek [3], Daniela-Eugenia Malliga [4], Manfred Lamprecht [5,6] and Daniele Del Rio [1,7,*]**

[1]    The Laboratory of Phytochemicals in Physiology, Human Nutrition Unit, Department of Food & Drug, University of Parma, 43125 Parma, Italy; letizia.bresciani@unipr.it (L.B.); daniela.martini@unipr.it (D.M.); pedromiguel.menaparreno@unipr.it (P.M.); michele.tassotti@studenti.unipr.it (M.T.); giacomo.brigati@studenti.unipr.it (G.B.); furio.brighenti@unipr.it (F.B.)
[2]    Department of Food & Drug, University of Parma, 43124 Parma, Italy; luca.calani@unipr.it
[3]    Institute of Pathophysiology and Immunology, Medical University of Graz, A-8010 Graz, Austria; sandra.holasek@medunigraz.at
[4]    Division of Cardiac Surgery, Department of Surgery, Medical University of Graz, A-8010 Graz, Austria; daniela-eugenia.martin@medunigraz.at
[5]    Institute of Physiological Chemistry, Medical University of Graz, A-8010 Graz, Austria; manfred.lamprecht@medunigraz.at
[6]    Green Beat—Institute of Nutrient Research and Sport Nutrition, 8042 Graz, Austria
[7]    The Need for Nutrition Education/Innovation Programme (NNEdPro), Global Centre for Nutrition and Health, St John's Innovation Centre, Cambridge CB4 0WS, UK
[*]    Correspondence: daniele.delrio@unipr.it; Tel.: +39-0521-903-830

Received: 30 January 2017; Accepted: 23 February 2017; Published: 26 February 2017

**Abstract:** The market of plant-based nutraceuticals and food supplements is continuously growing due to the increased consumer demand. The introduction of new products with relevant nutritional characteristics represents a new way of providing bioactive compounds and (poly)phenols to consumers, becoming a strategy to ideally guarantee the health benefits attributed to plant foodstuffs and allowing the increase of daily bioactive compound intake. A paramount step in the study of nutraceuticals is the evaluation of the bioavailability and metabolism of their putatively active components. Therefore, the aim of the present study was to investigate the absorption profile of the (poly)phenolic compounds contained in three different plant-based food supplements, made of 36 different plant matrices, which were consumed by 20 subjects in an open one-arm study design. Blood samples were collected at baseline and 1, 2, 5, and 10 h after capsule intake. Twenty quantifiable metabolites deriving from different (poly)phenolic compounds were identified. Results showed that the consumption of the three capsules allowed the effective absorption of several (poly)phenolic compounds and metabolites appearing at different times in plasma, thereby indicating different absorption profiles. The capsules thus ensured potential health-promoting molecules to be potentially available to target tissues and organs.

**Keywords:** fruit and vegetables; capsules; (poly)phenolic compounds; absorption

## 1. Introduction

Daily consumption of five portions or at least 400 g of fruits and vegetables is promoted in many national and international dietary guidelines and by public policies [1,2]. An adequate consumption of fruit and vegetables has been associated with human health promotion thanks to their role in chronic disease prevention [3]. Conversely, it has been estimated that up to 2635 million deaths per year can be attributable to low fruit and vegetable consumption [4]. In detail, several scientific studies report the correlation between fruit and vegetable consumption with a reduction in all-cause mortality [5], a decrease in overall cancer risk [6], and prevention of metabolic diseases like type II diabetes [7,8]. Many national nutrition surveys have shown that the minimum population goal of 400 g of fruit and vegetables per day established by FAO/WHO is not easily met, especially in selected groups of population such as teenagers [9,10]. However, nowadays, consumers are more aware of the health benefits associated with a healthy lifestyle, including high consumption of fruit and vegetables, increasing their will to buy products rich in bioactive compounds [11]. In this context, consumer health demands have boosted the market of plant-based nutraceuticals and food supplements, encouraging the introduction of new products with relevant nutritional characteristics. These products represent new ways of providing bioactive compounds to consumers, becoming a relevant strategy to ideally guarantee the health benefits attributed to plant foodstuffs [12] and allowing the increase of daily bioactive compound intake.

The nutritional relevance of fruit and vegetables on human health could be attributed to their dietary fiber content, mainly soluble, as well as to a large range of micronutrients, including carotenoids, vitamins (mainly vitamin C, and folate), and minerals (as potassium, calcium, and magnesium). In addition, fruit and vegetables are well-recognized sources of non-nutrient bioactive compounds, also called "phytochemicals", among which (poly)phenolic compounds are the predominant and the most investigated [13–17]. The term (poly)phenol includes a number of different chemical structures, including flavonoids and related compounds, but also refers to hydroxycinnamates and phenolic acids, which have only one phenolic ring [18].

A growing amount of experimental research is trying hard to demonstrate the beneficial role of (poly)phenols in humans, trying to unravel the biological mechanisms behind the many proposed effects. Daily consumption of (poly)phenols has been related to reduction of inflammation, hypertension, risk of cardiovascular, metabolic, neurodegenerative diseases, and cancer [18–22]. An essential part of the scientific research in vivo is represented by the investigation of the absorption, metabolism and bioavailability of (poly)phenolic compounds after human intake. In fact, the large structure variety of this class of phytochemicals, together with the food matrices, complex human metabolic pathways and the role of human intestinal microbiota, can deeply influence the metabolism of (poly)phenol compounds, and as a consequence, the availability of their potentially beneficial metabolites to the human body's internal compartments.

The aim of the present study was to investigate the absorption profile of the (poly)phenolic compounds contained in three different plant-based food supplements, made of 36 different vegetal matrices, recently characterized for their (poly)phenol content [23], designed to integrate and increase the daily intake of dietary phenolics. The supplements have been previously shown to exert wide biological effects in diverse health conditions [24–28].

## 2. Materials and Methods

### 2.1. Subjects

The sample size of our study was based on the number of volunteers usually recruited for bioavailability studies involving (poly)phenolic compounds. However, seven subjects would have provided sufficient power ($\alpha$ error of 0.05, 80% power) to detect a minimum increase of 40 nmol/L in 2 h in the absorption kinetics of flavan-3-ols, based on available published data [29]. Twenty participants were recruited from the Graz region (comprising a radius of 50 km around the center of Graz, Austria) to take part in the study. Selected participants were 9 males (m) and 11 females (f) with the following characteristics: age 34.3 ± 9.9 (m) and 32.9 ± 9.1 (f), weight 71.9 ± 11.7 (m) and 63.6 ± 9.4 (f) kg, height 174 ± 9 (m) and 167 ± 9 (f) cm and BMI

23.2 ± 3.0 (m) and 22.8 ± 3.05 (f) (kg/m$^2$) (data expressed as mean ± SD). The volunteers had to meet all the inclusion and exclusion criteria. Subjects had to be non-smokers, with a BMI between 20 and 30 kg/m$^2$, not on medication, not premenopausal, following normal dietary habits (no specific diets, meals and food components.) and adhering to a wash-out period. Exclusion criteria included: not consuming more than four servings of fruits and vegetables per day, not having any type of food allergy or histamine intolerance, not displaying a high level of physical activity (defined as more than five training units/week), not having menstrual dysfunctions and not abusing alcohol.

All participants were informed about the purpose of the study via telephone calls or personal meetings. Subjects who wanted to join the study signed the informed consent form before their inclusion in the trial. Moreover, the selected subjects received a (poly)phenol-poor diet plan which they had to adhere to for 48 h before the first blood sampling. The list of permitted and forbidden foods is provided in Table S1. Relevant principles of Good Clinical Practice were followed throughout the study. The study was conducted according to the guidelines laid down in the Declaration of Helsinki, and all procedures involving human subjects were approved by the Ethics Committee of the Medical University of Graz, Austria, (EC-number: 27-507ex14/15). The trial was registered at www.clinicaltrials.gov (identifier No. NCT02587468).

### 2.2. Test Capsules

Capsules used for the study were provided by the Juice Plus Company/NSA LLC, Collierville, TN, USA and manufactured for Europe by Natural Alternatives International (NAI), Manno, Switzerland. The capsules contained powdered juice concentrate derived from 36 different fruits, vegetables, and berries including juice and pulp from different vegetal matrices, namely Juice PLUS+® Vineyard (a berry blend), Juice PLUS+® Fruit Blend and Juice PLUS+® Vegetable Blend, which were kindly supplied by the Juice PLUS+® company. In detail, the powder samples differed for their composition: Juice PLUS+® Vineyard (hereafter called "berry blend") contained 750 mg of dried powder blend of juice and pulp from grapes and berries (45.7%) including Concord grape, blueberry, cranberry, blackberry, bilberry, raspberry, redcurrant, blackcurrant, elderberry, in varying proportions, besides green tea, ginger root, grape seed, artichoke leaf powder, cocoa powder, and pomegranate powder. Juice PLUS+® Fruit Blend ("fruit blend") instead contained 750 mg of dried powder blend of juice and pulp (52%) of apple, orange, pineapple, cranberry, peach, acerola cherry, papaya, in varying proportions, beet root, date, and prune. Lastly, Juice PLUS+® Vegetable Blend ("vegetable blend") contained 750 mg of dried powder blend of juice and pulp (60%) of carrot, parsley, beet, kale, broccoli, cabbage, tomato, and spinach, in varying proportions, as well as sugar beet, garlic powder, oat, and rice bran. Moreover, the fruit and the vegetable powders were enriched with vitamins C, and folic acid) and with a natural carotenoid and tocopherol blend. The berry blend powder was enriched with vitamins C and folic acid as well as with a natural tocopherol blend.

### 2.3. Study Design

In an open one-arm study design, three capsules (one berry, fruit, and one vegetable blend), were consumed by each participant on one single occasion. Before the test meal, participants were asked to follow a two-week wash-out period avoiding all food supplements and dietetic products and all kinds of drugs/medications. Additionally, participants were asked to consume a (poly)phenol-poor diet 48 h before the test day. To facilitate participant adherence to the dietary restrictions, a list of permitted and forbidden foods was supplied. The day of the test, subjects visited the lab after an overnight fast, and after the baseline blood drawing (T$_0$), they received the three capsules (one of each blend), to be consumed with 250 mL of still water. Four additional blood samples were collected, at 1, 2, 5, and 10 h after capsule intake. After the 2 h blood sampling, the subjects consumed a standardized (poly)phenol-poor snack, including white bread, cheese, ham, milk, and water *ad libitum*, in accordance to Pereira-Caro [30]. For each blood drawing, 5 mL of venous EDTA-blood from the elbow were collected via vein catheter, in supine position. Blood was immediately centrifuged at 2500 g for ten minutes to separate the plasma, which was frozen at −70 °C until uHPLC/MS$^n$ analyses.

### 2.4. Chemicals

All chemicals and solvents were of analytical grade. 3-Hydroxybenzoic acid, protocatechuic acid, 3-hydroxyphenylpropionic acid, hippuric acid, dihydrocaffeic acid, ferulic acid, dihydroferulic acid, (+)-catechin, 3-caffeoylquinic acid, 5-caffeoylquinic acid, quercetin 3-glucuronide, (hydroxyphenyl)-γ-valeric acid, and pyrogallol were purchased from Sigma-Aldrich (St. Louis, MO, USA). Dihydrocaffeic acid 3-O-sulfate, ferulic acid 4′-O-sulfate, dihydroferulic acid 4′-O-sulfate, caffeic acid 4′-O-glucuronide, dihydrocaffeic acid 3-O-glucuronide, isoferulic acid 3-O-glucuronide were purchased from Toronto Research Chemicals (Toronto, ON, Canada). (3′-hydroxyphenyl)-γ-valerolactone, (4′-hydroxyphenyl)-γ-valerolactone, (3′,5′-dihydroxyphenyl)-γ-valerolactone, (3′,4′-dihydroxyphenyl)-γ-valerolactone, (3′,4′,5′-trihydroxyphenyl)-γ-valerolactone, phenyl-γ-valerolactone-4′-O-sulfate, phenyl-γ-valerolactone-3′-O-sulfate, (5′-hydroxyphenyl)-γ-valerolactone-3′-O-sulfate, (4′-hydroxyphenyl)-γ-valerolactone-3′-O-sulfate, phenyl-γ-valerolactone-3′-O-glucuronide, phenyl-γ-valerolactone-3′, 4′-di-O-sulfate, and (5′-hydroxyphenyl)-γ-valerolactone-3′-O-glucuronide were synthesized in house using the synthetic strategy previously outlined by Curti and colleagues [31] and following known procedures reported in the literature [32,33]. Feruloylglycine, 4-hydroxyhippuric acid, quercetin 3′-O-sulfate, hesperetin 3′-O-glucuronide, and hesperetin 7-O-glucuronide were kindly supplied by Professor Alan Crozier. Vanillic acid and (3-methoxy, 4-hydroxyphenyl)acetic acid were purchased from Alfa Aesar (Thermo Fisher (Kandel) GmbH, Postfach, Karlsruhe, Germany) and from Extrasynthese (Genay Cedex, France), respectively. Naringenin 4′-O-glucuronide and naringenin 7-O-glucuronide were purchased from Bertin Pharma (Montigny le Bretonneux, France). Ultrapure water from MilliQsystem (Millipore, Bedford, MA, USA) was used throughout the experiment.

### 2.5. Plasma Extraction

Plasma samples of all volunteers were extracted using a solid phase extraction (SPE) method as reported by Urpi-Sarda and colleagues, with some modifications [34]. Oasis® HLB Vac cartridges (1 cc, 30 mg sorbent, 30 μm particle size) (Waters, Milford, Massachusetts, MA, USA) were conditioned with 1 mL of methanol and equilibrated with 1 mL of water. An aliquot of 800 μL of plasma was added with 16 μL of o-phosphoric acid (2.5%) and then loaded into cartridges. The cartridges were washed with 1 mL of acidified water (0.1% formic acid) and finally eluted with 1 mL of methanol containing formic acid (1.5 mol/L). The eluates were evaporated overnight to dryness by means of a rotary speed-vacuum at room temperature and reconstituted with 80 μL of methanol/acidified water (0.1% formic acid) (50:50 *v*/*v*) prior uHPLC/MS$^n$ analysis.

### 2.6. UHPLC/MS$^n$ Analysis

Plasma extracts were analyzed by a UHPLC DIONEX Ultimate 3000 equipped with a triple quadrupole TSQ Vantage (Thermo Fisher Scientific Inc., San Josè, CA, USA) fitted with a heated-ESI (H-ESI) (Thermo Fisher Scientific Inc., San Josè, CA, USA) probe. Separations were carried out by means of a Kinetex EVO C18 (100 × 2.1 mm) column, 1.7 μm particle size (Phenomenex, Torrance, CA, USA).

For UHPLC, mobile phase A was acetonitrile containing 0.2% formic acid and mobile phase B was 0.2% formic acid in water. The gradient started with 5% A, isocratic conditions were maintained for 0.5 min, and reached 95% A after 6.5 min, followed by 1 min at 95%. The starting gradient was then immediately reestablished and maintained for 4 min to re-equilibrate the column. The flow rate was 0.4 mL/min, the injection volume was 5 μL, and the column temperature was set at 40 °C.

The applied mass spectrometry (MS) method consisted in the selective determination of each target precursor ion by the acquisition of characteristic product ions in selective reaction monitoring (SRM) mode (Table 1), applying a negative ionization.

**Table 1.** Spectrometric characteristics of the 92 monitored compounds, and standard compounds used for quantification of the 20 identified metabolites. Legend: SRM: selective reaction monitoring; ND: not detected.

| Compound | [M − H]⁻ | SRM Transition | S-Lens Value | Quantification |
|---|---|---|---|---|
| Catechol | 109 | 108, 81 | 68 | ND |
| Methylcatechol | 123 | 108, 81 | 68 | ND |
| Pyrogallol | 125 | 124, 81, 97 | 68 | ND |
| Hydroxybenzoic acid | 137 | 91, 93, 45 | 70 | ND |
| Hydroxyphenylacetic acid | 151 | 107 | 51 | ND |
| Dihydroxybenzoic acid | 153 | 108, 109 | 64 | ND |
| 3-(3'-Hydroxyphenyl)propionic acid | 165 | 119, 121 | 48 | ND |
| Vanillic acid | 167 | 152, 108, 123 | 60 | ND |
| Gallic acid | 169 | 125 | 68 | ND |
| Hippuric acid | 178 | 134 | 68 | Hippuric acid |
| (3'-Methoxy, 4'-hydroxyphenyl)acetic acid | 181 | 137 | 61 | ND |
| Dihydrocaffeic acid | 181 | 137, 119 | 64 | ND |
| Methylgallic acid | 183 | 168, 139 | 64 | ND |
| Catechol sulfate | 189 | 109, 81 | 70 | ND |
| (3'-Hydroxyphenyl)-γ-valerolactone | 191 | 147, 106 | 70 | ND |
| (4'-Hydroxyphenyl)-γ-valerolactone | 191 | 147, 173, 103, 107 | 70 | ND |
| Ferulic acid | 193 | 134, 178 | 71 | ND |
| (Hydroxyphenyl)-γ-valeric acid | 193 | 147, 149, 157, 175 | 72 | ND |
| 4-Hydroxyhippuric acid | 194 | 100, 150 | 72 | 4-Hydroxyhippuric acid |
| Dihydroferulic acid | 195 | 136 | 73 | ND |
| Syringic acid | 197 | 153, 182 | 73 | ND |
| Methylcatechol sulfate | 203 | 123, 108, 81 | 70 | ND |
| Pyrogallol sulfate | 205 | 125, 124, 81, 97 | 68 | Dihydrocaffeic acid 3-O-sulfate |
| (3',5'-Dihydroxyphenyl)-γ-valerolactone | 207 | 163, 123, 121 | 75 | ND |
| (3',4'-Dihydroxyphenyl)-γ-valerolactone | 207 | 163, 122 | 75 | ND |
| (3',5'-Dihydroxyphenyl)-γ-valeric acid | 209 | 101, 124, 147 | 63 | ND |
| (3',4'-Dihydroxyphenyl)-γ-valeric acid | 209 | 151, 165, 191, 194 | 63 | ND |
| Hydroxybenzoic acid sulfate | 217 | 137, 93, 45 | 70 | ND |
| Methyl-trihydroxybenzoic acid sulfate | 219 | 139, 124, 125, 81, 97 | 68 | Dihydroferulic acid 4'-O-sulfate |
| (3',4',5'-Trihydroxyphenyl)-γ-valerolactone | 223 | 179, 205, 138 | 75 | ND |
| Dihydroxybenzoic acid sulfate | 233 | 153, 108, 109 | 64 | Dihydrocaffeic acid 3-O-sulfate |
| Hydroxyphenylpropionic acid sulfate | 245 | 165, 121, 119 | 90 | Dihydrocaffeic acid 3-O-sulfate |
| Vanillic acid sulfate | 247 | 167, 152, 108, 123 | 90 | ND |
| Gallic acid sulfate | 249 | 169, 125 | 68 | ND |
| Feruloylglycine | 250 | 206, 134, 162, 191, 177 | 79 | Feruloylglycine |
| Dihydrocaffeic acid sulfate | 261 | 181, 137 | 96 | ND |
| Methylgallic acid sulfate | 263 | 183, 168, 125 | 68 | ND |
| Phenyl-γ-valerolactone-4'-O-sulfate | 271 | 191, 147 | 93 | ND |
| Phenyl-γ-valerolactone-3'-O-sulfate | 271 | 191, 147, 93, 80, 106 | 93 | Phenyl-γ-valerolactone-3'-O-sulfate |
| Ferulic acid sulfate | 273 | 193, 134, 178 | 92 | ND |
| Phenyl-γ-valeric acid-O-sulfate | 273 | 193, 175, 157, 149, 147 | 92 | ND |
| Dihydroferulic acid sulfate | 275 | 195, 136 | 75 | ND |
| (5'-Hydroxyphenyl)-γ-valerolactone-3'-O-sulfate | 287 | 207, 122, 163 | 96 | ND |
| (4'-hydroxyphenyl)-γ-valerolactone-3'-O-sulfate | 287 | 207, 109, 163 | 96 | (4'-Hydroxyphenyl)-γ-valerolactone-3'-O-sulfate |
| (Epi)catechin | 289 | 245, 203, 204.9 | 98 | ND |
| (Hydroxyphenyl)-γ-valeric acid-O-sulfate | 289 | 209, 191, 151, 147, 124, 101 | 92 | ND |
| Dihydroxyphenyl-γ-valerolactone-O-sulfate | 303 | 179, 223 | 90 | ND |
| Methyl(epi)catechin | 303 | 288, 245, 205 | 98 | ND |
| Hydroxybenzoic acid glucuronide | 313 | 137, 93, 45 | 70 | ND |
| (Methyl-hydroxyphenyl)-γ-valerolactone-O-sulfate | 317 | 222, 237 | 92 | ND |
| Dihydroxybenzoic acid glucuronide | 329 | 153, 108, 109 | 64 | ND |

Table 1. *Cont.*

| Compound | [M − H]⁻ | SRM Transition | S-Lens Value | Quantification |
|---|---|---|---|---|
| Gallic acid glucuronide | 345 | 169, 125 | 68 | ND |
| Apigenin sulfate | 349 | 269, 225 | 98 | ND |
| Naringenin sulfate | 351 | 271, 151 | 84 | ND |
| 3-Caffeoylquinic acid | 353 | 191, 179, 135 | 85 | ND |
| 5-Caffeoylquinic acid | 353 | 191 | 85 | ND |
| Caffeic acid glucuronide | 355 | 179, 135 | 87 | ND |
| Dihydrocaffeic acid glucuronide | 357 | 181, 137, 113 | 63 | ND |
| Kaempferol sulfate | 365 | 285, 257 | 90 | ND |
| Phenyl-γ-valerolactone-3′-O-glucuronide | 367 | 191, 113, 207 | 93 | ND |
| Phenyl-γ-valerolactone-3′,4′-di-O-sulfate | 367 | 287, 147 | 93 | ND |
| Ferulic acid glucuronide | 369 | 193, 178, 175 | 92 | Isoferulic acid 3′-O-glucuronide |
| (Epi)catechin sulfate | 369 | 289, 245, 203, 205 | 98 | ND |
| Dihydroxyphenyl-γ-valeric acid disulfate | 369 | 209, 191, 151, 147, 124 | 92 | ND |
| Diosmetin sulfate | 379 | 299, 284 | 90 | Quercetin 3′-O-sulfate |
| Quercetin 3′-sulfate | 381 | 301, 151, 179 | 83 | Quercetin 3′-O-sulfate |
| Hesperetin sulfate | 381 | 301, 151, 179 | 115 | Quercetin 3′-O-sulfate |
| (4′-hydroxyphenyl)-γ-valerolactone-3′-O-glucuronide | 383 | 207, 163 | 87 | (5′-hydroxyphenyl)-γ-valerolactone-3′-O-glucuronide |
| Methyl(epi)katechin sulfate | 383 | 303, 288, 245, 205 | 98 | ND |
| (Epi)gallocatechin sulfate | 385 | 305, 179, 221 | 98 | ND |
| Myricetin sulfate | 397 | 317, 316, 179 | 90 | ND |
| Dihydroxyphenyl-γ-valerolactone-O-glucuronide | 399 | 223, 175, 179 | 87 | ND |
| Methyl(epi)gallocatechin sulfate | 411 | 319, 304, 179, 221 | 98 | ND |
| Patuletin sulfate | 411 | 331, 316, 209 | 90 | ND |
| Spinacetin sulfate | 425 | 345, 330 | 90 | Quercetin 3′-O-sulfate |
| Apigenin glucuronide | 445 | 269, 225 | 90 | ND |
| Naringenin 4′-glucuronide | 447 | 271 151, 379, 119 | 112 | Naringenin 4′-O-glucuronide |
| Naringenin 7-glucuronide | 447 | 271, 151 | 84 | ND |
| Kaempferol glucuronide | 461 | 285, 257 | 90 | Quercetin 3-O-glucuronide |
| Phenyl-γ-valerolactone-3′,4′-O-sulfate-O-glucuronide | 463 | 163, 207, 287, 383 | 87 | ND |
| (Epi)catechin glucuronide | 465 | 289, 245, 205 | 98 | ND |
| Diosmetin glucuronide | 475 | 299, 284 | 90 | ND |
| Quercetin 3-glucuronide | 477 | 301, 151, 179 | 91 | Quercetin 3-O-glucuronide |
| Hesperetin 3′-glucuronide | 477 | 301, 113 | 115 | ND |
| Hesperetin 7-glucuronide | 477 | 301, 151 | 115 | Hesperetin 7-O-glucuronide |
| Methyl(epi)catechin glucuronide | 479 | 303, 288, 245, 205 | 98 | ND |
| Hydroxyphenyl-γ-valerolactone-O-sulfate-O-glucuronide | 479 | 303, 223, 175, 259 | 91 | ND |
| (Epi)gallocatechin glucuronide | 481 | 305, 179, 221 | 98 | ND |
| Myricetin glucuronide | 493 | 317, 316, 209 | 90 | Quercetin 3-O-glucuronide |
| Methyl(epi)gallocatechin glucuronide | 495 | 319, 304, 179, 221 | 98 | ND |
| Patuletin glucuronide | 507 | 331, 316, 209 | 90 | ND |
| Spinacetin glucuronide | 521 | 345, 330 | 90 | ND |

To optimize the method, all the available standard compounds were infused into the MS to set the best mass parameters and to check the actual fragmentation patterns. Finally, for all the analyses, the spray voltage was set at 3 kV, the vaporizer temperature at 300 °C, and the capillary temperature operated at 270 °C. The sheath gas flow was 60 units, and auxiliary gas pressure was set to 10 units. Ultrahigh purity argon gas was used for collision-induced dissociation (CID). The S-lens values were defined for each compound based on infusion parameter optimization (Table 1). Conversely, for compounds that were not available for infusion, the S-lens values were set using the values obtained for the chemically closest available standards. Quantification was performed with calibration curves of standards, when available (Table 1). Data processing was performed using Xcalibur software (Thermo Scientific Inc., Waltham, MA, USA). All data were expressed as mean values ± SEM.

## 3. Results

*(Poly)Phenolic Compound Absorption*

The capsules consumed in the present study were previously characterized for (poly)phenolic profile and quantified for their total phenolic content [23]. Capsules were made of 36 different plant matrices, and contained a wide array of different phenolic compounds, principally ellagitannins, flavan-3-ols, flavonols, and anthocyanins in berry blend capsules, flavones, flavonols, flavanones, and anthocyanins in fruit blend capsules, and flavones and flavonols in vegetable blend capsules.

Out of the 92 monitored molecules, 20 quantifiable metabolites were identified, or tentatively identified in plasma samples. All the quantified metabolites were found as conjugated compounds with sulfate, glucuronide or glycine moieties. Three glycine-conjugated metabolites, hippuric acid, 4-hydroxyhippuric acid, and feruloylglycine, were detected. A total of five metabolites were flavonol derivatives, including conjugates of quercetin, kaempferol, myricetin, and patuletin. Three metabolites were directly linked to flavanone metabolism, namely naringenin, and hesperetin derivatives, whereas only one flavone metabolite, namely diosmetin sulfate, was detected. Among flavan-3-ol derivatives, three conjugated phenyl-γ-valerolactones were detected. Finally, five metabolites were small phenolic derivatives, including hydroxyphenylpropionic acid sulfate, ferulic acid glucuronide, pyrogallol sulfate, dihydroxybenzoic acid sulfate, and methyl-trihydroxybenzoic acid sulfate. Generally, with the exception of hippuric acid, plasma levels of the quantified metabolites did not exceed the nanomolar range. Considering those metabolites for which the origin is strictly attributable to (poly)phenolic compounds contained in the capsules, the most abundant metabolites resulted in the low molecular weight phenolics which are usually produced in the colon by microbial transformation of flavonoids.

The glycine-conjugated metabolites are ubiquitous and could originate both by endogenous precursors [18,35] and by microbial metabolism of phenolic compounds [36–38]. Their potential endogenous origin justifies the high concentration at baseline (Figure S1).

Actually, the absorption curves of hippuric acid and 4-hydroxyhippuric acid did not show a notable concentration peak and their levels were basically constant during the study period. On the contrary, feruloylglycine exhibited a peak plasma concentration 2 h after consumption, indicating a stronger connection with the phenolic compounds introduced through the capsules, as only the capsules were consumed within the 2 h.

Looking to the other circulating metabolites appearing after capsule consumption, two metabolic phases could be easily distinguished. Conjugated metabolites appearing in the circulatory system within 1 or 2 h after capsule ingestion suggest an absorption in the first part of the gastro-intestinal tract. Native compounds are rapidly hydrolysed to release the aglycones, which are then conjugated by sulfotransferases (SULTs) and uridine-5′-diphosphate glucuronosyltransferases (UGTs) at both enterocyte and hepatic level before entering the systemic circulatory system [18]. Kaempferol glucuronide, quercetin glucuronide, quercetin sulfate, myricetin glucuronide, and diosmetin sulfate absorption curves are the expression of (poly)phenol metabolism in the first gastro-intestinal tract (Figure 1).

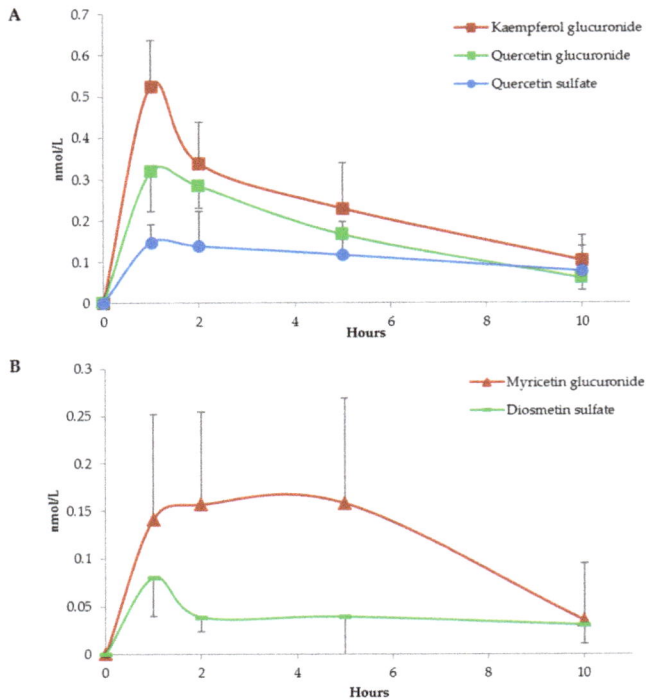

**Figure 1.** Absorption curves of kaempferol glucuronide, quercetin glucuronide, quercetin sulfate in graph (**A**); and myricetin glucuronide and diosmetin sulfate in graph (**B**). Data are expressed as mean values and bars represent standard error of means (SEM).

A concentration peak recorded between 5 and 10 h after test meal indicates, instead, a clear interaction between the indigested (poly)phenolic fraction and the colonic microbiota. The absorption profile outlined by patuletin sulfate and hesperetin sulfate likely represents a colonocyte level absorption and a subsequent conjugation at hepatic level (Figure 2). Actually, their plasmatic concentration reached a maximum level 5 h post capsule consumption.

Two quantified metabolites, namely naringenin glucuronide and hesperetin glucuronide, showed a double phase metabolism (Figure 3).

Probably, naringenin and hesperetin were partially cleaved in the first gastro-intestinal tract and rapidly absorbed and metabolized at intestinal/hepatic level, resulting in a first peak approximately 1 h after capsule ingestion. However, the peak between 5 and 10 h indicates a more important role of the colonic microbiota in flavanone metabolism [30]. Similarly, ferulic acid glucuronide absorption profile showed a double phase curve (Figure 3). Nevertheless, no ferulic acid was detected in the capsules [23], suggesting that this compound probably originated by catechol-*O*-methyltransferase (COMT) activity on other hydroxycinnamic acids present in the capsules [39].

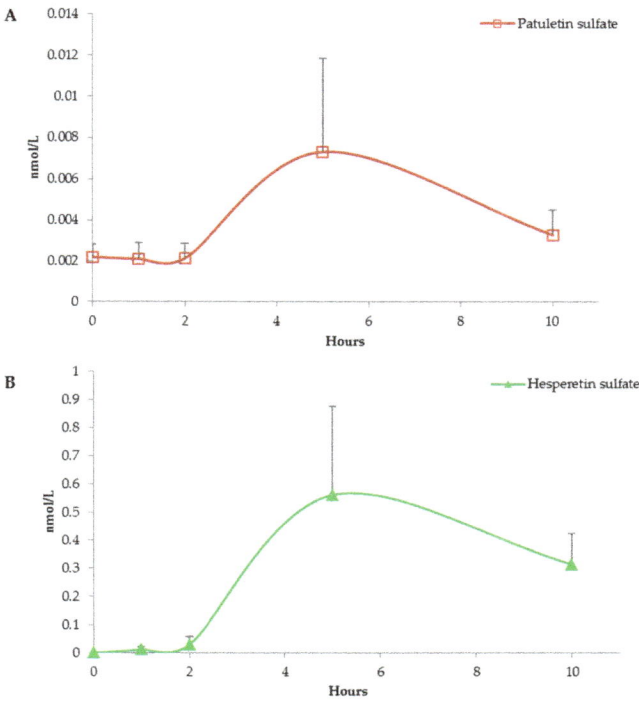

**Figure 2.** Absorption curves of patuletin sulfate in graph (**A**) and hesperetin sulfate in graph (**B**). Data are expressed as mean values and bars represent standard error of means (SEM).

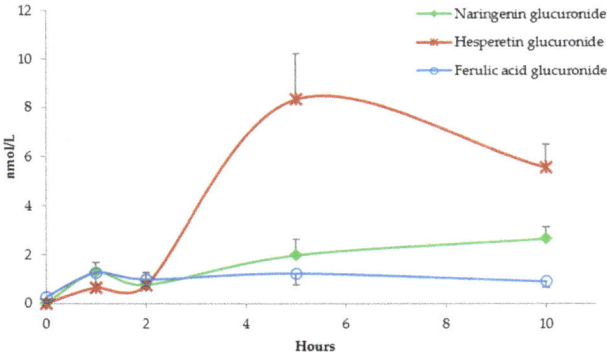

**Figure 3.** Absorption curves of naringenin glucuronide, hesperetin glucuronide, and ferulic acid glucuronide. Data are expressed as mean values and bars represent standard error of means (SEM).

Finally, most (poly)phenolic compounds passing unmodified and unabsorbed through the first gastro-intestinal tract become a suitable substrate for the locally hosted microbiota. Several modifications on native compounds have been reported to be catalyzed by microbial enzymes, resulting in the formation of low molecular weight compounds [40], which are efficiently absorbed by colonocytes before hepatic conjugation.

The three phenyl-γ-valerolactone derivatives, hydroxyphenylpropionic acid, pyrogallol, dihydroxybenzoic acid, and methyl-trihydroxybenzoic acid, having a peak concentration registered within 5 or 10 h, are typical metabolites generated by the host microbiota activity [41–43] (Figure 4).

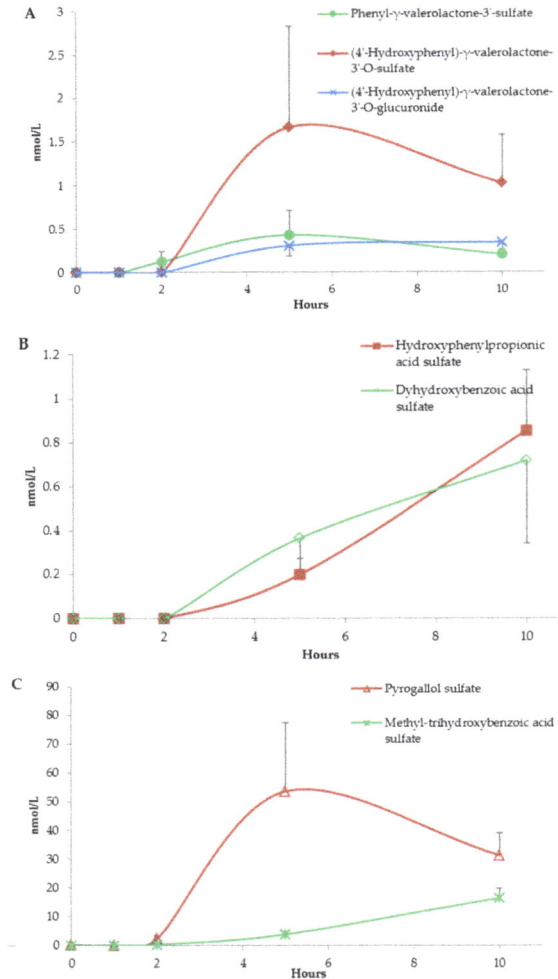

**Figure 4.** Absorption curves of phenyl-γ-valerolactone-3′-O-sulfate, (4′-hydroxyphenyl)-γ-valerolactone-3′-O-sulfate, and (4′-hydroxyphenyl)-γ-valerolactone-3′-O-glucuronide in graph (**A**); hydroxyphenylpropionic acid sulfate and (dihydroxybenzoic acid sulfate in graph (**B**); and pyrogallol sulfate and methyl-trihydroxybenzoic acid sulfate in graph (**C**). Data are expressed as mean values and bars represent standard error of means (SEM).

## 4. Discussion

In the present study, the absorption profile of (poly)phenolic compounds derived from the ingestion of Juice PLUS+® berry, fruit and vegetable blend capsules has been investigated. A total of 20 circulating metabolites have been identified, or tentatively identified, and quantified. As expected, detected metabolites derived from different (poly)phenols and appeared at different times in plasma. Flavonol metabolites principally originated in the first part of the gastro-intestinal tract, as previously reported by other authors. Feliciano and colleagues [41] reported a time to reach the maximum plasma concentration ($T_{max}$) for kaempferol 3-*O*-glucuronide and quercetin 3-*O*-glucuronide of about 2 h. An absorption curve similar to those reported in the present study for quercetin 3-glucuronide and quercetin 3-sulfate was reported by Mullen and colleagues, who highlighted a concentration peak between 1 and 2 h after onion ingestion [44]. To the best of our knowledge, this is the first study in which plasma concentrations of patuletin and myricetin metabolites have been reported, suggesting that other flavonols could be effectively absorbed and hence investigated for their potential bioactivity. Moreover, a new flavone metabolite at plasmatic level has been detected, namely diosmetin sulfate. Its early peak plasma level registered at 1 h is in contrast with scientific data previously reported for other flavones, like apigenin. The $T_{max}$ of apigenin (measured as aglycone after enzymatic hydrolysis) has been reported to be around 7 h after consumption of parsley [45]. The few human feeding studies involving flavones available so far reported a low bioavailability for this phytochemical [18,46], which could be ascribable to the low absorption of flavones, as demonstrated in the present investigation. Conversely, several scientific data are available for naringenin and hesperetin absorption, and all studies agree about the importance of colonic microbiota activity on this class of (poly)phenols [47–49]. The absorption curves observed in the present work confirm that flavanone metabolism principally occurs in the large intestine. Brett and colleagues reported a plasma concentration peak of flavanone conjugates 6 h after orange consumption [50], whereas the highest naringenin and hesperetin derivative urinary excretion has been reported within 2 and 10 h after orange juice consumption [30]. Flavan-3-ols were the most representative compounds in berry blend capsules [23]. However, no catechin monomer conjugates nor dimers or oligomeric proanthocyanidins were detected in plasma. However, in vivo studies have shown that both monomers and high molecular weight flavan-3-ols are effectively degraded by the gut microbiota into hydroxyphenyl-γ-valerolactones [51–53]. Many phenyl-γ-valerolactone derivatives have been detected after green tea [51,54], cocoa [34,55,56], wine [57] and almond [58] consumption. Partially compensating for the absence of flavan-3-ol monomers in plasma in the present study, three phenyl-γ-valerolactones were detected and quantified.

It was then demonstrated that phenyl-γ-valerolactones represent an intermediate step in the microbial metabolism of flavan-3-ols and that other low molecular weight compounds, such as phenylacetic, phenylpropionic, benzoic acids derivatives [59] and hippuric acid, which derive from benzoic acids [60], could be formed. Likewise, flavonols, flavones, and flavanones, could be degraded into smaller phenolics, namely phenylacetic, phenylpropionic, and benzoic acid derivatives [61]. Similarly, anthocyanins undergo an important colonic set of transformations, giving rise to low molecular weight metabolites. After glucosidic cleavage of the sugar moiety, cyanidin could be the precursor of caffeic acid, from which ferulic and isoferulic acids could be formed after COMT activity [62–64]. Ferulic acid may undergo further phase II metabolism, namely sulfation and glucuronidation, generating conjugated ferulic derivatives [39,65]. Feliciano and colleagues recently hypothesized that peonidin could also lead to the formation of ferulic acids [41]. Moreover, anthocyanins could be converted into small phenolics such as phenylpropionic, phenylacetic, benzoic acids, and pyrogallol [62,64,66].

Concerning pyrogallol, the high plasmatic concentration of pyrogallol sulfate between 5 and 10 h recorded in the present study is in agreement with a $T_{max}$ reported after cranberry consumption [41]. Gallic acid, which was present in the capsules, could have contributed to the formation of small metabolites [67], but also to other compounds like methylgallic acid [68], and, after phase II metabolism, to its 3-*O*-sulfate derivative [69].

It now appears clear that the extensive bioconversion of (poly)phenol compounds strictly depends on the characteristics of individual colonic microbiota, and differences in microbiota composition now allow to discriminate phenotypes associated with producers and non-producers of specific metabolites [67,70,71]. As a matter of fact, inter-individual differences in the intestinal ecology may lead to differences in bioavailability, linked to specific metabolite production and, ideally, to differences in health benefits [72]. In the present study, the absorption of phenolics and the production of their metabolites is accompanied by a considerable inter-individual variability, plausibly due to the interaction between these compounds and the gut microbiota of the host. A clear example of this large variability among participants concerns the circulating concentration of phenyl-γ-valerolactones resulting from the catabolic transformations of catechins and procyanidins, operated mainly by *Clostridium coccoides* and *Bifidobacterium* spp. [73]. By analyzing the absorption curves of each participants, five subjects resulted as abundant producers of phenyl-γ-valerolactones, whereas the remaining subjects produced only extremely small amounts of these compounds (data not shown), suggesting marked variations in the colonic microflora of the individual volunteers. The inter-individual variability can affect not only the quantity of metabolites but also the timing of their appearance. For instance, the wide bars observed in the curves of kaempferol glucuronide are ascribable to the fact that these metabolites disappeared after 5 and 10 h in almost all the participants with the only exception of two subjects, who showed a second, later peak, probably due to colonic absorption. Considering this large variability, there is an increased interest in stratifying future study participants based on their polyphenol-metabolizing phenotypes (i.e., metabotypes) [72], and the present study supports the hypothesis that this variability should be carefully considered as a confounder of in vivo studies evaluating health effects of these phytochemicals. Finally, considering all the circulating detected metabolites, excluding those compounds whose origin could be attributed to endogenous precursors, such as hippuric acid, 4-hydroxyhippuric acid, and feruloylglycine [18,35], a "global" curve could be depicted to summarize the totality of quantified phenolic metabolites at every specific time point (Figure 5). Observing this graph, some considerations can be drawn: (i) the absorption and metabolism of (poly)phenols in the first gastro-intestinal tract (1–2 h after capsule ingestion) is low when compared to what occurs in the colon (5–10 h after capsule consumption); (ii) the plasma curves of the phenolic metabolites clearly highlighted the deep interaction between these compounds and the gut microbiota; (iii) the beneficial effects attributed to the regular consumption of these capsules does not depend on very high concentration of phenolic metabolites circulating after their consumption. In fact, plasmatic metabolites rarely exceeded nanomolar concentrations, as previously reported [18,19]. However, the effect of the regular and long time intake of these products may modify the way our organism interacts with the contained phenolics, perhaps improving its ability to absorb some of them at small intestinal level. Moreover, a modulation of the colonic microbiota in the long run seems plausible, perhaps in the direction of improved transformations, leading to increased absorption of microbial metabolites. Finally, the large variability observed in this short acute absorption study should be taken into consideration in future interventions, as not all the recruited volunteers might deal with Juice PLUS+® phenolics in the same way.

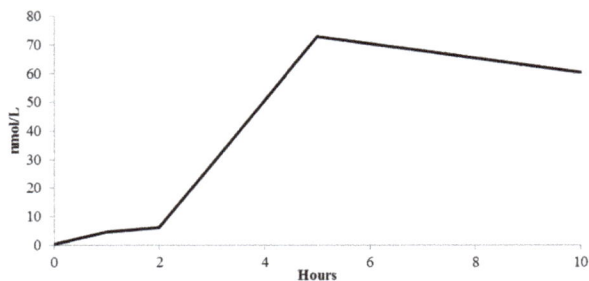

**Figure 5.** Total concentration of all circulating (poly)phenol metabolites, excluding hippuric acid, 4-hydroxyhippuric acid, and feruloylglycine. Data are expressed as mean values.

## 5. Conclusions

In conclusion, the consumption of Juice PLUS+® Vineyard, Fruit, Vegetable blend, containing 36 different fruits, vegetables, and berries, allowed the effective absorption of several (poly)phenolic compounds. The capsules therefore ensure potential health-promoting molecules to be potentially available to target tissues and organs, presumably becoming responsible for the previously observed health effects.

**Supplementary Materials:** The following are available online at http://www.mdpi.com/2072-6643/9/3/194/s1, Table S1: List of forbidden and permitted foods during the (poly)phenol-poor diet. Figure S1: Absorption curves of (a) hippuric acid, (b) 4-hydroxyhippuric acid, (c) feruloylglycine. Data are expressed as mean values and bars represent standard error of means (SEM).

**Acknowledgments:** Sponsor/Funder is Green Beat—Institute of Nutrient Research and Sports Nutrition, Petersbergenstrasse 95b, 8042 Graz, Austria.

**Author Contributions:** Manfred Lamprecht and Daniele Del Rio conceived and designed the experiments; Manfred Lamprecht, Daniela-Eugenia Malliga and Sandra Holasek performed the experiments; Daniela-Eugenia Malliga was the study physician, Letizia Bresciani and Giacomo Brigati analyzed the samples and the data; Pedro Mena, Michele Tassotti and Luca Calani contributed with materials and analysis tools; Letizia Bresciani and Daniela Martini wrote the paper; Furio Brighenti critically read and improved the manuscript.

**Conflicts of Interest:** Manfred Lamprecht is research consultant of The Juice Plus+® Company, NSA LLC.

## References

1. Agudo, A. Measuring intake of fruit and vegetables. In *Joint FAO/WHO Workshop on Fruit and Vegetables for Health, WHO/FAO, Kobe, Japan, 1–3 September 2004*; World Health Organization: Geneva, Switzerland, 2005.
2. World Health Organization. *European Action Plan for Food and Nutrition Policy 2007–2012*; World Health Organization: Copenhagen, Denmark, 2008.
3. Boeing, H.; Bechthold, A.; Bub, A.; Ellinger, S.; Haller, D.; Kroke, A.; Leschik-Bonnet, E.; Muller, M.J.; Oberritter, H.; Schulze, M.; et al. Critical review: Vegetables and fruit in the prevention of chronic diseases. *Eur. J. Nutr.* **2012**, *51*, 637–663. [CrossRef] [PubMed]
4. Lock, K.; Pomerleau, J.; Causer, L.; Altmann, D.R.; McKee, M. The global burden of disease attributable to low consumption of fruit and vegetables: Implications for the global strategy on diet. *Bull. WHO* **2005**, *83*, 100–108. [PubMed]
5. Leenders, M.; Sluijs, I.; Ros, M.M.; Boshuizen, H.C.; Siersema, P.D.; Ferrari, P.; Weikert, C.; Tjonneland, A.; Olsen, A.; Boutron-Ruault, M.C.; et al. Fruit and vegetable consumption and mortality: European prospective investigation into cancer and nutrition. *Am. J. Epidemiol.* **2013**, *178*, 590–602. [CrossRef] [PubMed]
6. Boffetta, P.; Couto, E.; Wichmann, J.; Ferrari, P.; Trichopoulos, D.; Bueno-de-Mesquita, H.B.; van Duijnhoven, F.J.; Buchner, F.L.; Key, T.; Boeing, H.; et al. Fruit and vegetable intake and overall cancer risk in the European Prospective Investigation into Cancer and Nutrition (EPIC). *J. Natl. Cancer Inst.* **2010**, *102*, 529–537. [CrossRef] [PubMed]
7. Bazzano, L.A.; Li, T.Y.; Joshipura, K.J.; Hu, F.B. Intake of fruit, vegetables, and fruit juices and risk of diabetes in women. *Diabetes Care* **2008**, *31*, 1311–1317. [CrossRef] [PubMed]
8. Mursu, J.; Virtanen, J.K.; Tuomainen, T.P.; Nurmi, T.; Voutilainen, S. Intake of fruit, berries, and vegetables and risk of type 2 diabetes in Finnish men: The Kuopio Ischaemic Heart Disease Risk Factor Study. *Am. J. Clin. Nutr.* **2014**, *99*, 328–333. [CrossRef] [PubMed]
9. Public Health England; Food Standards Agency. *Results of the National Diet and Nutrition Survey (NDNS) Rolling Programme for 2008 and 2009 to 2011 and 2012*; National Diet and Nutrition Survey (NDNS); Public Health England: London, UK, 2014.
10. Leclercq, C.; Arcella, D.; Piccinelli, R.; Sette, S.; Le Donne, C.; Turrini, A. The Italian National Food Consumption Survey INRAN-SCAI 2005–06: Main results in terms of food consumption. *Public Health Nutr.* **2009**, *12*, 2504–2532. [CrossRef] [PubMed]
11. Niva, M. 'All foods affect health': Understandings of functional foods and healthy eating among health-oriented Finns. *Appetite* **2007**, *48*, 384–393. [CrossRef] [PubMed]

12. Nile, S.H.; Park, S.W. Edible berries: Bioactive components and their effect on human health. *Nutrition* **2014**, *30*, 134–144. [CrossRef] [PubMed]

13. Murphy, M.M.; Barraj, L.M.; Herman, D.; Bi, X.; Cheatham, R.; Randolph, R.K. Phytonutrient intake by adults in the United States in relation to fruit and vegetable consumption. *J. Acad. Nutr. Diet.* **2012**, *112*, 222–229. [CrossRef] [PubMed]

14. Liu, R.H. Dietary bioactive compounds and their health implications. *J. Food Sci.* **2013**, *78* (Suppl. 1), A18–A25. [CrossRef] [PubMed]

15. Grosso, G.; Stepaniak, U.; Topor-Madry, R.; Szafraniec, K.; Pajak, A. Estimated dietary intake and major food sources of polyphenols in the Polish arm of the HAPIEE study. *Nutrition* **2014**, *30*, 1398–1403. [CrossRef] [PubMed]

16. Pérez-Jiménez, J.; Fezeu, L.; Touvier, M.; Arnault, N.; Manach, C.; Hercberg, S.; Galan, P.; Scalbert, A. Dietary intake of 337 polyphenols in French adults. *Am. J. Clin. Nutr.* **2011**, *93*, 1220–1228. [CrossRef] [PubMed]

17. Tresserra-Rimbau, A.; Medina-Remon, A.; Perez-Jimenez, J.; Martinez-Gonzalez, M.A.; Covas, M.I.; Corella, D.; Salas-Salvado, J.; Gomez-Gracia, E.; Lapetra, J.; Aros, F.; et al. Dietary intake and major food sources of polyphenols in a Spanish population at high cardiovascular risk: The PREDIMED study. *Nutr. Metab. Cardiovasc. Dis.* **2013**, *23*, 953–959. [CrossRef] [PubMed]

18. Del Rio, D.; Rodriguez-Mateos, A.; Spencer, J.P.; Tognolini, M.; Borges, G.; Crozier, A. Dietary (poly)phenolics in human health: Structures, bioavailability, and evidence of protective effects against chronic diseases. *Antioxid. Redox Signal.* **2013**, *18*, 1818–1892. [CrossRef] [PubMed]

19. Rodriguez-Mateos, A.; Vauzour, D.; Krueger, C.G.; Shanmuganayagam, D.; Reed, J.; Calani, L.; Mena, P.; del Rio, D.; Crozier, A. Bioavailability, bioactivity and impact on health of dietary flavonoids and related compounds: An update. *Arch. Toxicol.* **2014**, *88*, 1803–1853. [CrossRef] [PubMed]

20. Grosso, G.; Stepaniak, U.; Micek, A.; Stefler, D.; Bobak, M.; Pajak, A. Dietary polyphenols are inversely associated with metabolic syndrome in Polish adults of the HAPIEE study. *Eur. J. Nutr.* **2016**. [CrossRef] [PubMed]

21. Liu, Y.J.; Zhan, J.; Liu, X.L.; Wang, Y.; Ji, J.; He, Q.Q. Dietary flavonoids intake and risk of type 2 diabetes: A meta-analysis of prospective cohort studies. *Clin. Nutr.* **2014**, *33*, 59–63. [CrossRef] [PubMed]

22. Grosso, G.; Godos, J.; Lamuela-Raventos, R.; Ray, S.; Micek, A.; Pajak, A.; Sciacca, S.; D'Orazio, N.; del Rio, D.; Galvano, F. A comprehensive meta-analysis on dietary flavonoid and lignan intake and cancer risk: Level of evidence and limitations. *Mol. Nutr. Food Res.* **2016**. [CrossRef] [PubMed]

23. Bresciani, L.; Calani, L.; Cossu, M.; Mena, P.; Sayegh, M.; Ray, S.; del Rio, D. (Poly)phenolic characterization of three food supplements containing 36 different fruits, vegetables and berries. *PharmaNutrition* **2015**, *3*, 11–19. [CrossRef]

24. Lamprecht, M.; Obermayer, G.; Steinbauer, K.; Cvirn, G.; Hofmann, L.; Ledinski, G.; Greilberger, J.F.; Hallstroem, S. Supplementation with a juice powder concentrate and exercise decrease oxidation and inflammation, and improve the microcirculation in obese women: Randomised controlled trial data. *Br. J. Nutr.* **2013**, *110*, 1685–1695. [CrossRef] [PubMed]

25. De Spirt, S.; Sies, H.; Tronnier, H.; Heinrich, U. An encapsulated fruit and vegetable juice concentrate increases skin microcirculation in healthy women. *Skin Pharmacol. Physiol.* **2012**, *25*, 2–8. [CrossRef] [PubMed]

26. Roll, S.; Nocon, M.; Willich, S.N. Reduction of common cold symptoms by encapsulated juice powder concentrate of fruits and vegetables: A randomised, double-blind, placebo-controlled trial. *Br. J. Nutr.* **2011**, *105*, 118–122. [CrossRef] [PubMed]

27. Nantz, M.P.; Rowe, C.A.; Nieves, C., Jr.; Percival, S.S. Immunity and antioxidant capacity in humans is enhanced by consumption of a dried, encapsulated fruit and vegetable juice concentrate. *J. Nutr.* **2006**, *136*, 2606–2610. [PubMed]

28. Plotnick, G.D.; Corretti, M.C.; Vogel, R.A.; Hesslink, R., Jr.; Wise, J.A. Effect of supplemental phytonutrients on impairment of the flow-mediated brachial artery vasoactivity after a single high-fat meal. *J. Am. Coll. Cardiol.* **2003**, *41*, 1744–1749. [CrossRef]

29. Ottaviani, J.I.; Momma, T.Y.; Heiss, C.; Kwik-Uribe, C.; Schroeter, H.; Keen, C.L. The stereochemical configuration of flavanols influences the level and metabolism of flavanols in humans and their biological activity in vivo. *Free Radic. Biol. Med.* **2011**, *50*, 237–244. [CrossRef] [PubMed]

30. Pereira-Caro, G.; Borges, G.; van der Hooft, J.; Clifford, M.N.; Del Rio, D.; Lean, M.E.; Roberts, S.A.; Kellerhals, M.B.; Crozier, A. Orange juice (poly)phenols are highly bioavailable in humans. *Am. J. Clin. Nutr.* **2014**, *100*, 1378–1384. [CrossRef] [PubMed]

31. Curti, C.; Brindani, N.; Battistini, L.; Sartori, A.; Pelosi, G.; Mena, P.; Brighenti, F.; Zanardi, F.; del Rio, D. Catalytic, Enantioselective Vinylogous Mukaiyama Aldol Reaction of Furan-Based Dienoxy Silanes: A Chemodivergent Approach to γ-Valerolactone Flavan-3-ol Metabolites and δ-Lactone Analogues. *Adv. Synth. Catal.* **2015**. [CrossRef]

32. Liu, Y.; Lien, I.F.; Ruttgaizer, S.; Dove, P.; Taylor, S.D. Synthesis and protection of aryl sulfates using the 2,2,2-trichloroethyl moiety. *Org. Lett.* **2004**, *6*, 209–212. [CrossRef] [PubMed]

33. Zhang, M.; Jagdmann, G.E., Jr.; Van Zandt, M.; Sheeler, R.; Beckett, P.; Schroeter, H. Chemical synthesis and characterization of epicatechin glucuronides and sulfates: Bioanalytical standards for epicatechin metabolite identification. *J. Nat. Prod.* **2013**, *76*, 157–169. [CrossRef] [PubMed]

34. Urpi-Sarda, M.; Monagas, M.; Khan, N.; Llorach, R.; Lamuela-Raventos, R.M.; Jauregui, O.; Estruch, R.; Izquierdo-Pulido, M.; Andres-Lacueva, C. Targeted metabolic profiling of phenolics in urine and plasma after regular consumption of cocoa by liquid chromatography-tandem mass spectrometry. *J. Chromatogr. A* **2009**, *1216*, 7258–7267. [CrossRef] [PubMed]

35. Kern, S.M.; Bennett, R.N.; Mellon, F.A.; Kroon, P.A.; Garcia-Conesa, M.T. Absorption of hydroxycinnamates in humans after high-bran cereal consumption. *J. Agric. Food Chem.* **2003**, *51*, 6050–6055. [CrossRef] [PubMed]

36. Bresciani, L.; Scazzina, F.; Leonardi, R.; Dall'Aglio, E.; Newell, M.; Dall'Asta, M.; Melegari, C.; Ray, S.; Brighenti, F.; del Rio, D. Bioavailability and metabolism of phenolic compounds from wholegrain wheat and aleurone-rich wheat bread. *Mol. Nutr. Food Res.* **2016**, *60*, 2343–2354. [CrossRef] [PubMed]

37. Roowi, S.; Mullen, W.; Edwards, C.A.; Crozier, A. Yoghurt impacts on the excretion of phenolic acids derived from colonic breakdown of orange juice flavanones in humans. *Mol. Nutr. Food Res.* **2009**, *53* (Suppl. 1), S68–S75. [CrossRef] [PubMed]

38. Mulder, T.P.; Rietveld, A.G.; van Amelsvoort, J.M. Consumption of both black tea and green tea results in an increase in the excretion of hippuric acid into urine. *Am. J. Clin. Nutr.* **2005**, *81* (Suppl. 1), 256S–260S. [PubMed]

39. Del Rio, D.; Stalmach, A.; Calani, L.; Crozier, A. Bioavailability of coffee chlorogenic acids and green tea flavan-3-ols. *Nutrients* **2010**, *2*, 820–833. [CrossRef] [PubMed]

40. Ozdal, T.; Sela, D.A.; Xiao, J.; Boyacioglu, D.; Chen, F.; Capanoglu, E. The Reciprocal Interactions between Polyphenols and Gut Microbiota and Effects on Bioaccessibility. *Nutrients* **2016**, *8*, 78. [CrossRef] [PubMed]

41. Feliciano, R.P.; Boeres, A.; Massacessi, L.; Istas, G.; Ventura, M.R.; Nunes Dos Santos, C.; Heiss, C.; Rodriguez-Mateos, A. Identification and quantification of novel cranberry-derived plasma and urinary (poly)phenols. *Arch. Biochem. Biophys.* **2016**, *599*, 31–41. [CrossRef] [PubMed]

42. Ou, K.; Sarnoski, P.; Schneider, K.R.; Song, K.; Khoo, C.; Gu, L. Microbial catabolism of procyanidins by human gut microbiota. *Mol. Nutr. Food Res.* **2014**, *58*, 2196–2205. [CrossRef] [PubMed]

43. Dall'Asta, M.; Calani, L.; Tedeschi, M.; Jechiu, L.; Brighenti, F.; del Rio, D. Identification of microbial metabolites derived from in vitro fecal fermentation of different polyphenolic food sources. *Nutrition* **2012**, *28*, 197–203. [CrossRef] [PubMed]

44. Mullen, W.; Edwards, C.A.; Crozier, A. Absorption, excretion and metabolite profiling of methyl-, glucuronyl-, glucosyl- and sulpho-conjugates of quercetin in human plasma and urine after ingestion of onions. *Br. J. Nutr.* **2006**, *96*, 107–116. [CrossRef] [PubMed]

45. Meyer, H.; Bolarinwa, A.; Wolfram, G.; Linseisen, J. Bioavailability of apigenin from apiin-rich parsley in humans. *Ann. Nutr. Metab.* **2006**, *50*, 167–172. [CrossRef] [PubMed]

46. Tang, D.; Chen, K.; Huang, L.; Li, J. Pharmacokinetic properties and drug interactions of apigenin, a natural flavone. *Expert Opin. Drug Metab. Toxicol.* **2017**, *13*, 323–330. [CrossRef] [PubMed]

47. Zeng, X.; Bai, Y.; Peng, W.; Su, W. Identification of Naringin Metabolites in Human Urine and Feces. *Eur. J. Drug Metab. Pharmacokinet.* **2016**. [CrossRef] [PubMed]

48. Pereira-Caro, G.; Ludwig, I.A.; Polyviou, T.; Malkova, D.; Garcia, A.; Moreno-Rojas, J.M.; Crozier, A. Identification of Plasma and Urinary Metabolites and Catabolites Derived from Orange Juice (Poly)phenols: Analysis by High-Performance Liquid Chromatography-High-Resolution Mass Spectrometry. *J. Agric. Food Chem.* **2016**, *64*, 5724–5735. [CrossRef] [PubMed]

49.  Aschoff, J.K.; Riedl, K.M.; Cooperstone, J.L.; Hogel, J.; Bosy-Westphal, A.; Schwartz, S.J.; Carle, R.; Schweiggert, R.M. Urinary excretion of Citrus flavanones and their major catabolites after consumption of fresh oranges and pasteurized orange juice: A randomized cross-over study. *Mol. Nutr. Food Res.* **2016**, *60*, 2602–2610. [CrossRef] [PubMed]

50.  Brett, G.M.; Hollands, W.; Needs, P.W.; Teucher, B.; Dainty, J.R.; Davis, B.D.; Brodbelt, J.S.; Kroon, P.A. Absorption, metabolism and excretion of flavanones from single portions of orange fruit and juice and effects of anthropometric variables and contraceptive pill use on flavanone excretion. *Br. J. Nutr.* **2009**, *101*, 664–675. [CrossRef] [PubMed]

51.  Del Rio, D.; Calani, L.; Cordero, C.; Salvatore, S.; Pellegrini, N.; Brighenti, F. Bioavailability and catabolism of green tea flavan-3-ols in humans. *Nutrition* **2010**, *26*, 1110–1116. [CrossRef] [PubMed]

52.  Van der Hooft, J.J.; de Vos, R.C.; Mihaleva, V.; Bino, R.J.; Ridder, L.; de Roo, N.; Jacobs, D.M.; van Duynhoven, J.P.; Vervoort, J. Structural elucidation and quantification of phenolic conjugates present in human urine after tea intake. *Anal. Chem.* **2012**, *84*, 7263–7271. [CrossRef] [PubMed]

53.  Ottaviani, J.I.; Kwik-Uribe, C.; Keen, C.L.; Schroeter, H. Intake of dietary procyanidins does not contribute to the pool of circulating flavanols in humans. *Am. J. Clin. Nutr.* **2012**, *95*, 851–858. [CrossRef] [PubMed]

54.  Calani, L.; Del Rio, D.; Luisa Callegari, M.; Morelli, L.; Brighenti, F. Updated bioavailability and 48 h excretion profile of flavan-3-ols from green tea in humans. *Int. J. Food Sci. Nutr.* **2012**, *63*, 513–521. [CrossRef] [PubMed]

55.  Wiese, S.; Esatbeyoglu, T.; Winterhalter, P.; Kruse, H.P.; Winkler, S.; Bub, A.; Kulling, S.E. Comparative biokinetics and metabolism of pure monomeric, dimeric, and polymeric flavan-3-ols: A randomized cross-over study in humans. *Mol. Nutr. Food Res.* **2015**, *59*, 610–621. [CrossRef] [PubMed]

56.  Urpi-Sarda, M.; Monagas, M.; Khan, N.; Lamuela-Raventos, R.M.; Santos-Buelga, C.; Sacanella, E.; Castell, M.; Permanyer, J.; Andres-Lacueva, C. Epicatechin, procyanidins, and phenolic microbial metabolites after cocoa intake in humans and rats. *Anal. Bioanal. Chem.* **2009**, *394*, 1545–1556. [CrossRef] [PubMed]

57.  Appeldoorn, M.M.; Vincken, J.P.; Aura, A.M.; Hollman, P.C.; Gruppen, H. Procyanidin dimers are metabolized by human microbiota with 2-(3,4-dihydroxyphenyl)acetic acid and 5-(3,4-dihydroxyphenyl)-gamma-valerolactone as the major metabolites. *J. Agric. Food Chem.* **2009**, *57*, 1084–1092. [CrossRef] [PubMed]

58.  Bartolome, B.; Monagas, M.; Garrido, I.; Gomez-Cordoves, C.; Martin-Alvarez, P.J.; Lebron-Aguilar, R.; Urpi-Sarda, M.; Llorach, R.; Andres-Lacueva, C. Almond (Prunus dulcis (Mill.) D.A. Webb) polyphenols: From chemical characterization to targeted analysis of phenolic metabolites in humans. *Arch. Biochem. Biophys.* **2010**, *501*, 124–133. [CrossRef] [PubMed]

59.  Zhang, L.; Wang, Y.; Li, D.; Ho, C.T.; Li, J.; Wan, X. The absorption, distribution, metabolism and excretion of procyanidins. *Food Funct.* **2016**. [CrossRef] [PubMed]

60.  Pan, P.; Skaer, C.W.; Stirdivant, S.M.; Young, M.R.; Stoner, G.D.; Lechner, J.F.; Huang, Y.W.; Wang, L.S. Beneficial Regulation of Metabolic Profiles by Black Raspberries in Human Colorectal Cancer Patients. *Cancer Prev. Res. (Phila.)* **2015**, *8*, 743–750. [CrossRef] [PubMed]

61.  Serra, A.; Macià, A.; Romero, M.-P.; Reguant, J.; Ortega, N.; Motilva, M.-J. Metabolic pathways of the colonic metabolism of flavonoids (flavonols, flavones and flavanones) and phenolic acids. *Food Chem.* **2012**, *130*, 383–393. [CrossRef]

62.  Ludwig, I.A.; Mena, P.; Calani, L.; Borges, G.; Pereira-Caro, G.; Bresciani, L.; del Rio, D.; Lean, M.E.; Crozier, A. New insights into the bioavailability of red raspberry anthocyanins and ellagitannins. *Free Radic. Biol. Med.* **2015**, *89*, 758–769. [CrossRef] [PubMed]

63.  De Ferrars, R.M.; Cassidy, A.; Curtis, P.; Kay, C.D. Phenolic metabolites of anthocyanins following a dietary intervention study in post-menopausal women. *Mol. Nutr. Food Res.* **2014**, *58*, 490–502. [CrossRef] [PubMed]

64.  de Ferrars, R.M.; Czank, C.; Zhang, Q.; Botting, N.P.; Kroon, P.A.; Cassidy, A.; Kay, C.D. The pharmacokinetics of anthocyanins and their metabolites in humans. *Br. J. Pharmacol.* **2014**, *171*, 3268–3282. [CrossRef] [PubMed]

65.  Stalmach, A.; Mullen, W.; Barron, D.; Uchida, K.; Yokota, T.; Cavin, C.; Steiling, H.; Williamson, G.; Crozier, A. Metabolite profiling of hydroxycinnamate derivatives in plasma and urine after the ingestion of coffee by humans: Identification of biomarkers of coffee consumption. *Drug Metab. Dispos.* **2009**, *37*, 1749–1758. [CrossRef] [PubMed]

66.  Gonzalez-Barrio, R.; Edwards, C.A.; Crozier, A. Colonic catabolism of ellagitannins, ellagic acid, and raspberry anthocyanins: In vivo and in vitro studies. *Drug Metab. Dispos.* **2011**, *39*, 1680–1688. [CrossRef] [PubMed]

67. Selma, M.V.; Espin, J.C.; Tomas-Barberan, F.A. Interaction between phenolics and gut microbiota: Role in human health. *J. Agric. Food Chem.* **2009**, *57*, 6485–6501. [CrossRef] [PubMed]
68. Margalef, M.; Pons, Z.; Bravo, F.I.; Muguerza, B.; Arola-Arnal, A. Plasma kinetics and microbial biotransformation of grape seed flavanols in rats. *J. Funct. Foods* **2015**, *12*, 478–488. [CrossRef]
69. Pimpao, R.C.; Dew, T.; Figueira, M.E.; McDougall, G.J.; Stewart, D.; Ferreira, R.B.; Santos, C.N.; Williamson, G. Urinary metabolite profiling identifies novel colonic metabolites and conjugates of phenolics in healthy volunteers. *Mol. Nutr. Food Res.* **2014**, *58*, 1414–1425. [CrossRef] [PubMed]
70. Rodriguez-Mateos, A.; Cifuentes-Gomez, T.; Gonzalez-Salvador, I.; Ottaviani, J.I.; Schroeter, H.; Kelm, M.; Heiss, C.; Spencer, J.P. Influence of age on the absorption, metabolism, and excretion of cocoa flavanols in healthy subjects. *Mol. Nutr. Food Res.* **2015**, *59*, 1504–1512. [CrossRef] [PubMed]
71. Mennen, L.I.; Sapinho, D.; Ito, H.; Galan, P.; Hercberg, S.; Scalbert, A. Urinary excretion of 13 dietary flavonoids and phenolic acids in free-living healthy subjects - variability and possible use as biomarkers of polyphenol intake. *Eur. J. Clin. Nutr.* **2008**, *62*, 519–525. [CrossRef] [PubMed]
72. Tomas-Barberan, F.A.; Selma, M.V.; Espin, J.C. Interactions of gut microbiota with dietary polyphenols and consequences to human health. *Curr. Opin. Clin. Nutr. Metab. Care* **2016**, *19*, 471–476. [CrossRef] [PubMed]
73. Marin, L.; Miguelez, E.M.; Villar, C.J.; Lombo, F. Bioavailability of dietary polyphenols and gut microbiota metabolism: Antimicrobial properties. *Biomed. Res. Int.* **2015**, *2015*, 905215. [CrossRef] [PubMed]

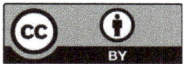

*nutrients*

MDPI

*Article*

# Association between Coffee Consumption and Its Polyphenols with Cardiovascular Risk Factors: A Population-Based Study

**Andreia Machado Miranda \*, Josiane Steluti, Regina Mara Fisberg and Dirce Maria Marchioni**

Department of Nutrition, School of Public Health, University of São Paulo, São Paulo 01246-904, Brazil; jsteluti@gmail.com (J.S.); rfisberg@usp.br (R.M.F.); marchioni@usp.br (D.M.M.)
\* Correspondence: andreia.am.miranda@gmail.com; Tel.: +55-11-3061-7856

Received: 26 January 2017; Accepted: 10 March 2017; Published: 14 March 2017

**Abstract:** Epidemiological studies have examined the effect of coffee intake on cardiovascular disease, but the benefits and risks for the cardiovascular system remain controversial. Our objective was to evaluate the association between coffee consumption and its polyphenols on cardiovascular risk factors. Data came from the "Health Survey of São Paulo (ISA-Capital)" among 557 individuals, in São Paulo, Brazil. Diet was assessed by two 24-h dietary recalls. Coffee consumption was categorized into <1, 1–3, and ≥3 cups/day. Polyphenol intake was calculated by matching food consumption data with the Phenol-Explorer database. Multiple logistic regression models were used to assess the associations between cardiovascular risk factors (blood pressure, total cholesterol, low-density lipoprotein cholesterol (LDL-c), high-density lipoprotein cholesterol (HDL-c), triglycerides, fasting glucose, and homocysteine) and usual coffee intake. The odds were lower among individuals who drank 1–3 cups of coffee/day to elevated systolic blood pressure (SBP) (Odds Ratio (OR) = 0.45; 95% Confidence Interval (95% CI): 0.26, 0.78), elevated diastolic blood pressure (DBP) (OR = 0.44; 95% CI: 0.20, 0.98), and hyperhomocysteinemia (OR = 0.32; 95% CI: 0.11, 0.93). Furthermore, significant inverse associations were also observed between moderate intake of coffee polyphenols and elevated SBP (OR = 0.46; 95% CI: 0.24, 0.87), elevated DBP (OR = 0.51; 95% CI: 0.26, 0.98), and hyperhomocysteinemia (OR = 0.29; 95% CI: 0.11, 0.78). In conclusion, coffee intake of 1–3 cups/day and its polyphenols were associated with lower odds of elevated SBP, DBP, and hyperhomocysteinemia. Thus, the moderate consumption of coffee, a polyphenol-rich beverage, could exert a protective effect against some cardiovascular risk factors.

**Keywords:** coffee consumption; coffee polyphenol intake; cardiovascular risk factors; representative sample

---

## 1. Introduction

Cardiovascular diseases (CVD) are considered to be the leading global cause of death, accounting for 17.3 million deaths per year, which is predicted to rise to more than 23.6 million by 2030 [1]. The main causes of CVD involve non-modifiable risk factors, in addition to the metabolic risk factors, that are targeted together with the behavioral risk factors, such as unhealthy diets (rich in salt, saturated fat, and calories) [2]. However, there are still food items whose role is controversial, such as coffee.

Coffee has been considered an important dietary factor, because it is one of the most popular and widely consumed nonalcoholic beverages in the world. Finland is the largest coffee consumer market, followed by Brazil. In Brazil, the average coffee consumption is 5.9 kg per capita [3], with an estimated prevalence of intake of 79%, i.e., the second-most consumed food in the country [4].

Coffee beverage, a mixture of several pharmacologically-bioactive compounds, including caffeine, phenolic acids, and the diterpene alcohols, cafestol and kahweol, can also have long term effects on risk factors for CVD, such as blood pressure, plasma concentrations of cholesterol and homocysteine, and the incidence of type 2 diabetes mellitus [5–7].

Caffeine, a central nervous system stimulant and psychoactive substance, has been positively associated with blood pressure [8,9], systemic vascular resistance and unfavorable effects on endothelial function [9], serum lipids concentration [10], and insulin resistance [11]. Other prospective studies, however, have generally not supported adverse risk effects on CVD associated with coffee consumption [12–14]. The major beneficial properties of coffee seem to depend on its content of phenolic acids, which demonstrates protective roles in the cardiovascular system [15]. This cardiovascular protection has been demonstrated in vivo, and can be explained by various mechanisms, including their anti-inflammatory properties [16], the strong antioxidant capacity [17] related to nitric oxide (NO) bioavailability, as well as low-density lipoprotein (LDL) oxidation, and antithrombotic properties through endothelial protection [18].

Contrary to earlier studies focused on caffeine, existing evidence is suggesting that coffee may exert a beneficial effect toward cardiovascular-related outcomes, together with all-cause and cancer mortality [19]. However, the public debate about reducing or increasing the risk of CVD by drinking coffee is still relevant due to the previous contrasting findings on cardiovascular effects. Additionally, its effects on CVD might have considerable public health and clinical implications [12].

Therefore, the current study aimed to assess the association between usual coffee consumption and coffee polyphenol intake on cardiovascular risk factors, e.g., systolic and diastolic blood pressure, total cholesterol, low-density lipoprotein cholesterol (LDL-c), high-density lipoprotein cholesterol (HDL-c), triglyceride, fasting plasma glucose, and homocysteine, in a representative sample of individuals aged 20 years or older in São Paulo City.

## 2. Materials and Methods

### 2.1. Study Population

Data were retrieved from the "Health Survey of São Paulo (ISA-Capital)", a cross-sectional population-based study designed to assess the health and nutritional status of non-institutionalized individuals residing in São Paulo City in Southeastern Brazil, between 2008 and 2009.

A complex probabilistic sampling, by conglomerates, based on census tracts and households that had already been drawn in the National Household Sample Survey 2005 (PNAD 2005) was used. The drawing was systematic, and eight study domains were defined: less than one year old; one to 11 years old, and three more age groups by sex: 12 to 19 years (adolescents), 20 to 59 years (adults), and 60 years or over (older adults). A minimum sample size of 300 in each of the six domains was estimated to be needed based on a prevalence of 0.5 with a standard error of 0.07 at a 5% significance level and a design effect of 1.5.

A total of 2691 individuals, aged 12 years or over, were selected to answer questions about diet, life conditions, and sociodemographic information. Thereby, only 1662 individuals of the initial sample agreed to participate. Of those, 750 subjects provided a blood sample for biochemical analysis, completed two 24-h dietary recalls (24 HR), anthropometric data, as well as arterial blood pressure measurements. For the present study, only adults and older adults were included, totaling a final sample of 557 individuals.

The study protocol was reviewed and approved by the Ethics Committee at the School of Public Health, University of São Paulo (Approval Number: 003.0.162.000-08). A written informed consent form was obtained from all participants.

### 2.2. Dietary Assessment

The dietary intake was measured by two 24 HR. The first 24 HR was administered at households by trained interviewers using the multiple pass method [20]; the second 24 HR was performed by telephone using the automated multiple pass method [21]. The multiple pass method, automated or not, is structured in five steps: (1) a quick list, where participants list all of the foods and beverages consumed uninterruptedly; (2) a forgotten list, where participants are asked about commonly consumed forgotten foods, such as candies, coffees, and sodas; (3) time and location of food and beverage intake; (4) detailing cycle, that is, a description of the way of preparation and amounts consumed; and (5) a final review, which verifies whether a certain food consumed during the day was not previously recorded. The sampling days covered all the days of the week and seasons. Dietary data were entered into the Nutrition Data System for Research software (version 2007, University of Minnesota, Minneapolis, MN, USA), which is mainly based on data from the food composition table published by the United States Department for Agriculture (USDA).

The multiple source method (MSM), a statistical modeling technique, was used to estimate the usual dietary intake of polyphenols and nutrients and to remove within-person variation. In the first step, the probability of eating the food on a random day for each individual was estimated by a logistic regression model. Secondly, the usual amount of food or nutrient intake is estimated by a linear regression model. Finally, the resulting numbers from step one and two are multiplied by each other to estimate the usual daily intake for each individual [22].

### 2.2.1. Assessment of Coffee Consumption

In the 24 HR, the participants reported if they consumed coffee on the day before the interview and, thereafter, a question about the method of coffee preparation (filtered, instant, espresso, or other), and whether additional items were typically added to the coffee (none, milk, sugar, artificial sweetener, etc.) were probed. Daily coffee intake (in mL) was categorized, according to the standard cup size used in the study (50 mL), into three categories: <1 cup/day, 1–3 cups/day, and ≥3 cups/day. The category of <1 cup/day of coffee was used as the reference group.

### 2.2.2. Estimation of Polyphenol Intake from Coffee

Data on the polyphenol content in foods were obtained from the Phenol-Explorer database [23] that presents data on the content of 502 polyphenols in 452 foods [24].

The polyphenol intake was calculated by matching usual food intake data from the 24HR with the polyphenol content in foods from the Phenol-Explorer database. The individual polyphenol intake from each food was calculated by multiplying the content of each polyphenol by the daily consumption of each food, including coffee. The total polyphenol intake was the sum of all individual polyphenol intakes from all food sources reported in the 24 HR. Other details on the estimation of polyphenol intakes are available elsewhere in previous publications [25].

For the present study, the classes of polyphenols ingested from coffee included the phenolic acids, especially hydroxycinnamic acids (4-caffeoylquinic acid, 5-caffeoylquinic acid, 3-caffeoylquinic acid, 5-feruloylquinic acid, caffeic acid), alkylmethoxyphenols (4-ethylguaiacol, 4-vinylguaiacol), and others (catechol, pyrogallol, phenol). The coffee polyphenols were categorized into three categories: <101 mg/day (corresponding to <1 cup coffee/day), 101–337 mg/day (corresponding to 1–3 cups/day), and ≥337 mg/day (corresponding to ≥3 cups/day).

### 2.3. Demographic and Lifestyle Characteristics

Sociodemographic and lifestyle characteristics included age, sex, household per capita income, smoking status, alcohol drinking, and the use of medicines.

The physical activity included energy expenditure in leisure time by reporting type and duration of activity according to the predetermined questionnaire items of the long version of the International Physical Activity Questionnaire (IPAQ) [26], validated in Brazil. The physical activity level was categorized as daily low, moderate and high. In the current study, physical activity was grouped in two categories: low and moderate/high. More details for levels of physical activity proposed by IPAQ are available online [27].

The smoking status was categorized as nonsmoker and current smoker or former smoker.

## 2.4. Anthropometric Measurements

Anthropometric measurements were obtained in participant homes by a trained nursing assistant following the procedures recommended by the WHO [28]. Body weight (kg) was measured using a calibrated digital scale (Tanita®, model HD-313, Tanita Corporation of America, Inc., Arlington Heights, IL, USA). Height (cm) was measured with a portable wall-mounted stadiometer (Seca®, model 208, Seca Brazil, São Paulo, Brazil). Body mass index (BMI) was calculated by dividing weight (kilograms) by the square of the height (meters).

## 2.5. Outcome Measurements

### 2.5.1. Blood Pressure (BP)

During the home visit, BP was measured using an automatic blood pressure monitor (Omron HEM-712C, Omron Health Care, Inc., Vernon Hills, IL, USA) handled by a nursing technician, according to the recommendations of the V Brazilian Guidelines on Hypertension [29]. Participants were considered to have high BP if they had systolic (SBP) and/or diastolic (DBP) higher or equal to 140 mmHg and 90 mmHg, respectively, according to the national and international recommendations [29,30].

### 2.5.2. Blood Samples

The blood samples were collected by venipuncture after 12-h of overnight fasting by a nursing assistant, using a standardized protocol.

Serum total cholesterol (TC) and fractions, LDL-c and HDL-c, as well as triglyceride (TG), were determined by enzymatic-colorimetric method (Roche Diagnostics GmbH, Mannheim, Germany). We considered the cut-off point value for elevated TC level $\geq$200 mg/dL, for elevated LDL-c >100 mg/dL, reduced HDL-c <40 mg/dL in males or <50 mg/dL in females, and elevated TG $\geq$150 mg/dL [31].

Fasting plasma glucose (FPG) was measured by enzymatic-colorimetric glucose oxidase procedure using the kit gluco-quant Glucose/HK (GLU Roche/Hitachi 1,447,513; Roche Diagnostics GmbH, Mannheim, Germany). The cut-off value for elevated fasting glucose level was $\geq$100 mg/dL [31].

The immunoassay method of chemiluminescence microparticles using the ARCHITECT Homocysteine Reagent Kit (Abbott Diagnostics Division, Abbott Park, Lake Forest, IL, USA) was used to analyze the plasma concentrations of homocysteine. We selected the value of plasma homocysteine >16 $\mu$mol/L for older adults and a value >12 $\mu$mol/L for adults, as cut-off point for categorization in hyperhomocysteinemia [32].

## 2.6. Statistical Analysis

The characteristics of the study participants were described by coffee consumption categories, and presented as medians and interquartile range (IQR) for continuous variables, and frequencies and percentages for categorical variables. The variables were examined for normality (Kolmogorov-Smirnov test). Differences between coffee consumption categories were tested by Kruskall-Wallis test for continuous variables, and by the Chi-square test for categorical variables.

The associations between the independent variables (categories of usual coffee consumption and coffee polyphenol intake) and the following dependent variables (i.e., SBP, DBP, FPG, serum TC, LDL-c, HDL-c, TG, and homocysteine) were tested by multiple logistic regression analysis.

Two models were fitted for each independent variable. The first model was the crude model (unadjusted). The second model (adjusted), corresponding to models 1, 2, 3, and 4, was adjusted for classic potential confounders (i.e., age, sex, race, BMI, smoking status, alcohol consumption, physical activity level, household per capita income, intake of caffeine, added sugars, total energy intake, and saturated fat), and additionally adjusted for particular variables hypothesized to be associated with each cardiovascular risk factor, according to the literature. Thus, model 1 corresponded to both

SBP and DBP was additionally adjusted for sodium intake, and antihypertensive drugs; model 2 corresponded to fasting plasma glucose was additionally adjusted for hypoglycemic drugs; model 3 corresponded to TC, LDL-c, HDL-c, and TG was additionally adjusted for monounsaturated fat, polyunsaturated fat, and hypolipidemic medicines; and lastly model 4 corresponded to homocysteine was additionally adjusted for folate, B6, and B12 vitamins.

All analyses were conducted using the appropriate sample weights to account for the complex survey design. For all analyses, Stata® statistical software package version 12 (StataCorp LLC, College Station, TX, USA) was used and a $p$-value < 0.05 was considered statistically significant.

## 3. Results

The final study population had a mean age of 45.1 years, mostly women (54.2%), self-declared white (61.1%), non-smokers (58.4%), insufficiently active (77.7%), and non-obese (74.5%).

The mean of coffee consumption for the whole population was 143.4 mL/day. A minority of participants consumed espresso coffee ($n = 7$), and there were no decaffeinated coffee consumers in the current study population. Furthermore, the median total intake of polyphenols was 363.9 mg/day. Coffee provided 247.0 mg/day of polyphenols, which represented approximately 68% of the total intake.

The sociodemographic, biochemical, and dietary characteristics of the studied population according to coffee consumption categories are shown in Table 1. Coffee drinking was higher in older adults than in adults, and among current smokers than in non-smokers. Differences were also observed between the usual coffee consumption and polyphenols intake from coffee, and caffeine intake. A further significant difference by coffee consumption was found with prevalence of DBP.

The associations between coffee consumption categories and cardiovascular risk factors are presented in Table 2. The adjusted models demonstrated lower odds for SBP, DBP, and homocysteine in individuals that were consuming 1–3 cups of coffee per day, than in individuals who drank less than 1 cup of coffee per day to elevated SBP (Odds Ratio (OR) 0.45, 95% Confidence Interval (95% CI): 0.26, 0.78); elevated DBP (OR 0.44, 95% CI: 0.20, 0.98), and hyperhomocysteinemia (OR 0.32, 95% CI: 0.11, 0.93). For those subjects with higher consumption (≥3 cups/day), the association was not significant for any cardiovascular risk factors.

Table 3 shows the association between the same cardiovascular risk factors and categories of coffee polyphenols in this population. After adjustment for potential confounding factors, OR showed that a moderate intake of coffee polyphenols (101 to 337 mg/day) was inversely associated with elevated SBP (OR 0.46, 95% CI: 0.24, 0.87), elevated DBP (OR 0.51, 95% CI: 0.26, 0.98), and hyperhomocysteinemia (OR 0.29, 95% CI: 0.11, 0.78).

Table 1. General characteristics of the Health Survey of São Paulo (ISA-Capital) population according to category of coffee consumption. São Paulo, Brazil, 2008/09.

| Characteristics | Coffee Consumption, Cups per Day | | | | p-Value [a] |
| --- | --- | --- | --- | --- | --- |
| | <1 | 1–3 | ≥3 | Total | |
| **No. of subjects** | 193 | 185 | 179 | 557 | |
| **Sociodemographic** | | | | | |
| Age (years), median (IQR) | 40 (29.0, 53.0) | 44 (33.0, 57.0) | 47 (36.0, 57.0) | 61 (44.0, 70.5) | 0.013 [1] |
| Sex, n (%) | | | | | 0.360 [2] |
| Male | 64 (40.9) | 71 (50.2) | 71 (47.0) | 206 (45.8) | |
| Female | 129 (59.1) | 114 (49.8) | 108 (53.0) | 351 (54.2) | |
| Race, n (%) | | | | | 0.918 [2] |
| White | 120 (63.0) | 109 (58.1) | 117 (62.1) | 346 (61.1) | |
| Black | 14 (5.8) | 18 (6.5) | 9 (6.4) | 41 (6.2) | |
| Others | 59 (31.2) | 58 (35.4) | 53 (31.5) | 170 (32.7) | |
| Household *per capita* income, n (%) | | | | | 0.851 [2] |
| <1 MW | 80 (34.6) | 83 (37.5) | 68 (38.3) | 231 (36.7) | |
| ≥1 MW | 113 (65.4) | 102 (62.5) | 111 (61.7) | 326 (63.3) | |
| Physical activity level, n (%) | | | | | 0.608 [2] |
| Low | 157 (74.1) | 161 (80.5) | 152 (79.2) | 470 (77.7) | |
| Moderate/High | 36 (25.9) | 23 (19.5) | 27 (20.8) | 86 (22.3) | |
| Smoking status, n (%) | | | | | 0.034 [2] |
| Non-smoker | 114 (65.6) | 96 (56.1) | 97 (52.1) | 307 (58.4) | |
| Smoker | 79 (34.4) | 82 (43.9) | 89 (47.9) | 250 (41.6) | |
| Body Mass Index (kg/m$^2$), median (IQR) | 25.2 (23.2, 29.1) | 24.9 (22.7, 28.6) | 26.7 (23.7, 30.8) | 26.5 (23.6, 30.5) | 0.307 [1] |
| **Biochemical** | | | | | |
| SBP (mm Hg), n (%) | | | | | 0.089 [2] |
| Normal | 133 (80.1) | 130 (87.2) | 119 (77.3) | 382 (81.5) | |
| Elevated | 60 (19.9) | 55 (12.8) | 60 (22.7) | 175 (18.5) | |
| DBP (mm Hg), n (%) | | | | | 0.045 [2] |
| Normal | 163 (85.3) | 168 (91.5) | 144 (81.8) | 465 (86.2) | |
| Elevated | 30 (14.7) | 27 (8.5) | 35 (18.2) | 92 (13.8) | |

Table 1. *Cont.*

| Characteristics | Coffee Consumption, Cups per Day | | | | p-Value [a] |
|---|---|---|---|---|---|
| | <1 | 1–3 | ≥3 | Total | |
| FPG (mg/dL), n (%) | | | | | 0.177 [2] |
| Normal | 167 (90.9) | 154 (86.0) | 158 (92.5) | 479 (89.8) | |
| Elevated | 26 (9.1) | 31 (14.0) | 21 (7.4) | 78 (10.2) | |
| TC (mg/dL), n (%) | | | | | 0.061 [2] |
| Normal | 118 (69.0) | 98 (58.7) | 88 (54.0) | 304 (61.1) | |
| Elevated | 75 (31.0) | 87 (41.3) | 91 (46.0) | 253 (38.9) | |
| LDL-c (mg/dL), n (%) | | | | | 0.098 [2] |
| Normal | 63 (36.2) | 46 (26.6) | 31 (20.5) | 140 (28.2) | |
| Elevated | 130 (63.8) | 139 (73.4) | 148 (79.5) | 417 (71.8) | |
| HDL-c (mg/dL), n (%) | | | | | 0.466 [2] |
| Normal | 150 (68.7) | 133 (61.1) | 129 (61.2) | 412 (64.0) | |
| Elevated | 43 (31.3) | 52 (38.9) | 50 (38.8) | 145 (36.0) | |
| TG (mg/dL), n (%) | | | | | 0.565 [2] |
| Normal | 135 (74.2) | 123 (69.5) | 116 (66.8) | 374 (70.4) | |
| Elevated | 58 (25.8) | 62 (30.5) | 63 (33.2) | 183 (29.6) | |
| Homocysteine (µmol/L) | | | | | 0.350 [2] |
| Normal | 163 (88.0) | 162 (93.4) | 156 (89.9) | 481 (90.3) | |
| Elevated | 30 (12.0) | 23 (6.6) | 23 (10.1) | 76 (9.7) | |
| **Dietetic** | | | | | |
| Coffee polyphenol intake (mg/day), median (IQR) | 66.6 (0, 147.4) | 261.6 (225.3, 297.3) | 408.4 (351.8, 546.1) | 247.0 (145.9, 346.7) | <0.001 [1] |
| Caffeine intake (mg/day), median (IQR) | 44.7 (24.0, 67.1) | 91.3 (80.2, 100.6) | 147.3 (117.3, 173.3) | 92.4 (60.8, 125.2) | <0.001 [1] |
| Alcohol intake (g/day), median (IQR) | 0.1 (0.0, 1.2) | 0.2 (0.0, 2.3) | 0.3 (0.0, 3.2) | 0.2 (0.0, 2.1) | 0.412 [1] |
| Sodium intake (mg/day), median (IQR) | 2986.1 (2526.5, 3848.9) | 3260.0 (2563.4, 3895.6) | 3015.9 (2567.4, 3677.5) | 2863.4 (2342.0, 3472.7) | 0.995 [1] |
| Total energy intake (kcal/day), median (IQR) | 1679.4 (1354.4, 2013.8) | 1712.8 (1382.3, 2152.6) | 1671.1 (1361.8, 2010.2) | 1543.9 (1243.8, 1887.9) | 0.615 [1] |

Abbreviations: DBP: Diastolic blood pressure; FPG: Fasting plasma glucose; HDL-c: High-density lipoprotein cholesterol; IQR: Interquartile Range; LDL-c: Low-density lipoprotein cholesterol; MW: Minimum Wage; SBP: Systolic blood pressure; TC: Total cholesterol; TG: Triglyceride. Comparisons across categories were performed using the [1] Kruskall-Wallis test; [2] chi-squared. [a] p-value < 0.05 was considered statistically significant. The sample weight was considered for statistical analysis.

**Table 2.** Association between cardiovascular risk factors and categories of coffee consumption in Health Survey of São Paulo (ISA-Capital) population. São Paulo, Brazil, 2008/09.

| Cardiovascular Risk Factors | Coffee Consumption, cups per Day | | |
|---|---|---|---|
| | <1 | 1-3 | ≥3 |
| **Elevated SBP** (≥140 mm Hg) | | | |
| OR crude (unadjusted) | 1.00 | 0.58 (0.33, 1.05) | 1.17 (0.63, 2.21) |
| OR adjusted [1] | 1.00 | 0.45 (0.26, 0.78) | 0.81 (0.41, 1.61) |
| **Elevated DBP** (≥90 mm Hg) | | | |
| OR crude (unadjusted) | 1.00 | 0.54 (0.24, 1.22) | 1.30 (0.66, 2.54) |
| OR adjusted [1] | 1.00 | 0.44 (0.20, 0.98) | 0.89 (0.45, 1.75) |
| **Increased FPG** (≥100 mg/dL) | | | |
| OR crude (unadjusted) | 1.00 | 1.64 (0.82, 3.24) | 0.81 (0.34, 1.92) |
| OR adjusted [2] | 1.00 | 1.39 (0.60, 3.23) | 0.72 (0.22, 2.26) |
| **Increased TC** (≥200 mg/dL) | | | |
| OR crude (unadjusted) | 1.00 | 1.57 (0.86, 2.85) | 1.89 (1.22, 2.93) |
| OR adjusted [3] | 1.00 | 1.46 (0.76, 2.80) | 1.45 (0.94, 2.22) |
| **Increased LDL-c** (>100 mg/dL) | | | |
| OR crude (unadjusted) | 1.00 | 1.56 (0.76, 3.20) | 2.20 (1.12, 4.32) |
| OR adjusted [3] | 1.00 | 1.46 (0.68, 3.12) | 2.07 (0.92, 4.67) |
| **Reduced HDL-c** (<40 mg/dL men; <50 mg/dL women) | | | |
| OR crude (unadjusted) | 1.00 | 1.40 (0.77, 2.54) | 1.39 (0.75, 2.59) |
| OR adjusted [3] | | 1.67 (0.87, 3.20) | 1.77 (0.80, 3.94) |
| **Increased TG** (≥150 mg/dL) | | | |
| OR crude (unadjusted) | 1.00 | 1.26 (0.59, 2.71) | 1.43 (0.73, 2.80) |
| OR adjusted [3] | 1.00 | 1.26 (0.59, 2.63) | 1.35 (0.61, 2.98) |
| **Increased Homocysteine** (>12 μmol/L adults; >16 μmol/L older adults) | | | |
| OR crude (unadjusted) | 1.00 | 0.52 (0.16, 1.43) | 0.82 (0.35, 1.94) |
| OR adjusted [4] | 1.00 | 0.32 (0.11, 0.93) | 0.43 (0.19, 1.01) |

Odds ratio (OR) and 95% Confidence Interval (95% CI) were calculated by using multivariate logistic regression. Models were adjusted for age, sex, race, body mass index (BMI), smoking, alcohol, physical activity, household per capita income, intake of caffeine, added sugars, total energy intake, and saturated fat: [1] additionally adjusted for sodium intake, and antihypertensive drugs; [2] additionally adjusted for hypoglycemic drugs; [3] additionally adjusted for monounsaturated fat, polyunsaturated fat, and hypolipidemic drugs; [4] additionally adjusted for vitamins folate, B6, and B12. Abbreviations: DBP: Diastolic blood pressure; FPG: Fasting plasma glucose; HDL-c: High-density lipoprotein cholesterol; LDL-c: Low-density lipoprotein cholesterol; SBP: Systolic blood pressure; TC: Total cholesterol; TG: Triglyceride.

**Table 3.** Association between cardiovascular risk factors and categories of coffee polyphenol intake in Health Survey of São Paulo (ISA-Capital) population. São Paulo, Brazil, 2008/09.

| Cardiovascular Risk Factors | Polyphenol Intake from Coffee, mg per Day [a] | | |
|---|---|---|---|
| | <101 | 101–337 | ≥337 |
| **Elevated SBP** (≥140 mm Hg) | | | |
| OR crude (unadjusted) | 1.00 | 0.55 (0.30, 1.02) | 0.94 (0.52, 1.73) |
| OR adjusted [1] | 1.00 | 0.46 (0.24, 0.87) | 0.72 (0.35,1.45) |
| **Elevated DBP** (≥90 mm Hg) | | | |
| OR crude (unadjusted) | 1.00 | 0.52 (0.26, 1.06) | 0.86 (0.45, 1.65) |
| OR adjusted [1] | 1.00 | 0.51 (0.26, 0.98) | 0.70 (0.39, 1.27) |
| **Increased FPG** (≥100 mg/dL) | | | |
| OR crude (unadjusted) | 1.00 | 1.77 (0.97, 3.23) | 0.66 (0.28, 1.58) |
| OR adjusted [2] | 1.00 | 1.98 (0.87, 4.54) | 0.71 (0.23, 2.20) |
| **Increased TC** (≥200 mg/dL) | | | |
| OR crude (unadjusted) | 1.00 | 0.96 (0.54, 1.72) | 1.35 (0.92, 1.98) |
| OR adjusted [3] | 1.00 | 0.83 (0.44, 1.57) | 1.07 (0.71, 1.59) |
| **Increased LDL-c** (>100 mg/dL) | | | |
| OR crude (unadjusted) | 1.00 | 1.05 (0.49, 2.25) | 1.80 (0.86, 3.75) |
| OR adjusted [3] | 1.00 | 0.99 (0.45, 2.17) | 1.67 (0.70, 4.03) |
| **Reduced HDL-c** (<40 mg/dL men; <50 mg/dL women) | | | |
| OR crude (unadjusted) | 1.00 | 1.31 (0.78, 2.18) | 1.31 (0.74, 2.31) |
| OR adjusted [3] | 1.00 | 1.27 (0.70, 2.31) | 1.51 (0.74, 3.07) |
| **Increased TG** (≥150 mg/dL) | | | |
| OR crude (unadjusted) | 1.00 | 0.87 (0.45, 1.71) | 1.00 (0.52, 1.92) |
| OR adjusted [3] | 1.00 | 0.72 (0.36, 1.45) | 0.86 (0.41, 1.78) |
| **Increased Homocysteine** (>12 μmol/L adults; >16 μmol/L older adults) | | | |
| OR crude (unadjusted) | 1.00 | 0.52 (0.18, 1.51) | 0.84 (0.40,1.81) |
| OR adjusted [4] | 1.00 | 0.29 (0.11, 0.78) | 0.59 (0.31, 1.11) |

Odds ratio (OR) and 95% CI were calculated by using multivariate logistic regression. Models were adjusted for age, sex, race, BMI, smoking, alcohol, physical activity, household per capita income, intake of caffeine, added sugars, total energy intake, saturated fat, and other polyphenol intake (except polyphenols from coffee). [1] additionally adjusted for sodium intake, and antihypertensive drugs; [2] additionally adjusted for hypoglycemic drugs; [3] additionally adjusted for monounsaturated fat, polyunsaturated fat, and hypolipidemic drugs; [4] additionally adjusted for vitamins folate, B6, and B12. [a] < 101 mg/day (corresponding to <1 cup coffee/day), 101–337 mg/day (corresponding to 1–3 cups/day), and ≥ 337 mg/day (corresponding to ≥3 cups/day). Abbreviations: DBP: Diastolic blood pressure; FPG: Fasting plasma glucose; HDL-c: High-density lipoprotein cholesterol; LDL-c: Low-density lipoprotein cholesterol; SBP: Systolic blood pressure; TC: Total cholesterol; TG: Triglyceride.

## 4. Discussion

The current study found that a moderate coffee consumption (1 to 3 cups per day), which corresponds to a coffee polyphenol intake of 101–337 mg/day, had a beneficial effect on cardiovascular risk factors, such as, elevated SBP, elevated DBP, and hyperhomocysteinemia.

Previous epidemiological studies on the benefits of coffee consumption on the cardiovascular system have provided inconsistent and conflicting results [33]. In this way, some studies suggested a positive association between coffee consumption and risk of CVD [34,35], whereas others reported no association [36,37], or even an inverse association [12–14]. Therefore, these controversial findings may be due to the different types of studies, with different designs performed in distinct populations. Additionally, inconsistent and conflicting results may be related to the various confounding dietary factors, different forms of brewing coffee and the daily amount consumed.

Numerous risk factors for CVD have been described in the literature, and elevated BP is a recognized and well-established risk factor for coronary heart disease and stroke. A large number of epidemiological studies on the effect of coffee or caffeine on BP has been published, but they have provided conflicting results, and the effect of chronic coffee consumption on BP is still unclear [9,38]. A meta-analysis of randomized controlled clinical trials has concluded that regular coffee consumption slightly increases systolic and diastolic BP [8]. Interestingly, Noordzij et al. [8] showed that the BP elevations were larger in the studies using caffeine than in the studies on coffee consumption. In agreement with these findings, another recent systematic review and meta-analysis reports that BP elevations appeared to be significant only for caffeine but not for coffee consumption [9]. The prevailing explanation for such effect is that caffeine antagonizes endogenous adenosine, resulting in vasoconstriction and elevated total peripheral vascular resistance [39]. Moreover, although these results suggesting that caffeine acutely increasing BP, its effects may be somehow attenuated if ingested as coffee, so, it seems that other compounds in the coffee could potentially counterbalance the pressor effect of caffeine [8]. Coffee is a drink with a very complex chemical composition, rich in BP-lowering minerals (that is, potassium and magnesium) and antioxidant compounds (phenolic acids) that may outweigh the hypertensive effects of caffeine [40]. The beneficial effects of these other components in the cardiovascular system, may help explain the lack of association between long-term coffee consumption and increase BP or CVD risk in large cohort studies [9].

It was observed in our study that moderate coffee drinking was associated with lower odds of elevated SBP and DBP, especially due to the presence of polyphenols. The high content of phenolic compounds in coffee, especially due to the group of hydroxycinnamic acids (caffeic, chlorogenic, feluric, and p-coumaric acids), exhibits a strong antioxidant activity, and protects against atherothrombosis or atherosclerotic lesion development through endothelial protection (attenuates oxidative stress, improved NO bioavailability, and decreased E-selectin, intercellular adhesion molecule-1 (ICAM-1), and vascular cell adhesion protein-1 (VCAM-1) expression, among others) [18,41]. In this context, investigations during the last decade have implied that chlorogenic acid consumption can have a significant lowering effect on BP [42,43]. This hypotensive effect might involve nitric oxide (NO)-mediated vasodilation, and improvement of endothelial function. In this way, the dietary intake of chlorogenic acids may hold promise for providing a non-pharmacological approach for the prevention and treatment of high BP [42].

Increased concentrations of total plasma homocysteine have been associated with an increased risk of cardiovascular disease [6,41]. Therefore, modifiable factors can influence homocysteine levels. Besides folate intake i.e., the most important dietary determinant of plasma total homocysteine concentration, coffee consumption has an effect on total homocysteine levels in the general population [44].

A positive association, in a dose-dependent manner between homocysteine concentrations and coffee consumption, was reported in a cross-sectional study [44] and has confirmed in randomized controlled trials [45,46]. Grubben et al. [45] have suggested that 10% higher concentration of homocysteine is associated with very high intake of unfiltered coffee (1 L/day), but it is not clear whether the serum lipid fraction, i.e., cholesterol-raising diterpenes present exclusively in unfiltered coffee, is the only factor responsible for the increase in homocysteine concentration. Although the authors were not able to conclude whether this association depends on the brewing method, it seems that unfiltered coffee is more likely to increase total homocysteine than filtered coffee. They speculated that the effect of coffee, mediated by caffeine, on increased plasma homocysteine concentrations could be due to a decrease in blood vitamin B6 concentration, a vitamin related to homocysteine metabolism, whose deficit results in higher production of homocysteine. Additionally, chlorogenic acid, a polyphenol that is present in coffee, may also be partly responsible for the increase of the homocysteine production through increased methylation reactions [47].

On the other hand, moderate coffee consumption among healthy subjects did not significantly increase the homocysteine concentration [48], and a population based-study described that coffee was no longer associated with plasma homocysteine after adjustment for plasma folate concentration [49]. In addition, Mursu et al. [50] found similar results and showed that the consumption of filtered coffee has neither short- nor long-term detectable effects on lipid peroxidation nor on plasma homocysteine concentrations in healthy non-smoking men. More recently, according to Corrêa et al. [51] in Brazilian population, no changes were observed for plasma total homocysteine, after the consumption of three or four cups of paper-filtered coffee per day. The inconsistencies between the above-mentioned epidemiological studies suggest that not all types of coffee brew have the same effect on plasma homocysteine concentrations or that the effect is spurious.

In the current study, we reported that individuals who were consuming more than three cups of filtered coffee per day had lower odds (even not significant) for hyperhomocysteinemia, and moderate consumption of filtered coffee and the polyphenols intake from coffee were inversely associated with hyperhomocysteinemia. A possible hypothesis for this finding is that caffeic acid inhibited hyperhomocysteinemia, elicited leukocyte rolling and adhesion, decreased reactive oxygen species production and activation of cyclooxygenase-2 (COX-2) in endothelial cells. Additionally, caffeic acid was seen to reduce the expression of adhesion molecules such as E-selectin and ICAM-1 on endothelium and integrin CD11b/CD18 (Mac-1 (macrophage-1 antigen)) on leukocytes caused by hyperhomocysteinemia [52,53]. However, the biological mechanisms involved on the effect of coffee consumption on homocysteine concentrations are still unclear and need further investigation.

In addition, coffee consumption has also been associated with alterations in circulating lipids, particularly higher serum TC and LDL-c concentrations, in some observational studies, but not in all [5,6,41]. There are two distinct reasons for these findings. The reason in favor of coffee consumption is that the antioxidants included in coffee might reduce lipid oxidation. The topic has been insufficiently investigated, with two small studies reporting protective (unfiltered coffee for one week) and neutral (filtered coffee for three weeks) effects [6]. The unfavorable reason is that unfiltered coffee is rich in the cholesterol-raising oils (diterpenes, kahweol and cafestol), which contribute significantly to the increase in TC, LDL-c and TG [54]. In contrast to unfiltered coffee, consumption of filtered coffee had no substantial effects on blood lipids [41,55], because the brewing releases oil droplets containing diterpenes from ground coffee beans, and the oil is retained by a paper filter [6,41]. In the present study, we found no association between coffee consumption and serum lipids (cholesterol profiles, and triglyceride levels), perhaps due to the fact that the traditional brewing method of coffee in Brazil is filtering. Thus, our study corroborated and supported this information.

To our knowledge, this is the first study in Brazil to investigate the association between usual coffee consumption and its polyphenols and the main cardiovascular risk factors, and the most important merit of our study is the emphasis of the role of moderate coffee consumption through its relation with BP and homocysteine in decreasing risk of CVD.

However, some limitations of this study should be considered when interpreting results. Firstly, our study is of a cross-sectional nature, which does not allow definitive establishment of causal inference. Furthermore, several confounders in multivariate models were controlled, but other unknown or unmeasured confounders (such as genetic information) may exist. This should be the focus of future studies. Further research, especially coming from randomized clinical trials, is warranted to confirm our findings and establish the biological basis of coffee's potential preventive effects on CVD.

## 5. Conclusions

Our study shows that moderate coffee consumption and its polyphenols were associated with lower odds of elevated SBP and DBP, and hyperhomocysteinemia in this population. Therefore, moderate coffee consumption, a polyphenol-rich beverage, could provide beneficial effects against clinical cardiovascular risk factors.

**Acknowledgments:** We would like to thank all of the volunteers involved in this research for their valuable cooperation. Furthermore, we also thank Maria Cecilia Goi Porto Alves from the Health Institute, State Government of Sao Paulo. The authors also would like to express their gratitude for financial support from Sao Paulo Research Foundation (FAPESP) and the Brazilian National Counsel of Technological and Scientific Development (CNPq).

**Author Contributions:** A.M.M. was responsible for the design of the present study, data analysis, drafted, and wrote the manuscript, and has the primary responsibility for the final content. J.S. participated in data analysis and reviewed the final version of manuscript. R.M.F. participated in design, critical analysis, and final review. D.M.M. led the team and participated in the study design and conception, data analysis, manuscript conception, critical analysis, and final review. All authors read and approved the final manuscript.

**Conflicts of Interest:** The authors declare that they have no conflict of interest. The founding sponsors had no role in the design of the study; in the collection, analyses, or interpretation of data, in the writing of the manuscript, and in the decision to publish the results.

**Financial Disclosure:** A.M.M. received scholarship from the Sao Paulo Research Foundation (FAPESP) (grant number 2014/04540-2). D.M.M. had financial support from Sao Paulo Research Foundation (FAPESP) (grant number 2009/15831-0) and received research productivity scholarship from the Brazilian National Council for Scientific and Technological Development (CNPq) (grant number 306029/2011-1). All funding agencies had no role in the design, analysis, or writing of this article.

## References

1. Mozaffarian, D.; Benjamin, E.J.; Go, A.S.; Arnett, D.K.; Blaha, M.J.; Cushman, M.; Dai, S.; De Simone, G.; Ferguson, T.B.; Ford, E.; et al. Heart disease and stroke statistics-2015 update: A report from the American Heart Association. *Circulation* **2015**, *131*, e29–e322. [CrossRef] [PubMed]
2. World Health Organization (WHO). *Global Atlas on Cardiovascular Disease Prevention and Control*; WHO: Geneva, Switzerland, 2011.
3. International Coffee Organization. Trade Statistics. Available online: http://www.ico.org/profiles_e.asp (accessed on 20 February 2017).
4. Souza, A.M.; Pereira, R.A.; Yokoo, E.M.; Levy, R.B.; Sichieri, R. Alimentos mais consumidos no Brasil: Inquérito Nacional de Alimentação 2008–2009 (Most consumed foods in Brazil: National Dietary Survey 2008–2009). *Rev. Saúde Publica* **2013**, *47*, 190S–199S.
5. O'Keefe, J.H.; Bhatti, S.K.; Patil, H.R.; DiNicolantonio, J.J.; Lucan, S.C.; Lavie, C.J. Effects of habitual coffee consumption on cardiometabolic disease, cardiovascular health, and all-cause mortality. *J. Am. Coll. Cardiol.* **2013**, *62*, 1043–1051. [CrossRef] [PubMed]
6. Cano-Marquina, A.; Tarín, J.J.; Cano, A. The impact of coffee on health. *Maturitas* **2013**, *75*, 7–21. [CrossRef] [PubMed]
7. Ding, M.; Bhupathiraju, S.N.; Chen, M.; van Dam, R.M.; Hu, F.B. Caffeinated and Decaffeinated Coffee Consumption and Risk of Type 2 Diabetes: A systematic review and a dose-response meta-analysis. *Diabetes Care* **2014**, *37*, 569–586. [CrossRef] [PubMed]
8. Noordzij, M.; Uiterwaal, C.S.P.M.; Arends, L.R.; Kok, F.J.; Grobbee, D.E.; Geleijnse, J.M. Blood pressure response to chronic intake of coffee and caffeine: A meta-analysis of randomized controlled trials. *J. Hypertens.* **2005**, *23*, 921–928. [CrossRef] [PubMed]
9. Mesas, A.E.; Leon-Muñoz, L.M.; Rodriguez-Artalejo, F.; Lopez-Garcia, E. The effect of coffee on blood pressure and cardiovascular disease in hypertensive individuals: A systematic review and meta-analysis. *Am. J. Clin. Nutr.* **2011**, *94*, 1113–1126. [CrossRef] [PubMed]

10. Rodrigues, I.M.; Klein, L.C. Boiled or filtered coffee? Effects of coffee and caffeine on cholesterol, fibrinogen and C-reactive protein. *Toxicol. Rev.* **2006**, *25*, 55–69. [CrossRef] [PubMed]

11. Whitehead, N.; White, H. Systematic review of randomized controlled trials of the effects of caffeine or caffeinated drinks on blood glucose concentrations and insulin sensitivity in people with diabetes mellitus. *J. Hum. Nutr. Diet.* **2013**, *26*, 111–125. [CrossRef] [PubMed]

12. Wu, J.N.; Ho, S.C.; Zhou, C.; Ling, W.H.; Chen, W.Q.; Wang, C.L.; Chen, Y.-M. Coffee consumption and risk of coronary heart diseases: A meta-analysis of 21 prospective cohort studies. *Int. J. Cardiol.* **2009**, *137*, 216–225. [CrossRef] [PubMed]

13. Ding, M.; Satija, A.; Bhupathiraju, S.N.; Hu, Y.; Sun, Q.; Han, J.; Lopez-Garcia, E.; Willett, W.; van Dam, R.M.; Hu, F.B. Association of Coffee Consumption with Total and Cause-Specific Mortality in Three Large Prospective Cohorts. *Circulation* **2015**, *132*, 2305–2315. [CrossRef] [PubMed]

14. Ding, M.; Bhupathiraju, S.N.; Satija, A.; van Dam, RM.; Hu, F.B. Long-term coffee consumption and risk of cardiovascular disease: A systematic review and a dose-response meta-analysis of prospective cohort studies. *Circulation* **2014**, *129*, 643–659. [CrossRef] [PubMed]

15. Guo, X.; Tresserra-Rimbau, A.; Estruch, R.; Martínez-González, M.; Medina-Remón, A.; Castañer, O.; Corella, D.; Salas-Salvadó, J.; Lamuela-Raventós, R.M. Effects of Polyphenol, Measured by a Biomarker of Total Polyphenols in Urine, on Cardiovascular Risk Factors After a Long-Term Follow-Up in the PREDIMED Study. *Oxid. Med. Cell. Longev.* **2016**. [CrossRef] [PubMed]

16. Kempf, K.; Herder, C.; Erlund, I.; Kolb, H.; Martin, S.; Carstensen, M.; Koenig, W.; Sundvall, J.; Bidel, S.; Kuha, S.; et al. Effects of coffee consumption on subclinical inflammation and other risk factors for type 2 diabetes: A clinical trial. *Am. J. Clin. Nutr.* **2010**, *91*, 950–957. [CrossRef] [PubMed]

17. Natella, F.; Nardini, M.; Giannetti, I.; Dattilo, C.; Scaccini, C. Coffee drinking influences plasma antioxidant capacity in humans. *J. Agric. Food Chem.* **2002**, *50*, 6211–6216. [CrossRef] [PubMed]

18. Fuentes, E.; Palomo, I. Mechanisms of endothelial cell protection by hydroxycinnamic acids. *Vasc. Pharmacol.* **2014**, *63*, 155–161. [CrossRef] [PubMed]

19. Grosso, G.; Micek, A.; Godos, J.; Sciacca, S.; Pajak, A.; Martínez-González, M.A.; Giovannucci, E.L.; Galvano, F. Coffee consumption and risk of all-cause, cardiovascular, and cancer mortality in smokers and non-smokers: A dose-response meta-analysis. *Eur. J. Epidemiol.* **2016**, *31*, 1191–1205. [CrossRef] [PubMed]

20. Guenther, P.M.; DeMaio, T.J.; Ingwersen, L.A.; Berline, M. The multiple-pass approach for the 24 h recall in the Continuing Survey of Food Intakes by Individuals (CSFII) 1994 ± 1996. In Proceedings of the International Conference on Dietary Assessment Methods, Boston, MA, USA, January 1995.

21. Blanton, C.A.; Moshfegh, A.J.; Baer, D.J.; Kretsch, M.J. The USDA Automated Multiple-Pass Method accurately estimates group total energy and nutrient intake. *J. Nutr.* **2006**, *136*, 2594–2599. [PubMed]

22. Harttig, U.; Haubrock, J.; Knueppel, S.; Boeing, H.; Consortium EFCOVAL. The MSM program: Web-based statistics package for estimating usual dietary intake using the Multiple Source Method. *Eur. J. Clin. Nutr.* **2011**, *65*, S87–S91. [CrossRef] [PubMed]

23. Scalbert, A. Phenol-Explorer: Database on Polyphenol Content in Foods. Available online: http://phenol-explorer.eu/ (accessed on 28 September 2015).

24. Pérez-Jiménez, J.; Neveu, V.; Vos, F.; Scalbert, A. Systematic analysis of the content of 502 polyphenols in 452 foods and beverages: An application of the Phenol-Explorer database. *J. Agric. Food Chem.* **2010**, *58*, 4959–4969. [CrossRef] [PubMed]

25. Miranda, A.M.; Steluti, J.; Fisberg, R.M.; Marchioni, D.M. Dietary intake and food contributors of polyphenols in adults and elderly adults of Sao Paulo: A population-based study. *Br. J. Nutr.* **2016**, *115*, 1061–1070. [CrossRef] [PubMed]

26. Craig, C.L.; Marshall, A.L.; Sjostrom, M.; Bauman, A.E.; Booth, M.L.; Ainsworth, B.E.; Pratt, M.; Ekelund, U.; Yngve, A.; Sallis, J.F.; et al. International physical activity questionnaire: 12-country reliability and validity. *Med. Sci. Sports Exerc.* **2003**, *35*, 1381–1395. [CrossRef] [PubMed]

27. The IPAQ Group. International Physical Activity Questionnaire. Available online: http://www.ipaq.ki.se (accessed on 12 October 2016).

28. World Health Organization (WHO). *Physical Status: The Use E Interpretation of Anthropometry*; WHO: Geneva, Switzerland, 1995.

29. Sociedade Brasileira de Cardiologia; Sociedade Brasileira de Hipertensão; Sociedade Brasileira de Nefrologia. V Diretrizes brasileiras de hipertensão arterial. *Arq. Bras. Cardiol.* **2007**, *89*, e24–e79.

30. Chobanian, A.V.; Bakris, G.L.; Black, H.R.; Cushman, W.C.; Green, L.A.; Izzo, J.L., Jr. The Seventh Report of the Joint National Committee on Detection, Evaluation, and Treatment of High Blood Pressure. The JNC 7 Report. *JAMA* **2003**, *289*, 2560–2571. [CrossRef] [PubMed]
31. Expert Dyslipidemia Panel of the International Atherosclerosis Society. An International Atherosclerosis Society Position Paper: Global recommendations for the management of dyslipidemia-full report. *J. Clin. Lipidol.* **2014**, *8*, 29–60.
32. Refsum, H.; Smith, A.D.; Ueland, P.M.; Nexo, E.; Clarke, R.; McPartlin, J.; Johnston, C.; Engbaek, F.; Schneede, J.; McPartlin, C.; et al. Facts and recommendations about total homocysteine determinations: An expert opinion. *Clin. Chem.* **2004**, *50*, 3–32. [CrossRef] [PubMed]
33. Butt, M.S.; Sultan, M.T. Coffee and its consumption: Benefits and risks. *Crit. Rev. Food Sci. Nutr.* **2011**, *51*, 363–373. [CrossRef] [PubMed]
34. Liu, J.; Sui, X.; Lavie, C.J.; Hebert, J.R.; Earnest, C.P.; Zhang, J.; Blair, S.N. Association of coffee consumption with all-cause and cardiovascular disease mortality. *Mayo Clin. Proc.* **2013**, *88*, 1066–1074. [CrossRef] [PubMed]
35. Grioni, S.; Agnoli, C.; Sieri, S.; Pala, V.; Ricceri, F.; Masala, G.; Saieva, C.; Panico, S.; Mattiello, A.; Chiodini, P.; et al. Espresso coffee consumption and risk of coronary heart disease in a large Italian Cohort. *PLoS ONE* **2015**, *10*, e0126550. [CrossRef] [PubMed]
36. Floegel, A.; Pischon, T.; Bergmann, M.M.; Teucher, B.; Kaaks, R.; Boeing, H. Coffee consumption and risk of chronic disease in the European Prospective Investigation into Cancer and Nutrition (EPIC)-Germany study. *Am. J. Clin. Nutr.* **2012**, *95*, 901–908. [CrossRef] [PubMed]
37. Lopez-Gracia, E.; Van Dam, R.M.; Willett, W.C.; Rimm, E.B.; Manson, J.E.; Stampfer, M.J.; Rexrode, K.M.; Hu, F.B. Coffee consumption and coronary heart disease in men and women. *Circulation* **2006**, *113*, 2045–2053. [CrossRef] [PubMed]
38. Riksen, N.P.; Rongen, G.A.; Smits, P. Acute and long-term cardiovascular effects of coffee: Implications for coronary heart disease. *Pharmacol. Ther.* **2009**, *121*, 185–191. [CrossRef] [PubMed]
39. Echeverri, D.; Montes, F.R.; Cabrera, M.; Galán, A.; Prieto, A. Caffeine's vascular mechanisms of action. *Int. J. Vasc. Med.* **2010**, *2010*, 834060. [CrossRef] [PubMed]
40. Godos, J.; Pluchinotta, F.R.; Marventano, S.; Buscemi, S.; Li Volti, G.; Galvano, F.; Grosso, G. Coffee components and cardiovascular risk: Beneficial and detrimental effects. *Int. J. Food Sci. Nutr.* **2014**, *21*, 1–12. [CrossRef] [PubMed]
41. Ranheim, T.; Halvorsen, B. Coffee consumption and human health-beneficial or detrimental?-Mechanisms for effects of coffee consumption on different risk factors for cardiovascular disease and type 2 diabetes mellitus. *Mol. Nutr. Food Res.* **2005**, *49*, 274–284. [CrossRef] [PubMed]
42. Zhao, Y.; Wang, J.; Ballevre, O.; Luo, H.; Zhang, W. Antihypertensive effects and mechanisms of chlorogenic acids. *Hypertens. Res.* **2012**, *35*, 370–374. [CrossRef] [PubMed]
43. Mubarak, A.; Bondonno, C.P.; Liu, A.H.; Considine, M.J.; Rich, L.; Mas, E.; Croft, K.D.; Hodgson, J.M. Acute effects of chlorogenic acid on nitric oxide status, endothelial function, and blood pressure in healthy volunteers: A randomized trial. *J. Agric. Food Chem.* **2012**, *60*, 9130–9136. [CrossRef] [PubMed]
44. De Bree, A.; Verschuren, W.M.; Blom, H.J.; Kromhout, D. Lifestyle factors and plasma homocysteine concentrations in a general population sample. *Am. J. Epidemiol.* **2001**, *154*, 150–154. [CrossRef] [PubMed]
45. Grubben, M.J.; Boers, G.H.; Blom, H.J.; Broekhuizen, R.; de Jong, R.; van Rijt, L.; de Ruijter, E.; Swinkels, D.W.; Nagengast, F.M.; Katan, M.B. Unfiltered coffee increases plasma homocysteine concentrations in healthy volunteers: A randomized trial. *Am. J. Clin. Nutr.* **2000**, *71*, 480–484. [PubMed]
46. Urgert, R.A.; van Vliet, T.; Zock, P.L.; Katan, M.B. Heavy coffee consumption and plasma homocysteine: A randomized controlled trial in healthy volunteers. *Am. J. Clin. Nutr.* **2000**, *72*, 1107–1110. [PubMed]
47. Olthof, M.R.; Hollman, P.C.; Zock, P.L.; Katan, M.B. Consumption of high doses of chlorogenic acid, present in coffee, or of black tea increases total homocysteine concentrations in humans. *Am. J. Clin. Nutr.* **2001**, *73*, 532–538. [PubMed]
48. Esposito, F.; Morisco, F.; Verde, V.; Ritieni, A.; Alezio, A.; Caporaso, N.; Fogliano, V. Moderate coffee consumption increases plasma glutathione but not homocysteine in healthy subjects. *Aliment. Pharmacol. Ther.* **2003**, *17*, 595–601. [CrossRef] [PubMed]

49. Saw, S.M.; Yuan, J.M.; Ong, C.N.; Arakawa, K.; Lee, H.P.; Coetzee, G.A.; Yu, M.C. Genetic, dietary and other lifestyle determinants of plasma homocysteine concentrations in middle-aged and older Chinese men and women in Singapore. *Am. J. Clin. Nutr.* **2001**, *73*, 232–239. [PubMed]

50. Mursu, J.; Voutilainen, S.; Nurmi, T.; Alfthan, G.; Virtanen, J.K.; Rissanen, T.H.; Happonen, P.; Nyyssönen, K.; Kaikkonen, J.; Salonen, R.; et al. The effects of coffee consumption on lipid peroxidation and plasma total homocysteine concentrations: A clinical trial. *Free Radic. Biol. Med.* **2005**, *38*, 527–534. [CrossRef] [PubMed]

51. Corrêa, T.A.; Rogero, M.M.; Mioto, B.M.; Tarasoutchi, D.; Tuda, V.L.; César, L.A.; Torres, E.A. Paper-filtered coffee increases cholesterol and inflammation biomarkers independent of roasting degree: A clinical trial. *Nutrition* **2013**, *29*, 977–981. [CrossRef] [PubMed]

52. Zhao, H.P.; Feng, J.; Sun, K.; Liu, Y.Y.; Wei, X.H.; Fan, J.Y.; Huang, P.; Mao, X.-W.; Zhou, Z.; Wang, C.-S.; et al. Caffeic acid inhibits acute hyperhomocysteinemia-induced leukocyte rolling and adhesion in mouse cerebral venules. *Microcirculation* **2012**, *19*, 233–244. [CrossRef] [PubMed]

53. Moon, M.K.; Lee, Y.J.; Kim, J.S.; Kang, D.G.; Lee, H.S. Effect of caffeic acid on tumor necrosis factor-alpha-induced vascular inflammation in human umbilical vein endothelial cells. *Biol. Pharm. Bull.* **2009**, *32*, 1371–1377. [CrossRef] [PubMed]

54. Cai, L.; Ma, D.; Zhang, Y.; Liu, Z.; Wang, P. The effect of coffee consumption on serum lipids: A meta-analysis of randomized controlled trials. *Eur. J. Clin. Nutr.* **2012**, *66*, 872–877. [CrossRef] [PubMed]

55. Rebello, S.A.; van Dam, R.M. Coffee consumption and cardiovascular health: Getting to the heart of the matter. *Curr. Cardiol. Rep.* **2013**, *15*, 403. [CrossRef] [PubMed]

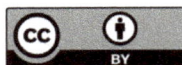

**nutrients**

MDPI

*Article*

# Gelidium elegans Regulates the AMPK-PRDM16-UCP-1 Pathway and Has a Synergistic Effect with Orlistat on Obesity-Associated Features in Mice Fed a High-Fat Diet

Jia Choi [†], Kui-Jin Kim [†], Eun-Jeong Koh and Boo-Yong Lee *

Department of Food Science and Biotechnology, College of Life Science, CHA University, Seongnam, Kyeonggi 463-400, Korea; wldk3176@gmail.com (J.C.); Kuijin.Kim@cha.ac.kr (K.-J.K.); kej763@naver.com (E.-J.K.)
* Correspondence: bylee@cha.ac.kr; Tel.: +82-31-881-7155
† These authors contributed equally to this work.

Received: 26 January 2017; Accepted: 28 March 2017; Published: 30 March 2017

**Abstract:** The incidence of obesity is rising at an alarming rate throughout the world and is becoming a major public health concern with incalculable social and economic costs. *Gelidium elegans* (GENS), also previously known as *Gelidium amansii*, has been shown to exhibit anti-obesity effects. Nevertheless, the mechanism by which GENS is able to do this remains unclear. In the present study, our results showed that GENS prevents high-fat diet (HFD)-induced weight gain through modulation of the adenosine monophosphate-activated protein kinase (AMPK)-PR domain-containing16 (PRDM16)-uncoupling protein-1 (UCP-1) pathway in a mice model. We also found that GENS decreased hyperglycemia in mice that had been fed a HFD compared to corresponding controls. We also assessed the beneficial effect of the combined treatment with GENS and orlistat (a Food and Drug Administration-approved obesity drug) on obesity characteristics in HFD-fed mice. We found that in HFD-fed mice, the combination of GENS and orlistat is associated with more significant weight loss than orlistat treatment alone. Moreover, our results demonstrated a positive synergistic effect of GENS and orlistat on hyperglycemia and plasma triglyceride level in these animals. Thus, we suggest that a combination therapy of GENS and orlistat may positively influence obesity-related health outcomes in a diet-induced obese population.

**Keywords:** *Gelidium elegans*; *Gelidium amansii*; high-fat diet-induced obese mice; hyperglycemia; obesity

## 1. Introduction

Obesity is a global health concern that has reached epidemic proportions [1]. Obesity is caused by body fat accumulation in adipose tissue due to abnormalities in energy metabolism. It is associated with a number of metabolic diseases such as diabetes, cardiovascular disease, and low chronic inflammation [2,3]. Although pharmaceutical treatment of obesity costs approximately $ 2 trillion per year [4], the population of obese individuals is rapidly growing worldwide, indicating that prevention or intervention of obesity may be difficult due to the complex multisystem pathophysiology [5]. Clinical guidelines from several countries recommend pharmacological agents such as orlistat for obese patients [6,7]. Orlistat is a Food and Drug Administration (FDA)-approved medicine for the treatment of obesity in the United States. It is an inhibitor of intestinal lipase that decreases dietary fat absorption [8].

Although orlistat treatment helps to reduce weight [9,10], it is now generally believed that physical activity and a healthy diet may prevent weight gain and obesity by maintaining energy balance and efficiently burning excessive energy [11]. Increasing consumption of fruits, vegetables, and edible plants and decreasing consumption of high-calorie foods leads to a decrease in weight gain and stabilization of weight in participants [12]. The bioactive compounds present in these food categories that are implicated in obesity prevention include resveratrol, curcumin, conjugated linoleic acid, and omega-3 fatty acids [13–16].

Recent studies have indicated that seaweeds and their derivatives may also have potential therapeutic implications for obesity [17,18]. In particular, *Gelidium elegans* (GENS), previously known as *Gelidium amansii*, has been shown to have nutraceutical activities such as anti-adipogenesis and anti-obesity effects [19–21]. However, the mechanism by which GENS is able to achieve its anti-obesity effects remains to be clearly defined. We have previously demonstrated that GENS has the potential to alter adipocyte phenotypes to beige-like adipocytes in vitro [22]. This suggests that GENS may act as an energy expenditure enhancer by stimulating the PR domain-containing16 (PRDM16)/peroxisome proliferator-activated receptor gamma coactivator 1 alpha (PGC1α)/uncoupling protein-1 (UCP-1) pathway in vivo. We therefore aimed to determine the molecular mechanism of GENS and the efficacy of the combination therapy of GENS and orlistat on weight gain, blood biochemistry and gene expression changes in high-fat diet (HFD)-induced obese mice.

## 2. Materials and Methods

### 2.1. Materials

GENS extract was obtained from NEWTREE Inc. (Seongnam, Kyeonggi, Korea). The composition of GENS extract is described in Table 1. The following antibodies were purchased from Santa Cruz Biotechnology (Dallas, TX, USA): CCAAT/enhancer binding protein alpha (C/EBPα, SC-61), diacylglycerol O-acyltransferase-1 (DGAT-1, SC-32861), fatty acid synthase (FAS, SC-20140), peroxisome proliferator activated receptor gamma (PPARγ, SC-7273), glyceraldehyde 3-phosphate dehydrogenase (GAPDH, SC-25778), sterol regulatory element binding protein-1 (SREBP-1, SC-366), and uncoupling proteins-1 (UCP-1, SC-6529). PR domain-containing16 (PRDM16, ab106410) were obtained from Abcam (Cambridge, MA, USA). Phospho-adenosine monophosphate-activated protein kinase (p-AMPK, CS-2603s), AMPK (CS-2603s), phospho-acetyl-CoA carboxylase (p-ACC, CS-3661s), and ACC (CS-3662s) were purchased from Cell Signaling Technology (Bedford, MA, USA). Orlistat and metformin were purchased from Cayman Chemical Company (Ann Arbor, MI, USA). Glucose and methylcellulose were purchased from Sigma (Sigma, St. Louis, MO, USA). All chemicals and reagents used were of analytical and obtained from commercial sources.

**Table 1.** The composition of *Gelidium elegans* (GENS) extract [23].

| Component | GENS Extract |
| --- | --- |
| Carbohydrate | 47.6% |
| Crude protein | 16.7% |
| Moisture | 5.1% |
| Crude ash | 24.1% |
| Total polyphenols | 8.79 mg per 1 g |

### 2.2. Animal Husbandry and Maintenance

Male ICR mice (5 weeks old) were purchased form Orient Bio Co. (Gapyeong, Kyeonggi, Korea) and maintained in the animal facility at CHA University, Seongnam, Kyeonggi, Korea. The project was approved by the Institutional Animal Care and Use committee of CHA University (IACUC Approval Number 150071). Male mice were individually housed for 1 week under a 12-h light/dark cycle in temperature (20–24 °C) and humidity (44.5%–51.8%). After a 1-week adaptation period, mice were randomly divided into six groups (*n* = 6 per group). Mice were fed for 7 weeks with either 60% HFD (Central Lab Animal Inc., Seoul, Korea) or NIH-07 rodent chow diet (Zeigler Brothers, Gardners, PA, USA). GENS (50, 200 mg/kg/day) and/or orlistat (20 mg/kg/day) or an equal volume of vehicle (1.0% methylcellulose, HFD and chow diet group) were orally administered to the mice by gavage every day for 7 weeks. During the experiment period, and survival rates were investigated daily. The body weight, food intake, and water consumption were recorded weekly.

### 2.3. Concentration of Blood Glucose

The blood glucose concentration was measured from mice tail vein after 12 h (dark-period) of fasting every week, using a glucose analyzer (GlucoDr, Allmedicus, Kyeonggi, Korea).

### 2.4. Intraperitoneal Glucose Tolerance Test (IPGTT)

Mice were fasted for 12 h (dark-period) before IPGTT experiments, and glucose (1.0 g/kg body weight) was administered by intraperitoneal injection), as previously described [24]. Blood samples were collected from tail vein at 30, 60, and 90 min to assess in vivo glucose clearance. Blood glucose levels were determined immediately using a glucometer (G-Doctor, Allmedicus, Anyang, Korea).

### 2.5. Biochemical Analysis

Mice were sacrificed by $CO_2$ asphyxiation and cervical dislocation. Blood collected by direct cardiac puncture in an ethylenediaminetetraacetic acid (EDTA)-coated tube aseptically. Blood was allowed to clot for 1 h at room temperature and then plasma was isolated by centrifuging the blood at $13,000 \times g$ for 15 min at 4 °C to collect plasma. The plasma samples were collected and stored at −80 °C. Plasma triglycerides (TG) and high-density lipoprotein (HDL)-cholesterol levels were measured by enzymatically commercial kits (Roche, Mannheim, Germany), Plasma insulin levels were measured by enzymatically commercial kit (Wako Pure Chemical. Ltd., Osaka, Japan). The hepatic TG content was determined using a commercially available TG quantification kit (Cayman Chemical Company, Ann Arbor, MI, USA).

### 2.6. Organ Weight

Mice were euthanized using $CO_2$ and cervical dislocation. Heart, lung, kidney, spleen, liver, abdominal fat, and subcutaneous fat were removed and weighed carefully.

### 2.7. Tissue Samples Preparation for Oil Red O

Hepatic tissues were fixed in 4% paraformaldehyde, embedded in using tissue freezing medium, optimum cutting temperature (OCT) (Cell Path Ltd., Newtown, UK). To detect fat deposition in the liver, frozen sections of 6 μm for liver were rinsed with distilled water, stained with 0.18% Oil red O (Sigma, St. Louis, MO, USA) with 60% 2-propanol (Sigma, St. Louis, MO, USA) for 20 min at 37 °C, and then rinsed with distilled water and examined under light microscopy with Nikon Eclipse E600 (Nikon, Tokyo, Japan).

### 2.8. Western Blot Analysis

For protein extraction, frozen tissues were homogenized in specific lysis buffer (PRO-PREP; iNtRON Biotechnology Inc., Seoul, Korea) containing protease with phosphatase inhibitor cocktail 2 and 3 (Sigma, St. Louis, MO, USA). The lysates were clarified by centrifugation at $12,000 \times g$ for 20 min at 4 °C. The protein concentration of clarified supernatants was determined by the Bradford assay (Bio Legend, San Diego, CA, USA). Protein samples (30 μg) were separated by sodium dodecyl sulfate polyacrylamide gel electrophores (SDS-PAGE), and transferred onto polyvinylidene fluoride (PVDF) membranes (Bio-Rad, Hercules, CA, USA), as previously described [25]. The membranes were probed with each antibodies and visualized using an enhanced chemiluminescence substrate. The signals were detected with LAS image software (Fuji, New York, NY, USA).

*2.9. Quantitative Reverse Transcription Polymerase Chain Reaction (Quantitative RT-PCR) Analysis*

Mouse liver RNA was extracted by using TRIzol reagent (Invitrogen, Carlsbad, CA, USA). Total RNA was reverse transcribed with the Maxime PCR premix Kit (iNtRON Biotechnology, Seongnam, Korea). Quantitative RT-PCR using SYBR Green 2× master mix kit (m.biotech., Inc., Seoul, Korea) was run in hexaplicate on a CFX96 Touch real-Time PCR Detection System (Bio-Rad, Hercrules, CA, USA). The 18s was used for the relative quantization of the target genes based on the comparative ΔΔ threshold cycle (Ct) method, as previously described [26]. Primer sequences are shown in Table 2.

**Table 2.** Sequence identification and primers used for quantitative reverse transcription (RT)-PCR analysis of specific messenger RNA.

| Gene | Primer Sequence (5′ to 3′) |
|---|---|
| **HMG-CoA reductase** | Forward GCGACTATGAGCGTGAACAA<br>Reverse TGGAGATCATGTGCTGCTTC |
| **LDLR** | Forward TGTGGAGCTCATCCTCTGTG<br>Reverse CACATGGTGTGAGGTTCCTG |
| **18s** | Forward CCATCCAATCGGTAGTAGCG<br>Reverse GTAACCCGTTGAACCCCATT |

HMG-CoA: hydoxymethylglutaryl-CoA; LDLR: low-density lipoprotein receptor.

*2.10. Statistical Analysis*

All statistical analyses were performed using the Statistical Package for Social Sciences version 12.0 (SPSS, Chicago, IL, USA). One-way analysis of variance (ANOVA) was used for comparisons among group. Significant differences between the mean values were assessed using Duncan's test. All values are presented as the mean ± standard deviation (SD) values. The $p$-value in the multiple comparison results (e.g., a, b, c, and d) indicate significant differences among the groups, $p < 0.05$.

## 3. Results

*3.1. Effect of GENS on Changes in Body Weight, Blood Glucose, Insulin, TG, and Gene Expression in Abdominal White Adipose Tissue in HFD-Fed Mice*

Changes in the body weight of mice fed with chow diet or HFD with the absence or presence of GENS were measured once a week during the experimental period. The introduction of GENS at 50 and 200 mg/kg/day strongly prevented this weight gain and resulted in low amounts of subcutaneous fat and abdominal fat in the mice, as shown in Figure 1A–C. Although the total food intake and average water consumption were not significantly different among the group (Figure 1D and Table 3), the group with HFD alone showed a continuous increase in body weight compared to the chow diet group.

**Table 3.** Effect of supplementation with GENS on water consumption in chow diet and HFD-induced obese mice for 7 weeks.

| Group | Water Consumption (mL) | | | | | | |
|---|---|---|---|---|---|---|---|
| | 1 Week | 2 Weeks | 3 Weeks | 4 Weeks | 5 Weeks | 6 Weeks | 7 Weeks |
| Chow diet | 129.5 ± 0.7 [a] | 125.0 ± 0.0 [a] | 117.0 ± 4.2 [a] | 124.5 ± 0.7 [a] | 117.0 ± 9.9 | 130.5 ± 2.1 [a] | 119.0 ± 11.3 |
| HFD | 130.0 ± 1.4 [a] | 103.5 ± 6.4 [ab] | 93.5 ± 2.1 [b] | 90.5 ± 2.1 [b] | 77.5 ± 0.7 | 114.5 ± 5.0 [a] | 118.5 ± 7.9 |
| HFD+GENS 50 * | 99.0 ± 7.1 [b] | 106.5 ± 3.5 [b] | 89.0 ± 11.3 [b] | 91.0 ± 0.0 [b] | 97.0 ± 1.4 | 96.0 ± 7.1 [b] | 104.5 ± 20.5 |
| HFD+GENS 200 * | 110.5 ± 0.7 [b] | 95.5 ± 3.5 [b] | 90.0 ± 0.0 [b] | 106.0 ± 4.2 [a,b] | 82.5 ± 15.0 | 91.0 ± 2.8 [b] | 99.5 ± 0.7 |

* (mg/kg/day), Data are mean ± SD ($n = 6$).

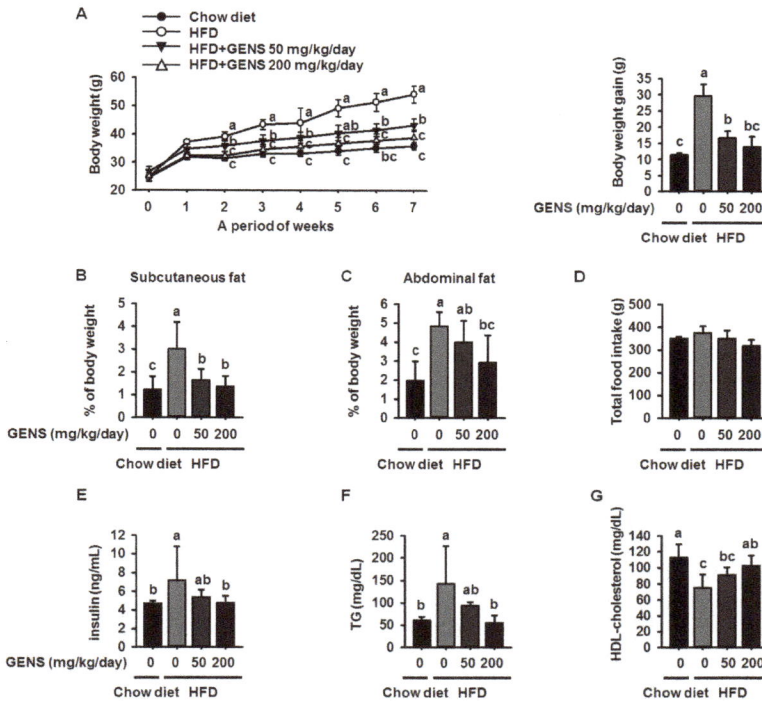

**Figure 1.** Effect of GENS on body weight change (**A**); subcutaneous fat (**B**); abdominal fat (**C**); total food intake (**D**); serum levels of insulin (**E**); levels of serum triglycerides (TG) (**F**); and high-density lipoprotein (HDL)-cholesterol concentration (**G**) in high-fat diet (HFD)-fed mice. Five-week-old mice were maintained with or without GENS (50 and 200 mg/kg/day) under HFD for 7 weeks. Data are mean ± SD ($n = 6$).

In addition, we observed that the HFD increased the average weight of the liver, subcutaneous fat and abdominal fat compared to the chow diet in mice (Table 4). However, the average weight of the heart, lungs, spleen, and kidney were not affected. Obesity is initially characterized by excess adipose tissue mass and hyperglycemia [27,28].

**Table 4.** Effect of GENS on organ weight in chow diet and HFD-induced obese mice for 7 weeks.

| Group | Organ Weight (g) | | | |
|---|---|---|---|---|
| | **Chow Diet** | | **HFD** | |
| **Variables** | **GENS 0 \*** | **GENS 0 \*** | **GENS 50 \*** | **GENS 200 \*** |
| Liver | 1.6 ± 0.1 [c] | 1.9 ± 0.3 [a] | 1.5 ± 0.2 [b] | 1.5 ± 0.1 [b,c] |
| Subcutaneous fat | 0.7 ± 0.4 [b] | 2.8 ± 0.6 [a] | 1.6 ± 0.5 [b] | 1.3 ± 0.6 [b] |
| Abdominal fat | 0.5 ± 0.2 [b] | 1.6 ± 0.6 [a] | 0.8 ± 0.2 [b] | 0.6 ± 0.3 [b] |
| Heart | 0.3 ± 0.1 | 0.3 ± 0.1 | 0.2 ± 0.0 | 0.2 ± 0.0 |
| Lung | 0.3 ± 0.0 | 0.3 ± 0.1 | 0.3 ± 0.0 | 0.3 ± 0.0 |
| Kidney | 0.7 ± 0.1 | 0.7 ± 0.1 | 0.7 ± 0.0 | 0.7 ± 0.0 |
| Spleen | 0.1 ± 0.0 | 0.2 ± 0.0 | 0.1 ± 0.0 | 0.1 ± 0.0 |

\* (mg/kg/day), Data are mean ± SD ($n = 6$).

Finding an effective treatment for hyperglycemia is one of the top priorities in obesity-associated disease research [29]. Moreover, it has been suggested that hyperglycemia in certain types of health conditions is associated with an increased risk of obesity development [30,31].

We therefore investigated whether HFD causes hyperglycemia in our experimental system and whether GENS is able to prevent HFD-mediated hyperglycemia in vivo. As shown in Table 5, the fasting blood glucose level in all group of mice before the treatment was within the normal range (126.0 ± 3.2 mg/dL). We observed that the blood glucose level was significantly increased after 2 weeks of HFD compared to mice fed a chow diet and remained constant for 7 weeks.

In contrast, administration of GENS dramatically prevented this increase in HFD-fed mice. Moreover, hyperglycemia is characterized by an increase in insulin and TG levels in blood serum. Therefore, the level of serum insulin and TG were also measured as shown in Figure 1E,F. The levels of serum insulin and TG in HFD-fed mice were significantly increased as compared to chow diet. However, GENS group dramatically decreased insulin and TG level in blood serum, indicating that GENS may efficiently ameliorate HFD-induced hyperglycemia in these animals. Moreover, it is well known that obesity is frequently associated with low levels of serum HDL-cholesterol [32]. As shown Figure 1G, the HDL-cholesterol in the HFD group were decreased as compared to chow diet. In contrast, administration of GENS significantly increased HDL-cholesterol level in blood serum. Our results thus provide preliminary evidence that GENS has potential as a preventive agent for diet-induced obesity and hyperglycemia.

**Table 5.** Effect of supplementation with GENS on fasting glucose level in chow diet and HFD-induced obese mice for 7 weeks.

| Group | Blood Glucose (mg/dL) | | | | | | |
|---|---|---|---|---|---|---|---|
| | 1 Week | 2 Weeks | 3 Weeks | 4 Weeks | 5 Weeks | 6 Weeks | 7 Weeks |
| Chow diet | 123.0 ± 20.3 | 108.7 ± 11.1 [c] | 103.3 ± 15.8 [c] | 115.5 ± 16.4 [c] | 110.7 ± 18.3 [c] | 100.5 ± 11.6 [c] | 105.5 ± 13.3 [c] |
| HFD | 121.8 ± 5.1 | 185.8 ± 28.0 [a] | 172.7 ± 26.5 [a] | 190.2 ± 39.2 [a] | 161.8 ± 10.7 [a] | 167.8 ± 17.6 [a] | 169.5 ± 22.4 [a] |
| HFD + GENS 50 * | 133.5 ± 12.3 | 156.0 ± 13.7 [a,b] | 140.2 ± 14.9 [b] | 143.0 ± 12.5 [b,c] | 143.3 ± 15.0 [a,b] | 144.3 ± 13.5 [a,b] | 131.3 ± 18.2 [b,c] |
| HFD + GENS 200 * | 142.2 ± 39.4 | 142.7 ± 24.4 [b] | 134.0 ± 14.1 [b] | 149.0 ± 7.0 [b] | 138.8 ± 12.9 [a,b] | 127.7 ± 21.1 [bc] | 139.7 ± 21.6 [b] |

* (mg/kg/day), Data are mean ± SD ($n = 6$).

### 3.2. Effect of GENS on Adipogenic Factors and IPGTT in HFD-Fed Mice

We then analyzed the adipose tissues of HFD-fed mice to confirm how GENS regulated the observed changes. To clarify whether GENS suppress the development of adipose tissue, we analyzed crucial markers of adipogenesis, including C/EBPα and PPARγ [33], by western blotting. As shown in Figure 2A, there was a 5.5-fold increase in the C/EBPα protein level in the adipose tissue of mice fed HFD for 7 weeks compared to that of mice fed a chow diet. There was also a significant elevation of the PPARγ protein expression in the adipose tissue of HFD-fed mice compared to a chow diet. In contrast, GENS at 200 mg/kg/day almost completely suppressed the expression of C/EBPα and PPARγ protein. This result is consistent with recent research, thereby suggesting that the consumption of edible seaweed GENS may result in a lower weight gain through the inhibition of adipose tissue development [19].

Hyperglycemia is characterized by an excessive amount of blood glucose and is often observed in the obese [34,35]. Also, impaired glucose tolerance is a pre-diabetic state of hyperglycemia that is associated with insulin resistance [36]. As shown Figure 2B, the 1.0 g/kg glucose control group reached a glucose level of 142.5 ± 14.2 mg/dL at 30 min. On the other hand, the groups that received 50 or 200 mg/kg GENS had a significantly suppressed rise in blood glucose, with glucose levels of 137.8 ± 25.7 mg/dL and 121.5 ± 24.8 mg/dL at 30 min, respectively. In comparison with the 1.0 g/kg glucose control group, the group that was administered 200 mg/kg GENS significantly decreased their blood glucose levels, by approximately 14.7% at 30 min. At 60 min, the 1.0 g/kg glucose level of the control group reached 100.5 ± 18.6 mg/dL. On the other hand, the groups that received 200 mg/kg GENS had a significantly suppressed the rise in blood glucose, with glucose levels of 90.8 ± 18.0 mg/dL, when compared to the 1.0 g/kg glucose control group at 60 min.

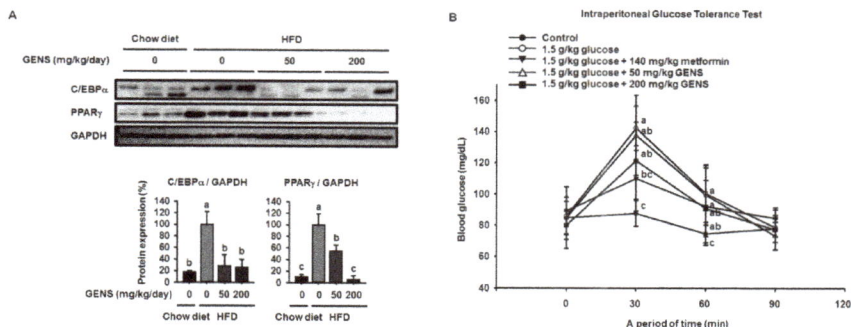

**Figure 2.** Effect of GENS on key adipogenic factors in HFD-fed mice of white adipose tissue and glucose tolerance. Five-week-old mice were maintained with or without GENS (50 and 200 mg/kg/day) under HFD for 7 weeks. Each parameter was measured by western blot analysis with C/EBPα and PPARγ. The protein expression level was normalized against GAPDH. Protein level was quantified using Image J software (**A**). Five groups of male mice (5 weeks old) were fasted for 12 h (dark-period). After 12-h fasting, mice were administered 1.0 g/kg glucose by intraperitoneal injection. The first group received only Phosphate Buffered Saline (PBS), the second group received 1.0 g/kg glucose, the third group received 1.0 g/kg glucose + 140 mg/kg metformin and the fourth and fifth group received 1.0 g/kg glucose + GENS (50 and 200 mg/kg). Blood glucose levels were measured at the indicated times (0, 30, 60, and 90 min) (**B**). Data are mean ± SD (n = 6).

### 3.3. GENS Represses Hepatic Lipogenesis via the Activation of Thermogenesis-Associated Pathway in HFD-Fed Mice

Because previous studies reported that HFD resulted in increases in hepatic lipogenesis and/or non-alcoholic fatty liver [37,38], we also examined the effect of GENS on hepatic lipogenesis in the hepatic tissues of mice. The levels of lipid droplets were evaluated by the combined use of Oil Red O with classic hematoxylin and eosin (H&E) stains in formalin-fixed paraffin-embedded liver tissues. As shown in Figure 3A, Oil Red O staining of liver sections confirmed the abundance of lipid in HFD-fed mice compared to mice fed a chow diet, while GENS prevented hepatic lipogenesis in HFD-fed mice. As shown in Figure 3B, the hepatic TG contents in HFD-fed mice were significantly increased compared to chow diet-fed mice. On the other hand, the group that was administered 50 and 200 mg/kg GENS had significantly suppressed hepatic TG contents, by approximately 28.8% and 26.1%, respectively.

Several studies have demonstrated that SREBP-1 plays an important role in modulating the transcription of genes involved in hepatic lipogenesis, including FAS, ACC, and stearoyl-CoA desaturase1 (SCD1) [39,40]. As shown in Figure 3D, HFD-fed mice markedly enhanced the expression of the SREBP-1 compared to mice fed a chow diet. In contrast, GENS reduced the expression of SREBP-1 in a dose-dependent manner in HFD-fed mice. SREBP-1 regulated transcription of genes such as hydoxymethylglutaryl-CoA (HMG-CoA) reductase and low-density lipoprotein receptor (LDLR) encoding many other enzymes in the cholesterol biosynthetic pathway [41]. We further investigated the effect of GENS on the SREBP-1 downstream target genes that contribute to the intracellular TG synthesis. ACC, DGAT-1, and FAS are downstream target genes of SREBP-1 and play a crucial role in TG synthesis and lipid accumulation [42]. As shown in Figure 3C, the expression of HMG-CoA reductase and LDLR mRNA were notably increased in HFD-fed mice compared to mice fed a chow diet. On the other hand, the GENS group markedly downregulated the expression of HMG-CoA reductase and LDLR mRNA compared to HFD-fed mice. As shown in Figure 3D, the expression levels of the genes DGAT-1 and FAS in HFD-fed mice increased notably compared to mice fed a chow diet. In contrast, the expression of the SREBP-1 downstream target genes ACC, DGAT-1, and FAS were markedly downregulated in the GENS group compared to HFD-fed mice.

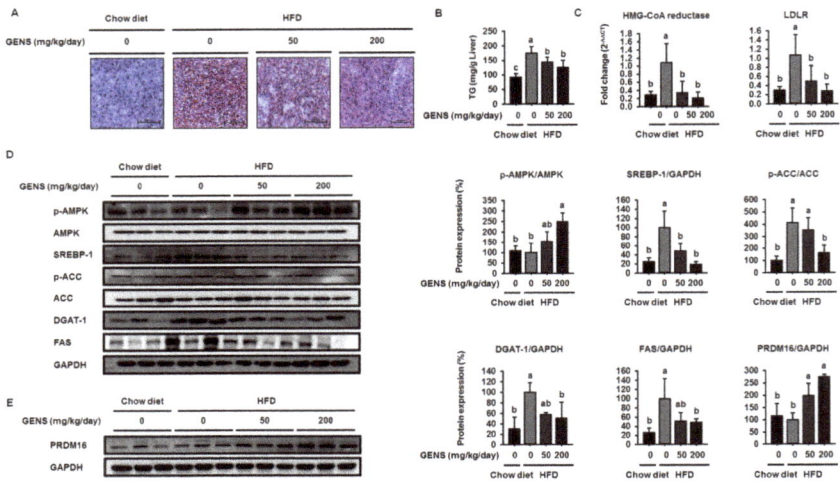

**Figure 3.** GENS represses hepatic lipogenesis and cholesterol factors in HFD-fed mice. Five-week-old mice were maintained with or without GENS (50 and 200 mg/kg/day) under HFD for 7 weeks. Each parameter was measured by western blot analysis with specific antibodies. The liver sections stained with Oil red O (**A**); Hepatic TG content (**B**); Expression levels of HMG-CoA reductase and LDLR genes were determined by quantitative RT-PCR in liver samples (**C**); p-AMPK, AMPK, SREBP-1, p-ACC, ACC, DGAT-1, and FAS (**D**); PRDM16 (**E**). The protein expression level was normalized against AMPK, ACC, and GAPDH. Protein level was quantified using Image J software. Data are mean ± SD (*n* = 6).

The phosphorylation of AMPK inhibits the expression of SREBP-1 to attenuate hepatic lipogenesis [43]. To determine whether GENS decreased the expression of SREBP-1 through the phosphorylation of AMPK, we examined the AMPK protein by western blot. We observed that HFD slightly decreased the phosphorylation of AMPK compared to chow diet, while GENS stimulated the HFD-induced reduction of AMPK phosphorylation. AMPK is a multiple nutrient sensor and a key energy balance interactor of thermogenic transcription factors including PRDM16 [44,45]. Therefore, our findings indicated that GENS could prevent hepatic lipogenesis via the activation of thermogenesis and energy expenditure.

PRDM16 is a zinc finger protein that has been proposed to regulate brown adipocyte differentiation, thermogenesis and energy expenditure in adipose tissue and skeletal muscles [36,37]. PRDM16 induces the cellular production of the PGC1α protein, which gives the mitochondria its energy expenditure phenotype [38]. We thus proceeded to investigated if GENS was responsible for the increase in PRDM16 expression. As shown in Figure 3E, HFD with GENS increased the expression of PRDM16 in the mice, whereas HFD alone had no effect on the expression of PRDM16 compared to chow diet. These results suggested that GENS is responsible for the increase in expression of PRDM16, probably via the thermogenesis pathway in brown adipose tissue.

### 3.4. GENS Stimulates the Expression of PRDM16 and UCP-1 Protein in Brown Adipose Tissue and Suppresses Hyperglycemia in HFD-Fed Mice

To further assess the role of GENS in the development of brown adipose tissue, we investigated thermogenesis-associated proteins in this tissue. As shown in Figure 4, HFD-fed mice had a lower level of AMPK phosphorylation compared to mice fed a chow diet, while GENS prevented this HFD-induced reduction.

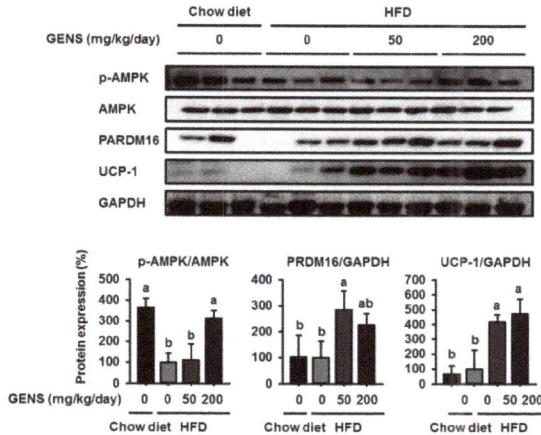

**Figure 4.** Effect of GENS on energy expenditure protein expression in brown adipose tissue of HFD-fed mice. Five-week-old mice were maintained with or without GENS (50 and 200 mg/kg/day) under HFD for 7 weeks. Each parameter was measured by western blot analysis with p-AMPK, PRDM16, and uncoupling protein-1 (UCP-1). The protein expression level was normalized against AMPK and GAPDH. Protein level was quantified using Image J software. Data are mean ± SD (*n* = 6).

Although there was no difference in the expression of PRDM16 and UCP-1 between mice fed a chow diet and those fed a HFD, we found GENS significantly enhanced the expression of PRDM16 and UCP-1 in brown adipose tissue compared to the corresponding controls. These results suggested that GENS acts as a critical regulator of thermogenesis and the development of brown adipose tissue.

### 3.5. Effect of Combination of GENS and Orlistat on Body Weight, Organ Weight, Insulin, TG, and HDL-Cholesterol in HFD-Fed Mice

Our data illustrated a potential mechanism for a thermogenic effect of GENS, suggesting that combination therapy with GENS and orlistat may produce a strong synergistic effect on weight gain prevention in vivo. Based on the above dose response in HFD-fed mice and on previous literature, dosages of 50 mg/kg/day of GENS and 20 mg/kg/day of orlistat were chosen. Orlistat was administered alone or in combination with GENS for 7 weeks in HFD-fed mice. As shown in Figure 5A, orlistat significantly suppressed body weight change compared to HFD-fed mice, and a combination of GENS and orlistat showed a synergistic effect on body weight change.

In particular, the calculation of total body weight gain revealed that orlistat reduced weight gain by approximately 20.4% compared to HFD-fed mice (Figure 5B). Moreover, GENS and orlistat exhibited better prevention of weight gain in terms of amounts of subcutaneous fat and abdominal fat accumulation in the mice, as shown in Figure 5C,D. In addition, the combination inhibited weight gain compared to HFD-fed mice given orlistat alone. We also observed that serum HDL-cholesterol levels were 84 ± 14.6 mg/dL, 88.6 ± 11.9 mg/dL, and 109.6 ± 17.8 mg/dL in HFD-fed mice, HFD-fed mice treated with orlistat, and HFD-fed treated with GENS + orlistat, respectively. In comparison with

HFD-fed mice, mice receiving a combination of GENS and orlistat showed significantly increased serum HDL-cholesterol levels, by approximately 30.5%. (Figure 5E). However, total food intake and average water consumption were not significantly different among the group (Figure 5F and Table 6).

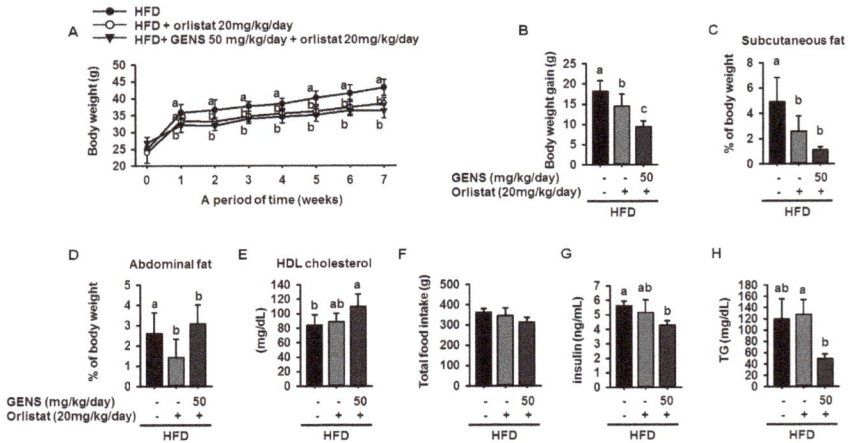

**Figure 5.** Synergistic effect of GENS and orlistat on weight change (**A**); body weight gain (**B**); subcutaneous fat (**C**); abdominal fat (**D**); HDL-cholesterol concentration (**E**); total food intake (**F**); serum levels of insulin (**G**); and serum levels of TG (**H**) in HFD-fed mice. Five-week-old mice were maintained with or without GENS (50 and 200 mg/kg/day) under HFD for 7 weeks. Data are mean $\pm$ SD ($n$ = 6).

**Table 6.** Combination effect of GENS and orlistat on water consumption in HFD-fed mice.

| Group | Water Consumption (mL) | | | | | | |
|---|---|---|---|---|---|---|---|
| | 1 Week | 2 Weeks | 3 Weeks | 4 Weeks | 5 Weeks | 6 Weeks | 7 Weeks |
| Chow diet | 138.5 ± 13.4 | 119.5 ± 7.7 | 112.5 ± 10.6 [a] | 111.0 ± 19.8 | 105.0 ± 26.8 [a] | 128.5 ± 0.7 [a] | 125.0 ± 2.8 |
| HFD | 130.0 ± 1.4 | 108.0 ± 0.0 | 93.00 ± 2.83 [b] | 105.5 ± 2.1 | 81.0 ± 4.2 [b] | 116.0 ± 7.0 [b] | 121.5 ± 9.2 |
| HFD + orlistat 20 * | 112.5 ± 23.3 | 113.5 ± 16.2 | 97.0 ± 9.9 [b] | 108.5 ± 7.6 | 92.0 ± 11.6 [b] | 101.0 ± 0.0 [c] | 115.0 ± 0.0 |
| HFD + GENS 50 * + orlistat 20 * | 121.0 ± 1.41 | 121.5 ± 0.7 | 95.0 ± 4.2 [b] | 99.5 ± 2.1 | 99.5 ± 2.1 [b] | 90.5 ± 3.5 [c] | 118.0 ± 5.6 |

* (mg/kg/day), Data are mean $\pm$ SD ($n$ = 6).

Notably, blood glucose analysis (Table 5) showed consistently that hyperglycemia was initiated at 2 weeks after beginning a HFD and persisted until 7 weeks (Table 7). These data indicated that GENS and orlistat possibly stimulated insulin secretion in the bloodstream. Therefore, we have measured the level of insulin among the group. As shown Figure 5G, the combination of GENS and orlistat significantly suppressed the level of insulin by approximately 24.1% and 8.4% compared to HFD-fed mice or HFD-fed mice with orlistat, suggesting that combination of GENS and orlistat ameliorated impaired insulin homeostasis in HFD-fed mice.

Although there was an insignificant change in the blood glucose level at 20 mg/kg/day orlistat, combined treatment with GENS and orlistat significantly inhibited the elevation of blood glucose level at 6 and 7 weeks in HFD-fed mice. Furthermore, even though combined treatment with GENS and orlistat did not have any synergistic effect on blood glucose level (Table 7), these mice showed a significant decrease in plasma TG content compared to HFD-fed mice with or without orlistat alone (Figure 5H).

**Table 7.** Combination effect of supplementation with GENS and orlistat on fasting glucose level in HFD-induced obese mice for 7 weeks.

| Group | Blood Glucose (mg/dL) | | | | | | |
|---|---|---|---|---|---|---|---|
| | 1 Week | 2 Weeks | 3 Weeks | 4 Weeks | 5 Weeks | 6 Weeks | 7 Weeks |
| Chow diet | 125.3 ± 23.9 | 115.8 ± 25.2 [b] | 118.0 ± 20.0 [b] | 120.0 ± 14.0 [b] | 113.2 ± 7.6 [b] | 108.2 ± 15.0 [b] | 116.5 ± 11.7 [b] |
| HFD | 123.3 ± 12.2 | 171.2 ± 30.7 [a] | 145.3 ± 31.8 [a] | 136.0 ± 21.5 [b] | 132.0 ± 16.5 [a,b] | 129.2 ± 18.7 [a,b] | 148.2 ± 29.9 [a] |
| HFD + orlistat 20 * | 122.0 ± 21.2 | 132.8 ± 31.6 [a,b] | 135.0 ± 16.8 [a,b] | 169.8 ± 24.5 [a] | 146.7 ± 18.2 [b] | 142.2 ± 23.2 [a] | 143.5 ± 18.3 [a] |
| HFD + GENS 50 * + orlistat 20 * | 116.7 ± 15.9 | 133.5 ± 34.0 [a,b] | 156.0 ± 15.1 [a,b] | 143.3 ± 24.3 [a,b] | 124.0 ± 27.0 [a,b] | 135.8 ± 33.5 [a,b] | 126.8 ± 7.1 [a,b] |

* (mg/kg/day), Data are mean ± SD (*n* = 6).

### 3.6. Effect of Combination of GENS and Orlistat on White Adipose Tissue and Hepatic Lipogenesis in HFD-Fed Mice

To further elucidate the molecular mechanism of the synergistic effect of GENS and orlistat on white adipose tissue and hepatic lipogenesis, we used western blot to evaluate the expression of C/EBPα and PPARγ in white adipose tissue and SREBP-1, AMPK, and PRDM16 in hepatic tissue. We noticed that high levels of C/EBPα and PPARγ were expressed in HFD-fed mice in the presence or absence of orlistat, as shown in Figure 6A. In contrast, combined treatment of GENS and orlistat reduced the expression of C/EBPα and PPARγ compared to the corresponding control.

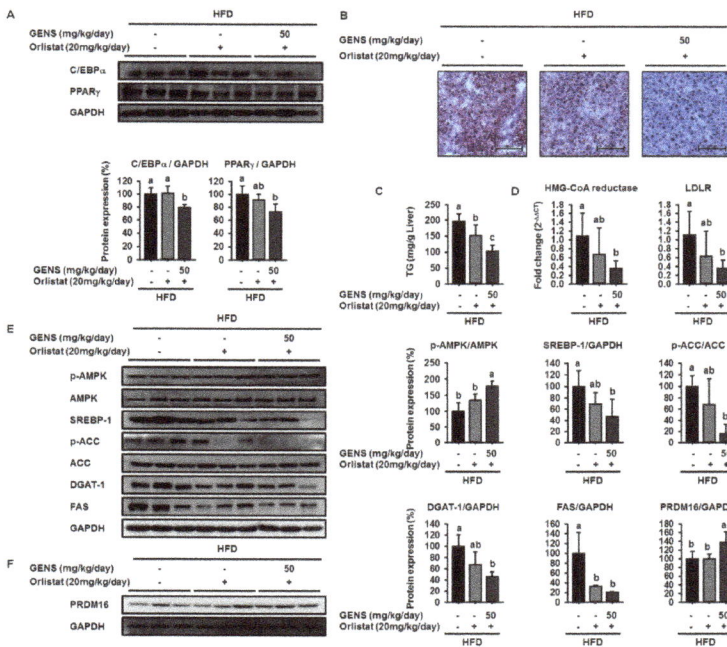

**Figure 6.** Combination effect of GENS and orlistat on white adipose tissue and hepatic lipogenesis and cholesterol synthesis-associated genes in HFD-fed mice. Five-week-old mice were maintained with or without orlistat (20 mg/kg/day) and GENS (50 mg/kg/day) under HFD for 7 weeks. Each parameter was measured by western blot analysis with C/EBPα and PPARγ (**A**); The liver sections stained with Oil red O (**B**); Hepatic TG content (**C**); Expression levels of HMG-CoA reductase and LDLR genes were determined by quantitative RT-PCR in liver samples (**D**); p-AMPK, AMPK, SREBP-1, p-ACC, ACC, DGAT-1, FAS (**E**) and PRDM16 (**F**). The protein expression level was normalized against AMPK, ACC, and GAPDH. Protein level was quantified using Image J software. Data are mean ± SD (*n* = 6).

To examine whether the combination of GENS and orlistat synergistically inhibited hepatic lipogenesis, we also performed Oil red O staining of formalin-fixed paraffin-embedded liver from HFD-fed mice. As shown in Figure 6B, Oil red O staining revealed that the combination of GENS and orlistat efficiently decreased hepatic lipogenesis.

In agreement with this observation, in mice fed with HFD, liver weights were 78.6% lower in orlistat-treated mice and 70.9% lower in those receiving a combination of GENS and orlistat compared to mice that were fed a HFD alone (Table 8). Moreover, in mice fed with HFD, liver TG contents were 58.8% lower in those receiving a combination of GENS and orlistat compared to HFD-fed mice (Figure 6C). The combination of GENS and orlistat dramatically decreased the expression of HMG-CoA reductase and LDLR in HFD-fed mice (Figure 6D). In addition, western blot analysis revealed that the combination of GENS and orlistat synergistically increased the phosphorylation of AMPK and decreased the expression of SREBP-1, ACC, DGAT-1, and FAS in HFD-fed mice, as shown in Figure 6E.

**Table 8.** Effect of GENS and/or orlistat on organ weight in HFD-induced obese mice for 7 weeks.

| Group | Organ Weight (g) | | | |
|---|---|---|---|---|
| | Chow Diet | | HFD | |
| Variables | GENS 0 * | GENS 0 * | Orlistat 20 * | HFD + GENS 50 * + Orlistat 20 * |
| Liver | 1.6 ± 0.0 [b] | 2.0 ± 0.2 [a] | 1.6 ± 0.1 [b] | 1.4 ± 0.1 [c] |
| Subcutaneous fat | 0.7 ± 0.3 [a,b] | 1.1 ± 0.6 [a] | 0.9 ± 0.3 [a,b] | 0.5 ± 0.1 [b] |
| Abdominal fat | 1.2 ± 0.6 [b] | 2.0 ± 0.5 [a] | 1.8 ± 0.5 [a] | 1.0 ± 0.3 [b] |
| Heart | 0.2 ± 0.0 | 0.3 ± 0.1 | 0.2 ± 0.0 | 0.3 ± 0.0 |
| Lung | 0.3 ± 0.0 | 0.3 ± 0.0 | 0.3 ± 0.0 | 0.3 ± 0.0 |
| Kidney | 0.7 ± 0.1 | 0.7 ± 0.2 | 0.7 ± 0.0 | 0.7 ± 0.1 |
| Spleen | 0.2 ± 0.0 | 0.1 ± 0.0 | 0.2 ± 0.0 | 0.1 ± 0.0 |

* (mg/kg/day), Data are mean ± SD ($n = 6$).

We also found that orlistat alone did not change the expression of PRDM16, but rather the combination of GENS and orlistat significantly induced the expression of PRDM16, thereby indicating that orlistat can contribute to inhibiting lipid metabolism but does not affect thermogenesis (Figure 6F). We sought to further investigate of the effect of combination of GENS and orlistat on thermogenesis-associated proteins in brown adipose tissue by western blot. Consistent with the above observations, we found that orlistat alone induced a statistically insignificant increase in the AMPK phosphorylation, PRDM16, and UCP-1 expression, whereas the combination of GENS and orlistat dramatically elevated AMPK phosphorylation and the expression of PRDM16 and UCP-1 (Figure 7). These results suggested that orlistat plays the role of a negative regulator of lipogenesis, while GENS synergistically acts as an enhancer of thermogenesis and subsequently inhibits the progression of adipogenesis and changes in circulating TG content from hematogenous spread in HFD-fed mice in the presence of orlistat.

To further analyze whether GENS and orlistat plays a role in systemic glucose sensitivity, we performed IPGTT. As shown Figure 7B, the 1.0 g/kg glucose control group reached a glucose level of 138.7 ± 23.7 mg/dL at 30 min. On the other hand, the groups that received combination group (20 mg/kg orlistat + 50 mg/kg GENS) had a significantly suppressed rise in blood glucose, with glucose levels of 125.8 ± 8.9 mg/dL at 30 min. In comparison with the 1.0 g/kg glucose control group, the group that was administered combination group (20 mg/kg orlistat + 50 mg/kg GENS) significantly decreased their blood glucose levels by approximately 9.3% at 30 min. In the current study, our result showed GENS improved glucose homeostasis in vivo. Moreover, the group that was administered 200 mg/kg GENS and combination group (20 mg/kg orlistat + 50 mg/kg GENS) had a significant decrease in blood glucose levels after glucose loading.

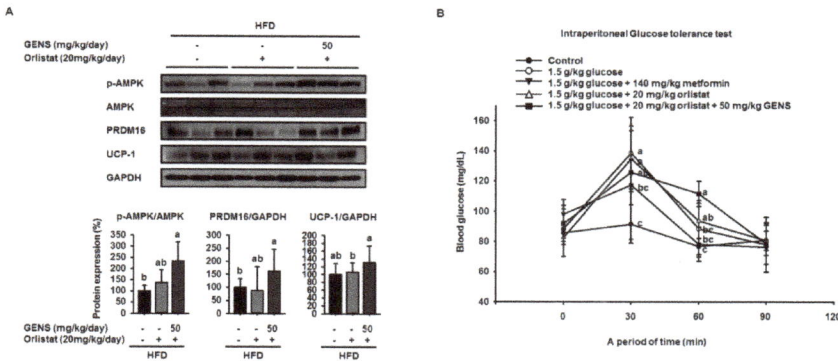

**Figure 7.** Combination effect of GENS and orlistat on energy expenditure-associated protein expression in brown adipose tissue of HFD-fed mice. Five-week-old mice were maintained with or without orlistat (20 mg/kg/day) and GENS (50 mg/kg/day) under HFD for 7 weeks. Protein extracts from brown adipose tissue were assayed for p-AMPK, PRDM16, and UCP-1 by western blot analysis with specific antibodies. The protein expression level was normalized against GAPDH (**A**). Protein level was quantified using Image J software. Five groups of male mice (5 weeks old) were fasted for 12 h (dark-period). After 12-h fasting, mice were administered 1.0 g/kg glucose by intraperitoneal injection. The first group received only PBS, the second group received 1.0 g/kg glucose, third groups received 1.0 g/kg glucose + 140 mg/kg metformin, the fourth group received 1.0 g/kg glucose + 20 mg/kg orlistat and the fifth group received 1.0 g/kg glucose + 20 mg/kg orlistat + 50 mg/kg GENS. Blood glucose levels were measured at the indicated times (0, 30, 60, and 90 min) (**B**). Data are mean $\pm$ SD ($n$ = 6).

## 4. Discussion

Here, we showed that GENS is sufficient to inhibit multiple characteristics of obesity, including weight gain, adipose tissue mass, hepatic lipogenesis, and hyperglycemia, in the HFD-induced obese mouse model. Notably, GENS altered energy metabolism by stimulating the expression of known thermogenesis regulator molecules such as PRDM16 and UCP-1. Moreover, we demonstrated that combined treatment with GENS and orlistat attenuated the plasma TG content and body weight gain in HFD-fed mice. In obesity, excessive energy intake promotes an increase in the storage of lipids in adipose tissue [39], thus resulting in an increase in adipose tissue mass through the formation of new adipocytes and an increase in the size of adipocytes [40]. These events involve cellular and molecular changes including morphological modifications of a number of critical adipogenic transcription factors, such as C/EBPα and PPARγ [28]. HFD can activate the expression of C/EBPα and PPARγ in tissues and cause hyperglycemia resulting from diet-induced early insulin resistance through hematogenous spread [41]. The elevated C/EBPα and PPARγ expression and increased hyperglycemia in obese mice was ameliorated by the intake of fruits, vegetables, and edible seaweed and/or its derivatives. This suggests the natural dietary substances can attenuate characteristics associated with obesity [12,46–48].

Our previous study, as well as recent studies, suggested that GENS may exert a protective effect on adipogenesis in adipocytes in vitro [49] and in adipose tissue mass in vivo by regulating C/EBPα and PPARγ proteins [19]. Consistent with previous results, our results showed that GENS decreased the expression of C/EBPα and PPARγ in white adipose tissue in HFD-fed mice.

Diet-induced hepatic lipogenesis is associated with non-alcohol-induced fatty liver (NAFLD), a disease state that is a crucial factor in insulin resistance and early-stage diabetes [50]. Prior studies have suggested that GENS has the potential to ameliorate hepatic lipid accumulation and plasma TG content in rats that have been fed a high fructose diet [51].

However, these studies did not provide molecular mechanisms for how GENS regulates these processes. In this study, we demonstrated that GENS suppressed hepatic lipogenesis through modulation of the AMPK-SREBP-1 pathway in HFD-fed mice. In regulating energy metabolism, AMPK stimulates the interaction between PGC1α and PRDM16 resulting in increased mitochondrial biogenesis, thermogenesis, and energy expenditure [52]. Interestingly, we noticed that in HFD-fed mice treated with GENS, PRDM16 in the liver was significantly increased, indicating that GENS may elevate mitochondrial biogenesis or thermogenesis via activation of the thermogenic factor PRDM16 in these animals.

It has been previously demonstrated that HFD induces hepatic lipogenesis, leading to hyperglycemia [53]. In this study, we revealed that hyperglycemia was induced in HFD-fed mice, whereas GENS significantly prevented HFD-mediated hyperglycemia. Although we could not address the detailed mechanism of the interaction between hepatic lipogenesis and hyperglycemia, we speculate that mitochondrial function such as biogenesis and thermogenesis might be involved in the link in these processes.

We hypothesized that if the anti-obesity effects of GENS were mainly due to the affect thermogenesis, GENS might alter the expression of thermogenesis-associated protein in brown adipose tissue. Thus, we analyzed the expression of thermogenic genes in brown adipose tissue, and our results revealed that levels of the most important thermogenesis-associated proteins AMPK, PRDM16, and UCP-1 were dramatically increased. Previous work has demonstrated that AMPK increases the expression of Sirt1 and enhances mitochondrial biogenesis through the regulation of PGC1α [54]. It is well known that PRDM16 plays a crucial role in controlling the expression of UCP-1 in brown adipocytes [55]. Therefore, we postulated that GENS may stimulate thermogenesis or energy expenditure through the AMPK-PRDM16-UCP-1 pathway in HFD-fed mice.

Orlistat has been used to promote weight loss and plasma TG content normalization in NAFLD and obesity patients [56,57]. It has also been reported as a specific intestinal lipase that breaks down TG, thus resulting in a decrease in fat absorption [58]. As orlistat treatment can promote the inhibition of dietary fat absorption and fatty acid synthesis, we utilized a different mechanism of activity than GENS to assess whether the combination of low-dose GENS and orlistat affected obesity characteristics in HFD-fed mice. We found that the combination was effective in weight-gain prevention in HFD-fed mice. More importantly, the combined treatment with low-dose GENS and orlistat significantly inhibited the expression of C/EBPα and PPARγ in white adipose tissue. It was reasonable to assume that the beneficial effect of GENS and orlistat on adipose tissue mass in HFD-fed mice was through the inhibition of adipogenesis since there was a significant difference in this variable between the HFD group, the orlistat group, and the low-dose GENS + orlistat group. As the highest level of reduction in hyperglycemia and plasma TG content was achieved with the combination of low-dose GENS and orlistat in HFD-fed mice, this combination seems ideal to reduce obesity features. In addition, we noticed that in these mice, the thermogenic genes AMPK, PRDM16, and UCP-1 were also synergistically activated by the combination treatment. This might indicate that an active UCP-1 protein is a heat generator that in mice contributes to loss of energy in the form of heat. The animal study was performed at 20–24 °C, whereas thermoneutrality for mice is 28–30 °C. Therefore, the UCP-1 protein would be expected to be active in the mice housed under the conditions used in the present study. As the GENS mice had less adipose tissue, both subcutaneous and abdominal, they also have less insulating material. This could mean that these mice had to generate more heat through UCP-1 activation. Obviously, this would contribute to less adipose tissue mass as observed, but the mechanism could be independent of any effect of GENS or orlistat. Under these circumstances, a reduced fat absorption would contribute to less available energy, and hence accentuate the mobilization of fatty acids from white adipose tissue for UCP-1 heat generation. Although the mechanisms of action of GENS and orlistat are distinct, we have provided partial evidence that GENS and orlistat can act synergistically in HFD-fed mice.

## 5. Conclusions

It is known that the incidence of overweight and obesity is responsible for increased abnormalities in multiple signaling pathways, including adipogenesis, lipolysis, and energy expenditure-associated pathways [59,60], and can cause hyperglycemia and NAFLD. In this study, we provided evidence to suggest that in HFD-fed mice, thermogenesis is activated in response to GENS consumption, possibly through the AMPK-PRDM16-UCP-1 pathway.

This results in the modulation of hepatic lipogenesis as reflected by altered AMPK-PRDM16-UCP-1 pathway and suppression of white adipose tissue mass expansion. Moreover, we postulated that combination of GENS and orlistat is associated with more significant weight loss than the orlistat alone in HFD-fed mice. In particular, our results demonstrated a synergistic effect between GENS and orlistat on hyperglycemia and hepatic lipogenesis in HFD-fed mice. Therefore, we suggest that combination therapy with GENS and orlistat may positively influence the outcomes related to obesity characteristics in a diet-induced obese population.

**Acknowledgments:** This research was partially supported by Basic Science Research Program through the National Research Foundation of Korea (NRF) funded by the Ministry of Education (2016R1D1A1A09917209). The funders had no role in study design, data collection and analysis, decision to publish, or preparation of the manuscript.

**Author Contributions:** Jia Choi, Kui-Jin Kim, and Boo-Yong Lee conceived and designed the study; Jia Choi and Eun-Jeong Koh performed the experiments; Jia Choi and Kui-Jin Kim analyzed the data; Jia Choi and Kui-Jin Kim wrote the paper and edited the paper.

**Conflicts of Interest:** The authors declare no conflict of interest.

## References

1. World Health Organization. *Obesity: Preventing and Managing the Global Epidemic*; World Health Organization: Geneva, Switzerland, 2000.
2. Farmer, S.R. Regulation of ppargamma activity during adipogenesis. *Int. J. Obes.* **2005**, *29* (Suppl. 1), S13–S16. [CrossRef] [PubMed]
3. Dandona, P.; Aljada, A.; Bandyopadhyay, A. Inflammation: The link between insulin resistance, obesity and diabetes. *Trends Immunol.* **2004**, *25*, 4–7. [CrossRef] [PubMed]
4. Dobbs, R.; Sawers, C.; Thompson, F.; Manyika, J.; Woetzel, J.R.; Child, P.; McKenna, S.; Spatharou, A. *Overcoming Obesity: An Initial Economic Analysis*; McKinsey Global Institute: Tamil Nadu, India, 2014.
5. Roberts, D.L.; Dive, C.; Renehan, A.G. Biological mechanisms linking obesity and cancer risk: New perspectives. *Annu. Rev. Med.* **2010**, *61*, 301–316. [CrossRef] [PubMed]
6. Lau, D.C.; Douketis, J.D.; Morrison, K.M.; Hramiak, I.M.; Sharma, A.M.; Ur, E. Obesity Canada Clinical Practice Guidelines Expert Panel. *Can. Med. Assoc. J.* **2007**, *176*, S1–S13. [CrossRef] [PubMed]
7. Pi-Sunyer, F.X.; Becker, D.M.; Bouchard, C.; Carleton, R.; Colditz, G.; Dietz, W.; Foreyt, J.; Garrison, R.; Grundy, S.; Hansen, B. Clinical guidelines on the identification, evaluation, and treatment of overweight and obesity in adults. *Am. J. Clin. Nutr.* **1998**, *68*, 899–917.
8. Heck, A.M.; Yanovski, J.A.; Calis, K.A. Orlistat, a new lipase inhibitor for the management of obesity. *Pharmacotherapy* **2000**, *20*, 270–279. [CrossRef] [PubMed]
9. Rossner, S.; Sjostrom, L.; Noack, R.; Meinders, E.; Noseda, G. Weight loss, weight maintenance, and improved cardiovascular risk factors after 2 years treatment with orlistat for obesity. *Obes. Res.* **2000**, *8*, 49–61. [CrossRef] [PubMed]
10. Heymsfield, S.B.; Segal, K.R.; Hauptman, J.; Lucas, C.P.; Boldrin, M.N.; Rissanen, A.; Wilding, J.P.; Sjöström, L. Effects of weight loss with orlistat on glucose tolerance and progression to type 2 diabetes in obese adults. *Arch. Intern. Med.* **2000**, *160*, 1321–1326. [CrossRef] [PubMed]

11. Kumanyika, S.K.; Obarzanek, E.; Stettler, N.; Bell, R.; Field, A.E.; Fortmann, S.P.; Franklin, B.A.; Gillman, M.W.; Lewis, C.E.; Poston, W.C.; et al. Population-based prevention of obesity the need for comprehensive promotion of healthful eating, physical activity, and energy balance: A scientific statement from american heart association council on epidemiology and prevention, interdisciplinary committee for prevention (formerly the expert panel on population and prevention science). *Circulation* **2008**, *118*, 428–464. [PubMed]

12. Epstein, L.H.; Gordy, C.C.; Raynor, H.A.; Beddome, M.; Kilanowski, C.K.; Paluch, R. Increasing fruit and vegetable intake and decreasing fat and sugar intake in families at risk for childhood obesity. *Obes. Res.* **2001**, *9*, 171–178. [CrossRef] [PubMed]

13. Szkudelska, K.; Szkudelski, T. Resveratrol, obesity and diabetes. *Eur. J. Pharmacol.* **2010**, *635*, 1–8. [CrossRef] [PubMed]

14. Ejaz, A.; Wu, D.; Kwan, P.; Meydani, M. Curcumin inhibits adipogenesis in 3t3-l1 adipocytes and angiogenesis and obesity in c57/bl mice. *J. Nutr.* **2009**, *139*, 919–925. [CrossRef] [PubMed]

15. Blankson, H.; Stakkestad, J.A.; Fagertun, H.; Thom, E.; Wadstein, J.; Gudmundsen, O. Conjugated linoleic acid reduces body fat mass in overweight and obese humans. *J. Nutr.* **2000**, *130*, 2943–2948. [PubMed]

16. Ruzickova, J.; Rossmeisl, M.; Prazak, T.; Flachs, P.; Sponarova, J.; Vecka, M.; Tvrzicka, E.; Bryhn, M.; Kopecky, J. Omega-3 pufa of marine origin limit diet-induced obesity in mice by reducing cellularity of adipose tissue. *Lipids* **2004**, *39*, 1177–1185. [CrossRef] [PubMed]

17. Miyashita, K. The carotenoid fucoxanthin from brown seaweed affects obesity. *Lipid Technol.* **2009**, *21*, 186–190. [CrossRef]

18. Maeda, H.; Tsukui, T.; Sashima, T.; Miyashita, K. Seaweed carotenoid, fucoxanthin, as a multi-functional nutrient. *Asia Pac. J. Clin. Nutr.* **2008**, *17*, 196–199. [PubMed]

19. Kang, M.-C.; Kang, N.; Kim, S.-Y.; Lima, I.S.; Ko, S.-C.; Kim, Y.-T.; Kim, Y.-B.; Jeung, H.-D.; Choi, K.-S.; Jeon, Y.-J. Popular edible seaweed, gelidium amansii prevents against diet-induced obesity. *Food Chem. Toxicol.* **2016**, *90*, 181–187. [CrossRef] [PubMed]

20. Yang, T.-H.; Yao, H.-T.; Chiang, M.-T. Red algae (gelidium amansii) reduces adiposity via activation of lipolysis in rats with diabetes induced by streptozotocin-nicotinamide. *J. Food Drug Anal.* **2015**, *23*, 758–765. [CrossRef]

21. Seo, M.-J.; Lee, O.-H.; Choi, H.-S.; Lee, B.-Y. Extract from edible red seaweed (gelidium amansii) inhibits lipid accumulation and ros production during differentiation in 3t3-l1 cells. *Prev. Nutr. Food Sci.* **2012**, *17*, 129–135. [CrossRef] [PubMed]

22. Choi, J.; Kim, K.-J.; Koh, E.-J.; Lee, B.-Y. Altered gelidium elegans extract-stimulated beige-like phenotype attenuates adipogenesis in 3t3-l1 cells. *J. Food Nutr. Res.* **2016**, *4*, 448–453.

23. Kim, K.-J.; Choi, J.; Lee, B.-Y. Evaluation of the genotoxicity of a *Gelidium elegans* extract in vitro and in vivo. *J. Food Nutr. Res.* **2016**, *4*, 653–657.

24. Wang, Z.; Oh, E.; Clapp, D.W.; Chernoff, J.; Thurmond, D.C. Inhibition or ablation of p21-activated kinase (pak1) disrupts glucose homeostatic mechanisms in vivo. *J. Biol. Chem.* **2011**, *286*, 41359–41367. [CrossRef] [PubMed]

25. Harlow, E.D.; Lane, D. *Using Antibodies: A Laboratory Manual*; Cold Spring Harbor Laboratory Press: Cold Spring Harbor, NY, USA, 1999.

26. Morelli, A.; Filippi, S.; Comeglio, P.; Sarchielli, E.; Chavalmane, A.K.; Vignozzi, L.; Fibbi, B.; Silvestrini, E.; Sandner, P.; Gacci, M.; et al. Acute vardenafil administration improves bladder oxygenation in spontaneously hypertensive rats. *J. Sex. Med.* **2010**, *7*, 107–120. [CrossRef] [PubMed]

27. Dubuc, P.U. The development of obesity, hyperinsulinemia, and hyperglycemia in ob/ob mice. *Metabolism* **1976**, *25*, 1567–1574. [CrossRef]

28. Newcomer, J.W. Metabolic syndrome and mental illness. *Am. J. Manag. Care* **2007**, *13*, S170–S177. [PubMed]

29. European Diabetes Policy Group. A desktop guide to type 2 diabetes mellitus. In *Diabet. Med.*; 1999; Volume 16, pp. 716–730.

30. Hillier, T.A.; Pedula, K.L.; Schmidt, M.M.; Mullen, J.A.; Charles, M.-A.; Pettitt, D.J. Childhood obesity and metabolic imprinting the ongoing effects of maternal hyperglycemia. *Diabetes Care* **2007**, *30*, 2287–2292. [CrossRef] [PubMed]

31. Watkins, M.L.; Rasmussen, S.A.; Honein, M.A.; Botto, L.D.; Moore, C.A. Maternal obesity and risk for birth defects. *Pediatrics* **2003**, *111*, 1152–1158. [PubMed]

32. Arai, T.; Yamashita, S.; Hirano, K.-I.; Sakai, N.; Kotani, K.; Fujioka, S.; Nozaki, S.; Keno, Y.; Yamane, M.; Shinohara, E.; et al. Increased plasma cholesteryl ester transfer protein in obese subjects. A possible mechanism for the reduction of serum hdl cholesterol levels in obesity. *Arterioscler. Thromb.* **1994**, *14*, 1129–1136. [CrossRef] [PubMed]

33. Hu, E.; Tontonoz, P.; Spiegelman, B.M. Transdifferentiation of myoblasts by the adipogenic transcription factors ppar gamma and c/ebp alpha. *Proc. Natl. Acad. Sci. USA* **1995**, *92*, 9856–9860. [CrossRef] [PubMed]

34. Laakso, M. Hyperglycemia and cardiovascular disease in type 2 diabetes. *Diabetes* **1999**, *48*, 937–942. [CrossRef] [PubMed]

35. Ikemoto, S.; Takahashi, M.; Tsunoda, N.; Maruyama, K.; Itakura, H.; Ezaki, O. High-fat diet-induced hyperglycemia and obesity in mice: Differential effects of dietary oils. *Metabolism* **1996**, *45*, 1539–1546. [CrossRef]

36. Nathan, D.M.; Davidson, M.B.; DeFronzo, R.A.; Heine, R.J.; Henry, R.R.; Pratley, R.; Zinman, B. Impaired fasting glucose and impaired glucose tolerance. *Diabetes Care* **2007**, *30*, 753–759. [CrossRef] [PubMed]

37. Yang, L.; Zhang, Y.; Wang, L.; Fan, F.; Zhu, L.; Li, Z.; Ruan, X.; Huang, H.; Wang, Z.; Huang, Z.; et al. Amelioration of high fat diet induced liver lipogenesis and hepatic steatosis by interleukin-22. *J. Hepatol.* **2010**, *53*, 339–347. [CrossRef] [PubMed]

38. Carmiel-Haggai, M.; Cederbaum, A.I.; Nieto, N. A high-fat diet leads to the progression of non-alcoholic fatty liver disease in obese rats. *FASEB J.* **2005**, *19*, 136–138. [CrossRef] [PubMed]

39. Horton, J.D.; Goldstein, J.L.; Brown, M.S. Srebps: Activators of the complete program of cholesterol and fatty acid synthesis in the liver. *J. Clin. Investig.* **2002**, *109*, 1125–1131. [CrossRef] [PubMed]

40. Yahagi, N.; Shimano, H.; Hasty, A.H.; Matsuzaka, T.; Ide, T.; Yoshikawa, T.; Amemiya-Kudo, M.; Tomita, S.; Okazaki, H.; Tamura, Y.; et al. Absence of sterol regulatory element-binding protein-1 (srebp-1) ameliorates fatty livers but not obesity or insulin resistance inlep ob/lep ob mice. *J. Biol. Chem.* **2002**, *277*, 19353–19357. [CrossRef] [PubMed]

41. Brown, M.S.; Goldstein, J.L. The srebp pathway: Regulation of cholesterol metabolism by proteolysis of a membrane-bound transcription factor. *Cell* **1997**, *89*, 331–340. [CrossRef]

42. Harris, C.A.; Haas, J.T.; Streeper, R.S.; Stone, S.J.; Kumari, M.; Yang, K.; Han, X.; Brownell, N.; Gross, R.W.; Zechner, R.; et al. Dgat enzymes are required for triacylglycerol synthesis and lipid droplets in adipocytes. *J. Lipid Res.* **2011**, *52*, 657–667. [CrossRef] [PubMed]

43. Li, Y.; Xu, S.; Mihaylova, M.M.; Zheng, B.; Hou, X.; Jiang, B.; Park, O.; Luo, Z.; Lefai, E.; Shyy, J.Y.-J.; et al. Ampk phosphorylates and inhibits srebp activity to attenuate hepatic steatosis and atherosclerosis in diet-induced insulin-resistant mice. *Cell Metab.* **2011**, *13*, 376–388. [CrossRef] [PubMed]

44. Hardie, D.G. Ampk—Sensing energy while talking to other signaling pathways. *Cell Metab.* **2014**, *20*, 939–952. [CrossRef] [PubMed]

45. Kajimura, S.; Seale, P.; Tomaru, T.; Erdjument-Bromage, H.; Cooper, M.P.; Ruas, J.L.; Chin, S.; Tempst, P.; Lazar, M.A.; Spiegelman, B.M. Regulation of the brown and white fat gene programs through a prdm16/ctbp transcriptional complex. *Genes Dev.* **2008**, *22*, 1397–1409. [CrossRef] [PubMed]

46. Kang, J.H.; Tsuyoshi, G.; Han, I.S.; Kawada, T.; Kim, Y.M.; Yu, R. Dietary capsaicin reduces obesity-induced insulin resistance and hepatic steatosis in obese mice fed a high-fat diet. *Obesity* **2010**, *18*, 780–787. [CrossRef] [PubMed]

47. Maeda, H.; Hosokawa, M.; Sashima, T.; Murakami-Funayama, K.; Miyashita, K. Anti-obesity and anti-diabetic effects of fucoxanthin on diet-induced obesity conditions in a murine model. *Mol. Med. Rep.* **2009**, *2*, 897–902. [CrossRef] [PubMed]

48. Jayaprakasam, B.; Olson, L.K.; Schutzki, R.E.; Tai, M.-H.; Nair, M.G. Amelioration of obesity and glucose intolerance in high-fat-fed c57bl/6 mice by anthocyanins and ursolic acid in cornelian cherry (cornus mas). *J. Agric. Food Chem.* **2006**, *54*, 243–248. [CrossRef] [PubMed]

49. Jeon, H.J.; Seo, M.J.; Choi, H.S.; Lee, O.H.; Lee, B.Y. *Gelidium elegans*, an edible red seaweed, and hesperidin inhibit lipid accumulation and production of reactive oxygen species and reactive nitrogen species in 3t3-l1 and raw264.7 cells. *Phytother. Res.* **2014**, *28*, 1701–1709. [CrossRef] [PubMed]

50. Gregor, M.F.; Hotamisligil, G.S. Inflammatory mechanisms in obesity. *Annu. Rev. Immunol.* **2011**, *29*, 415–445. [CrossRef] [PubMed]

51.  Liu, H.-C.; Chang, C.-J.; Yang, T.-H.; Chiang, M.-T. Long-term feeding of red algae (*Gelidium amansii*) ameliorates glucose and lipid metabolism in a high fructose diet-impaired glucose tolerance rat model. *J. Food Drug Anal.* **2016**. [CrossRef]

52.  Zhang, H.; Zhang, S.; Jiang, C.; Li, Y.; Xu, G.; Xu, M.; Wang, X. Intermedin/adrenomedullin 2 polypeptide promotes adipose tissue browning and reduces high-fat diet-induced obesity and insulin resistance in mice. *Int. J. Obes.* **2016**, *40*, 852–860. [CrossRef] [PubMed]

53.  Lin, J.; Yang, R.; Tarr, P.T.; Wu, P.-H.; Handschin, C.; Li, S.; Yang, W.; Pei, L.; Uldry, M.; Tontonoz, P.; et al. Hyperlipidemic effects of dietary saturated fats mediated through pgc-1β coactivation of srebp. *Cell* **2005**, *120*, 261–273. [CrossRef] [PubMed]

54.  Fernandez-Marcos, P.J.; Auwerx, J. Regulation of pgc-1alpha, a nodal regulator of mitochondrial biogenesis. *Am. J. Clin. Nutr.* **2011**, *93*, 884S–890S. [CrossRef] [PubMed]

55.  Seale, P.; Kajimura, S.; Yang, W.; Chin, S.; Rohas, L.M.; Uldry, M.; Tavernier, G.; Langin, D.; Spiegelman, B.M. Transcriptional control of brown fat determination by prdm16. *Cell Metab.* **2007**, *6*, 38–54. [CrossRef] [PubMed]

56.  Zelber-Sagi, S.; Kessler, A.; Brazowsky, E.; Webb, M.; Lurie, Y.; Santo, M.; Leshno, M.; Blendis, L.; Halpern, Z.; Oren, R. A double-blind randomized placebo-controlled trial of orlistat for the treatment of nonalcoholic fatty liver disease. *Clin. Gastroenterol. Hepatol.* **2006**, *4*, 639–644. [CrossRef] [PubMed]

57.  Van Gaal, L.; Broom, J.; Enzi, G.; Toplak, H. Efficacy and tolerability of orlistat in the treatment of obesity: A 6-month dose-ranging study. *Eur. J. Clin. Pharmacol.* **1998**, *54*, 125–132. [CrossRef] [PubMed]

58.  Kiortsis, D.; Filippatos, T.; Elisaf, M. The effects of orlistat on metabolic parameters and other cardiovascular risk factors. *Diabetes Metab.* **2005**, *31*, 15–22. [CrossRef]

59.  Spiegelman, B.M.; Flier, J.S. Adipogenesis and obesity: Rounding out the big picture. *Cell* **1996**, *87*, 377–389. [CrossRef]

60.  Hamilton, M.T.; Hamilton, D.G.; Zderic, T.W. Role of low energy expenditure and sitting in obesity, metabolic syndrome, type 2 diabetes, and cardiovascular disease. *Diabetes* **2007**, *56*, 2655–2667. [CrossRef] [PubMed]

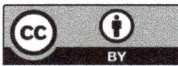

*nutrients*

MDPI

*Article*

# Genistein Ameliorates Ischemia/Reperfusion-Induced Renal Injury in a SIRT1-Dependent Manner

Wei-Fang Li [1], Kang Yang [1], Ping Zhu [2], Hong-Qian Zhao [1], Yin-Hong Song [1], Kuan-Can Liu [3,4,5,]* and Wei-Feng Huang [1,]*

[1]  Medical College, China Three Gorges University, Yichang 443002, China; lwf199023@163.com (W.-F.L.); yangkang0218@126.com (K.Y.); 15271506793@163.com (H.-Q.Z.); syh728@126.com (Y.-H.S.)
[2]  Department of Medicine, the First College of Clinical Medical Science, China Three Gorges University, Yichang 443002, China; topgan2000@163.com
[3]  Institute for Laboratory Medicine, Fuzhou General Hospital, PLA, Fuzhou 350025, China
[4]  Department of Medicine, Columbia University Medical Center, New York, NY 10032, USA
[5]  Dongfang Hospital, Xiamen University, Fuzhou 350025, China
*  Correspondence: liukuancan@163.com (K.-C.L.); huangweifeng@ctgu.edu.cn (W.-F.H.); Tel.: +86-591-2285-9490 (K.-C.L.); +86-717-639-7438 (W.-F.H.)

Received: 6 February 2017; Accepted: 17 April 2017; Published: 20 April 2017

**Abstract:** Renal ischemia/reperfusion (I/R) injury continues to be a complicated situation in clinical practice. Genistein, the main isoflavone found in soy products, is known to possess a wide spectrum of biochemical and pharmacological activities. However, the protective effect of genistein on renal I/R injury has not been well investigated. In the current study, we explore whether genistein exhibits its renal-protective effects through SIRT1 (Sirtuin 1) in I/R-induced mice model. We found the treatment of genistein significantly reduced renal I/R-induced cell death, simultaneously stimulating renal cell proliferation. Meanwhile, SIRT1 expression was up-regulated following the administration of genistein in renal region. Furthermore, pharmacological inhibition or shRNA-mediated depletion of SIRT1 significantly reversed the protective effect of genistein on renal dysfunction, cellular damage, apoptosis, and proliferation following I/R injury, suggesting an indispensible role of the increased SIRT1 expression and activity in this process. Meanwhile, the reduced p53 and p21 expression and increased PCNA (Proliferating Cell Nuclear Antigen) expression were blocked after the depletion of SIRT1 compared with the genistein treatment group in the renal I/R process. Hence, our results provided further experimental basis for the potential use of genistein for the treatment of kidney disease with deficiency of SIRT1 activity.

**Keywords:** genistein; SIRT1; renal ischemia-reperfusion

## 1. Introduction

Renal I/R injury is a major cause of acute kidney injury (AKI), which is a clinical condition of frequent occurrence and high mortality [1,2]. I/R injury can increasingly develop into AKI in many clinical settings, such as kidney transplantation, renal artery angioplasty, sepsis, and partial nephrectomy, or by the action of vasoconstrictor drugs and certain hypotensive states [3]. There are many factors that likely contribute to I/R-induced renal injury. However, the exact molecular mechanisms underlying renal I/R injury are not completely understood. Various pharmaceuticals have been identified for the treatment of renal I/R injury in the laboratory, such as AICAR (5-amino-4-imidazolecarboxamide riboside-1-b-D-ribofuranoside), yohimbine, and pioglitazone [4–6]. However, these are limited, and few renal protectants have been successfully translated into clinical applications. Therefore, it is critical and urgent to develop safe and effective drugs for treating IR-induced renal injury.

SIRT1, an NAD$^+$ (nicotinamide adenosine denucleotide)-dependent protein deacetylase, exerts cytoprotective effects through multiple mechanisms, such as anti-apoptosis, anti-oxidative, and anti-inflammation effects and the regulation of mitochondrial biogenesis and autophagy [7]. Many studies have shown that SIRT1 can regulate multiple physiological processes, including gene transcription, glucose homeostasis, cellular stress response, and immune response through its capability of deacetylating various factors. The target proteins of deacetylation by SIRT1 include histones, transcriptional regulators (p53; forkhead box O transcription factors, FoxOs; Nuclear factor κB, NF-κB; hypoxia-inducible factors 2α, hypoxia-inducible factors 2α, HIF 2α), enzymes (acetyl-CoA synthase1, AceCS1), and other signaling molecules such as peroxisome proliferator activated receptor γ co-activator 1α (PGC1-α), thus affecting crucial cellular pathways in physiological and pathological processes [8]. The renal protected effects of SIRT1 have been demonstrated in various kidney diseases [9]. For example, SIRT1 preserves podocyte function by tuning claudin-1, which is a key regulator of albuminuria and glomerular function [10]. He et al. [11] have reported that SIRT1 protects the kidney medulla from oxidative stress-induced cellular injury by regulating the induction of COX2 (cytochrome c oxidase subunit II). In addition, in mesangial cells, SIRT1 can prevent oxidative stress-induced apoptosis by the deacetylation of p53 [12]. SIRT1 inhibits TGF β1 (transforming growth factor β1)-induced apoptosis in glomerular mesangial cells via Smad7 deacetylation [13]. Recent studies have suggested that SIRT1 protects against I/R-induced renal injury by attenuating apoptosis and promoting regeneration [14]. The protection caused by SIRT1 is closely involved in the inhibition of the p53 signaling pathway. Specific deletion of p53 in the proximal tubule cells protects kidneys from I/R-induced renal functional and histologic deterioration [15,16]. Moreover, caloric restriction has been shown to provide protection against I/R-induced renal injury [17]. SIRT1 expression is strongly influenced by calorie restriction. While multiple genes respond to caloric restriction, SIRT1 is at least thought to be involved in the health benefits attributed to long-term caloric restriction [7].

Genistein (4′,5,7-trihydroxyisoflavone), the most extensively studied soy isoflavone thus far, is a polyphenolic non-steroidal compound commonly used as a dietary supplement. Because genistein possesses oestrogen-like biological activity, its biological effects have been explored in conditions such as cancer, inflammation, and apoptosis [18]. Previously, we also found that genistein inhibited cancer stem cell-like properties and reduced the chemoresistance of gastric cancer [19]. Genistein has been reported to protect against I/R-induced cerebral injury in the rat [20], and it has a protective role on I/R-induced small intestine injury [21]. Additionally, Canyilmaz, E. et al. demonstrated that the administration of genistein protects mice against radiation-induced nephrotoxicity [22]. It is of particular relevance that the physiological activity of genistein as a phytoestrogen is closely related to SIRT1 activity [23]. Genistein has multiple beneficial properties, including low toxicity, it has potential in clinical treatment. However, the role and potential mechanism of genistein in I/R-induced kidney injury remains unknown.

In this study, we aimed to determine the role of genistein in I/R-induced kidney injury and then dissect the exact mechanism responsible for the treatment of I/R-induced kidney injury. Thus, it will be helpful for us to establish guidance for the treatment of I/R-induced kidney injury.

## 2. Materials and Methods

### 2.1. Experimental Animals, I/R, Genistein Treatment, and SIRT1 Inhibition

Seven- to nine-week-old BALB/c mice were supplied by the China Three Gorges University Laboratory Animal Center, and they were housed in an air-conditioned room with 12-h light and dark cycles. All of the experiments were carried out in accordance with NIH Guidelines for the Care and Use of Laboratory Animals. The animals were kept in sterile cages (maximum of five per cage) and fed standard rodent chow and allowed free access to water ad libitum. All of the experimental protocols were approved by our School of Medicine Animal Care and Use Committee. An animal's ability to drink water, feed, ambulate, and its general appearance were evaluated after operation. They were monitored three times in 24 h after genistein treatment.

An established model of the renal I/R-induced injury was established previously [24]. Briefly, an abdominal midline incision was made, and right nephrectomy was performed under anesthesia. Mice were anaesthetized using 100 mg/kg ketamine and 0.75 mg/kg chlorpromazine intraperitoneally. Left renal ischemia was induced by clamping renal pedicles for 45 min with microvascular clamps and then subjected to reperfusion. Mice in the sham group underwent right nephrectomy and were treated as indicated in the specific experiment. The mice were hydrated with warm saline during the operation, and the body temperature was maintained constantly at 37 °C using a heating pad until awake. The wounds were sutured after removal of the clips, and the animals were allowed to recover.

Genistein (Sigma Aldrich, St. Louis, MO, USA; dissolved in 0.9% sodium chloride containing 1% dimethyl sulphoxide) was given (intravenous injection, i.v.) 30 min before the induction of ischaemia. For the pharmacological inhibition of SIRT1 activity, mice were treated (i.v.) with Sirtinol (Sigma Aldrich, St. Louis, MO, USA; 1 mg/kg dissolved in 0.9% sodium chloride containing 1% dimethyl sulfoxide) 60 min before the induction of ischemia. The others received the same volume of vehicle. For the inhibition of SIRT1 by lentivirus, a 31-gauge needle was used to inject 100 μL of ultracentrifugation-purified lentivirus (lentivirus, LV; LV-control or LV-shSIRT1, ≈3 × $10^7$ TU) at the lower pole of the left kidneys parallel to the long axis and was slowly removed 72 h later [25]; then, induction of ischemia was performed.

For the dose-dependent analyses of genistein effects on I/R-induced renal injury, mice were randomized into five groups ($n = 6$/group): (1) sham group; (2) I/R group; (3) G5 group; (4) G10 group; and (5) G15 group. In the sham group, mice received the same volume of vehicle without I/R; in the I/R group, mice received the same volume of vehicle with I/R; in the G5 group, mice were pre-treated with 5 mg/kg genistein following I/R; in the G10 group, mice were pre-treated with 10 mg/kg genistein following I/R; in the G15 group, mice were treated with 15 mg/kg genistein. The mice were decapitated after 24 h of reperfusion, and blood samples were collected for the analysis of biochemical measurements. The kidneys were excised and then washed with ice-cold saline for further analysis.

For the time-dependent analyses of the genistein effects on I/R renal-induced injury, mice were randomized into three groups ($n = 24$/group): (1) sham group; (2) I/R group; and (3) G15 group. In the sham group, mice received the same volume of vehicle without I/R; in the G15 group, mice were pre-treated with 15 mg/kg genistein following I/R. Six mice in each group were decapitated at 12, 24, 48, and 72 h of the reperfusion period, and blood samples were collected for the analysis of biochemical measurements. The kidneys were excised and then washed with ice-cold saline for further analysis.

For the inhibition of SIRT1 by Sirtinol, mice were randomized into four groups ($n = 6$/group): (1) vehicle group; (2) Sirtinol group; (3) G15 group; and (4) Sirtinol + G15 group. Ischemia was induced in all groups. In the vehicle group, mice received the same volume of vehicle; in the Sirtinol group, mice were pre-treated with 1 mg/kg Sirtinol; in the G15 group, mice were pre-treated with 15 mg/kg genistein; in the Sirtinol + G15 group, mice were treated with 15 mg/kg genistein and 1 mg/kg Sirtinol. Sirtinol and genistein were administered as described above. The mice were decapitated after 24 h of reperfusion and blood samples were collected for the analysis of biochemical measurements. The kidneys were excised and then washed with ice-cold saline for the further analysis.

For the inhibition of SIRT1 by lentivirus carrying shRNA targeting SIRT1, mice were randomized into four groups ($n = 6$/group): (1) LV-control group; (2) LV-shSIRT1 group; (3) G15 group; and (4) LV-shSIRT1 + G15 group. Ischemia was induced in all of the groups. In the LV-control group, mice were injected with lentivirus carrying scrambled shRNA and were pre-treated with the same volume of vehicle; in the LV-shSIRT1 group, mice were injected with lentivirus carrying SIRT1 shRNA; in the G15 group, mice were injected with lentivirus carrying scrambled shRNA and were pre-treated with 15 mg/kg genistein; in the G15 + LV-shSIRT1 group, mice were injected with lentivirus carrying SIRT1 shRNA and were pre-treated with 15 mg/kg genistein. Lentivirus injection and genistein treatment were performed as described above. The mice were decapitated at 24 h of the reperfusion period, and trunk blood samples were collected for the analysis of biochemical measurements. The kidneys were excised and then were washed with ice-cold saline for further analysis.

## 2.2. Biochemical Determinations

Serum was obtained from blood samples to measure blood urea nitrogen (BUN) and serum creatinine (Scr) using an automatic biochemistry analyzer (Hitachi 7060, Tokyo, Japan) after reperfusion.

## 2.3. Kidney Histology

For histological examination, the kidneys were fixed in 4% paraformaldehyde, embedded in paraffin, sectioned at 4-μm thickness, and stained with hematoxylin and eosin (H&E). Tubular injury was scored on a scale of 0–4 based on the percentage of tubules with necrosis, dilatation, cast formation and cell lysis: 0, no damage; 1, 5%–25%; 2, 25%–50%; 3, 50%–75%; and 4, >75%. The morphological changes from the cross-sectional area cortex and outer medulla were evaluated by a pathologist according to the acute tubular necrosis (ATN) scoring system in a blinded manner [26].

## 2.4. Immunohistochemistry

For immunohistochemical (IHC) studies, 4-μm-thick sections were microwaved in 0.01 mol/L sodium citrate (pH 6.0) three times for 5 min each. The primary antibodies used were anti-SIRT1 (1:100; Abcam, Cambridge, UK), anti-cleaved caspase-3 (Cell Signaling Technology, Danvers, MA, USA) and anti-PCNA (1:200; Santa Cruz, Dallas, TX, USA), respectively. IHC was performed using the UltrasensitiveTM SP (Mouse/Rabbit) IHC kit (Mai-xin Biotechnology Co., Fuzhou, China). Images were acquired using a digital camera (Olympus, Tokyo, Japan) at 400× magnification, and the results were analyzed by Image-Pro Plus 6.0 (Media Cybernetics, Rockville, MD, USA). The results were defined as the number of positive cells/total number of cells.

## 2.5. TUNEL Assay

Apoptosis detection was performed using the terminal deoxynucleotidyl transferase-mediated digoxigenindeoxyuridine nick-end labelling (TUNEL) assay (Roche Diagnostics, Mannheim, Germany) according to the protocols of the manufacturer. Briefly, samples were incubated in equilibration buffer for 5 min, followed by incubation in the labelling reaction reagent for 1 h at 37 °C, and DNA fragments in apoptotic cells were recognized. The positive cellular counts of staining were assessed at 400× magnification using five randomly selected fields, and the apoptosis index was expressed as the percentage of positive cells in high-power fields. Data were averaged.

## 2.6. Western Blotting

Proteins from kidney samples were isolated using lysis buffer followed by centrifugation. Western blot analysis of the proteins in mouse kidneys was performed according to standard protocols. Immunoblotting was performed using anti-SIRT1 antibody (1:5000; Abcam, Cambridge, UK), anti-cleaved caspase-3 antibody (1:1000; Cell Signaling Technology, Danvers, MA, USA), anti-pro-caspase-3 antibody (1:1000; Zen BioScience, Chengdu, China), anti-PCNA antibody (1:2000; Santa Cruz, Dallas, TX, USA), anti-p53 antibody (1:1000; Santa Cruz, Dallas, TX, USA), anti-acetyl-p53 antibody (K381) (1:1000; Abcam, Cambridge, UK), and anti-p21 antibody (1:2000; Santa Cruz, Dallas, TX, USA). The blots were detected using the Immobilon Western Chemiluminescent HRP Substrate kit (Millipore, Danvers, MA, USA) followed by exposure to Kodak-X-Omat film (Shanghai, China).

*2.7. Statistical Analysis*

All of the statistical analyses were performed using GraphPad Prism 5.0 software. The values are expressed as the mean ± SEM (standard error of the mean). Pair-wise comparisons were performed using Student's *t*-test (two-tailed), and multiple-group comparisons were performed using one-way ANOVA with Bonferroni's post-hoc test. A *p*-value < 0.05 was considered significant.

## 3. Results

*3.1. Genistein Protects the Kidney Against I/R Injury*

Renal I/R injury increased the Scr (serum creatinine) and BUN (blood urea nitrogen) levels to 1.8 ± 0.1 and 218.4 ± 9.7 mg/dL, respectively, from the levels in the sham group (0.3 ± 0.02 and 25.3 ± 1.7 mg/dL, respectively; Figure 1a, *p* < 0.05). The genistein-pretreated group showed significant reduction in the elevated Scr and BUN levels in a dose-dependent manner. Genistein at the dose of 15 mg/kg significantly decreased the Scr (0.5 ± 0.05 mg/dL, *p* < 0.05) levels and BUN (56.1 ± 5.4 mg/dL, *p* < 0.05) levels compared with those of the I/R group.

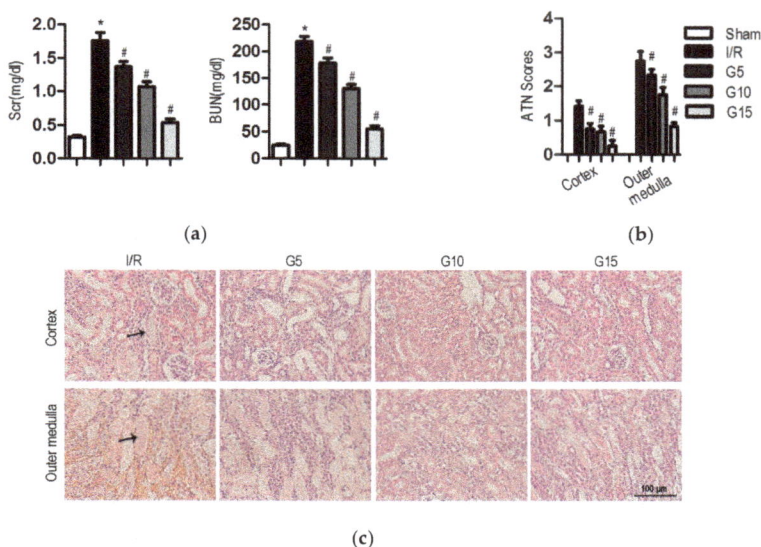

**Figure 1.** Effect of genistein on kidney injury following I/R injury. In the sham group, mice received the same volume of vehicle without I/R; in the I/R group, mice received the same volume of vehicle with I/R; in the G5 group, mice were pre-treated with 5 mg/kg genistein following I/R; in the G10 group, mice were pre-treated with 10 mg/kg genistein following I/R; and in the G15 group, mice were treated with 15 mg/kg genistein following I/R. The mice were decapitated after 24 h of reperfusion for further analysis. The data were expressed as the mean ± SEM; *n* = 6; * *p* < 0.05 vs. Sham; # *p* < 0.05 vs. I/R. (a) The Scr levels and BUN levels were examined 24 h after surgery; (b) A semi-quantitative assessment of the lesion was performed by a pathologist in a blinded manner according to the ATN–scoring system. Each tubular segment visible in the cortex and the outer medulla was evaluated; (c) Representative images of the cortex and outer medulla in different groups stained with H&E. Original magnification, 400×. The black arrows indicate the areas of I/R-induced tissue damages.

To investigate the effect of genistein on I/R-induced renal tubular damage, kidney sections were stained with H&E. Tubular dilatation, necrosis, brush border loss, and cast formation were evident in the I/R group. However, after pre-treatment with genistein, the damage was limited to mild swelling of the tubular epithelial cells, and less histological damage was observed with the H&E stain (Figure 1c). Pretreatment with genistein significantly reduced the tubular necrosis score in both the cortex and medulla compared with the score in sections from mice with I/R injury (Figure 1b).

To further explore the protective effects of genistein on I/R-induced renal injury, mice were treated with 15 mg/kg genistein or vehicle 30 min before the induction of ischemia, followed by 12, 24, 48, and 72 h of reperfusion. Genistein treatment led to a significant decrease in the elevated Scr and BUN levels in the I/R group of mice at 12, 24, 48, and 72 h post I/R injury (Figure A1). Genistein treatment at 48 h post I/R injury had returned the Scr and BUN levels to those of the sham group. Examination of the cortical and outer-medullary regions of the kidneys confirmed the results of the aforementioned functional studies (Figure A2).

### 3.2. Genistein Increases SIRT1 Expression in Renal Cells after Renal I/R-Induced Injury

Previous studies have demonstrated that the regulation of SIRT1 by naturally occurring dietary polyphenols is beneficial in the therapeutic intervention of various diseases [27]. To determine whether SIRT1 is also involved in the protective effect of genistein, we analyzed the protein and mRNA expression in renal tissues. No significant differences occurred in SIRT1 expression between the I/R group and the sham group (Figures 2a and A3). Interestingly, pre-treatment with 10 and 15 mg/kg genistein dramatically increased the expression of SIRT1 protein and mRNA (Figures 2a and A3, $p < 0.05$). The mRNA and protein levels of SIRT1 in the 15 mg/kg genistein-treated group were 2.3- and 1.6-fold higher than those in the I/R group ($p < 0.05$), respectively. The upregulation of SIRT1 protein was further confirmed by the IHC assay (Figure 2b). The results showed that pre-treatment with 15 mg/kg genistein significantly increased SIRT1 expression in the renal cortex and outer medulla compared with that in the I/R group. These data indicate that SIRT1 may contribute to the protective effects of genistein on tubular damage and the loss of renal function in I/R injury.

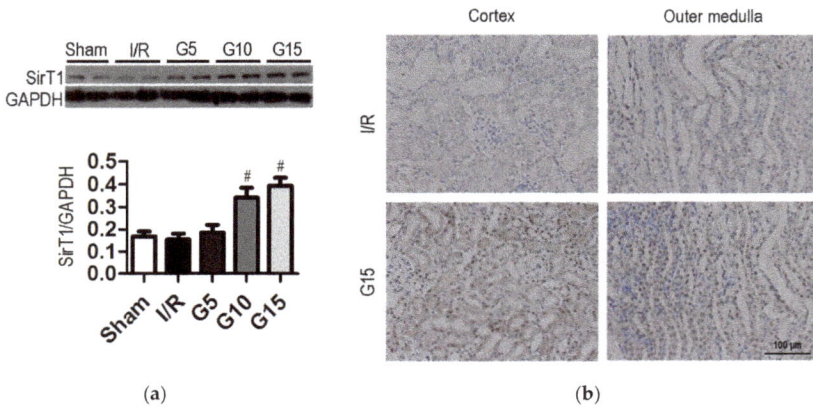

**Figure 2.** Effect of genistein on SIRT1 expression following I/R injury. Mice were treated as described in Figure 1. The data were expressed as the mean ± SEM; $n = 6$; $^{\#} p < 0.05$ vs. I/R. (**a**) Western blots analysis for SIRT1 expression in mouse kidney tissues. Densitometric analysis of the SIRT1 expression by Image-Pro Plus 6.0. GAPDH was calibrated; (**b**) Representative images of SIRT1 expression in the kidney, as determined by IHC. Original magnification, 400×. The black arrows indicate the positive cells.

### 3.3. Genistein Inhibits Apoptosis and Increases Proliferation after Renal I/R-Induced Injury

Several lines of experimental evidence have supported a crucial role for apoptosis in the pathogenesis of I/R-induced injury [28]. Apoptotic cells were detected in the kidney of all groups using terminal deoxynucleotidyl transferase-mediated dUTP nick-end labelling (TUNEL) staining. As shown in Figure 3a, mice with I/R injury had more TUNEL-positive cells predominantly in the tubules of the outer medulla than in the cortex region. Pre-treatment with genistein (5, 10, and 15 mg/kg) resulted in a significant decrease in the number of apoptotic cells (30.1% ± 2.0%, 17.3% ± 1.6%, and 8.7% ± 1.3%, respectively) compared with that in the I/R group (40.2% ± 2.3%) in the outer medulla regions (Figure 3a, $p < 0.05$). Meanwhile, the level of cleaved caspase-3 in the kidney treated with genistein (5, 10, and 15 mg/kg) was significantly lower than that in the I/R group (Figure 3b, $p < 0.05$). This finding is consistent with the TUNEL assay.

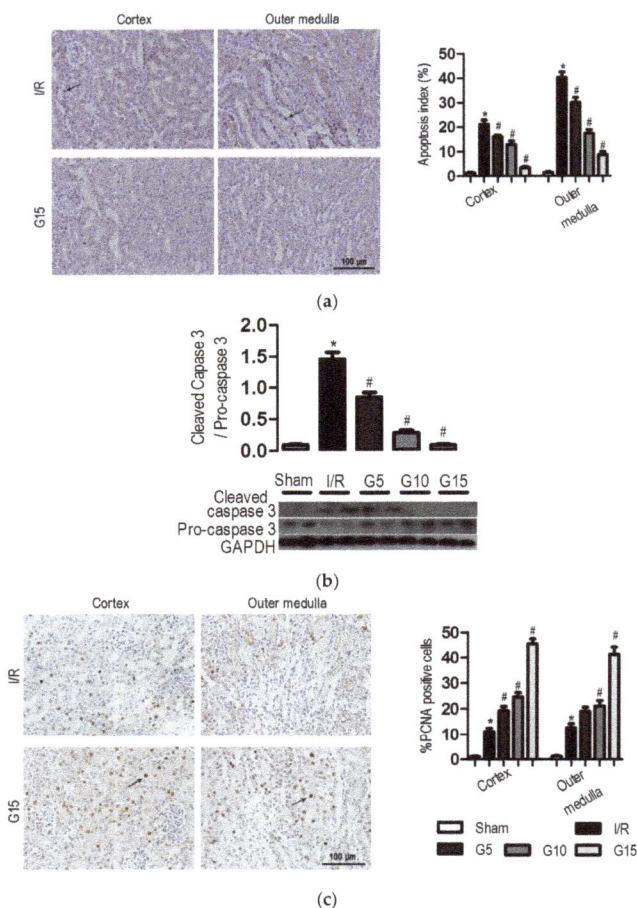

**Figure 3.** Effect of genistein on the cellular apoptosis and proliferation following I/R injury. Mice were treated as described in Figure 1. The data were expressed as the mean ± SEM; $n = 6$; * $p < 0.05$ vs. Sham; # $p < 0.05$ vs. I/R. (**a**) Representative photomicrograph of TUNEL-positive cells stained kidney tissues from the I/R and G15 groups and the percentage of positive cells is illustrated; (**b**) Cleaved caspase-3 and pro-caspase-3 expression was analyzed by western blotting; (**c**) Representative photomicrograph of PCNA-positive cells stained kidney tissues from the I/R and G15 groups and the percentage of positive cells is illustrated. Original magnification, 400×. The black arrows indicate the positive cells.

Renal cell proliferation was assessed using proliferating cell nuclear antigen (PCNA). Few PCNA-positive proliferating cells were detected in the kidneys of sham-operated mice. The number of PCNA-positive cells was significantly increased in the renal cortex (11.1% ± 1.3%) and outer medulla (12.6% ± 1.6%) following I/R (Figure 3c, $p < 0.05$). Pre-treatment with genistein (5, 10, and 15 mg/kg) resulted in a significant increase of the number of PCNA-positive cells in the kidney. The number of PCNA-positive cells for the 15 mg/kg genistein-treated group was significantly higher (45.4% ± 2.0% and 41.3% ± 2.8% for cortex and outer medulla) than that in I/R mice ($p < 0.05$). These results suggested that genistein inhibits apoptosis and promotes proliferation and then prevents the mice from I/R-induced renal injury.

### 3.4. The SIRT1 Inhibitor Abolishes the Protective Effects of Genistein on I/R-Induced Injury

To investigate whether SIRT1 is required for the renal-protective effects of genistein against I/R-induced injury, Sirtinol, a SIRT1 inhibitor, was administered 60 min before the induction of ischemia with or without genistein. Sirtinol preconditioning slightly aggravated I/R-induced renal injury. The Scr, BUN, and injury score in Sirtinol-treated mice exhibited higher levels than those of the vehicle mice, although no significant difference occurred between these two groups (Figure 4). Notably, Sirtinol abrogated the protective effect of genistein. The reduction of Scr and BUN in genistein-treated mice was inhibited by Sirtinol. Consistent with this result, the kidney of G15 + Sirtinol mice displayed severe and extensive injury, with widespread loss of the brush border, tubular dilation, and vacuolization (Figure 4).

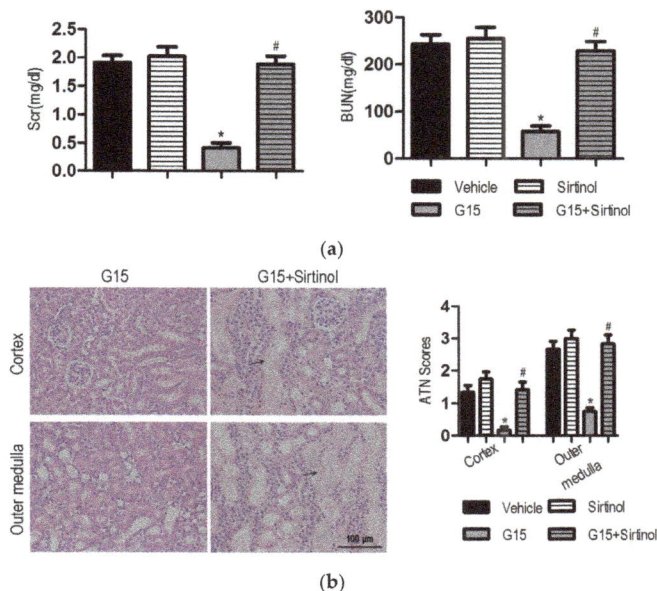

(a)

(b)

**Figure 4.** Sirtinol abolishes the protective effect of genistein on renal function and histology in I/R-induced injury. In the vehicle group, mice received the same volume of vehicle; in the Sirtinol group, mice were pre-treated with 1 mg/kg Sirtinol; in the G15 group, mice were pre-treated with 15 mg/kg genistein; in the Sirtinol + G15 group, mice were treated with 15 mg/kg genistein and 1 mg/kg Sirtinol. Ischemia was induced in all of the groups. The mice were decapitated at 24 h of the reperfusion period for further analysis. The data were expressed as the mean ± SEM; $n = 6$; * $p < 0.05$ vs. Sham; # $p < 0.05$ vs. I/R. The Scr (**a, left**) levels and BUN (**a, right**) levels were examined 24 h after reperfusion. (**b, left**) Representative images of the cortex and outer medulla from the G15 and G15 + Sirtinol groups stained with H&E. Original magnification, 400×. The black arrows indicate the areas of I/R-induced tissue damages. (**b, right**) A semi-quantitative assessment of the lesion was performed by a pathologist in a blinded manner according to the ATN–scoring system. Each tubular segment visible in the cortex and outer medulla was evaluated.

Similarly, tubular cell apoptosis was also determined by the TUNEL assay and analysis of cleaved caspase-3 expression. No significant difference occurred in the apoptosis and proliferation of tubular cells between Sirtinol-treated mice and I/R mice (Figures 5 and A4). Pre-treatment with Sirtinol abolished the protective effect of genistein on I/R-induced apoptosis (Figure 5a). In addition, the promoted effect of genistein on renal proliferation was abrogated by Sirtinol following I/R

(Figure 5b). Lower renal PCNA expression following I/R was also observed in Sirtinol-treated mice using immunoblotting (Figure A5), suggesting that the protective effects of genistein depend on SIRT1 activation in the kidney with I/R injury.

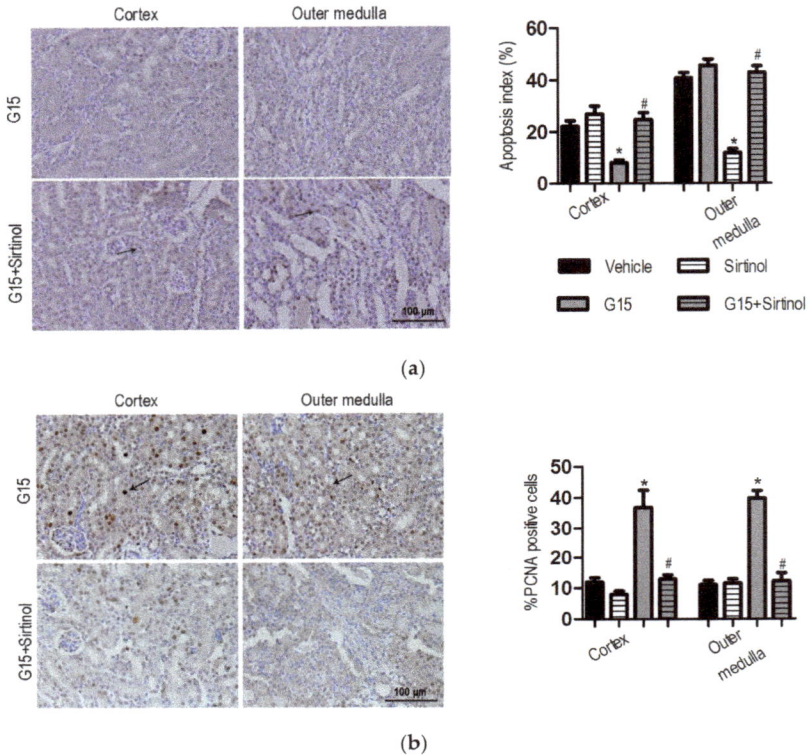

(a)

(b)

**Figure 5.** Mice were treated as described in Figure 4. The data were expressed as the mean ± SEM; *n* = 6; * *p* < 0.05 vs. Vehicle; # *p* < 0.05 vs. G15. (a) Representative photomicrograph of TUNEL-positive from the G15 and G15 + Sirtinol groups and the percentage of positive cells were illustrated; (b) Representative photomicrograph of PCNA-positive from the G15 and G15 + Sirtinol groups and the percentage of positive cells were illustrated. Original magnification, 400×. The black arrows indicate the positive cells.

### 3.5. SIRT1 Depletion Eliminates the Protective Effects of Genistein on I/R-Induced Injury

Because both SIRT1 and SIRT2 are inhibited by Sirtinol, the specific contribution of SIRT1 to the protective effects of genistein on I/R-induced injury was determined using shRNA-mediated knockdown with lentivirus. SIRT1 protein was significantly induced by genistein in kidneys injected with lentivirus carrying the scrambled shRNA cassette; however, its expression was significantly lower in I/R- and genistein-treated mice receiving lentivirus with the SIRT1 shRNA cassette (Figure A6). Knockdown of SIRT1 was verified by IHC analysis (Figure A7). Consistent with the result using the SIRT1 inhibitor Sirtinol, knockdown of SIRT1 with shRNA significantly reversed the effect of genistein on renal dysfunction (Figure 6a), cellular damage (Figure 6b), apoptosis (Figure A8), and proliferation (Figure A9) following I/R injury. Thus, the protective effects of genistein depend on SIRT1 expression in the kidney with I/R injury.

(a)

(b)

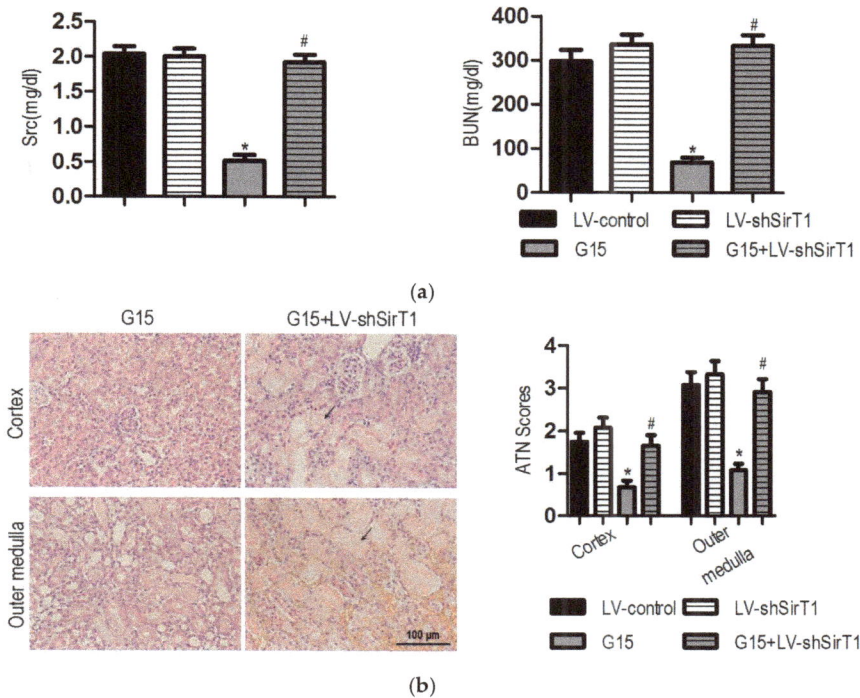

**Figure 6.** SIRT1 depletion abrogates the protective effect of genistein on renal function and histology in I/R-induced injury. In the LV-control, mice were injected with lentivirus carrying scrambled shRNA and pre-treated with the same volume of vehicle; in the LV-shSIRT1 group, mice were injected with lentivirus carrying SIRT1 shRNA; in the G15 group, mice were injected with lentivirus carrying scrambled shRNA and were pre-treated with 15 mg/kg genistein; in the LV-shSIRT1 + G15 group, mice were injected with lentivirus carrying SIRT1 shRNA and were pre-treated with 15 mg/kg genistein. Ischemia was induced in all of the groups. The mice were decapitated after 24 h of reperfusion for further analysis. The data were expressed as the mean $\pm$ SEM; $n = 6$; * $p < 0.05$ vs. Sham; # $p < 0.05$ vs. I/R. The Scr (**a**, **left**) levels and BUN (**a**, **right**) levels were examined 24 h after reperfusion. (**b**, **left**) Representative images of the cortex and outer medulla from G15 and G15 + LV-shSIRT1 groups stained with H&E. Original magnification, 400×. The black arrows indicate the areas of I/R-induced tissue damages. (**b**, **right**) Semi-quantitative assessment of the lesion was performed by a pathologist in a blinded manner according to the ATN-scoring system. Each tubular segment visible in the cortex and outer medulla was evaluated.

### 3.6. The Protective Effects of Genistein Is Associated with the SIRT1/p53 Axis

It has been reported that the expression of p53 is regulated by SIRT1, which then exerts its anti-apoptotic and proliferative effect, thereby contributing to the pathogenesis of ischemic renal injury [14]. Of interest is to investigate whether SIRT1/p53 axis contributes to the protective effects of genistein on I/R-induced injury [15,16]. Our western blot analyses revealed that SIRT1/p53 signaling was also involved in the protective effects of genistein: (1) genistein reduced the expression of p53 and; (2) no significant difference occurred in p53 between LV-shSIRT1-treated mice and LV-control mice; (3) by contrast, the reduction of p53 caused by genistein was significantly prevented by SIRT1 depletion; (4) in addition, the level of the cell cycle-related p21, a target of p53, was significantly inhibited in the kidneys of genistein-treated mice; (5) knock-down of SIRT1 with the shRNA cassette largely blocked the inhibitory effect of genistein on p21 expression; (6) there were inverse correlations between the expression of p53 and p21 and PCNA in the kidneys of different groups following I/R (Figure 7a,b). However, it did not significantly alter the acetylation status of p53 (Figure 7c). Taken together, all of these data strongly suggested that SIRT1/p53 is important for the protective effects of genistein on I/R-induced injury.

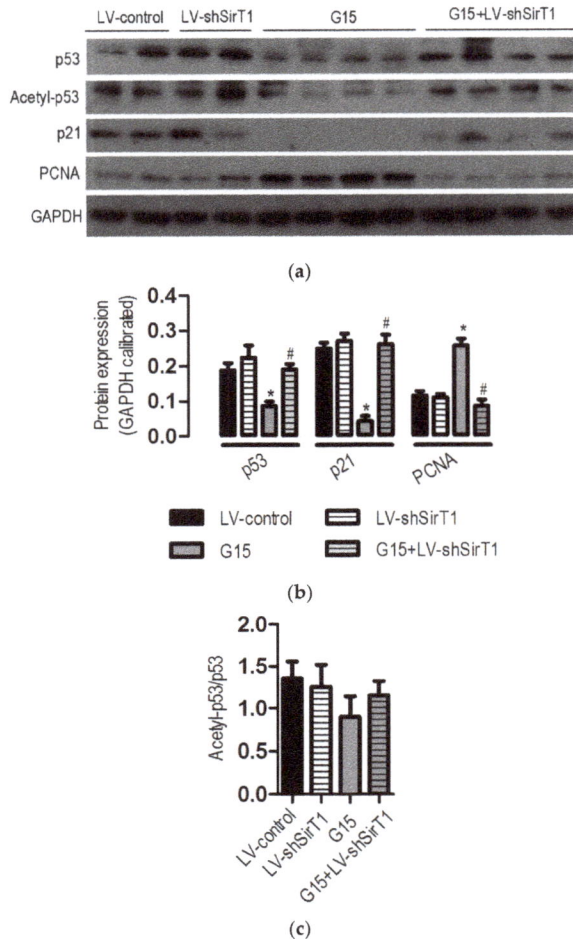

(a)

(b)

(c)

**Figure 7.** Effect of SIRT1 depletion on protein expression following I/R-induced renal injury. Mice were treated as described in Figure 6. The data were expressed as the mean ± SEM; $n = 6$; * $p < 0.05$ vs. LV-control; # $p < 0.05$ vs. G15. (**a**) Representative western blots for p53, Acetyl-p53, p21, and PCNA expression in mouse kidney tissues; (**b**) Densitometric analysis of p53, p21, and PCNA expression by Image-Pro Plus 6.0. GAPDH was calibrated; (**c**) Densitometric analysis of Acetyl-p53 expression by Image-Pro Plus 6.0. Total p53 was calibrated.

## 4. Discussion

Renal ischemia-reperfusion is a common cause of acute kidney injury (AKI), which is a common clinical complication characterized by an abrupt decrease in the glomerular filtration rate. Despite the improvement in therapeutic methods, including renal replacement therapy, the overall mortality of AKI is estimated to be 50% [2]. There are several pathologic processes contributing to AKI, including endothelial and epithelial cell death, intratubular obstruction, and changes in the local microvascular blood flow, as well as immunological and inflammatory processes. Therefore, the mechanisms underlying I/R damage to kidneys are most likely multifactorial and interdependent, involving hypoxia, inflammatory responses, and free radical damage [1]. Effective treatments for I/R-induced renal injury in clinics are still absent. It is crucial to screen effective drugs to treat I/R-induced renal injury. It is well established that the inhibition of apoptotic signalling and cell death is an effective measure to relieve I/R in a murine model. Pre-ischaemic activation of the A1 AR protects against I/R injury in vivo through mechanisms that reduce necrosis and apoptosis [29], and other studies have suggested that tubular cell regeneration and proliferation play an important role in the recovery of AKI [14,28]. As a plant-derived isoflavone, genistein is a polyphenolic non-steroidal compound, and its biological activity has been widely explored in cancer, inflammation, and apoptosis. Recently, it has been reported that genistein plays a neuro-protective role in ischemic insults [30]. As a member of the Sirtuin family, SIRT1 belongs to the typical class III histone deacetylases (HDAC). SIRT1 has been involved in influencing a wide range of cellular processes including aging, transcriptional reprogramming, apoptosis, inflammation, and stress resistance, as well as energy efficiency and alertness during low-calorie situations [7,31]. Moreover, it can also control circadian clocks and mitochondrial biogenesis, suggesting that SIRT1 is an important age-related protective factor against I/R-induced kidney injury. Activation of SIRT1 attenuated I/R-induced renal injury; conversely, the ablation of one allele of the SIRT1 gene significantly resulted in higher susceptibility to I/R-induced kidney injury. Furthermore, the kidney-specific overexpression of SIRT1 could also protect against cisplatin-induced AKI [32]. In this study, renal function and morphology were significantly recovered 24 h after renal I/R injury following pretreatment with genistein (5, 10, and 15 mg/kg). Meanwhile, renal function and morphology were markedly recovered at 12, 24, 48, and 72 h after renal I/R injury following pretreatment with 15 mg/kg genistein. These results strongly support that genistein is an effective agent for the treatment of I/R-induced kidney injury. Consistent with our results, anti-apoptosis activity caused by genistein is also the important mechanism for its neuro-protective role in ischemic insults [30]. In addition, we also showed that the protective roles of genistein in I/R-induced renal injury are associated with a higher cellular proliferation rate, which was evaluated by the PCNA level. All of these studies indicated that genistein and SIRT1 both have multiple roles in many physiological processes, suggesting that they may also contribute to the repair of renal ischemia/reperfusion (I/R) injury.

Previously, many studies have revealed the close relationship between genistein and SIRT1, and the expression of SIRT1 and its activity were stimulated by isoflavones such as resveratrol and quercetin [27]. However, the effect of genistein on SIRT1 expression and activity is seemingly controversial. On the one hand, genistein has been demonstrated to enhance SIRT1 expression and activity in C2C12 myotubes [23] and breast cancer T47D cells but not in MCF-7cells [33]. Moreover, genistein was found to increase AMPK (adenosine monophosphate activated protein kinase) activity in liver cells, which could trigger SIRT1 activity [34]. On the other hand, genistein has also been demonstrated to inhibit the expression of SIRT1 in prostate cancer cells [35]. A reasonable explanation for these phenomena is that genistein might have dual effects on SIRT1 expression and activity, and the effects depend on the different tissue contexts and dosage. Recently, one reporter provided another explanation for the phenomena. The modulation of the intrinsic gene expression by genistein could lead to a difference in radio-sensitivity in between cancerous and normal cells [36]. Interestingly, our study clearly demonstrated that the expression of SIRT1 was significantly increased 24 h after renal I/R injury following pretreatment with genistein (10 mg/kg and 15 mg/kg), and the inhibition of SIRT1 activity or expression abolished the protective effects of genistein on I/R-induced renal injury. Genistein treatment significantly reduced apoptosis and enhanced cellular proliferation rate, further supporting the protective effect of SIRT1. However, the inhibition of SIRT1 activity or its expression reduced the proliferation rate mediated by genistein. Moreover, a significant reduction in the p21 expression level occurred in genistein-treated mice. p21 is a cyclin-dependent kinase (CDK) inhibitor, and it might bind to and inhibit the activity of cyclin-CDK2 or cyclin-CDK4 complexes, thereby regulating cell cycle progression. Therefore, our study showed that genistein may exert its renal protective effects on renal I/R injury through its stimulation of SIRT1 expression or activity. SIRT1 expression or activity could be regulated directly or indirectly in vitro and in vivo. Hence, it is necessary to explore the definite mechanism regarding how SIRT1 expression and activity are regulated by genistein in renal cells.

As a tumor suppressor, p53 is involved in multiple essential cell functions, such as pausing the cell cycle, promoting senescence and apoptosis, and regulating cell metabolism. The participation of p53 has been reported in nephrotoxic injury and ischemic renal injury, and targeted deletion of p53 in the proximal tubule prevents ischemic renal injury. p53 expression is negatively associated with SIRT1 expression and activity after AKI [14]. Kidney-specific overexpression of SIRT1 protects against AKI [30]. Furthermore, genistein decreases cisplatin-induced renal injury by preventing p53 induction [37]. Those data indicate that p53 expression is closely related to SIRT1 expression or activity after AKI. To test the potential relationships between genistein, p53, and SIRT1, we examined the level of p53, acetylated p53, p21, and PCNA (a proliferation marker) [13], respectively. Our study demonstrated that p53 and p21 were significantly decreased 24 h after renal I/R injury, accompanied by the induction of SIRT1 following pretreatment with genistein. The pivotal role of SIRT1 was further supported by the finding that the inhibition of SIRT1 activity or expression significantly blocks the repression of p53 expression, and p21 following the use of genistein. Moreover, there was the inverse correlation between p53, p21, and PCNA expression. It has shown that enhanced SIRT1 activity can reduce p53 expression by deacetylating p53 and promoting its ubiquitination and proteasomal degradation [38]. Genistein caused a robust reduction in p53 abundance but had no measurable effect on p53 acetylation associated with upregulated SIRT1 expression. It is plausible that SIRT1 caused the deacetylation of p53, contributing to p53 degradation by genistein. Remarkably, many factors contribute to the stability of p53 expression. These findings suggest the existence of other SIRT1-dependent mechanisms that tune p53 expression by genistein. Together, these data indicated that the SIRT1/p53 axis plays an important role in the protective effects of genistein on I/R-induced renal injury. In addition to regulation of DNA synthesis, PCNA has far-reaching impacts on a myriad of cellular functions by interaction with many protein and various post-translational modifications [39]. The protective roles of genistein in I/R-induced renal injury are associated with a higher PCNA level, implying the cellular proliferation involved at least in part in the protective effects of genistein. Moreover, it has to make great efforts to explore the more enigmatic PCNA-dependent function in this process, including senescence and apoptosis. In this study, we found that genistein could protect against I/R-induced renal injury, and the reno-protective effects of genistein were associated with reduced apoptosis and a higher renal proliferation rate. Surprisingly, the upregulation of SIRT1 expression is closely correlated with improved function against kidney injury in genistein-receiving mice. Pharmacological inhibition of SIRT1 abolished the reno-protective effects of genistein, and knockdown of SIRT1 abrogated the beneficial effects of genistein on kidney injury following I/R. Additionally, increased SIRT1 lead to reduced expression of p53, reduced apoptosis, and a higher renal cellular proliferation rate and vice versa, suggesting genistein may promote cell survival and enhance renal cellular proliferation via SIRT1/p53 axis to provide reno-protection in I/R-induced renal injury (Figure 8). The major isoflavones in soybean are genistein and daidzein. Daidzein can behave similarly to genistein and both of them have been shown to protect from metabolic disease in a SIRT1-dependent manner [40]. Daidzein has been shown to induce the expression and activity of SIRT1 in renal cells [40]. In the light of the protective effects of SIRT1 in kidney, daidzein administration could ameliorate I/R-induced kidney injury by stimulating the expression and activity of SIRT1. This needs to be testified in future study.

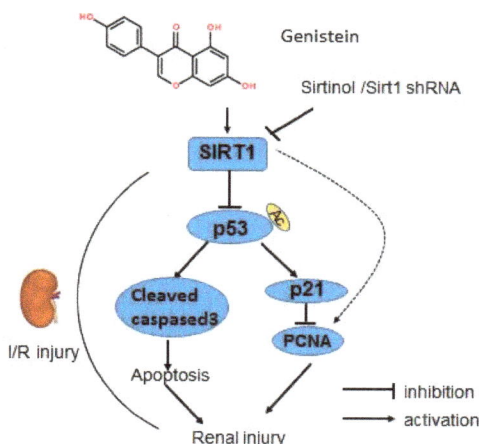

**Figure 8.** Proposed scheme for the roles of SIRT1, p53, and other molecules in the protective effect of genistein on I/R-induced renal injury. Genistein treatment significantly reduced renal I/R-induced cell death, simultaneously stimulating renal cell proliferation. Paralleling the protective effect of genistein against I/R-induced renal injury, SIRT1 expression was upregulated upon the administration of genistein. Genistein reduced p53, p21, and cleaved caspase-3 expression and increased PCNA expression. Pharmacological inhibition or shRNA-mediated depletion of SIRT1 significantly reversed the effect of genistein on renal dysfunction, cellular damage, apoptosis, and proliferation following I/R injury. The reduced p53, p21 expression, and increased PCNA expression were blunted after the depletion of SIRT1 compared with the genistein treatment group in the renal I/R process.

## 5. Conclusions

In summary, we confirmed that genistein possesses protective effects on renal ischemia-reperfusion injury and that the protective effect mainly depends on apoptosis inhibition and regeneration promotion accompanied by the increased expression of SIRT1, whereas inhibition of SIRT1 activity or expression blocked the protective effect. It is probable that genistein improves I/R-induced renal-injury in a SIRT1-dependent manner, making it a potential reagent for treatment of kidney disease with deficiency of SIRT1 activity. This need to be further verified using more in vivo and in vitro experiments.

**Acknowledgments:** This work was supported by National Natural Science Foundation of China (No. 81100281 to W.-F.H.), Medical and Health Research Project from Yichang Science and Technology Bureau (No. A15301-35 to W.-F.H.), the National Natural Science Foundation of China (No. 81302068 to K.-C.L.), the National High Technology Research and Development Program of China (863 Program, No. 2014AA020541 to K.-C.L.), and the Program for the Top Young Innovative Talents of Fujian Province (to K.-C.L.), and the International Collaborative Project of Fujian Province (No. 2017I0014 to K.-C.L.).

**Author Contributions:** W.-F.H. and K.-C.L. conceived and designed the experiments; W.-F.L. and K.Y. performed the experiments; W.-F.L., K.Y., P.Z., H.-Q.Z. and Y.-H.S. analyzed the data; W.-F.L. and K.Y. contributed reagents/materials/analysis tools; W.-F.H., K.-C.L. and W.-F.L. wrote the paper.

**Conflicts of Interest:** The authors declare no conflict of interest. The founding sponsors had no role in the design of the study; in the collection, analyses, or interpretation of data; in the writing of the manuscript, or in the decision to publish the results.

## Appendix A

*Appendix A.1. Lentivirus Preparation*

Lentiviruses were generated by cotransfecting subcofluent HEK293T cells with the lentiviral vectors (psh-control or psh-SIRT1) and packaging plasmids (pHR and pCMV-VSV-G) by calcium phosphate transfection. The targeted sequences for psh-SIRT1 and psh-control were 5'-AAGATGAAGTTGACCTCCTCA-3' and 5'-TTCTCCGAACGTGTCACGT-3', respectively. Viral supernatants were collected 48 h after transfection, centrifuged at $3000\times g$ for 15 min, and filtered through 0.45-μm filters (Millipore, Danvers, MA, USA). The concentrations of lentivirus were determined using ultracentrifugation approaches [41].

*Appendix A.2. Quantitative Real-Time RT-PCR*

Total RNA was extracted using TRIZOL Reagent (Invitrogen, Carlsbad, CA, USA) and was reverse transcribed with ReverTra Ace (Toyobo, Dalian, China) to produce cDNA. Real-time PCR was performed using SYBR (Synergy Brands) Green-based detection in StepOnePlus™ (ABI, Redlands, CA, USA) according to the manufacturer's instructions and using the following primer pairs: SIRT1 (NM_019812) (Forward: 5'-TGCTGGCCTAATAGACTTGCAA-3', Reverse: 5'-CAGGAACTAGAGGAC AAGACGTCA-3'); 18S rRNA (NR_003278) (Forward:5'-GGTCATAAGCTTGCGTTGATTAAG-3', Reverse: 5'-CTACGGAAACCTTGTTACGACTTT-3').

**Appendix B**

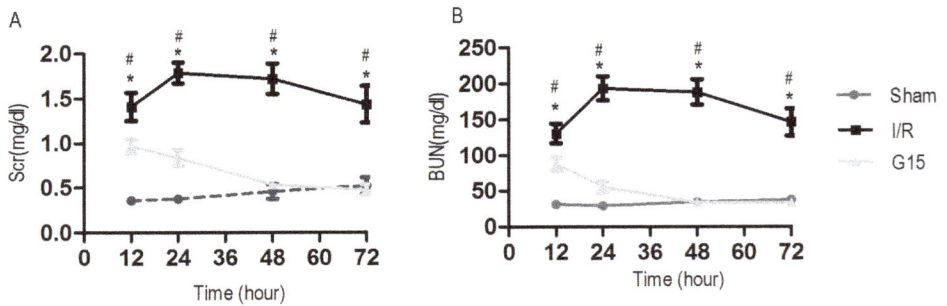

**Figure A1.** Effect of genistein on renal function at different time points. In the sham group, mice received the same volume of vehicle without I/R; in the I/R group, mice received the same volume of vehicle with I/R; in the G15 group, mice were treated with 15 mg/kg genistein. The mice were decapitated after 12, 24, 48, and 72 h of reperfusion for renal functional analysis. The data were expressed as the mean ± SEM; $n = 6$; * $p < 0.05$ vs. Sham; # $p < 0.05$ vs. I/R. The Scr (**A**) levels and BUN (**B**) levels were examined 12, 24, 48, and 72 h after reperfusion.

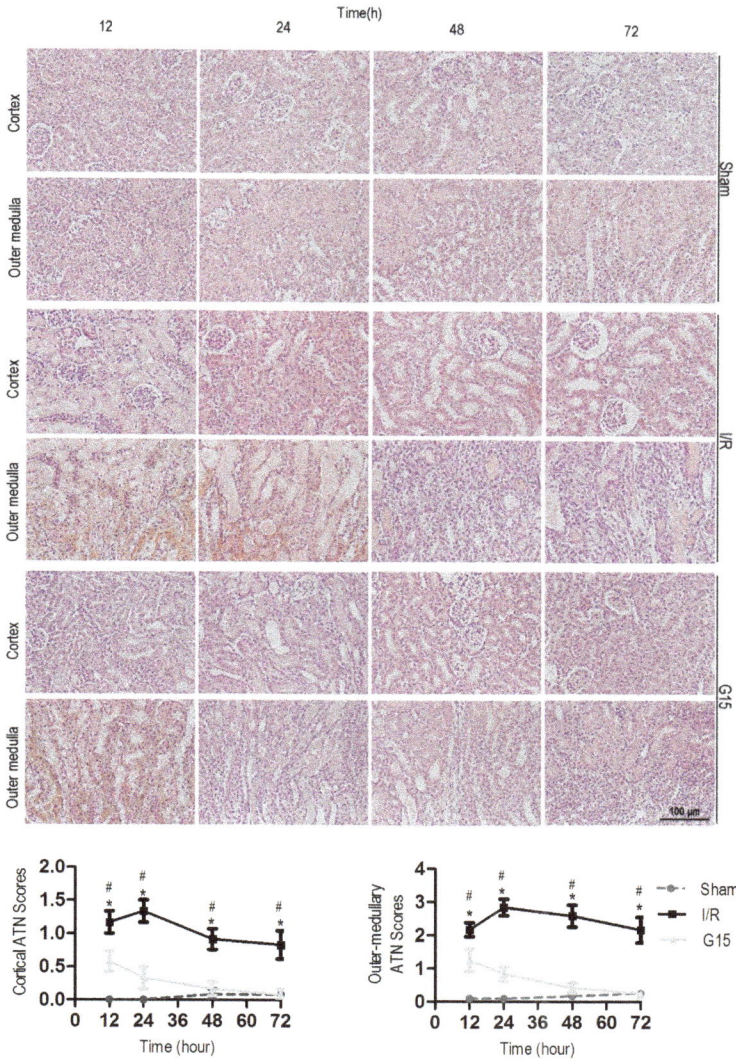

**Figure A2.** Effect of genistein on renal histology in I/R-induced injury at different time points. Mice were treated as described in supplemental Figure A1. The data were expressed as the mean $\pm$ SEM; $n = 6$; * $p < 0.05$ vs. Sham; [#] $p < 0.05$ vs. I/R. (**Top**) Representative images of the cortex and outer medulla at 12, 24, 48, and 72 h of the reperfusion period stained with H&E. Original magnification, 400$\times$; (**Bottom**) Semi-quantitative assessment of the lesion was performed by a pathologist in a blinded manner according to the ATN–scoring system. Each tubular segment visible in the cortex and outer medulla was evaluated.

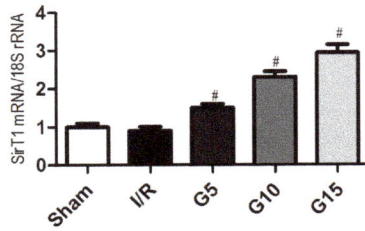

**Figure A3.** Effect of genistein on SIRT1 mRNA expression following I/R injury. In the sham group, mice received the same volume of vehicle without I/R; in the I/R group, mice received the same volume of vehicle with I/R; in the G5 group, mice were pre-treated with 5 mg/kg genistein following I/R; in the G10 group, mice were pre-treated with 10 mg/kg genistein following I/R; in the G15 group, mice were treated with 15 mg/kg genistein. The mice were decapitated at 24 h of the reperfusion period for further analysis. The data were expressed as the mean $\pm$ SEM; $n$ = 6; * $p < 0.05$ vs. Sham; # $p < 0.05$ vs. I/R. The SIRT1 mRNA levels for specific genes were normalized to 18S rRNA levels.

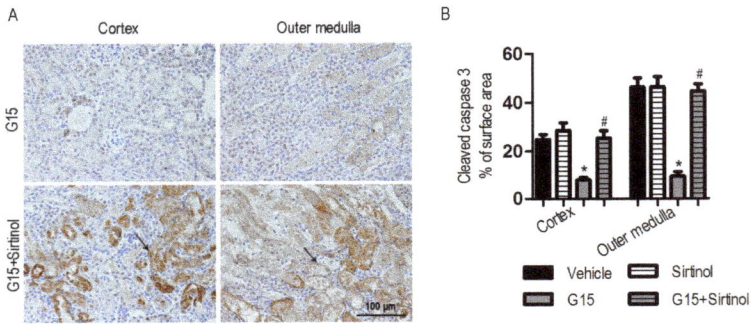

**Figure A4.** Sirtinol reverses the effect of genistein on apoptosis in I/R-induced acute renal injury. Mice were treated as described in supplemental Figure 4. The data were expressed as the mean $\pm$ SEM; $n$ = 6; * $p < 0.05$ vs. Vehicle; # $p < 0.05$ vs. G15. (**A**) Representative photomicrograph of cleaved caspase-3-stained kidney tissues from the G15 and G15 + Sirtinol groups. Original magnification, 400×; (**B**) Cleaved caspase-3-positive cells were counted, and the percentage of positive cells is illustrated. The black arrows indicate positive cells.

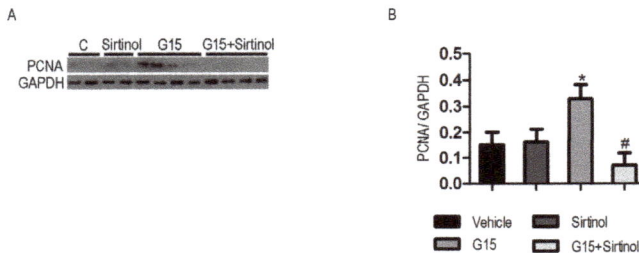

**Figure A5.** Sirtinol abrogates the effect of genistein on PCNA expression in I/R-induced acute renal injury. Mice were treated as described in supplemental Figure 4. The data were expressed as the mean $\pm$ SEM; $n$ = 6; * $p < 0.05$ vs. Vehicle; # $p < 0.05$ vs. G15. (**A**) Representative western blots for PCNA expression in mice kidney tissues; (**B**) Densitometric analysis of the PCNA expression by Image-Pro Plus 6.0. GAPDH was calibrated.

A

B

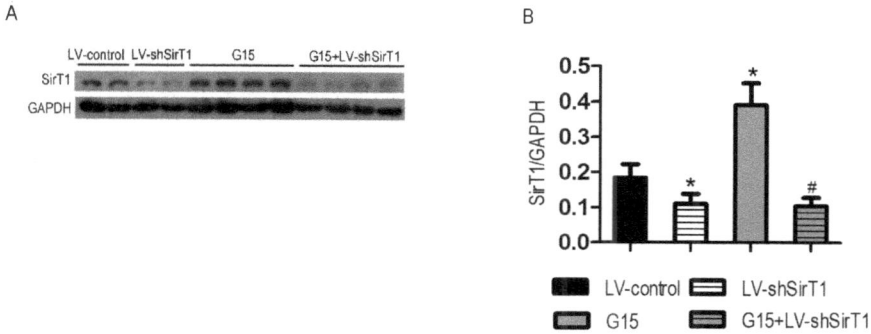

**Figure A6.** Western blot analyses demonstrating the knock-down of SIRT1 in kidney tissues. Seventy-two hours later after the injection of LV-control or LV-shSIRT1, genistein, or the same volume of vehicle. For the LV-control group and G15 groups, mice were pre-treated with vehicle; for the LV-shSIRT1 group, mice were pre-treated with vehicle; for the G15 and LV-shSIRT1 + G15 groups, mice were pre-treated with 15 mg/kg genistein. Ischemia was induced in all of the groups. The mice were decapitated after 24 h of reperfusion for the western blot analysis. The data were expressed as the mean ± SEM; $n$ = 6; * $p < 0.05$ vs. Sham; # $p < 0.05$ vs. I/R. (**A**) Representative western blots for SIRT1 expression in mouse kidney tissues; (**B**) Densitometric analysis of the SIRT1 expression by Image-Pro Plus 6.0. GAPDH was calibrated.

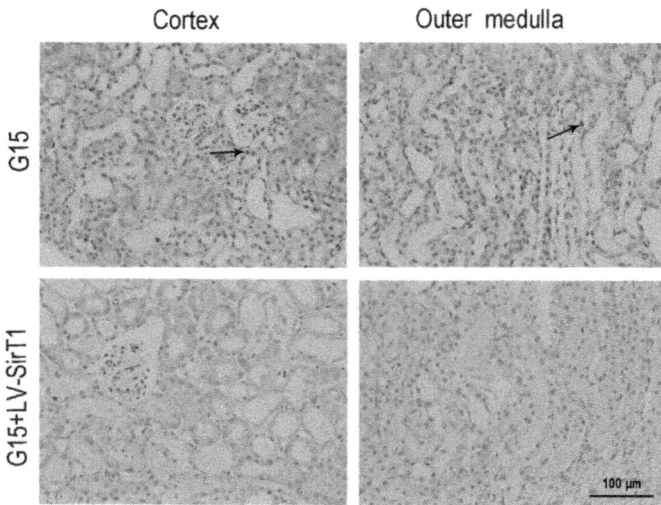

**Figure A7.** IHC analyses demonstrating the knock-down of SIRT1 in kidney tissues. Mice were treated as described in supplemental Figure 7. Representative photomicrograph of SIRT1-stained kidney tissues from the G15 and G15 + LV-shSIRT1 groups. Original magnification, 400×. The black arrows indicate positive cells.

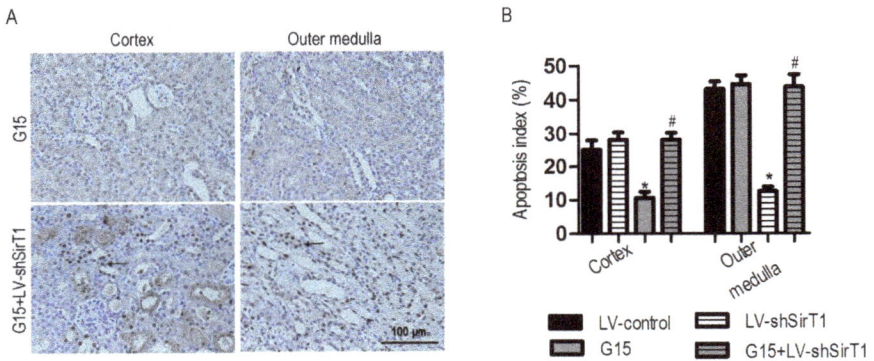

**Figure A8.** SIRT1 depletion reverses the effect of genistein on apoptosis in I/R-induced acute renal injury. Mice were treated as described in supplemental Figure 7. The data were expressed as the mean ± SEM; *n* = 6; * *p* < 0.05 vs. Sham; # *p* < 0.05 vs. I/R. (**A**) Representative photomicrograph of TUNEL-stained kidney tissues from the G15 and G15 + Sirtinol groups. Original magnification, 400×; (**B**) TUNEL-positive cells were counted and the percentage of positive cells is illustrated. The black arrows indicate positive cells.

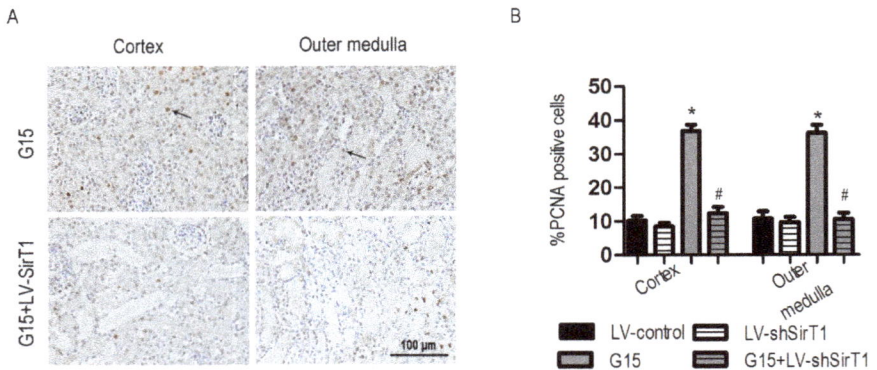

**Figure A9.** SIRT1 depletion reverses the increased effect of genistein on cellular proliferation in I/R-induced acute renal injury. Mice were treated as described in supplemental Figure 7. The data were expressed as the mean ± SEM; *n* = 6; * *p* < 0.05 vs. Sham; # *p* < 0.05 vs. I/R. (**A**) Representative photomicrograph of PCNA-stained kidney tissues from the G15 and G15 + Sirtinol groups. Original magnification, 400×; (**B**) PCNA-positive cells were counted, and the percentage of positive cells is illustrated. The black arrows indicate positive cells.

## References

1. Ichai, C.; Vinsonneau, C.; Souweine, B.; Armando, F.; Canet, E.; Clec'h, C.; Constantin, J.M.; Darmon, M.; Duranteau, J.; Gaillot, T.; et al. Acute kidney injury in the perioperative period and in intensive care units (excluding renal replacement therapies). *Ann. Intensive Care* **2016**, *6*, 48. [CrossRef] [PubMed]
2. Waikar, S.S.; Liu, K.D.; Chertow, G.M. Diagnosis, epidemiology and outcomes of acute kidney injury. *Clin. J. Am. Soc. Nephrol.* **2008**, *3*, 844–861. [CrossRef] [PubMed]
3. Gueler, F.; Gwinner, W.; Schwarz, A.; Haller, H. Long-term effects of acute ischemia and reperfusion injury. *Kidney Int.* **2004**, *66*, 523–527. [CrossRef] [PubMed]

4.  Lempiainen, J.; Finckenberg, P.; Levijoki, J.; Mervaala, E. AMPK activator AICAR ameliorates ischaemia reperfusion injury in the rat kidney. *Br. J. Pharmacol.* **2012**, *166*, 1905–1915. [CrossRef] [PubMed]

5.  Shimokawa, T.; Tsutsui, H.; Miura, T.; Nishinaka, T.; Terada, T.; Takama, M.; Yoshida, S.; Tanba, T.; Tojo, A.; Yamagata, M.; et al. Renoprotective effect of yohimbine on ischaemia/reperfusion-induced acute kidney injury through alpha2C-adrenoceptors in rats. *Eur. J. Pharmacol.* **2016**, *781*, 36–44. [CrossRef] [PubMed]

6.  Singh, A.P.; Singh, N.; Bedi, P.M. Pioglitazone ameliorates renal ischemia reperfusion injury through NMDA receptor antagonism in rats. *Mol. Cell. Biochem.* **2016**, *417*, 111–118. [CrossRef] [PubMed]

7.  Kelly, G. A review of the Sirtuin system, its clinical implications, and the potential role of dietary activators like resveratrol: Part 1. *Altern. Med. Rev.* **2010**, *15*, 245–263. [PubMed]

8.  Kumar, A.; Chauhan, S. How much successful are the medicinal chemists in modulation of SIRT1: A critical review. *Eur. J. Med. Chem.* **2016**, *119*, 45–69. [CrossRef] [PubMed]

9.  Wakino, S.; Hasegawa, K.; Itoh, H. Sirtuin and metabolic kidney disease. *Kidney Int.* **2015**, *88*, 691–698. [CrossRef] [PubMed]

10. Hasegawa, K.; Wakino, S.; Simic, P.; Sakamaki, Y.; Minakuchi, H.; Fujimura, K.; Hosoya, K.; Komatsu, M.; Kaneko, Y.; Kanda, T.; et al. Renal tubular SIRT1 attenuates diabetic albuminuria by epigenetically suppressing Claudin-1 overexpression in podocytes. *Nat. Med.* **2013**, *19*, 1496–1504. [CrossRef] [PubMed]

11. He, W.; Wang, Y.; Zhang, M.Z.; You, L.; Davis, L.S.; Fan, H.; Yang, H.C.; Fogo, A.B.; Zent, R.; Harris, R.C. SIRT1 activation protects the mouse renal medulla from oxidative injury. *J. Clin. Investig.* **2010**, *120*, 1056–1068. [CrossRef] [PubMed]

12. Kume, S.; Haneda, M.; Kanasaki, K.; Sugimoto, T.; Araki, S.; Isono, M.; Isshiki, K.; Uzu, T.; Kashiwagi, A.; Koya, D. Silent information regulator 2 (SIRT1) attenuates oxidative stress-induced mesangial cell apoptosis via p53 deacetylation. *Free. Radic. Biol. Med.* **2006**, *40*, 2175–2182. [CrossRef] [PubMed]

13. Kume, S.; Haneda, M.; Kanasaki, K.; Sugimoto, T.; Araki, S.; Isshiki, K.; Isono, M.; Uzu, T.; Guarente, L.; Kashiwagi, A.; et al. SIRT1 inhibits transforming growth factor beta-induced apoptosis in glomerular mesangial cells via Smad7 deacetylation. *J. Biol. Chem.* **2007**, *282*, 151–158. [CrossRef] [PubMed]

14. Fan, H.; Yang, H.C.; You, L.; Wang, Y.Y.; He, W.J.; Hao, C.M. The histone deacetylase, SIRT1, contributes to the resistance of young mice to ischemia/reperfusion-induced acute kidney injury. *Kidney Int.* **2013**, *83*, 404–413. [CrossRef] [PubMed]

15. Zhang, D.; Liu, Y.; Wei, Q.; Huo, Y.; Liu, K.; Liu, F.; Dong, Z. Tubular p53 regulates multiple genes to mediate AKI. *J. Am. Soc. Nephrol.* **2014**, *25*, 2278–2289. [CrossRef] [PubMed]

16. Ying, Y.; Kim, J.; Westphal, S.N.; Long, K.E.; Padanilam, B.J. Targeted deletion of p53 in the proximal tubule prevents ischemic renal injury. *J. Am. Soc. Nephrol.* **2014**, *25*, 2707–2716. [CrossRef] [PubMed]

17. Mitchell, J.R.; Verweij, M.; Brand, K.; van de Ven, M.; Goemaere, N.; van den Engel, S.; Chu, T.; Forrer, F.; Müller, C.; de Jong, M.; et al. Short-term dietary restriction and fasting precondition against ischemia reperfusion injury in mice. *Aging Cell* **2010**, *9*, 40–53. [CrossRef] [PubMed]

18. Banerjee, S.; Li, Y.; Wang, Z.; Sarkar, F.H. Multi-targeted therapy of cancer by genistein. *Cancer Lett.* **2008**, *269*, 226–242. [CrossRef] [PubMed]

19. Huang, W.; Wan, C.; Luo, Q.; Huang, Z.; Luo, Q. Genistein-inhibited cancer stem cell-like properties and reduced chemoresistance of gastric cancer. *Int. J. Mol. Sci.* **2014**, *15*, 3432–3443. [CrossRef] [PubMed]

20. Liang, H.W.; Qiu, S.F.; Shen, J.; Sun, L.N.; Wang, J.Y.; Bruce, I.C.; Xia, Q. Genistein attenuates oxidative stress and neuronal damage following transient global cerebral ischemia in rat hippocampus. *Neurosci. Lett.* **2008**, *438*, 116–120. [CrossRef] [PubMed]

21. Sato, Y.; Itagaki, S.; Oikawa, S.; Ogura, J.; Kobayashi, M.; Hirano, T.; Sugawara, M.; Iseki, K. Protective effect of soy isoflavone genistein on ischemia-reperfusion in the rat small intestine. *Biol. Pharm. Bull.* **2011**, *34*, 1448–1454. [CrossRef] [PubMed]

22. Canyilmaz, E.; Uslu, G.H.; Bahat, Z.; Kandaz, M.; Mungan, S.; Haciislamoglu, E.; Mentese, A.; Yoney, A. Comparison of the effects of melatonin and genistein on radiation-induced nephrotoxicity: Results of an experimental study. *Biomed. Rep.* **2016**, *4*, 45–50. [CrossRef] [PubMed]

23. Hirasaka, K.; Maeda, T.; Ikeda, C.; Haruna, M.; Kohno, S.; Abe, T.; Ochi, A.; Mukai, R.; Oarada, M.; Eshima-Kondo, S.; et al. Isoflavones derived from soy beans prevent MuRF1-mediated muscle atrophy in C2C12 myotubes through SIRT1 activation. *J. Nutr. Sci. Vitaminol.* **2013**, *59*, 317–324. [CrossRef] [PubMed]

24. Zheng, Y.; Lu, M.; Ma, L.; Zhang, S.; Qiu, M.; Wang, Y. Osthole ameliorates renal ischemia-reperfusion injury in rats. *J. Surg. Res.* **2013**, *183*, 347–354. [CrossRef] [PubMed]

25. Hao, S.; Bellner, L.; Zhao, H.; Ratliff, B.B.; Darzynkiewicz, Z.; Vio, C.P.; Ferreri, N.R. NFAT5 is protective against ischemic acute kidney injury. *Hypertension* **2014**, *63*, 46–52. [CrossRef] [PubMed]

26. Chung, S.; Yao, H.; Caito, S.; Hwang, J.W.; Arunachalam, G.; Rahman, I. Regulation of SIRT1 in cellular functions: Role of polyphenols. *Arch. Biochem. Biophys.* **2010**, *501*, 79–90. [CrossRef] [PubMed]

27. Havasi, A.; Borkan, S.C. Apoptosis and acute kidney injury. *Kidney Int.* **2011**, *80*, 29–40. [CrossRef] [PubMed]

28. Lee, H.T.; Gallos, G.; Nasr, S.H.; Emala, C.W. A1 adenosine receptor activation inhibits inflammation, necrosis, and apoptosis after renal ischemia-reperfusion injury in mice. *J. Am. Soc. Nephrol.* **2004**, *15*, 102–111. [CrossRef] [PubMed]

29. Migita, H.; Yoshitake, S.; Tange, Y.; Choijookhuu, N.; Hishikawa, Y. Hyperbaric Oxygen Therapy Suppresses Apoptosis and Promotes Renal Tubular Regeneration after Renal Ischemia/Reperfusion Injury in Rats. *Nephro-Urol. Mon.* **2016**, *8*, e34421. [CrossRef] [PubMed]

30. Cortina, B.; Torregrosa, G.; Castelló-Ruiz, M.; Burguete, M.C.; Moscardó, A.; Latorre, A.; Salom, J.B.; Vallés, J.; Santos, M.T.; Alborch, E. Improvement of the circulatory function partially accounts for the neuroprotective action of the phytoestrogen genistein in experimental ischemic stroke. *Eur. J. Pharmacol.* **2013**, *708*, 88–94. [CrossRef] [PubMed]

31. Imai, S. The NAD World: A new systemic regulatory network for metabolism and aging—SIRT1, systemic NAD biosynthesis, and their importance. *Cell Biochem. Biophys.* **2009**, *53*, 65–74. [CrossRef] [PubMed]

32. Hasegawa, K.; Wakino, S.; Yoshioka, K.; Tatematsu, S.; Hara, Y.; Minakuchi, H.; Sueyasu, K.; Washida, N.; Tokuyama, H.; Tzukerman, M.; et al. Kidney-specific overexpression of SIRT1 protects against acute kidney injury by retaining peroxisome function. *J. Biol. Chem.* **2010**, *285*, 13045–13056. [CrossRef] [PubMed]

33. Nadal-Serrano, M.; Pons, D.G.; Sastre-Serra, J.; Blanquer-Rosselló Mdel, M.; Roca, P.; Oliver, J. Genistein modulates oxidative stress in breast cancer cell lines according to ERalpha/ERbeta ratio: Effects on mitochondrial functionality, Sirtuins, uncoupling protein 2 and antioxidant enzymes. *Int. J. Biochem. Cell Biol.* **2013**, *45*, 2045–2051. [CrossRef] [PubMed]

34. Hsu, M.H.; Savas, U.; Lasker, J.M.; Johnson, E.F. Genistein, resveratrol, and 5-aminoimidazole-4-carboxamide-1-beta-D-ribofuranoside induce cytochrome P450 4F2 expression through an AMP-activated protein kinase-dependent pathway. *J. Pharmacol. Exp. Ther.* **2011**, *337*, 125–136. [CrossRef] [PubMed]

35. Kikuno, N.; Shiina, H.; Urakami, S.; Kawamoto, K.; Hirata, H.; Tanaka, Y.; Majid, S.; Igawa, M.; Dahiya, R. Genistein mediated histone acetylation and demethylation activates tumor suppressor genes in prostate cancer cells. *Int. J. Cancer* **2008**, *123*, 552–560. [CrossRef] [PubMed]

36. Liu, X.; Sun, C.; Liu, B.; Jin, X.; Li, P.; Zheng, X.; Zhao, T.; Li, F.; Li, Q. Genistein mediates the selective radiosensitizing effect in NSCLC A549 cells via inhibiting methylation of the keap1 gene promoter region. *Oncotarget* **2016**, *7*, 27267–27279. [CrossRef] [PubMed]

37. Sung, M.J.; Kim, D.H.; Jung, Y.J.; Kang, K.P.; Lee, A.S.; Lee, S.; Kim, W.; Davaatseren, M.; Hwang, J.T.; Kim, H.J.; et al. Genistein protects the kidney from cisplatin-induced injury. *Kidney Int.* **2008**, *74*, 1538–1547. [CrossRef] [PubMed]

38. Chen, Z.; Trotman, L.C.; Shaffer, D.; Lin, H.K.; Dotan, Z.A.; Niki, M.; Koutcher, J.A.; Scher, H.I.; Ludwig, T.; Gerald, W.; et al. Crucial role of p53-dependent cellular senescence in suppression of Pten-deficient tumorigenesis. *Nature* **2005**, *436*, 725–730. [CrossRef] [PubMed]

39. Rasbach, K.A.; Schnellmann, R.G. Isoflavones promote mitochondrial biogenesis. *J. Pharmacol. Exp. Ther.* **2008**, *325*, 536–543. [CrossRef] [PubMed]

40. Witko-Sarsat, V.; Ohayon, D. Proliferating cell nuclear antigen in neutrophil fate. *Immunol. Rev.* **2016**, *273*, 344–356. [CrossRef] [PubMed]

41. Reiser, J. Production and concentration of pseudotyped HIV-1-based gene transfer vectors. *Gene Ther.* **2000**, *7*, 910–913. [CrossRef] [PubMed]

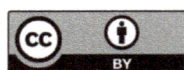

*nutrients*

MDPI

*Review*

# Association of Polyphenol Biomarkers with Cardiovascular Disease and Mortality Risk: A Systematic Review and Meta-Analysis of Observational Studies

**Johanna Rienks \*, Janett Barbaresko and Ute Nöthlings**

Department of Nutrition and Food Sciences, Nutritional Epidemiology, University of Bonn, Bonn 53115, Germany; j.barbaresko@uni-bonn.de (J.B.); noethlings@uni-bonn.de (U.N.)
\* Correspondence: johanna.rienks@uni-bonn.de; Tel.: +49-228-732020

Received: 24 March 2017; Accepted: 19 April 2017; Published: 22 April 2017

**Abstract:** Epidemiologic studies have suggested an inverse association between flavonoids and cardiovascular disease (CVD). However, the results might have been influenced by the use of dietary assessment methods, which are error prone. The aim of this paper was to systematically review and analyse the literature for evidence of associations between polyphenol biomarkers and CVD and mortality risk in observational studies. Eligible studies were identified through PubMed, Web of Science, and reference lists. Multivariable adjusted associations were extracted. Data were log-transformed and pooled using the random effects model. In total, eight studies were included, investigating 16 different polyphenol biomarkers in association with CVD and mortality. Blood and urine were used as biospecimens, and enterolactone, a lignan metabolite, was most often investigated. Three meta-analyses were conducted investigating the association between enterolactone, and all-cause and CVD mortality, and non-fatal myocardial infarction. A 30% and 45% reduced all-cause and CVD mortality risk were revealed at higher enterolactone concentrations. Furthermore, inverse associations were observed between polyphenol biomarkers and all-cause mortality, kaempferol, and acute coronary syndrome. There is evidence to suggest that enterolactone is associated with a lower CVD mortality risk. This emphasises the importance of the role of the microbiota in disease prevention. To strengthen the evidence, more studies are warranted.

**Keywords:** polyphenols; biomarkers; flavonoids; cardiovascular disease; mortality; observational; meta-analysis; enterolactone

---

## 1. Introduction

Cardiovascular diseases (CVD) are the leading cause of death worldwide [1]. By tackling modifiable lifestyle factors such as an unhealthy diet, most CVDs could in theory be prevented. A healthy diet containing plant-based foods [1] is abundant in bioactive compounds, such as polyphenols. Over 500 different heterogeneous molecular structures of polyphenols have been identified in plant foods [2]. Based on their structure, four groups of polyphenols can be distinguished, including flavonoids, phenolic acids, stilbenes, and lignans [3–5]. Of great interest to scientists is the group of flavonoids as their compounds are widely distributed in plant foods [6]. This group can be further classified into flavonols (main food sources: onions, curly kale, leeks, broccoli, apples, blueberries), flavanols (tea, grapes, cocoa), flavanones (citrus fruits), flavones (parsley, celery), anthocyanins (berries, black grapes), and isoflavones (soybeans) [3,7]. Also relatively abundant in plant foods are phenolic acids (coffee, outer part of fruits); however, with respect to disease risk, they have been investigated less often [5]. This is also the case for stilbenes, which are less dispersed in plant foods (wine, peanuts) [8]. Lignans, like flavonoids, have been investigated often and are found in linseed and cereals [5]. In the gut, lignans can be converted by microbiota to enterolactone (ENL) and enterodiol (END) [5], and can be detected in human biofluids.

The extensive research on polyphenols in animal and human studies has shown that these compounds possess a wide range of disease preventive properties including anti-inflammatory, antioxidant, and estrogenic activities [6]. However, because of the heterogeneity of findings across human studies, the role of polyphenols in CVD risk remains inconclusive. This might be due to the method used to assess the polyphenol intake. Most studies estimate polyphenol exposure of a participant's diet from food composition tables such as the USDA database [9] and Phenol-Explorer [2]. However, these tables might be of limited use because only a very restricted number of foods have been analysed for their polyphenol content using different analytical techniques [3]. Furthermore, polyphenol values in foods fluctuate as a result of climate, soil, ripeness, processing, and storage [3]. To overcome these measurement errors and provide more accurate measures of polyphenol exposure, the use of biomarkers has been suggested [10]. In large epidemiologic studies, mostly single samples of serum, plasma, or urine are collected. Considering the relatively short half-life of most compounds, habitual exposure is probably best reflected in 24-h urine. Zamora-Ros et al. [11] showed that the total urinary polyphenol excretion from 24-h urine was correlated with dietary intake. Furthermore, creatinine normalised spot urine proved to be a suitable biomarker when adjusted for factors modifying creatinine excretion [11].

The aims of the current study were to: (1) systematically review the literature for evidence of associations between polyphenol biomarkers and all-cause mortality, CVD mortality, and CVD incidence in observational studies; and (2) conduct meta-analyses of individual biomarkers of polyphenols and outcomes where possible. Isoflavone biomarkers and chronic disease and mortality were covered elsewhere [12].

## 2. Methods

This review was conducted according to the PRISMA guidelines [13] (Supplementary Table S1). A systematic search of the published literature was conducted in PubMed and Web of Science on 22 February 2017. The following search terms were used (both singular and plural): "biomarker", "plasma", "serum", "urine", "urinary", "excretion", "concentration", "level", with "polyphenol", "flavonoid", "flavone", "flavanone", "flavonol", "proanthocyanidin", "anthocyanin", "apigenin", "luteolin", "hesperetin", "hesperedin", "naringenin", "kaempferol", "quercetin", "tamarixetin", "matairesinol", "epicatechin", "epicatechin gallate", "coumestrol", "stilbene", "resveratrol", "tannin", "lignans", "enterolactone", "enterodiol", "enterolignan", "pinoresinol", "lariciresinol", "secoisolariciresinol", "matairesinol", "phenolic acid", "phytoestrogen", with "cardiovascular disease", "coronary heart disease", "heart disease", "CVD", "heart disease", "coronary artery disease", "myocardial infarction", "stroke", "cerebrovascular disease", "heart failure", "mortality", "death", "cardiovascular mortality", with "observational", "epidemiologic", "cohort", "longitudinal", "prospective", "case-control", "nested case-control", not "animals" (using MeSH terms in PubMed).

### 2.1. In- and Exclusion Criteria

Two authors (JR and JB) independently screened the titles and abstracts of the publications. A third acted as a moderator (UN), to remove any discrepancies. Articles were retained for review if the following inclusion criteria were met: (1) investigation of multiple, adjusted associations between polyphenol biomarker(s) and CVD risk or mortality; (2) use of an observational study design; (3) the study involved humans; and (4) the study was published in a scientific journal (conference abstracts and comments were excluded).

Articles were excluded if they met with at least one of the following criteria: (1) a dietary intervention was conducted prior to biospecimen sampling; or (2) only a dietary assessment method was used to assess polyphenol exposure. Finally, reference lists of all the included publications were screened to identify further articles meeting the inclusion criteria. No constraints were put on the language of the articles.

### 2.2. Data Extraction

From each article, the following details were extracted: first author, year of publication, country where the study was conducted, study design and cohort, characteristics of the participants (age, sex, number of cases/controls or cohort), follow-up time, specimen type, polyphenol biomarker(s), outcome(s), association measure, and confounding and matching variables.

### 2.3. Quality Assessment

The quality of the included studies was assessed using the Newcastle-Ottawa scale developed for non-randomised studies [14]. The scale appraised three aspects including the selection of the study groups, the comparability of the groups, and the ascertainment of either outcome or exposure from cohort or nested case-control studies, respectively. The maximum number of 'stars' awarded to each section was four, two, and three for selection, comparability, and outcome/exposure, respectively.

### 2.4. Statistical Analysis

Meta-analyses were conducted when at least two studies were available with a common exposure and outcome. This resulted in a total of three meta-analyses investigating the association between ENL, and all-cause and CVD mortality, and non-fatal myocardial infarction. For the meta-analyses, all effect sizes (HR, OR, RR) and 95% confidence intervals (CI) were log-transformed to maintain symmetry in the analysis. Standard errors were calculated from log CIs by subtracting the lower CI from the upper CI and subsequently dividing by 3.92. The $I^2$ statistic was calculated to test the percentage of variation across studies due to heterogeneity [15]. Heterogeneity was assumed to be present because of differences in the study design and population. Therefore, we used a random-effects model that assumes a distribution of the true effect size by allowing both between- and within study variation [16]. Pooled estimates were visualized in forest plots. Potential publication bias was investigated by a visual inspection of the funnel plot, whereby asymmetry illustrated publication bias, and was tested quantitatively with the Egger's test [17]. As CVD incidence and mortality differ between men and women, where possible, subgroup analyses were performed. The package 'meta' [18] in R [19] statistical software Version 3.3.2 was used to conduct the meta-analyses and 'metabias' was used to assess publication bias. A $p$-value < 0.05 was considered statistically significant.

## 3. Results

### 3.1. Search Results

After removing duplicates, 719 studies remained (Figure 1). The titles and abstracts were screened. Ten full-texts were read and in total eight observational studies [20–27] were identified that investigated polyphenol biomarkers in association with mortality or CVD. In total, 16 polyphenolic compounds were investigated (Table 1). Five studies investigated ENL [21–25], two END [22,23], and one total polyphenols [26], resveratrol [27], lignans [23], flavonoids [20], flavonols [20], flavanones [20], flavones [20], and phloretin [20]. Two studies solely investigated all-cause mortality [26,27], two studied all-cause and CVD mortality [23,25], two studied CVD incidence and mortality [20,21], and three CVD incidence [21,22,24]. The characteristics and results of the included studies are presented in Tables 2 and 3, respectively. The following biospecimens were used: two studies used 24 h urine [26,27], two used spot urine [20,23], three used serum [21,24,25], and one used plasma [22]. Six different study populations from five different countries were studied including Denmark, Finland, Italy, the Netherlands, and the USA. Four [23,25–27] studies had a prospective cohort study design, three [20,22,24] were nested case-control studies, and one [21] had a case-cohort design. All publications were of moderate to good quality with scores for both cohort and nested case-control studies ranging from five to eight stars (Supplementary Table S2).

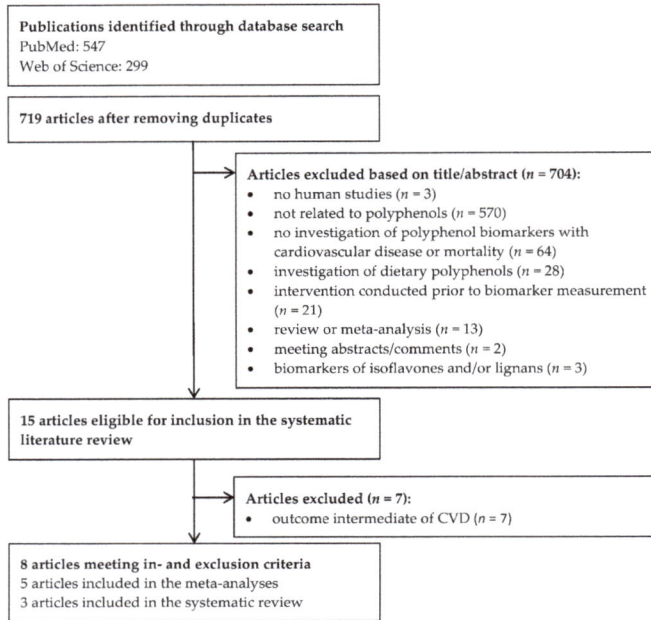

**Figure 1.** Flowchart of the study selection.

**Table 1.** Frequency of studies reporting on polyphenol biomarkers in association with mortality and cardiovascular disease (CVD).

| Polyphenolic Group Compound | Reference | Frequency of Investigation | Mortality | CVD Mortality | CVD Incidence |
|---|---|---|---|---|---|
| Total polyphenols | [26] | 1 | 1 | | |
| Total flavonoids | [20] | 1 | | | 1 |
| Total flavonols | | 1 | | | 1 |
| • Kaempferol | | 1 | | | 1 |
| • Quercetin | [20] | 1 | | | 1 |
| • Tamarixetin | | 1 | | | 1 |
| • Isorhamnetin | | 1 | | | 1 |
| Total flavanone | | 1 | | | 1 |
| • Naringenin | [20] | 1 | | | 1 |
| • Hesperetin | | 1 | | | 1 |
| Total flavone | [20] | | | | |
| • Apigenin | | 1 | | | 1 |
| Phloretin | [20] | 1 | | | 1 |
| Resveratrol | [27] | 1 | 1 | | |
| Lignans | [23] | 1 | 1 | 1 | |
| • Enterolactone | [21–25] | 5 | 2 | 3 | 3 |
| • Enterodiol | [22,23] | 2 | 1 | 1 | 1 |

**Table 2.** Characteristics of studies included in this systematic literature review investigating the association between polyphenol biomarkers and cardiovascular disease and mortality.

| Author (Year) Country | Design | Study Name | Specimen | Biomarker | Cases, n | Cohort, n (Sex % Women) | Age, Year | Follow-Up, y [1] | Outcome |
|---|---|---|---|---|---|---|---|---|---|
| Zamora-Ros et al. (2013) Italy [26] | ps | InCHIANTI | 24 h urine | POLY | 274 | 807 (58.7) | ≥65 | 12 | All-cause mortality |
| Semba et al. (2014) Italy [27] | ps | InCHIANTI | 24 h urine | RES | 268 | 783 (41.4) | ≥65 | 9 | All-cause mortality |
| Reger et al. (2016) USA [23] | ps | NHANES | Spot urine | ELIG, ENL, END | 108 290 | 5179 (52.4) | ≥18 | 5 | CVD mortality All-cause mortality |
| Vanharanta et al. (2003) Finland [25] | ps | KIHD | Serum | ENL | 70 103 242 | 1889 (0) | 42–60 | 12.2 | CHD mortality CVD mortality All-cause mortality |
| Kilkkinen et al. (2006) Finland [21] | caco | ATBC | Serum | ENL | 340 205 135 | 760 (0) | 50–69 | 11.1 | All CHD events Nonfatal MI Coronary death |
| Bredsdorff et al. (2013) Denmark [20] | ncc | DCH | Afternoon spot urine | flavonoids, phloretin, FLAVO, ISO, KAE, QUE, TAM, FLAVAN, HES, NAR, API | 393 | 786 (20.1) | 50–64 | 8 (TP) | Acute coronary syndrome |
| Kuijsten et al. (2009) The Netherlands [22] | ncc | Monitoring Project on CVD risk factors | Plasma | ENL, END | 236 | 519 (31.1) | 20–59 | 4.5 | Nonfatal MI |
| Vanharanta et al. (1999) Finland [24] | ncc | KIHD | Serum | ENL | 167 | 334 (0) | 42–60 | 10 | Acute coronary events |

[1] Mean or median (med) follow-up time, total study period (TP) was calculated, when follow-up time was not reported, by subtracting the year of last follow-up from the year of specimen collection. API, apigenin; ATBC, Alpha-Tocopherol, Beta-Carotene Cancer Prevention study; caco, case-cohort; CHD, coronary heart disease; CVD, cardiovascular disease; DCH, Diet Cancer and Health study; END, enterodiol; ENL, enterolactone; ELIG, enterolignan; FLAVAN, flavanones; FLAVO, flavonol; HES, hesperetin; InCHIANTI, Invecchiare in Chianti; ISO, isorhamnetin; KAE, kaempferol; KIHD, Kuopio Ischaemic Heart Disease Risk Factor Study MI, myocardial infarction; *n*, number; NAR, naringenin; ncc, nested case-control study; NHANES, National Health and Nutrition Examination Survey; POLY, polyphenols; ps, prospective study; QUE, quercetin; RES, resveratrol; TAM, tamarixetin; TP, total period.

**Table 3.** Results of the studies included in this systematic literature review of studies investigating the biomarkers of polyphenols with mortality and cardiovascular disease.

| Author Year, Country | Biomarker | Endpoint | Association (95% CI) of Extreme Quantiles | | P-trend | Confounders (C) and Matching (M) Variables |
|---|---|---|---|---|---|---|
| **All-cause mortality** | | | | | | |
| Zamora-Ros et al. (2013) Italy [26] | POLY | All-cause mortality | HR Q3/Q1 | 0.70 (0.49, 0.99) | 0.05 | C: age, sex, education, BMI, alcohol intake, smoking status, renal function, PA, CVD, DM, cancer, COPD, dementia, Parkinson's disease, energy intake only for TDPs |
| Semba et al. (2014) Italy [27] | RES | All-cause mortality | HR Q4/Q1 | 0.80 (0.54, 1.17) | 0.43 | C: age, sex, education, BMI, PA, total cholesterol, HDL, MMSE score, mean arterial BP, and chronic diseases: CHD, stroke, heart failure, cancer, DM, peripheral artery disease, chronic kidney disease |
| Reger et al. (2016) USA [23] | ELIG ENL END | All-cause mortality | HR Q3/Q1 | 0.65 (0.43, 0.96) 0.65 (0.44, 0.97) 0.98 (0.67, 1.43) | 0.019 0.014 0.85 | C: age, education, smoking status, BMI, total energy intake, sodium intake, urinary creatinine |
| Vanharanta et al. (2003) Finland [25] | ENL | All-cause mortality | HR Q4/Q1 | 0.76 (0.52, 1.12) | 0.09 | C: age, year of examination, year of serum ENL measurement, DM, hypertension, urinary excretion of nicotine metabolites, BMI, alcohol, LDL, HDL, dietary intake of fiber, folate, vitamins C and E, saturated fatty acids |
| **CVD incidence and mortality** | | | | | | |
| Bredsdorff et al. (2013) Denmark [20] | flavonoids phloretin FLAVO ISO KAE QUE TAM FLAVAN HES NAR API | Acute coronary syndrome | OR Q5/Q1 | 0.63 (0.37, 1.05) 0.87 (0.54, 1.39) 0.83 (0.50, 1.36) 0.72 (0.41, 1.25) 0.55 (0.32, 0.92) 0.94 (0.58, 1.51) 1.06 (0.65, 1.74) 0.68 (0.41, 1.12) 0.72 (0.43, 1.18) 0.63 (0.38, 1.02) 1.20 (0.73, 1.96) | 0.32 0.46 0.46 0.15 0.12 0.65 0.78 0.26 0.34 0.12 0.73 | C: period of analysis, BMI, waist circumference, smoking, hypertension, DM, alcohol, hypercholesterolemia, PA, level of school education M: sex, age, smoking, time specimen collection |

Table 3. *Cont.*

| Author Year, Country | Biomarker | Endpoint | Association (95% CI) of Extreme Quantiles | | P-trend | Confounders (C) and Matching (M) Variables |
|---|---|---|---|---|---|---|
| Kuijsten et al. (2009) the Netherlands [22] | ENL | Nonfatal MI | OR Q4/Q1 | 1.49 (0.85, 2.61) | 0.140 | C: current smoking, BMI, systolic blood pressure, total cholesterol, HDL cholesterol, ratio total/HDL cholesterol, current smoking, SBP, ratio total/HDL cholesterol |
| | END | | | 1.18 (0.67, 2.07) | 0.860 | M: age (5 years), sex, study center |
| Vanharanta et al. (1999) Finland [24] | ENL | Acute coronary events | OR Q4/Q1 | 0.35 (0.14, 0.88) | 0.01 | C: serum apolipoprotein B, dietary iron intake, fam hist of CHD, ischaemic findings on exercise test, dietary calcium intake, urinary excretion of nicotine metabolites, DM, SBP, maximum oxygen uptake M: age, examination year, place of residence |
| Kilkkinen et al. (2006) Finland [21] | ENL | All CHD events | RR Q5/Q1 | 0.63 (0.33, 1.11) | 0.07 | C: age, BMI, total and HDL cholesterol, DBP, SBP, alcohol intake, nr of smoking years and cigarettes smoked per day, hist of CHD and DM, fasting time, dietary factors |
| | | Nonfatal MI | | 0.67 (0.37, 1.23) | 0.10 | |
| | | Coronary death | | 0.57 (0.26, 1.25) | 0.18 | |
| Reger et al. (2016) USA [23] | ELIG | CVD mortality | HR Q3/Q1 | 0.48 (0.24, 0.97) | 0.07 | C: age, education, smoking status, BMI, total energy intake, sodium intake, urinary creatinine |
| | ENL | | | 0.54 (0.27, 1.07) | 0.10 | |
| | END | | | 0.71 (0.87, 1.78) | 0.52 | |
| Vanharanta et al. (2003) Finland [25] | ENL | CHD mortality | HR Q4/Q1 | 0.44 (0.20, 0.96) | 0.03 | C: age, year of examination, year of serum ENL measurement, DM, hypertension, urinary excretion of nicotine metabolites, BMI, alcohol, LDL, HDL, dietary intake of fiber, folate, vitamins C and E, saturated fatty acids |
| | | CVD mortality | | 0.55 (0.29, 1.01) | 0.04 | |

API, apigenin; BMI, body mass index; CHD, coronary heart disease; COPD, chronic obstructive pulmonary disease; CVD, cardiovascular disease; DBP, diastolic blood pressure; DM, diabetes mellitus; ELIG, enterolignan; END, enterodiol; ENL, enterolactone; fam hist, family history; FLAVA, flavanol; FLAVAN, flavanones; FLAVO, flavonol; ISO, isorhamnetin; HDL, high-density lipoprotein; HES, hesperetin; hist, history; HR, hazard ratio; ISO, isorhamnetin; KAE, kaempferol; LDL, low density lipoprotein; MMSE, mini-mental state examination; NAR, naringenin; OR, odds ratio; PA, physical activity; POLY, polyphenols; Q, quantile; QUE, quercetin; RES, resveratrol; RR, rate ratio; SBP, systolic blood pressure; TAM, tamarixetin; TDPs, total dietary polyphenols.

### 3.2. All-Cause Mortality

Four publications investigated all-cause mortality [23,25–27] (Table 3). The meta-analysis of two studies [23,25] revealed a 30% lower all-cause mortality risk at higher ENL concentrations (Figure 2A). Heterogeneity was not present and publication bias could not be indicated from the funnel plot. Furthermore, decreased mortality risks of 30%, 35%, and 35% were observed at higher total urinary polyphenol (TUP) [26], enterolignans [23], and ENL [23] concentrations, respectively. However, no associations were observed for resveratrol [27] and END [23].

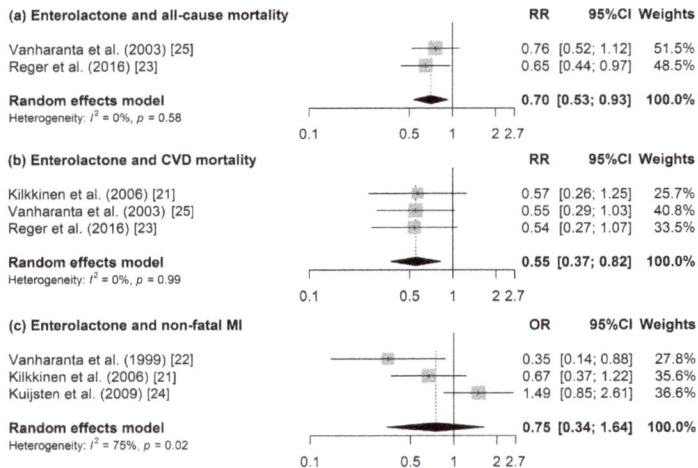

**(a) Enterolactone and all-cause mortality**

| | RR | 95%CI | Weights |
|---|---|---|---|
| Vanharanta et al. (2003) [25] | 0.76 | [0.52; 1.12] | 51.5% |
| Reger et al. (2016) [23] | 0.65 | [0.44; 0.97] | 48.5% |
| **Random effects model** | **0.70** | **[0.53; 0.93]** | **100.0%** |

Heterogeneity: $I^2 = 0\%$, $p = 0.58$

**(b) Enterolactone and CVD mortality**

| | RR | 95%CI | Weights |
|---|---|---|---|
| Kilkkinen et al. (2006) [21] | 0.57 | [0.26; 1.25] | 25.7% |
| Vanharanta et al. (2003) [25] | 0.55 | [0.29; 1.03] | 40.8% |
| Reger et al. (2016) [23] | 0.54 | [0.27; 1.07] | 33.5% |
| **Random effects model** | **0.55** | **[0.37; 0.82]** | **100.0%** |

Heterogeneity: $I^2 = 0\%$, $p = 0.99$

**(c) Enterolactone and non-fatal MI**

| | OR | 95%CI | Weights |
|---|---|---|---|
| Vanharanta et al. (1999) [22] | 0.35 | [0.14; 0.88] | 27.8% |
| Kilkkinen et al. (2006) [21] | 0.67 | [0.37; 1.22] | 35.6% |
| Kuijsten et al. (2009) [24] | 1.49 | [0.85; 2.61] | 36.6% |
| **Random effects model** | **0.75** | **[0.34; 1.64]** | **100.0%** |

Heterogeneity: $I^2 = 75\%$, $p = 0.02$

**Figure 2.** Forest of the association between enterolactone and (**a**) all-cause mortality; (**b**) CVD-mortality; and (**c**) non-fatal MI.

### 3.3. CVD Incidence and Mortality

In total, six studies investigated CVD incidence [20–22,24] or mortality [21,23,25]. Pooling data for CVD mortality, a 45% reduced risk was revealed when the highest and the lowest quantile of ENL concentration were compared (Figure 2B). Heterogeneity and publication bias were not present. In a subgroup analysis of men, a similar result was found (RR (95% confidence interval (CI): 0.56 (0.34, 0.91)). When stratifying by sex, a 47% reduced non-fatal MI risk was observed (RR (95% CI): 0.53 (0.29, 0.98)). Inverse associations were also found between ENL and CHD mortality [25], and kaempferol excretion and acute coronary syndrome (ACS) [20]; however, no associations were observed for the other polyphenols in this study [20], and between END and CVD mortality in another study [23].

In the meta-analysis of three studies on ENL [21,22,24], no statistically significant association was identified for non-fatal MI. Heterogeneity was high ($I^2$ = 75%) and there was no indication for publication bias according the Egger's test. END was not statistically significantly associated with nonfatal MI [22].

## 4. Discussion

To our knowledge, this is the first study to give a complete overview of the published evidence of associations between polyphenol biomarkers and CVD risk and mortality in human population-based studies. Only eight studies were found, allowing meta-analyses with only two or three studies comparing ENL and mortality, CVD-mortality, or CHD incidence. The meta-analyses of all-cause and CVD mortality revealed a 30% and 45% reduced risk at higher ENL levels, respectively. No associations were observed in meta-analyses for incident MI and ENL concentrations. Indeed, the microbiota-derived lignan metabolites ENL and END were most frequently investigated. Single findings were observed between TUP and all-cause mortality, and kaempferol and ACS.

### 4.1. Comparison with other Studies on Dietary Polyphenols

In line with the inverse association that was revealed in the present meta-analysis of all- cause mortality, is the 40% reduced risk observed for dietary lignans in Spanish community-dwelling elderly [28] and the 31% reduced risk for matairesinol found in elderly Dutch men [29]. No association was observed for total dietary lignans in this study [29]. In contrast to the reduced CVD mortality risk in the current meta-analysis, a prospective study from the Netherlands did not find an association with total dietary lignans; however, matairesinol again tended to be inversely associated [29].

No association was observed for total dietary polyphenols (TDP), as opposed to the statistically significant inverse association for TUP [26] in the same study. However, in a larger sample of a community-dwelling Spanish population, reduced risks of 37% and 52% were found for TDP and stilbenes (a group that includes resveratrol), respectively [28]. The result for stilbenes was not reflected in the resveratrol biomarker study [27] in the current review.

All in all, there seems to be some evidence from biomarker studies linking microbiota-derived lignan biomarkers to mortality endpoints, but overall, only a few studies were available.

In agreement with the null-finding for non-fatal MI, are the results from the EPIC-Prospect study [30]. The statistically significant reduced ACS risk of the kaempferol biomarker [20] is in line with the results of a meta-analysis [31] and a prospective Italian study [32]. The null associations found for flavonoid biomarkers and ACS [20] are consistent with a meta-analysis of total dietary flavonoids and their subgroups [31], dietary flavonols and flavanones, in two prospective studies [33,34], and flavones in three prospective studies [32–34]. In contrast, a statistically significant decreased CVD risk trend was observed for dietary dihydrochalcone intake [34] (class of phloretin [20]).

Evidence from biomarker studies is scarce and more studies on all compounds are warranted.

*4.2. Validity of the Biomarker Measure*

The main advantage of using biomarkers for an exposure assessment over dietary assessment methods is that these account for inter-individual differences in absorption, distribution, and metabolism [3]. Nevertheless, biomarker concentrations are influenced by several factors, of which some are known and others are yet to be determined. Treatment with antibiotics is a known factor that influences the formation of lignan metabolites [35]. The failure to account for antibiotic use is an important limitation of the studies included in the meta-analyses [21–25]. The number of antibiotic treatments and the time since the last treatment affect the microflora and were shown to result in lower ENL concentrations, even 12–16 months after treatment [35]. Since all of the studies included in the meta-analysis did not consider antibiotic use, their observed risks are likely to be attenuated. The included studies used single samples of blood and urine, which were predominantly sampled in a fasting state. This raises the question of which biomarker is better correlated with biological relevance, especially considering the potential differences between individuals. The absorption, peak plasma, metabolism, and excretion of polyphenols are likely to be determined by individual physiology. Therefore, a single sample may not provide a reliable marker for the total bioavailable concentration throughout time. Considering the relatively short half-lives of most polyphenolic compounds, 24 h urine should contain all of the ingested compounds and/or their metabolites and conjungates.

*4.3. Strengths and Limitations of the Present Review*

The main strength of the present study is the inclusion of several meta-analyses of polyphenol biomarkers. To our knowledge, these are the first meta-analyses of lignan biomarkers representing an internal dose. Although we only conducted meta-analyses on two (for all-cause mortality) and three (for CVD mortality and non-fatal MI) studies, a good overview of the level of consistency across the studies is provided.

All of the studies included in the meta-analysis of CVD-mortality used Cox proportional hazard models, either reporting HR or RR, which have the same meaning and are used interchangeably. Because the highest and lowest exposure quantiles were compared, a dose-response relationship could not be derived. Furthermore, the remaining three studies included in the systematic literature were slightly heterogeneous with regard to the polyphenol biomarker measured. However, this only emphasizes the complexity of the polyphenol exposure and the need to investigate the role of the individual polyphenols in cardiovascular disease and mortality. Another strength is that the quality of the included studies was judged to be moderate to good. Beside antibiotic use, another potential confounder, creatintine excretion, was only considered in the study by Reger et al. [23]. The failure to account for urinary creatinine excretion could result in an over- or underestimation of polyphenol concentrations, depending on the dilution of the urine. From the visual inspection of the funnel plots and interpretation of the Egger's test, publication bias was not present. However, significant heterogeneity was observed in the meta-analysis of MI. This was further explored in the sensitivity analysis. By excluding one study at a time, we observed that the study by Kuijsten et al. (2009) introduced the heterogeneity, as after exclusion, we found an $I^2$ of 25.6%. The heterogeneity could have resulted from sex differences, as the inclusion of men did result in an inverse association. Another explanation might be the difference in the biospecimens or the lower ENL concentrations in this study [22], where the cut-off in the highest quartile was >17.5 nmol/L. In comparison, ENL concentrations were much higher in the studies by Vanharanta et al. (1999) [24] and Kilkkinen et al. (2006) [21], namely >30.1 and >28.24 nmol/L, respectively. This could be simply explained by differences in dietary habits between the Netherlands and Finland, or because of the differences in biomarkers used to measure ENL. Furthermore, in addition to the search in two large databases and the articles' reference lists, a search in gray literature could have resulted in the identification of unpublished papers. Language bias was prevented by imposing no restrictions on language; in spite of this, no non-English written publications were retrieved that met the inclusion criteria. Interestingly, only one study [26] investigated polyphenol biomarkers and dietary polyphenols in the same study population. Therefore, the emerging question is whether these approaches would provide stronger results when biomarkers are measured in conjunction with dietary intake. The current review, however, suggests that the polyphenol biomarkers strongly reflect internal doses, which are not necessarily strongly associated with long-term intake due to the many factors influencing bioavailability [3,36].

## 5. Conclusions

A number of studies have been published reporting on the associations between polyphenol biomarkers, and all-cause, CVD mortality, and CVD risk. In the meta-analyses, inverse associations were revealed between ENL and all-cause and CVD mortality. Furthermore, in the systematic review, inverse associations were observed for TUP with all-cause mortality and ACS with kaempferol. For future research, comparability across studies should be improved to enable a quantitative analysis. Furthermore, it is recommended that groups investigate individual polyphenolic compounds and even metabolites instead of total polyphenols from different groups and classes. It might be worth considering collecting multiple biospecimen samples or 24 h urine samples that reflect circadian polyphenol exposure, although this might not be desirable in large cohort studies as it places a burden on the study participants.

**Supplementary Materials:** The following are available online at www.mdpi.com/2072-6643/9/4/415/s1, Table S1: PRISMA checklist, Table S2: Results of quality assessment of included studies using the Newcastle-Ottawa scale for non-randomised studies.

**Acknowledgments:** This research was supported by the German Academic Exchange Service (DAAD) (scholarship 91531364 to JR) and Diet Body Brain funded by the German Federal Ministry of Education and Research (BMBF) (grantnr: 01EA1410A).

**Author Contributions:** U.N. and J.R. conceived and designed the experiments; J.B. and J.R. conducted the literature search; J.R. analysed the data; U.N. and J.B. critically reviewed the manuscript for important intellectual content; J.R. wrote the paper.

## References

1.  World Health Organisation (WHO). Cardiovascular Diseases (CVDs). Available online: http://www.who.int/mediacentre/factsheets/fs317/en/ (accessed on 6 January 2017).
2.  Neveu, V.; Perez-Jimenez, J.; Vos, F.; Crespy, V.; du Chaffaut, L.; Mennen, L.; Knox, C.; Eisner, R.; Cruz, J.; Wishart, D.; et al. Phenol-explorer: An online comprehensive database on polyphenol contents in foods. *Database: J. Biol. Databases Curation* **2010**, *2010*, bap024. [CrossRef] [PubMed]
3.  Spencer, J.P.; Abd El Mohsen, M.M.; Minihane, A.M.; Mathers, J.C. Biomarkers of the intake of dietary polyphenols: Strengths, limitations and application in nutrition research. *Br. J. Nutr.* **2008**, *99*, 12–22. [CrossRef] [PubMed]
4.  Manach, C.; Williamson, G.; Morand, C.; Scalbert, A.; Remesy, C. Bioavailability and bioefficacy of polyphenols in humans. I. Review of 97 bioavailability studies. *Am. J. Clin. Nutr.* **2005**, *81*, 230S–242S. [PubMed]
5.  Manach, C.; Scalbert, A.; Morand, C.; Remesy, C.; Jimenez, L. Polyphenols: Food sources and bioavailability. *Am. J. Clin. Nutr.* **2004**, *79*, 727–747. [PubMed]
6.  Landete, J.M. Updated knowledge about polyphenols: Functions, bioavailability, metabolism, and health. *Crit. Rev. Food Sci. Nutr.* **2011**, *52*, 936–948. [CrossRef] [PubMed]
7.  Erdman, J.W., Jr.; Balentine, D.; Arab, L.; Beecher, G.; Dwyer, J.T.; Folts, J.; Harnly, J.; Hollman, P.; Keen, C.L.; Mazza, G.; et al. Flavonoids and heart health: Proceedings of the ilsi north america flavonoids workshop, May 31–June 1, 2005, Washington, DC. *J. Nutr.* **2007**, *137*, 718S–737S. [PubMed]
8.  Crozier, A.; Jaganath, I.B.; Clifford, M.N. Dietary phenolics: Chemistry, bioavailability and effects on health. *Nat. Prod. Rep.* **2009**, *26*, 1001–1043. [CrossRef] [PubMed]

9.  Bhagwat, S.; Haytowitz, D.B.; Wasswa-Kintu, S.I.; Holden, J.M. USDA develops a database for flavonoids to assess dietary intakes. *Procedia Food Sci.* **2013**, *2*, 81–86. [CrossRef]
10. Linseisen, J.; Rohrmann, S. Biomarkers of dietary intake of flavonoids and phenolic acids for studying diet-cancer relationship in humans. *Eur. J. Nutr.* **2008**, *47*, 60–68. [CrossRef] [PubMed]
11. Zamora-Ros, R.; Rabassa, M.; Cherubini, A.; Urpi-Sarda, M.; Llorach, R.; Bandinelli, S.; Ferrucci, L.; Andres-Lacueva, C. Comparison of 24-h volume and creatinine-corrected total urinary polyphenol as a biomarker of total dietary polyphenols in the invecchiare inchianti study. *Anal. Chim. Acta* **2011**, *704*, 110–115. [CrossRef] [PubMed]
12. Rienks, J.; Barbaresko, J.; Nöthlings, U. Association of isoflavone biomarkers with chronic disease and mortality risk: A systematic literature review and meta-analysis of observational studies. *Nutr. Rev.* **2017**. accepted.
13. Moher, D.; Liberati, A.; Tetzlaff, J.; Altman, D.G.; Group, P. Preferred reporting items for systematic reviews and meta-analyses: The prisma statement. *PLoS Med.* **2009**, *6*, e1000097. [CrossRef] [PubMed]
14. Wells, G.A.; Shea, B.; O'Connell, D.; Peterson, J.; Welch, V.; Tugwell, P. The Newcastle-Ottawa Scale (nos) for Assessing the Quality of Nonrandomised Studies in Meta-Analyses. Available online: http://www.ohri.ca/programs/clinical_epidemiology/oxford.asp (accessed on 1 July 2015).
15. Higgins, J.P.; Thompson, S.G.; Deeks, J.J.; Altman, D.G. Measuring inconsistency in meta-analyses. *BMJ (Clin. Res. Ed.)* **2003**, *327*, 557–560. [CrossRef] [PubMed]
16. DerSimonian, R.; Laird, N. Meta-analysis in clinical trials. *Controlled Clin. Trials* **1986**, *7*, 177–188. [CrossRef]
17. Egger, M.; Davey Smith, G.; Schneider, M.; Minder, C. Bias in meta-analysis detected by a simple, graphical test. *BMJ (Clin. Res. Ed.)* **1997**, *315*, 629–634. [CrossRef]
18. Schwarzer, G. Meta: General Package for Meta-Analysis. R Package Version 4.3-2. Available online: http://CRAN.R-project.org/package=meta (accessed on 17 February 2015).
19. R Core Team. R: A Language and Environment for Statistical Computing. R Foundation for Statistical Computing: Vienna, Austria. Available online: http://www.R-project.org/ (accessed on 1 January 2014).
20. Bredsdorff, L.; Obel, T.; Dethlefsen, C.; Tjonneland, A.; Schmidt, E.B.; Rasmussen, S.E.; Overvad, K. Urinary flavonoid excretion and risk of acute coronary syndrome in a nested case-control study. *Am. J. Clin. Nutr.* **2013**, *98*, 209–216. [CrossRef] [PubMed]
21. Kilkkinen, A.; Erlund, I.; Virtanen, M.J.; Alfthan, G.; Ariniemi, K.; Virtamo, J. Serum enterolactone concentration and the risk of coronary heart disease in a case-cohort study of finnish male smokers. *Am. J. Epidemiol.* **2006**, *163*, 687–693. [CrossRef] [PubMed]
22. Kuijsten, A.; Bueno-de-Mesquita, H.B.; Boer, J.M.A.; Arts, I.C.W.; Kok, F.J.; van't Veer, P.; Hollman, P.C.H. Plasma enterolignans are not associated with nonfatal myocardial infarction risk. *Atherosclerosis* **2009**, *203*, 145–152. [CrossRef] [PubMed]
23. Reger, M.K.; Zollinger, T.W.; Liu, Z.; Jones, J.; Zhang, J. Urinary phytoestrogens and cancer, cardiovascular, and all-cause mortality in the continuous national health and nutrition examination survey. *Eur. J. Nutr.* **2016**, *55*, 1029–1040. [CrossRef] [PubMed]
24. Vanharanta, M.; Voutilainen, S.; Lakka, T.A.; van der Lee, M.; Adlercreutz, H.; Salonen, J.T. Risk of acute coronary events according to serum concentrations of enterolactone: A prospective population-based case-control study. *Lancet* **1999**, *354*, 2112–2115. [CrossRef]
25. Vanharanta, M.; Voutilainen, S.; Rissanen, T.H.; Adlercreutz, H.; Salonen, J.T. Risk of cardiovascular disease-related and all-cause death according to serum concentrations of enterolactone: Kuopio ischaemic heart disease risk factor study. *Arch. Intern Med.* **2003**, *163*, 1099–1104. [CrossRef] [PubMed]
26. Zamora-Ros, R.; Rabassa, M.; Cherubini, A.; Urpi-Sarda, M.; Bandinelli, S.; Ferrucci, L.; Andres-Lacueva, C. High concentrations of a urinary biomarker of polyphenol intake are associated with decreased mortality in older adults. *J. Nutr.* **2013**, *143*, 1445–1450. [CrossRef] [PubMed]
27. Semba, R.D.; Ferrucci, L.; Bartali, B.; Urpi-Sarda, M.; Zamora-Ros, R.; Sun, K.; Cherubini, A.; Bandinelli, S.; Andres-Lacueva, C. Resveratrol levels and all-cause mortality in older community-dwelling adults. *JAMA Intern. Med.* **2014**, *174*, 1077–1084. [CrossRef] [PubMed]
28. Tresserra-Rimbau, A.; Rimm, E.B.; Medina-Remon, A.; Martinez-Gonzalez, M.A.; Lopez-Sabater, M.C.; Covas, M.I.; Corella, D.; Salas-Salvado, J.; Gomez-Gracia, E.; Lapetra, J.; et al. Polyphenol intake and mortality risk: A re-analysis of the predimed trial. *BMC Med.* **2014**, *12*, 77. [CrossRef] [PubMed]

29. Milder, I.E.; Feskens, E.J.; Arts, I.C.; Bueno-de-Mesquita, H.B.; Hollman, P.C.; Kromhout, D. Intakes of 4 dietary lignans and cause-specific and all-cause mortality in the zutphen elderly study. *Am. J. Clin. Nutr.* **2006**, *84*, 400–405. [PubMed]

30. Van der Schouw, Y.T.; Kreijkamp-Kaspers, S.; Peeters, P.H.M.; Keinan-Boker, L.; Rimm, E.B.; Grobbee, D.E. Prospective study on usual dietary phytoestrogen intake and cardiovascular disease risk in western women. *Circulation* **2005**, *111*, 465–471. [CrossRef] [PubMed]

31. Wang, X.; Ouyang, Y.Y.; Liu, J.; Zhao, G. Flavonoid intake and risk of CVD: A systematic review and meta-analysis of prospective cohort studies. *Br. J. Nutr.* **2014**, *111*, 1–11. [CrossRef] [PubMed]

32. Ponzo, V.; Goitre, I.; Fadda, M.; Gambino, R.; De Francesco, A.; Soldati, L.; Gentile, L.; Magistroni, P.; Cassader, M.; Bo, S. Dietary flavonoid intake and cardiovascular risk: A population-based cohort study. *J. Transl. Med.* **2015**, *13*, 218. [CrossRef] [PubMed]

33. Jacques, P.F.; Cassidy, A.; Rogers, G.; Peterson, J.J.; Dwyer, J.T. Dietary flavonoid intakes and cvd incidence in the framingham offspring cohort. *Br. J. Nutr.* **2015**, *114*, 1496–1503. [CrossRef] [PubMed]

34. Tresserra-Rimbau, A.; Rimm, E.B.; Medina-Remon, A.; Martinez-Gonzalez, M.A.; de la Torre, R.; Corella, D.; Salas-Salvado, J.; Gomez-Gracia, E.; Lapetra, J.; Aros, F.; et al. Inverse association between habitual polyphenol intake and incidence of cardiovascular events in the predimed study. *Nutr. Metab. Cardiovasc. Dis. (NMCD)* **2014**, *24*, 639–647. [CrossRef] [PubMed]

35. Kilkkinen, A.; Pietinen, P.; Klaukka, T.; Virtamo, J.; Korhonen, P.; Adlercreutz, H. Use of oral antimicrobials decreases serum enterolactone concentration. *Am. J. Epidemiol.* **2002**, *155*, 472–477. [CrossRef] [PubMed]

36. Potischman, N.; Freudenheim, J.L. Biomarkers of nutritional exposure and nutritional status: An overview. *J. Nutr.* **2003**, *133*, 873S–874S. [PubMed]

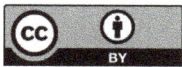

![nutrients logo]

*nutrients*

MDPI

*Article*

# Polyphenol Levels Are Inversely Correlated with Body Weight and Obesity in an Elderly Population after 5 Years of Follow Up (The Randomised PREDIMED Study)

Xiaohui Guo [1], Anna Tresserra-Rimbau [1,2], Ramón Estruch [2,3], Miguel A. Martínez-González [2,4,5], Alexander Medina-Remón [2,3], Montserrat Fitó [2,6], Dolores Corella [2,7], Jordi Salas-Salvadó [2,8], Maria Puy Portillo [2,9], Juan J. Moreno [1], Xavier Pi-Sunyer [10] and Rosa M. Lamuela-Raventós [1,2,*]

[1]   Department of Nutrition, Food Science and Gastronomy, XaRTA, INSA-UB, School of Pharmacy and Food Science, University of Barcelona, 08028 Barcelona, Spain; guoxiaohui1130@gmail.com (X.G.); annatresserra@ub.edu (A.T.-R.); jjmoreno@ub.edu (J.J.M.)
[2]   CIBEROBN Fisiopatología de la Obesidad y Nutrición, Instituto de Salud Carlos III, 28029 Madrid, Spain; restruch@clinic.ub.es (R.E.); mamartinez@unav.es (M.A.M.-G.); amedina@ub.edu (A.M.-R.); mfito@imim.es (M.F.); dolores.corella@uv.es (D.C.); jordi.salas@urv.cat (J.S.-S.); mariapuy.portillo@ehu.es (M.P.P.)
[3]   Department of Internal Medicine, Hospital Clínic, IDIBAPS, University of Barcelona, 08036 Barcelona, Spain
[4]   Department of Preventive Medicine and Public Health, School of Medicine & IdiSNA (Institute for Health Research), University of Navarra, 31080 Pamplona, Spain
[5]   Department of Nutrition, Harvard TH Chan School of Public Health, Boston, MA 02115, USA
[6]   Cardiovascular Risk and Nutrition Research Group (CARIN, Regicor Study Group), IMIM (Hospital del Mar Medical Research Institute), 08003 Barcelona, Spain
[7]   Department of Epidemiology, Preventive Medicine and Public Health, School of Medicine, University of Valencia, 46010 Valencia, Spain
[8]   Human Nutrition Unit, University Hospital of Sant Joan de Reus, Department of Biochemistry and Biotechnology, Faculty of Medicine and Health Sciences, IISPV, Rovira i Virgili University, 43201 Reus, Spain
[9]   Nutrition and Obesity Group, Department of Nutrition and Food Science, Faculty of Pharmacy and Lucio Lascaray Research Institute, University of País Vasco (UPV/EHU), 01006 Vitoria, Spain
[10]  New York Obesity Research Center, Department of Medicine and Institute of Human Nutrition, Columbia University, New York, NY 10032, USA; fxp1@columbia.edu
*   Correspondence: lamuela@ub.edu; Tel.: +34-934-034-843

Received: 17 March 2017; Accepted: 26 April 2017; Published: 3 May 2017

**Abstract:** Overweight and obesity have been steadily increasing in recent years and currently represent a serious threat to public health. Few human studies have investigated the relationship between polyphenol intake and body weight. Our aim was to assess the relationship between urinary polyphenol levels and body weight. A cross-sectional study was performed with 573 participants from the PREDIMED (Prevención con Dieta Mediterránea) trial (ISRCTN35739639). Total polyphenol levels were measured by a reliable biomarker, total urinary polyphenol excretion (TPE), determined by the Folin-Ciocalteu method in urine samples. Participants were categorized into five groups according to their TPE at the fifth year. Multiple linear regression models were used to assess the relationships between TPE and obesity parameters; body weight (BW), body mass index (BMI), waist circumference (WC), and waist-to-height ratio (WHtR). After a five years follow up, significant inverse correlations were observed between TPE at the 5th year and BW ($\beta = -1.004$; 95% CI: $-1.634$ to $-0.375$, $p = 0.002$), BMI ($\beta = -0.320$; 95% CI: $-0.541$ to $-0.098$, $p = 0.005$), WC ($\beta = -0.742$; 95% CI: $-1.326$ to $-0.158$, $p = 0.013$), and WHtR ($\beta = -0.408$; 95% CI: $-0.788$ to $-0.028$, $p = 0.036$) after adjustments for potential confounders. To conclude, a greater polyphenol intake may thus contribute to reducing body weight in elderly people at high cardiovascular risk.

*Nutrients* **2017**, *9*, 452

**Keywords:** overweight; obesity; polyphenol; urine; PREDIMED

## 1. Introduction

Overweight and obesity have been steadily increasing in recent years and currently represent a serious threat to public health [1]. In 2014, more than 1.9 billion adults were overweight worldwide, and of these over 600 million were obese [2]. With nearly three million adults dying each year as a result of being overweight or obese, the impact of obesity on morbidity, mortality, and health care costs is very high [3]. Lifestyle and dietary habits are key determinants in the prevalence of obesity [4–6].

Polyphenols, the most abundant antioxidants in nature, are widely distributed in plant-derived foods such as vegetables, fruits, seeds, coffee, wine, and tea [7]. Only a few human studies have reported a relationship between polyphenol intake and body weight, even though obesity is considered a major independent risk factor for various chronic diseases [8,9]. Evidence for the effects of polyphenols on obesity parameters in humans is inconsistent, possibly due to divergence among study designs, characteristics of the participants, and metabolic pathways. Although some intervention clinical trials with polyphenol-enriched food or polyphenol extracts do not show any effect on weight or waist circumference [10–12], other studies have reported that polyphenols reduce body weight and increase energy expenditure [13–16]. The oral bioavailability of polyphenols is particularly important because, after being modified and metabolized by enzymes, their concentration in tissues and biological fluids is quite low [9,12,15,17]. There is therefore a need for a biomarker to accurately reflect polyphenol concentration after their absorption and metabolism.

Polyphenol plasma levels or total urinary polyphenol excretion, considered in recent years as a reliable biomarker of total polyphenol intake, has been correlated with dietary polyphenol intake, and has been applied to explore associations between polyphenol intake and several chronic disease risk parameters [18–21]. Thus, the objective of the current study was to assess the associations between total polyphenol intake, measured by total urinary polyphenol excretion (TPE), and obesity parameters in an elderly population at high cardiovascular risk after five years of follow up.

## 2. Materials and Methods

The protocol for this trial and supporting Strengthening the Reporting of Observational studies in Epidemiology (STROBE) checklist are available as supporting information.

### 2.1. Ethics Statement

All participants provided informed consent. The Institutional Review Board (IRB) of the Hospital Clinic (Barcelona, Spain), accredited by the US Department of Health and Human Services (DHHS) update for Federal wide Assurance for the Protection of Human Subjects for International (Non-US) Institutions #00000738, approved the study protocol on 16 July 2002. The authors confirm that all ongoing and related trials for this drug/intervention are carried out following the rules of the Declaration of Helsinki of 1975 and registered (ISRCTN35739639).

### 2.2. Subjects

Participants were drawn from the PREDIMED Study ('Prevención con Dieta Mediterránea' (Prevention with the Mediterranean Diet), ISRCTN35739639). The information in the registry was delayed after recruitment began, to be sure about the feasibility of the study protocol; we started the trial as a 'pilot study' on October 2003, and, once we were sure that the intervention protocol worked, we decided to submit the study protocol for registration (date of application: 2 September 2005). The protocol and recruitment method are reported in detail elsewhere [22].

The present study looks at 573 participants that were recruited in two centers, the Clinic Hospital of Barcelona and the University of Valencia, both in Spain, and all were followed-up after more than five years. The period of recruitment was from 2003 to 2006, and the average follow up was 5.9 years.

## 2.3. Nutritional Measurements

The selected participants were asked to complete some questionnaires: a validated 137-item food frequency questionnaire (FFQ) to assess dietary habits [23]; a 47-item general questionnaire aimed to summarize information about lifestyle, health condition, education, history of illnesses, and medication use; a 14 point questionnaire evaluating the degree of adherence to the Mediterranean diet [24]; and a validated Spanish version of the Minnesota Leisure-Time Physical Activity Questionnaire to record physical activity [25]. Nutrient intake was adjusted by calories using the residual method [26]. All questionnaires were administered and repeated yearly during the follow up by trained staff in face-to-face interviews.

## 2.4. Urine Samples

Spot urine samples from the participants were collected and coded at the clinic by a technician and then immediately shipped to a central laboratory to be stored at $-80\ ^\circ C$ until analyzed.

## 2.5. TPE Measurements

The Folin-Ciocalteu method was applied to determine the content of TPE, using a clean-up procedure with solid phase extraction (SPE) performed in 96-well plate cartridges (Oasis MAX), which helped to remove urinary interferences. Finally, TPE was expressed as milligrams of gallic acid equivalent (GAE)/g of creatinine. All details have been previously described by Medina-Remón et al. [19].

## 2.6. Measurements

Weight and height were measured with calibrated scales and a wall-mounted stadiometer, respectively. Body mass index (BMI) was calculated as weight in kilograms divided by the square of height in meters. Waist circumference (WC) was measured midway between the lowest rib and the iliac crest. Waist-to-height ratio (WHtR) was calculated as the waist in centimeters divided by the height in meters. Blood pressure was determined in triplicate using a validated semi-automatic sphygmomanometer (Omron HEM-705CP, Tokyo, Japan) by trained nurses. Measurements were taken at three time points, separated by 2 min, while the participant was in a seated position after 5 min of rest [27]. Obesity is defined as BMI more than $30\ kg/m^2$.

## 2.7. Statistical Analysis

Results were expressed as mean $\pm$ SD for continuous variables or percentages for categorical variables. Kolmogorov and Levene tests were applied to examine the normality distribution and skewness. All participants, including total subjects, males, and females were divided into five categories according to their TPE at the fifth year of follow up. Changes in nutrient intakes and key food consumption according to the FFQs were assessed with yearly repeated-measures analysis during the follow up period. A Bonferroni post-hoc test and paired *t*-test were used to compare each variable within and between groups.

Multiple linear regression models were used to assess the relationship between anthropometric parameters (Body weight (BW), BMI, WC, and WHtR) and quintiles of TPE at the fifth year, adjusted for potential confounders, including sex, age, intervention groups, smoking status (never, current, former), family history of coronary heart disease (CHD), physical activity, hypertension, diabetes, dyslipidemia, marital status (single, married, widowed), education level (primary school, high school, university), medication used (antihypertensive drugs, vitamins, insulin, oral hypoglycemic drugs, aspirin, or other antiplatelet drug supplements taken in the last month), recruitment centers, 14 unit Mediterranean diet score, and energy intake at baseline. Multiple logistic regression analyses were used to calculate the odds ratio (OR) for quintiles of TPE and obesity (BMI > 30 kg/m$^2$). Models were adjusted for potential confounders as in linear regression analyses.

All analyses were performed using SPSS software V21.0 (SPSS Inc., Chicago, IL, USA,). All models were tested for the detection of outliers, multicollinearity, homoscedasticity, and normality and independence of errors. All statistical tests were two-tailed, and the significance level was $p < 0.05$. The detailed information of the participants is available as supporting information.

## 3. Results

A total of 650 subjects were randomly selected from two centers, the Hospital Clinic of Barcelona and the University of Valencia. From them, 38 were excluded because they did not meet the inclusion criteria during the intervention, and, after five years, 39 were excluded because their TPE concentrations were considered outliers, which was defined as any data point more than 1.5 interquartile ranges below the first quartile or above the third quartile; hence a total of 573 participants were finally included (Figure 1).

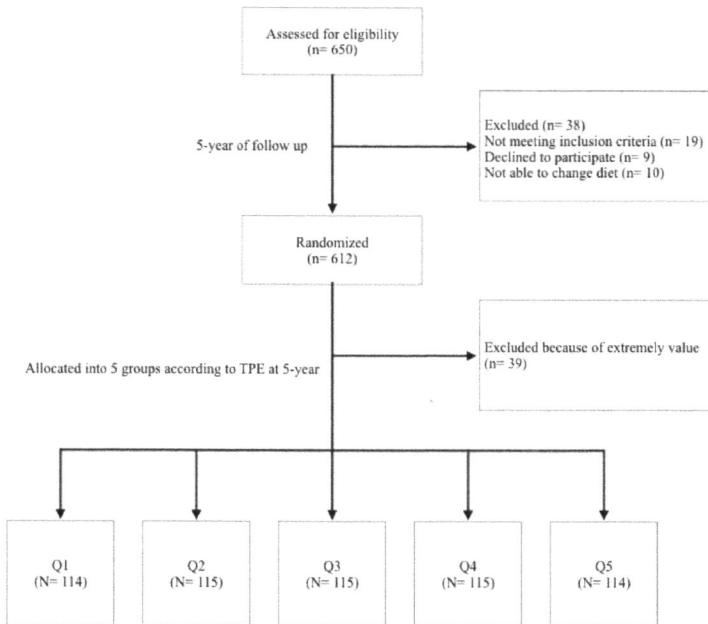

**Figure 1.** Flowchart of study participants.

The baseline characteristics of participants grouped by quintiles of TPE at baseline are shown in Table 1. There were a total of 277 men and 296 women with a mean age of 66.2 ± 6.1 years and 68.3 ± 5.4 years, respectively. Of those participants, 41.5% had diabetes, 80.5% had hypertension, 66.8% had dyslipidemia, 16.9% were current smokers, and 37.5% had a family history of CHD. Compared with participants with the lowest TPE, those with higher TPE were more likely to be women, older, less likely to smoke, and also had lower body weight. Q4 shows the lowest prevalence of hypertension.

**Table 1.** Baseline characteristics of participants according to quintiles of total urinary polyphenol excretion (TPE) at baseline.

| | TPE (mg GAE/g Creatinine) | | | | | |
| | Q1 | Q2 | Q3 | Q4 | Q5 | p |
| | (<76.55) | (76.56–95.20) | (95.21–119.18) | (119.19–145.86) | (>145.86) | |
|---|---|---|---|---|---|---|
| No. of subjects | 114 | 115 | 115 | 115 | 114 | - |
| Women, n (%) | 33 / 28 | 49 / 42.6 | 66 / 57.4 | 65 / 56.5 | 83 / 72.8 | <0.001 |
| Age (y), mean (SD) | 66.4 / 5.9 | 66.6 / 6.0 | 66.9 / 5.9 | 67.7 / 5.7 | 68.9 / 5.8 | 0.007 |
| Weight (kg), mean (SD) | 80.2 / 11.8 | 77.7 / 10.4 | 73.7 / 9.1 | 73.3 / 10.9 | 70.8 / 10.4 | <0.001 |
| BMI (kg/m²), mean (SD) | 29.8 / 2.9 | 29.5 / 3.2 | 29.1 / 3.1 | 28.9 / 3.6 | 28.8 / 3.4 | 0.080 |
| Systolic BP (mm Hg), mean (SD) | 150.9 / 16.9 | 153.9 / 19.5 | 149.9 / 17.0 | 151.8 / 19.5 | 150.4 / 15.9 | 0.454 |
| Diastolic BP (mm Hg), mean (SD) | 86.4 / 10.5 | 86.1 / 10.4 | 85.0 / 9.9 | 84.2 / 10.3 | 84.4 / 9.1 | 0.363 |
| Hypertension, n (%) | 93 / 81.6 | 102 / 88.7 | 94 / 81.7 | 79 / 68.7 | 93 / 81.6 | 0.004 |
| Diabetes, n (%) | 47 / 41.2 | 41 / 35.7 | 48 / 41.7 | 53 / 46.1 | 49 / 43.0 | 0.605 |
| Dyslipidemia, n (%) | 72 / 63.2 | 74 / 64.3 | 78 / 67.8 | 80 / 69.6 | 79 / 69.3 | 0.779 |
| Smoking status, n (%) | | | | | | 0.002 |
| Current | 32 / 28.1 | 22 / 19.1 | 16 / 13.9 | 18 / 15.7 | 9 / 7.9 | |
| Former | 26 / 22.8 | 25 / 21.7 | 24 / 20.9 | 31 / 27.0 | 20 / 17.5 | |
| Never | 56 / 49.1 | 68 / 59.1 | 75 / 65.2 | 66 / 57.4 | 85 / 74.6 | |
| Family history of CHD, n (%) | 39 / 34.2 | 42 / 36.5 | 45 / 39.1 | 41 / 35.7 | 48 / 42.1 | 0.95 |
| Medication, n (%) | | | | | | |
| Aspirin | 21 / 18.4 | 17 / 14.8 | 27 / 23.5 | 19 / 16.5 | 19 / 16.7 | 0.482 |
| Antihypertensive drugs | 87 / 76.3 | 90 / 78.3 | 82 / 71.3 | 71 / 61.7 | 84 / 73.7 | 0.049 |
| Hypolipidemic drugs | 40 / 35.1 | 45 / 39.1 | 50 / 43.5 | 53 / 46.1 | 51 / 44.7 | 0.426 |
| Insulin | 3 / 2.6 | 7 / 6.1 | 4 / 3.5 | 7 / 6.1 | 6 / 5.3 | 0.639 |
| Oral hypoglycemic drugs | 23 / 20.2 | 22 / 19.1 | 29 / 25.2 | 30 / 26.1 | 27 / 23.7 | 0.652 |
| Vitamin or minerals | 5 / 4.4 | 5 / 4.3 | 10 / 8.7 | 9 / 7.8 | 18 / 15.8 | 0.005 |
| Education level, n (%) | | | | | | 0.348 |
| University | 13 / 11.4 | 16 / 13.9 | 10 / 8.7 | 7 / 6.1 | 9 / 7.9 | |
| High school | 21 / 18.4 | 14 / 12.2 | 18 / 15.7 | 22 / 19.1 | 13 / 11.4 | |
| Primary school | 79 / 69.3 | 83 / 72.2 | 85 / 73.9 | 86 / 74.8 | 92 / 80.7 | |
| Marital status, n (%) | | | | | | 0.168 |
| Single | 7 / 6.1 | 5 / 4.3 | 4 / 3.5 | 3 / 2.6 | 6 / 5.3 | |
| Married | 96 / 84.2 | 93 / 80.9 | 93 / 80.9 | 88 / 76.5 | 80 / 70.2 | |
| Widowed | 10 / 8.8 | 14 / 12.2 | 16 / 13.9 | 24 / 20.9 | 25 / 21.9 | |
| Physical activity at leisure time (MET-min/d), mean (SD) | 267.5 / 222.5 | 302.7 / 256.3 | 233 / 172.9 | 283.7 / 271.3 | 261.7 / 247.3 | 0.237 |

TPE: total polyphenol excretion; GAE: gallic acid equivalent; BMI: body mass index; BP: blood pressure; CHD: coronary heart diseases. Data are given as means (SD) for continuous variables and percentages for categorical variables; $p < 0.05$ indicates statistical significance. * $p$-values calculated by analysis of variance or $\chi^2$ tests.

The comparison of total urinary polyphenol excretion between baseline and the fifth year of follow up by quintiles of TPE at the fifth year is shown in Figure 2. For the first two quintiles, TPE at baseline was significantly higher than at the fifth year. By contrast, TPE at the top two categories was higher than at baseline.

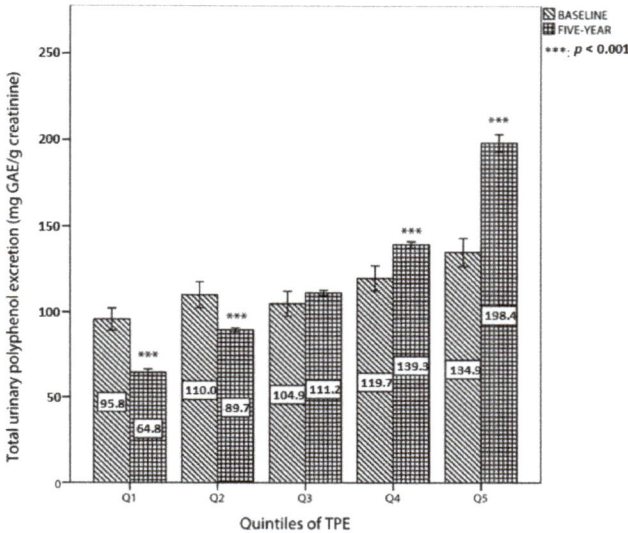

**Figure 2.** Total polyphenol excretion at baseline and at the fifth year of follow up by quintiles of TPE.

Table 2 summarizes information on key changes in food consumption during the intervention according to quintiles of TPE. As shown, at the end of the intervention, the consumption of most of the items belonging to a Mediterranean dietary pattern had increased significantly, including vegetables, fruits, fish, extra virgin olive oil, olive oil, nuts, coffee, and milk. However, the intake of wine decreased significantly, as well as intakes of cereals, meat, and pastries. Table 2 also shows changes in nutrient intake and degrees of adherence to a Mediterranean diet. Significant increments were observed in the consumption of total fat, fiber, polyunsaturated fatty acids (PUFA), monounsaturated fatty acids (MUFA), folic acid, potassium (K), and magnesium (Mg), while total carbohydrates, protein, cholesterol, sodium (Na), and saturated fatty acids (SFA) remained similar throughout.

**Table 2.** Changes in key food intake and nutrients according to the food frequency questionnaires (FFQs) after energy adjustment categorized by quintile of TPE at the fifth year [a].

| | | TPE (mg GAE/g Creatinine) | | | | | | | | | | p [b] | p [c] | | |
| | | Q1 (<79.02) | | Q2 (79.03–99.50) | | Q3 (99.51–124.53) | | Q4 (124.54–160.06) | | Q5 (>160.07) | | | | | |
| | | Mean | SD | Mean | SD | Mean | SD | Mean | SD | Mean | SD | ANOVA | TIME | GROUP | INTERACTION |
|---|---|---|---|---|---|---|---|---|---|---|---|---|---|---|---|
| Vegetables (g/day) | baseline | 302.6 | 126.5 | 295.2 | 122.6 | 283.3 | 114.1 | 312.9 | 142.4 | 297.0 | 107.0 | 0.484 | <0.001 | 0.916 | 0.440 |
| | changes | 47.7** | 131.5 | 53.1** | 130.2 | 76.3** | 150.4 | 46.0** | 162.3 | 59.0** | 131.6 | 0.514 | | | |
| Fruits (g/day) | baseline | 328.9 | 184.8 | 361.6 | 179.7 | 358.6 | 182.3 | 389.5 | 162.5 | 394.5 | 189.3 | 0.064 | <0.001 | 0.051 | 0.530 |
| | changes | 89.1** | 220.1 | 82.9** | 222.7 | 111.0** | 220.6 | 80.6** | 208.4 | 67.9** | 194.8 | 0.658 | | | |
| Legumes (g/day) | baseline | 18.5 | 8.4 | 19.3 | 7.4 | 20.0 | 9.2 | 19.2 | 7.2 | 19.0 | 6.6 | 0.634 | 0.446 | 0.251 | 0.045 |
| | changes | 0.3 | 10.7 | 1.7 | 11.3 | -3.2 | 29.1 | -1.0 | 8.5 | 1.0 | 8.3 | 0.160 | | | |
| Cereals (g/day) | baseline | 246.8 | 83.8 | 246.3 | 81.2 | 232.8 | 74.2 | 242.9 | 71.9 | 237.7 | 61.9 | 0.636 | <0.001 | 0.530 | 0.386 |
| | changes | -22.2* | 91.1 | -21.7** | 85.1 | -14.5 | 91.5 | -31.4** | 80.1 | -25.6** | 77.5 | 0.673 | | | |
| Milk (g/day) | baseline | 322.8 | 191.3 | 370.1 | 202.2 | 365.8 | 210.0 | 354.5 | 203.7 | 422.5 | 231.6 | 0.010 | 0.005 | 0.009 | 0.728 |
| | changes | 38.3 | 207.4 | 21.4 | 200.9 | 10.3 | 198.6 | 40.2* | 188.3 | 20.6 | 208.9 | 0.776 | | | |
| Meat (g/day) | baseline | 138.1 | 50.4 | 136.2 | 43.9 | 145.6 | 56.5 | 139.3 | 41.7 | 141.6 | 47.1 | 0.613 | <0.001 | 0.198 | 0.983 |
| | changes | -9.9 | 52.1 | -13.9** | 44.6 | -12.1* | 52.5 | -13.8** | 51.5 | -11.7* | 47.7 | 0.975 | | | |
| Fish (g/day) | baseline | 92.0 | 39.6 | 92.5 | 36.9 | 90.4 | 38.0 | 97.0 | 41.3 | 93.0 | 39.0 | 0.787 | 0.005 | 0.970 | 0.481 |
| | changes | 8.2* | 40.4 | 6.2 | 42.2 | 11.5** | 44.2 | 4.2 | 39.4 | 7.3 | 43.3 | 0.764 | | | |
| Pastries (g/day) | baseline | 29.6 | 32.1 | 23.6 | 22.4 | 24.1 | 24.7 | 23.9 | 22.4 | 26.6 | 26.5 | 0.379 | 0.006 | 0.291 | 0.920 |
| | changes | -4.8 | 32.4 | -3.0 | 29.4 | -4.3 | 27.2 | -3.2 | 24.3 | -3.9 | 29.2 | 0.991 | | | |
| EVOO (g/day) | baseline | 22.7 | 25.6 | 20.5 | 22.4 | 22.6 | 23.6 | 22.9 | 23.7 | 22.8 | 23.3 | 0.960 | <0.001 | 0.961 | 0.626 |
| | changes | 24.9** | 29.6 | 27.6** | 27.6 | 25.4** | 28.2 | 26.4** | 30.1 | 26.9** | 25.6 | 0.955 | | | |
| Olive oil (g/day) | baseline | 45.4 | 18.2 | 46.3 | 17.5 | 45.3 | 13.5 | 46.3 | 14.5 | 44.2 | 16.8 | 0.791 | <0.001 | 0.575 | 0.161 |
| | changes | 7.8** | 17.6 | 10.5** | 14.2 | 9.8** | 16.8 | 9.3** | 18.7 | 11.2** | 15.3 | 0.654 | | | |
| Nuts (g/day) | baseline | 10.7 | 14.2 | 11.2 | 12.6 | 10.0 | 12.7 | 10.0 | 13.6 | 10.9 | 14.0 | 0.904 | <0.001 | 0.634 | 0.192 |
| | changes | 3.1 | 16.4 | 5.3** | 17.1 | 5.5** | 15.8 | 9.5** | 17.3 | 4.2** | 11.5 | 0.039 | | | |
| Wine (g/day) | baseline | 104.9 | 144.8 | 97.0 | 138.3 | 103.9 | 171.5 | 98.2 | 136.2 | 81.2 | 125.6 | 0.739 | 0.013 | 0.647 | 0.984 |
| | changes | -8.4 | 124.2 | -13.3 | 129.4 | -17.1 | 111.3 | -18.1* | 95.3 | -14.5 | 91.9 | 0.971 | | | |
| Tea (mL) | baseline | 4.8 | 14.5 | 4.6 | 15.1 | 6.4 | 17.0 | 5.2 | 12.5 | 7.6 | 21.1 | 0.605 | 0.401 | 0.479 | 0.172 |
| | changes | 0.1 | 16.6 | -1.9 | 14.5 | -1.8 | 16.7 | 3.2 | 24.9 | -2.0 | 22.4 | 0.204 | | | |
| Coffee (mL) | baseline | 39.1 | 58.4 | 36.7 | 52.4 | 30.7 | 43.0 | 35.0 | 47.1 | 30.9 | 43.0 | 0.717 | 0.002 | 0.546 | 0.098 |
| | changes | -11.5* | 50.1 | -1.8 | 50.2 | -7.3* | 36.8 | -13.1** | 47.0 | 3.7 | 51.3 | 0.048 | | | |
| Total carbohydrates (g/day) | baseline | 237.5 | 43.2 | 242.1 | 38.0 | 237.0 | 41.7 | 235.8 | 36.3 | 239.7 | 34.8 | 0.682 | 0.769 | 0.114 | 0.025 |
| | changes | 4.5 | 78.6 | -10.3 | 71.6 | 5.7 | 72.4 | -13.2* | 68.1 | -0.4 | 64.6 | 0.166 | | | |
| Protein (g/day) | baseline | 90.3 | 43.2 | 94.9 | 38.0 | 89.7 | 41.7 | 88.5 | 36.3 | 92.5 | 34.8 | 0.682 | 0.274 | 0.307 | 0.474 |
| | changes | 2.3 | 47.6 | -3.0 | 41.4 | 6.1 | 46.9 | 2.5 | 40.9 | 4.6 | 39.6 | 0.592 | | | |

Table 2. Cont.

| | | TPE (mg GAE/g Creatinine) | | | | | | | | | | | $p^{b}$ | $p^{c}$ | | |
| | | Q1 (<79.02) | | Q2 (79.03–99.50) | | Q3 (99.51–124.53) | | Q4 (124.54–160.06) | | Q5 (>160.07) | | ANOVA | TIME | GROUP | INTERACTION |
| | | Mean | SD | Mean | SD | Mean | SD | Mean | SD | Mean | SD | | | | |
| Total Fat (g/day) | baseline | 100.4 | 13.6 | 100.9 | 12.7 | 102.8 | 13.7 | 102.7 | 12.9 | 104.5 | 13.6 | 0.132 | | | |
| | changes | 10.0** | 30.8 | 9.2** | 28.5 | 10.9** | 28.0 | 8.5** | 26.9 | 9.4** | 31.5 | 0.980 | <0.001 | 0.235 | 0.981 |
| Fiber (g/day) | baseline | 24.2 | 6.0 | 24.5 | 6.5 | 24.2 | 6.5 | 25.8 | 5.8 | 25.5 | 5.6 | 0.256 | | | |
| | changes | 1.1 | 8.2 | 1.4 | 9.7 | 3.2** | 8.4 | 0.2 | 8.2 | 1.0 | 7.8 | 0.107 | 0.006 | 0.632 | 0.013 |
| Alcohol (g/day) | baseline | 13.5 | 5.6 | 13.6 | 5.2 | 13.7 | 5.3 | 13.3 | 4.7 | 14.2 | 4.9 | 0.780 | | | |
| | changes | -0.2 | 17.8 | -1.6 | 15.0 | -1.2 | 16.7 | -1.9 | 14.4 | -3.2* | 14.2 | 0.707 | 0.032 | 0.961 | 0.765 |
| SFA (g/day) | baseline | 24.9 | 11.2 | 24.2 | 9.7 | 24.5 | 8.3 | 25.7 | 9.1 | 23.9 | 9.9 | 0.663 | | | |
| | changes | -0.5 | 12.9 | -0.1 | 10.6 | 0.7 | 9.8 | -1.5 | 11.1 | 1.6 | 11.3 | 0.301 | 0.541 | 0.772 | 0.266 |
| MUFA (g/day) | baseline | 52.1 | 16.8 | 51.3 | 15.4 | 52.4 | 16.0 | 53.6 | 14.5 | 52.4 | 15.0 | 0.828 | | | |
| | changes | 6.0** | 20.3 | 7.5** | 19.2 | 7.4** | 17.5 | 4.8** | 18.1 | 7.1** | 19.0 | 0.798 | <0.001 | 0.941 | 0.694 |
| PUFA (g/day) | baseline | 15.6 | 5.2 | 15.4 | 5.7 | 15.5 | 5.8 | 16.0 | 5.2 | 15.5 | 5.5 | 0.887 | | | |
| | changes | 3.0** | 7.7 | 3.1** | 7.8 | 3.4** | 7.1 | 3.4** | 8.1 | 4.2** | 8.9 | 0.800 | <0.001 | 0.575 | 0.670 |
| Folic acid (µg/day) | baseline | 379.3 | 89.5 | 373.3 | 90.5 | 369.8 | 76.5 | 394.4 | 98.8 | 394.2 | 85.7 | 0.152 | | | |
| | changes | 42.7** | 91.3 | 46.5** | 99.7 | 65.7** | 92.6 | 39.2** | 91.6 | 38.7** | 100.4 | 0.196 | <0.001 | 0.447 | 0.086 |
| Cholesterol (mg/day) | baseline | 354.9 | 92.4 | 340.0 | 92.2 | 351.4 | 93.3 | 353.5 | 81.6 | 359.1 | 95.5 | 0.505 | | | |
| | changes | 0.2 | 115.0 | 11.9 | 101.3 | 11.4 | 109.2 | -3.5 | 105.5 | 15.2 | 112.6 | 0.644 | 0.234 | 0.406 | 0.329 |
| Na (mg/day) | baseline | 2331.2 | 570.5 | 2254.1 | 499.7 | 2272.1 | 480.3 | 2286.1 | 491.3 | 2298.5 | 447.1 | 0.815 | | | |
| | changes | -64.0 | 941.6 | -83.1 | 728.6 | 10.6 | 730.0 | -184.2** | 713.4 | 10.8 | 752.6 | 0.306 | 0.257 | 0.258 | 0.319 |
| K (mg/day) | baseline | 4130.5 | 769.6 | 4218.7 | 756.2 | 4208.9 | 696.0 | 4312.6 | 808.1 | 4410.2 | 748.0 | 0.069 | | | |
| | changes | 379.8** | 1070.7 | 286.0** | 1042.2 | 497.3** | 1007.2 | 249.1* | 1116.2 | 268.1* | 1100.4 | 0.389 | <0.001 | 0.246 | 0.067 |
| Mg (mg/day) | baseline | 355.0 | 64.0 | 361.1 | 68.6 | 356. | 56.6 | 368.6 | 58.2 | 374.8 | 61.9 | 0.147 | | | |
| | changes | 30.7** | 97.9 | 26.8** | 99.2 | 42.9** | 87.9 | 22.0** | 87.3 | 23.9* | 95.9 | 0.481 | <0.001 | 0.474 | 0.056 |
| P-14 score | baseline | 8.9 | 1.8 | 9.0 | 1.8 | 9.2 | 1.9 | 8.8 | 1.9 | 9.1 | 1.8 | 0.441 | | | |
| | changes | 1.6** | 2.5 | 1.8** | 1.9 | 1.7** | 2.1 | 1.9** | 2.0 | 1.6** | 2.1 | 0.626 | <0.001 | 0.370 | 0.571 |
| Energy intake (Kcal/day) | baseline | 2508.8 | 582.3 | 2285.5 | 578.5 | 2338.5 | 463.0 | 2262.2 | 510.7 | 2191.7 | 470.7 | <0.001 | | | |
| | changes | -25.9 | 627.6 | 32.0 | 497.4 | 100.2* | 503.9 | 8.9 | 564.0 | 157.8** | 520.1 | 0.089 | 0.034 | <0.001 | 0.234 |

TPE: total polyphenol excretion; GAE: gallic acid equivalent; EVOO: Extra Virgin Olive Oil; SFA: saturated fatty acids; MUFA: monounsaturated fatty acids; PUFA: polyunsaturated fatty acids; Na: sodium; K: potassium; Mg: magnesium; p-14: 14 item dietary score test to appraise adherence of participants to the Mediterranean diet (it includes questions about consumption of fruits, vegetables, meat, fish, carbonic beverages, legumes, nuts, olive oil, wine, and culinary methods) [28]. [a] Data are given as means (SD); [a] Data were analyzed by one-way ANOVA. [c] Data analyzed by significance. Values with asterisks are statistically different from baseline by paired-samples t-test (* $p < 0.05$; ** $p < 0.01$). [b] Data analyzed by one-way ANOVA. [c] Data analyzed by repeated-measures two-factor ANOVA.

The associations between TPE and obesity indexes were analyzed by linear regression models (Table 3). For total participants, significant inverse associations were found between quintiles of TPE at the fifth year and BW ($\beta = -1.004$; $p = 0.002$), BMI ($\beta = -0.320$; $p = 0.005$), WC ($\beta = -0.742$; $p = 0.013$), and WHtR ($\beta = -0.408$; $p = 0.036$) after adjustment for potential confounders. For males, inverse associations were found in BW ($\beta = -0.959$; $p = 0.039$) and BMI ($\beta = -0.301$; $p = 0.034$), while, for females, only an inverse association was found in BMI ($\beta = -0.332$; $p = 0.046$) after a full adjustment.

**Table 3.** Multiple linear regression analyses with obesity indexes and quintiles of TPE at the fifth year for male, female, and total participants.

| | | | β | SE | Beta | Significance | 95% CI | |
|---|---|---|---|---|---|---|---|---|
| BW (kg) | Male | Model 1 | −1.446 | 0.440 | −0.195 | 0.001 | −2.313 | −0.580 |
| | | Model 2 | −1.259 | 0.440 | −0.170 | 0.005 | −2.126 | −0.392 |
| | | Model 3 | −0.959 | 0.461 | −0.131 | 0.039 | −1.868 | −0.050 |
| | Female | Model 1 | −1.103 | 0.415 | −0.153 | 0.008 | −1.920 | −0.287 |
| | | Model 2 | −0.756 | 0.414 | −0.105 | 0.069 | −1.571 | 0.058 |
| | | Model 3 | −0.757 | 0.431 | −0.107 | 0.080 | −1.606 | 0.091 |
| | Total | Model 1 | −2.350 | 0.331 | −0.285 | <0.001 | −3.000 | −1.700 |
| | | Model 2 | −1.070 | 0.315 | −0.130 | 0.001 | −1.689 | −0.451 |
| | | Model 3 | −1.004 | 0.320 | −0.124 | 0.002 | −1.634 | −0.375 |
| BMI (kg/m$^2$) | Male | Model 1 | −0.405 | 0.135 | −0.179 | 0.003 | −0.670 | −0.139 |
| | | Model 2 | −0.370 | 0.136 | −0.164 | 0.007 | −0.639 | −0.102 |
| | | Model 3 | −0.301 | 0.141 | −0.135 | 0.034 | −0.579 | −0.023 |
| | Female | Model 1 | −0.344 | 0.156 | −0.127 | 0.028 | −0.652 | −0.037 |
| | | Model 2 | −0.296 | 0.160 | −0.110 | 0.064 | −0.611 | 0.018 |
| | | Model 3 | −0.332 | 0.165 | −0.123 | 0.046 | −0.657 | −0.007 |
| | Total | Model 1 | −0.295 | 0.104 | −0.118 | 0.005 | −0.499 | −0.090 |
| | | Model 2 | −0.328 | 0.110 | −0.131 | 0.003 | −0.544 | −0.111 |
| | | Model 3 | −0.320 | 0.113 | −0.129 | 0.005 | −0.541 | −0.098 |
| WC (cm) | Male | Model 1 | −0.769 | 0.364 | −0.127 | 0.036 | −1.487 | −0.052 |
| | | Model 2 | −0.786 | 0.369 | −0.130 | 0.034 | −1.513 | −0.059 |
| | | Model 3 | −0.516 | 0.378 | −0.087 | 0.173 | −1.260 | 0.228 |
| | Female | Model 1 | −0.546 | 0.409 | −0.078 | 0.183 | −1.351 | 0.259 |
| | | Model 2 | −0.527 | 0.419 | −0.075 | 0.209 | −1.351 | 0.297 |
| | | Model 3 | −0.701 | 0.434 | −0.101 | 0.108 | −1.556 | 0.154 |
| | Total | Model 1 | −1.500 | 0.296 | −0.208 | <0.001 | −2.082 | −0.918 |
| | | Model 2 | −0.721 | 0.293 | −0.100 | 0.014 | −1.296 | −0.147 |
| | | Model 3 | −0.742 | 0.297 | −0.104 | 0.013 | −1.326 | −0.158 |
| WHtR (cm/m) | Male | Model 1 | −0.340 | 0.220 | −0.093 | 0.124 | −0.773 | 0.094 |
| | | Model 2 | −0.385 | 0.223 | −0.105 | 0.085 | −0.823 | 0.054 |
| | | Model 3 | −0.258 | 0.229 | −0.072 | 0.261 | −0.710 | 0.193 |
| | Female | Model 1 | −0.246 | 0.276 | −0.052 | 0.374 | −0.789 | 0.298 |
| | | Model 2 | −0.332 | 0.282 | −0.070 | 0.240 | −0.887 | 0.223 |
| | | Model3 | −0.501 | 0.294 | −0.106 | 0.089 | −1.079 | 0.078 |
| | Total | Model 1 | −0.298 | 0.178 | −0.070 | 0.094 | −0.648 | 0.051 |
| | | Model 2 | −0.367 | 0.189 | −0.087 | 0.052 | −0.739 | 0.004 |
| | | Model 3 | −0.408 | 0.194 | −0.097 | 0.036 | −0.788 | −0.028 |

BW: body weight; BMI: body mass index; WC: waist circumference; WHtR: waist-to-height ratio. TPE: total polyphenol excretion (mg GAE/g creatinine). β: Non-standardized coefficient (regression line coefficient); SE: Standard error; Beta: Standardized coefficient; CI: Confidence interval; $p$: two-sided test of significance. Model 1, unadjusted; Model 2 was adjusted for sex (only for total participants), age, and intervention groups; Model 3 adjusted as in Model 2 plus smoking status (never, current, former), family history of CHD, physical activity, hypertension, diabetes, dyslipidemia, marital status (single, married, divorced, widowed), education level (primary school, high school, university), medication used (antihypertensive drugs, vitamins, insulin, oral hypoglycemic drugs, aspirin, or other antiplatelet drug supplements taken in the last month), recruitment centers, 14 unit Mediterranean diet score, and energy intake at baseline.

Table 4 shows the odds ratio (OR) and a 95% CI for obesity according to the quintile of TPE at the fifth year. In fully adjusted models, for total participants in the category of highest TPE had a lower prevalence of obesity (OR = 0.346, 95% CI = 0.176 to 0.178; $p$-trend = 0.039) than those in the lowest category. For males, compared with the reference group, the top quintile group (Q5) showed significant reduction in the prevalence of obesity (OR = 0.340, 95% CI = 0.146 to 0.792 in Model 2).

**Table 4.** Multivariate adjusted odds ratios (95% confidence interval (CI)) for prevalent obesity (213 cases) after a five years follow up.

|  |  | Q1 | Q2 | 95% CI | | Q3 | 95% CI | | Q4 | 95% CI | | Q5 | 95% CI | | *p* |
|---|---|---|---|---|---|---|---|---|---|---|---|---|---|---|---|
| Male | Model 1 | 1 (ref.) | 0.531 | 0.244 | 1.155 | 0.545 | 0.250 | 1.188 | 0.488 | 0.223 | 1.070 | 0.313 | 0.135 | 0.722 | 0.095 |
| (90 case) | Model 2 | 1 (ref.) | 0.559 | 0.254 | 1.229 | 0.571 | 0.260 | 1.254 | 0.520 | 0.235 | 1.148 | 0.340 | 0.146 | 0.792 | 0.159 |
|  | Model 3 | 1 (ref.) | 0.586 | 0.243 | 1.416 | 0.588 | 0.238 | 1.452 | 0.511 | 0.204 | 1.283 | 0.387 | 0.146 | 1.029 | 0.418 |
| Female | Model 1 | 1 (ref.) | 0.934 | 0.454 | 1.924 | 0.791 | 0.384 | 1.628 | 0.643 | 0.310 | 1.333 | 0.429 | 0.200 | 0.919 | 0.195 |
| (123 case) | Model 2 | 1 (ref.) | 1.041 | 0.497 | 2.182 | 0.844 | 0.403 | 1.768 | 0.769 | 0.361 | 1.638 | 0.493 | 0.226 | 1.078 | 0.352 |
|  | Model 3 | 1 (ref.) | 1.257 | 0.538 | 2.934 | 0.748 | 0.317 | 1.764 | 0.595 | 0.244 | 1.450 | 0.461 | 0.181 | 1.170 | 0.223 |
| Total | Model 1 | 1 (ref.) | 0.639 | 0.375 | 1.089 | 0.769 | 0.454 | 1.302 | 0.664 | 0.390 | 1.129 | 0.450 | 0.259 | 0.782 | 0.073 |
| (213 case) | Model 2 | 1 (ref.) | 0.597 | 0.344 | 1.035 | 0.691 | 0.400 | 1.192 | 0.618 | 0.350 | 1.091 | 0.383 | 0.211 | 0.694 | 0.036 |
|  | Model 3 | 1 (ref.) | 0.604 | 0.332 | 1.100 | 0.720 | 0.399 | 1.300 | 0.560 | 0.298 | 1.054 | 0.346 | 0.176 | 0.678 | 0.039 |

Quintiles for males: Q1 < 70.61; Q2: 70.62–88.94; Q3: 88.95–108.61; Q4: 108.62–137.11; Q5 > 137.11; Quintiles for females: Q1 < 91.67; Q2: 91.68–113.96; Q3: 113.97–138.28; Q4: 138.29–181.01; Q5 > 181.01; Quintiles for total: Q1 < 79.02; Q2: 79.03–99.50; Q3: 99.51–124.53; Q4: 124.54–160.06; Q5 > 160.06. TPE is expressed as mg GAE/g creatinine. Obesity was defined as BMI > 30 kg/m². Model 1, unadjusted; Model 2 was adjusted for sex (only for total participants), age, and intervention groups; Model 3 adjusted as in Model 2 plus smoking status (never, current, former), family history of CHD, physical activity, hypertension, diabetes, dyslipidemia, marital status (single, married, divorced, widowed), education level (primary school, high school, university), medication used (antihypertensive drugs, vitamins, insulin, oral hypoglycemic drugs, aspirin or other antiplatelet drug supplements taken in the last month) recruitment centers, 14 unit Mediterranean diet score, and energy intake at baseline.

Table 5 shows the incidence of obesity after five years of intervention, conducted in subjects without obesity at baseline and adjusted for TPE and BW at baseline and other co-variables. The results show significant reduction in the incidence of obesity (odds ratio (OR) = 0.095, 95% confidence interval (CI) 0.018 to 0.498; *p*-trend, 0.018) at the end of the follow up after adjustments.

**Table 5.** Association between TPE after five years of follow up and the incidence of obesity (39 new-onset case).

|  | Q1 | Q2 | 95% CI | | Q3 | 95% CI | | Q4 | 95% CI | | Q5 | 95% CI | | *p* |
|---|---|---|---|---|---|---|---|---|---|---|---|---|---|---|
| Model 1 | 1 (ref.) | 0.912 | (0.337 | 2.468) | 0.676 | (0.253 | 1.810) | 0.351 | (0.142 | 0.866) | 0.406 | (0.164 | 1.005) | 0.054 |
| Model 2 | 1 (ref.) | 0.454 | (0.185 | 1.115) | 0.235 | (0.072 | 0.767) | 0.285 | (0.093 | 0.868) | 0.145 | (0.037 | 0.558) | 0.014 |
| Model 3 | 1 (ref.) | 0.382 | (0.146 | 1.001) | 0.193 | (0.055 | 0.676) | 0.272 | (0.084 | 0.885) | 0.119 | (0.028 | 0.505) | 0.014 |
| Model 4 | 1 (ref.) | 0.366 | (0.126 | 1.062) | 0.156 | (0.040 | 0.612) | 0.218 | (0.054 | 0.881) | 0.095 | (0.018 | 0.498) | 0.018 |

Model 1, unadjusted; Model 2 was adjusted for baseline TPE and baseline BW; Model 3 was adjusted as in Model 2 plus sex, age, and intervention groups; Model 4 was adjusted as in Model 3 plus smoking status (never, current, former), family history of CHD, physical activity, hypertension, diabetes, dyslipidemia, marital status (single, married, divorced, widowed), education level (primary school, high school, university), medication used (antihypertensive drugs, vitamins, insulin, oral hypoglycemic drugs, aspirin, or other antiplatelet drug supplements taken in the last month) recruitment centers, 14 unit Mediterranean diet score, and energy intake at baseline.

Table 6 shows the associations between TPE at the fifth year and changes in anthropometric parameters, analyzed by linear regression models. For total participants, inverse associations were found between changes in BW ($\beta = -0.363$; $p = 0.024$) and BMI ($\beta = -0.145$; $p = 0.023$) and TPE in the fifth year after adjustment. For males, there was not any inverse association, while for females, inverse associations were found for changes in BW ($\beta = -0.568$; $p = 0.008$) and BMI ($\beta = -0.221$; $p = 0.017$) after adjustment.

**Table 6.** Multiple linear regression analyses with changes in anthropometric parameters and quintiles of TPE at the fifth year.

| | | | β | SE | Beta | p | 95% CI | |
|---|---|---|---|---|---|---|---|---|
| Changes in BW | Male | Model 1 | −0.098 | 0.211 | −0.028 | 0.642 | −0.514 | 0.318 |
| (kg) | | Model 2 | −0.229 | 0.217 | −0.066 | 0.294 | −0.657 | 0.199 |
| | | Model 3 | −0.186 | 0.217 | −0.053 | 0.393 | −0.614 | 0.242 |
| | | Model 4 | −0.037 | 0.233 | −0.011 | 0.872 | −0.495 | 0.421 |
| | Female | Model 1 | −0.648 | 0.193 | −0.193 | 0.001 | −1.027 | −0.269 |
| | | Model 2 | −0.664 | 0.196 | −0.197 | 0.001 | −1.049 | −0.279 |
| | | Model 3 | −0.573 | 0.197 | −0.17 | 0.004 | −0.961 | −0.185 |
| | | Model 4 | −0.568 | 0.213 | −0.169 | 0.008 | −0.987 | −0.149 |
| | Total | Model 1 | −0.429 | 0.142 | −0.125 | 0.003 | −0.709 | −0.149 |
| | | Model 2 | −0.539 | 0.15 | −0.157 | <0.001 | −0.835 | −0.244 |
| | | Model 3 | −0.436 | 0.153 | −0.127 | 0.005 | −0.737 | −0.135 |
| | | Model 4 | −0.363 | 0.161 | −0.108 | 0.024 | −0.68 | −0.047 |
| Changes in BMI | Male | Model 1 | −0.04 | 0.075 | −0.033 | 0.589 | −0.187 | 0.107 |
| (kg/m²) | | Model 2 | −0.087 | 0.077 | −0.07 | 0.259 | −0.238 | 0.064 |
| | | Model 3 | −0.072 | 0.077 | −0.059 | 0.348 | −0.224 | 0.079 |
| | | Model 4 | −0.019 | 0.082 | −0.016 | 0.817 | −0.18 | 0.142 |
| | Female | Model 1 | −0.256 | 0.083 | −0.177 | 0.002 | −0.419 | −0.092 |
| | | Model 2 | −0.262 | 0.084 | −0.181 | 0.002 | −0.428 | −0.096 |
| | | Model 3 | −0.223 | 0.085 | −0.154 | 0.009 | −0.391 | −0.056 |
| | | Model 4 | −0.221 | 0.092 | −0.153 | 0.017 | −0.402 | −0.04 |
| | Total | Model 1 | −0.176 | 0.056 | −0.13 | 0.002 | −0.286 | −0.065 |
| | | Model 2 | −0.215 | 0.059 | −0.159 | <0.001 | −0.331 | −0.098 |
| | | Model 3 | −0.172 | 0.06 | −0.128 | 0.005 | −0.291 | −0.054 |
| | | Model 4 | −0.145 | 0.064 | −0.109 | 0.023 | −0.27 | −0.02 |
| Changes in WC | Male | Model 1 | −0.066 | 0.233 | −0.017 | 0.776 | −0.525 | 0.392 |
| (cm) | | Model 2 | −0.209 | 0.241 | −0.054 | 0.386 | −0.684 | 0.265 |
| | | Model 3 | −0.17 | 0.242 | −0.044 | 0.484 | −0.647 | 0.307 |
| | | Model 4 | −0.108 | 0.249 | −0.029 | 0.666 | −0.599 | 0.383 |
| | Female | Model 1 | −0.34 | 0.275 | −0.072 | 0.217 | −0.88 | 0.2 |
| | | Model 2 | −0.325 | 0.28 | −0.069 | 0.247 | −0.877 | 0.227 |
| | | Model 3 | −0.31 | 0.286 | −0.066 | 0.279 | −0.872 | 0.253 |
| | | Model 4 | −0.42 | 0.311 | −0.089 | 0.178 | −1.033 | 0.192 |
| | Total | Model 1 | −0.237 | 0.181 | −0.055 | 0.190 | −0.592 | 0.118 |
| | | Model 2 | −0.302 | 0.192 | −0.070 | 0.118 | −0.680 | 0.076 |
| | | Model 3 | −0.252 | 0.198 | −0.059 | 0.203 | −0.640 | 0.136 |
| | | Model 4 | −0.269 | 0.207 | −0.063 | 0.195 | −0.676 | 0.138 |
| Changes in WHtR | Male | Model 1 | −0.066 | 0.233 | −0.017 | 0.776 | −0.525 | 0.392 |
| (cm/m) | | Model 2 | −0.209 | 0.241 | −0.054 | 0.386 | −0.684 | 0.265 |
| | | Model 3 | −0.17 | 0.242 | −0.044 | 0.484 | −0.647 | 0.307 |
| | | Model 4 | −0.108 | 0.249 | −0.029 | 0.666 | −0.599 | 0.383 |
| | Female | Model 1 | −0.202 | 0.179 | −0.066 | 0.262 | −0.555 | 0.152 |
| | | Model 2 | −0.194 | 0.183 | −0.063 | 0.29 | −0.555 | 0.166 |
| | | Model 3 | −0.184 | 0.187 | −0.06 | 0.325 | −0.552 | 0.183 |
| | | Model 4 | −0.262 | 0.204 | −0.085 | 0.199 | −0.663 | 0.139 |
| | Total | Model 1 | −0.142 | 0.114 | −0.052 | 0.216 | −0.367 | 0.083 |
| | | Model 2 | −0.184 | 0.122 | −0.068 | 0.131 | −0.424 | 0.055 |
| | | Model 3 | −0.155 | 0.125 | −0.057 | 0.215 | −0.401 | 0.091 |
| | | Model 4 | −0.167 | 0.131 | −0.062 | 0.203 | −0.426 | 0.091 |

TPE: total polyphenol excretion; GAE: gallic acid equivalent; BW: body weight; BMI: body mass index. WC: waist circumference; WHtR: waist-to-height ratio. Model 1, unadjusted; Model 2 was adjusted for baseline TPE and baseline BW; Model 3 was adjusted as in Model 2 plus sex (only for total participants), age, and intervention groups; Model 4 was adjusted as in Model 3 plus smoking status (never, current, former), family history of CHD, physical activity, hypertension, diabetes, dyslipidemia, marital status (single, married, divorced, widowed), education level (primary school, high school, university), medication used (antihypertensive drugs, vitamins, insulin, oral hypoglycemic drugs, aspirin, or other antiplatelet drug supplements taken in the last month) recruitment centers, 14 unit Mediterranean diet score, and energy intake at baseline.

Changes in obesity parameters for male, female, and total participants between baseline and end of follow up were observed (Table S1). For total participants, subjects in the highest TPE category had the lowest BW (70.29 ± 10.25 kg) and BMI (28.40 ± 3.75 kg/m²) after the intervention. Inversely, those participants in the first quintile of TPE had significantly higher WC (101.41 ± 9.35 cm) and WHtR (61.80 ± 5.15) compared with baseline values. For males, there was a significant inverse trend among quintiles and BW and BMI both at baseline and the fifth year. Also a significant reduction was observed comparing the top quintile with the bottom quintile both at baseline and the fifth year. For females, there was a significant reduction of BW and BMI in the top quintile groups after five years of intervention.

Table S2 shows the associations between changes in anthropometric parameters and changes in TPE over five years with linear regression models. For total participants, inverse associations were found between changes in BW (β = −0.355; *p* = 0.036), BMI (β = −0.139; *p* = 0.037) and TPE five years after adjustment. For males, there was not any inverse association, while, for females, inverse associations were found for changes in BW (β = −0.723; *p* = 0.003), BMI (β = −0.283; *p* = 0.006), and WC (β = −0.701; *p* = 0.046) after adjustment.

## 4. Discussion

In this five years study conducted in elderly participants at high cardiovascular risk, a higher total polyphenol intake, expressed as TPE, was inversely associated with weight parameters including BW, BMI, WC, and WHtR, as well as with the prevalence of obesity after a five years follow up, suggesting that polyphenols could be considered an independent contributor to the weight loss effects of a Mediterranean diet.

Several PREDIMED sub-trials have reported a range of mechanisms for the weight loss effects of a Mediterranean diet, including a high ingestion of dietary fiber, antioxidants, unsaturated fatty acids, extra virgin olive oil, nuts, and moderate wine consumption [29–35]. The reduction we observed in weight parameters might be partly attributed to the intake of the aforementioned food items; however, in the fully adjusted models, we removed their effects by adjusting for adherence to the Mediterranean diet (14 unit MedDiet questionnaire). Furthermore, even though the intake of these foods increased after five years of follow up, none of them showed significant differences within quintile categories at the end of the intervention; therefore, polyphenol intake could be considered an independent factor.

The present findings are consistent with previous reports on the inverse associations between polyphenol intake and weight parameters. A 16 years longitudinal study from the Netherlands associated a higher intake of total flavonols/flavones and catechins with a lower increase in BMI [36]. Other supporting evidence showed a significant decrease of 1.9 cm in WC and 1.2 kg in BW after supplementation of catechin-rich green tea for 90 days, although at a much higher dose than habitual intakes [37]. Two 12 week intervention studies also demonstrated the anti-obesity effects of green tea intake, finding a considerable reduction in BW, BMI, WC, and total abdominal fat area [38,39]. Another clinical trial indicated that consumption of normal or high-polyphenolic orange juice reduced body weight in obese or overweight adults, demonstrating an inverse association between polyphenol intake and body weight [10]. On the contrary, the effect of daily decaffeinated green tea intake on weight and body composition were tested among a group population in overweight breast cancer survivors. Results showed a slight but not significant increasing in weight loss after the intervention [40]. Compared with Asian populations, Caucasians show inconsistent results: a study showed no effects on body weight with long-term green tea extract supplementation [11]; another study with relapsing-remitting multiple sclerosis patients using one of the main green tea polyphenols, (-)epigal-locatechin-3-gallate, after three months of consumption showed greater muscle metabolism improvement in males than females [41]; supplementation with resveratrol exerted significant effects on energy metabolism in obese subjects, while another two findings showed ineffectiveness in nonobese women and obese men [42–44]. The results are inconsistent probably because of the different doses of polyphenol intakes, sex-specific effects, sample sizes, or length of duration.

The Mediterranean diet could be considered rich in polyphenol content because it is characterized by a high consumption of fruit and vegetables, virgin olive oil, legumes, and nuts and a moderate consumption of wine [45]. Results from a meta-analysis of 16 randomized controlled trials with a

Mediterranean diet showed an average reduction in participant weight of 1.75 kg and a reduction in BMI of 0.57 kg/m$^2$, as well as a greater reduction in BW of 3.88 kg under conditions of energy restriction, suggesting that adherence to a Mediterranean diet helps to control weight [46]. The PREDIMED, the European Prospective Investigation into Cancer and Nutrition (EPIC-Spain) cohort and the Seguimiento Universidad de Navarra (SUN) cohort, also in Spain, have shown in the long-term a significantly lower risk of overweightness/obesity associated with better Mediterranean diet adherence [34,47,48]. We observed a 1.22 kg decrease in BW and 0.50 in BMI in the highest TPE quintile, which partly agrees with previous studies reporting a similar reduction in body weight parameters.

Indexes of abdominal obesity, namely WC and WHtR, were significantly lower in the highest TPE quintile. These parameters are more accurate discriminators of cardiovascular risk than BMI due to the closer relationship between cardiovascular disease and abdominal obesity [49]. In agreement with our findings, in a PREDIMED study, and several other studies, the Mediterranean diet was negatively associated with WC and WHtR [50–52]. Additionally, two feeding trials with green tea polyphenol extracts also showed beneficial effects on abdominal obesity parameters [39,53].

Our results indicate the weight loss effect of polyphenols is higher in females than males. There are several possible reasons to explain the observed results: first, the prevalence of obesity is higher in women than men, and weight loss tends to be lower in obese individuals [54]. In the current study, at baseline, the prevalence of obesity was 32.9% for males and 44.9% for females, which is in line with another elderly population in United States [55]. Second, a higher TPE increment was observed when comparing females and males after five years, which may potentially explain the difference in weight loss effectiveness. Third, self-characteristics concerning males and females may also contribute to the difference. Women tend to have higher concentrations of leptin, an appetite regulation hormone that helps to reduce energy intake [56]. Evidence shows a significant inverse association between polyphenol intakes and plasma leptin levels, indicating higher polyphenol intake responses to better weight loss effectiveness [10]. Furthermore, individual differences in the composition of the gut microbiota may also contribute to differences in bioavailability and polyphenolic metabolites, further influencing the weight loss effectiveness [57].

We also found less gain in WC in males, after five years of intervention. The observation could be primarily explained by the greater percentage of muscle mass and mineral mass in males compared with females. Waist circumference is affected by age, body weight, body composition, and fat distribution [58]. Various types of polyphenol help to reduce visceral fat [9]. Additionally, since waist circumference increases with age, it is worth noting that the average age is older in females in our population, which could be considered another possible explanation.

Potential explanations of the observed inverse association between polyphenol intake and weight loss likely involve several mechanisms due to the diversity of polyphenol chemical structures, complex metabolic pathways, and oral bioavailability. Excess adipose mass and adipose tissue expansion results from adipocyte hypertrophy and hyperplasia [59]. Common plausible mechanisms include the suppression of fat absorption and anabolic pathways; inhibition of adipogenesis and lipogenesis; stimulation of catabolic pathways with increment of lipolysis, apoptosis of mature adipocytes, and acid β-oxidation; reduction of chronic inflammatory response relative to adiposity; and increment in energy expenditure through up-regulating uncoupling protein (UCP1-3) [8,9]. However, knowledge of the anti-obesity effects of polyphenols is limited and only a few specific compounds have been analyzed in this context. For instance, it has been demonstrated that resveratrol, widely present in red grapes and red wine, exerts an anti-obesity action by reducing adipogenesis and increasing apoptosis in mature adipocytes and inhibiting fat accumulation processes and stimulating lipolytic and oxidative pathways in vivo studies and clinical trials [43,60,61]. Contrary results have been observed with anthocyanins, water-soluble plant pigments in blue, purple, and red fruits. On one hand, they seem to significantly reduce body weight. This effect may be due to the suppression of lipid synthesis, the up-regulation of adiponectin, which enhances insulin sensitivity, and the reduction in of serum triglycerides and leptin levels [8,62]. However, two clinical trials showed non-significant reduction trends in body weight after supplementation with food rich in anthocyanins [63,64]. The anti-obesity effects of flavonoids, which are a large group of polyphenols found in a wide range of Mediterranean diet foods [65,66], have been mainly attributed to improvement in adipocyte functionality and fat oxidation [67]. Also playing a key role in weight control is the down-regulation of a variety of pro-inflammatory adipocytokines, particularly tumor necrosis factor alpha (TNF-$\alpha$) [68]. A clinical trial indicates that the inhibition of intestinal fat absorption may contribute to the weight loss after an ingestion of a green tea beverage enriched with catechins [69]. In summary, even though the intake of some specific polyphenols has been associated with body weight management, there is still not enough evidence for the effect of total polyphenols or some classes of polyphenols, and further studies are needed to explore the mechanisms involved as well as potential synergistic effects among them.

The association between weight loss and improvement in cardiovascular risk factors has been widely discussed. Numerous studies indicate that polyphenol intake reduces cardiovascular risk factors [70,71]. A previous study found a significant improvement in cardiovascular risk factors, with a 5–10% of weight loss after one year [72]. We also found protective effects on cardiovascular risk factors, including diastolic blood pressure, glucose concentration, and triglycerides concentration, with the same population after five years of intervention [73]. A randomized study conducted in healthy participants, feed with apple polyphenol, also supported that an improvement in cardiovascular risk factor helps to regulate fat metabolism [74].

Some limitations of this study should be noted. First, given that the study was conducted among elderly subjects at high cardiovascular risk, the results cannot be extrapolated to the general population. Second, even though we adjusted for major potential confounders, we still cannot exclude residual confounding from measurements. Third, even though WC and WHtR may reflect abdominal obesity more accurately, they cannot differentiate between fat distribution in visceral adipose tissue and subcutaneous abdominal adipose tissue; hence we cannot conclude if a reduction in abdominal obesity parameters is beneficial to visceral or subcutaneous fat mass or both [75]. Another limitation is the lack of specific measurements of polyphenol metabolism in vivo.

The present study also has several strengths. Its main strong point is the use of TPE, a biomarker of polyphenol intake, which could provide more precise data than measuring total polyphenol intake through self-reported information in FFQs or databases. Another strength is its prospective design. Only a few studies have analyzed the association between total polyphenol intake and weight control, and the current work is the first to associate anti-obesity effects with total polyphenol intake in individuals at high cardiovascular risk [8,76]. In addition, the long-term duration of the intervention provides more robust results compared with other short-term trials.

## 5. Conclusions

In summary, with five years of follow up, the present study shows that polyphenol levels expressed as TPE in urine were inversely associated with BW, BMI, WC, and WHtR in an elderly population at high cardiovascular risk. Therefore, we confirmed that a long-term polyphenol-rich diet contributes to body weight loss, which can offer protection from several chronic diseases. For future research, similar studies should be conducted in the general population, and specific mechanisms need to be explored by further clinical trials.

**Supplementary Materials:** The following are available online at www.mdpi.com/2072-6643/9/5/452/s1, Table S1: Comparisons of obesity indexes, Table S2: Multiple linear regression analyses with changes in anthropometric parameters and changes in quintiles of TPE over five years, File S1: STROBE checklist, File S2: Protocol of the PREDIMED study, File S3: Database of participants.

**Acknowledgments:** We thank all the participants of the PREDIMED study. This work was supported in part by CICYT (AGL2016-79113-R), the Instituto de Salud Carlos III, ISCIII (CIBEROBN) from the Spanish Ministry of Economy and Competivity (MEC), and Generalitat de Catalunya (GC) 2014 SGR 773. X.G. received support from China Scholarship Council (CSC). Alexander Medina-Remón thanks the 'Juan de la Cierva' postdoctoral program (JCI-2012-13463) from MEC.

**Author Contributions:** R.M.L.-R., A.T.-R. and R.E. conceived and designed the experiments; A.T.-R., A.M.-R. and X.G. performed the experiments; X.G., A.T.-R. and A.M.-R. analyzed the data; A.T.-R., R.E., D.C., M.A.M.-G. and M.F. contributed reagents/materials/analysis tools; and X.P.-S., A.T.-R. and R.M.L.-R. wrote the paper. All authors agreed with the manuscript's results and conclusions.

**Conflicts of Interest:** The authors declare no conflict of interest. The founding sponsors had no role in the design of the study; in the collection, analyses, or interpretation of data; in the writing of the manuscript; or in the decision to publish the results.

## References

1.  Ng, M.; Fleming, T.; Robinson, M.; Thomson, B.; Graetz, N.; Margono, C.; Mullany, E.C.; Biryukov, S.; Alfonso, R.; Ali, M.K.; et al. Global, regional, and national prevalence of overweight and obesity in children and adults during 1980–2013: A systematic analysis for the Global Burden of Disease Study 2013. *Lancet* **2014**, *384*, 766–781. [CrossRef]

2.  World Health Organization. Obesity and Overweight. Available online: http://www.who.int/mediacentre/factsheets/fs311/en (accessed on 2 August 2016).

3.  Directorate-General for Health and Consumers. *Strategy for Europe on Nutrition, Overweight and Obesity Related Health Issues*; Implementation Progress Report; European Commission: Brussels, Belgium, December 2010.

4.  Fitch, A.; Everling, L.; Fox, C.; Goldberg, J.; Heim, C.; Johnson, K.; Kaufman, T.; Kennedy, E.; Kestenbaun, C.; Leslie, D.; et al. Prevention and Management of Obesity for Adults. ICSI Health Care Guideline, 2013. Available online: https://www.healthpartners.com/ucm/groups/public/@hp/@public/documents/documents/cntrb_037112.pdf (accessed on 2 August 2016).

5.  Malik, V.S.; Willett, W.C.; Hu, F.B. Global obesity: Trends, risk factors and policy implications. *Nat. Rev. Endocrinol.* **2013**, *9*, 13–27. [CrossRef] [PubMed]

6.  Ross, R.; Blair, S.; de Lannoy, L.; Després, J.-P.; Lavie, C.J. Changing the endpoints for determining effective obesity management. *Prog. Cardiovasc. Dis.* **2015**, *57*, 330–336. [CrossRef] [PubMed]

7.  Scalbert, A.; Williamson, G. Dietary intake and bioavailability of polyphenols. *J. Nutr.* **2000**, *130*, 2073–2085.

8.  Meydani, M.; Hasan, S.T. Dietary polyphenols and obesity. *Nutrients* **2010**, *2*, 737–751. [CrossRef] [PubMed]

9.  Wang, S.; Moustaid-Moussa, N.; Chen, L.; Mo, H.; Shastri, A.; Su, R.; Bapat, P.; Kwun, I.; Shen, C.L. Novel insights of dietary polyphenols and obesity. *J. Nutr. Biochem.* **2014**, *25*, 1–18. [CrossRef] [PubMed]

10. Rangel-Huerta, O.D.; Aguilera, C.M.; Martin, M.V.; Soto, M.J.; Rico, M.C.; Vallejo, F.; Tomas-Barberan, F.; Perez-de-la-Cruz, A.J.; Gil, A.; Mesa, M.D. Normal or high polyphenol concentration in orange juice affects antioxidant activity, blood pressure, and body weight in obese or overweight adults. *J. Nutr.* **2015**, *145*, 1808–1816. [CrossRef] [PubMed]

11. Janssens, P.L.H.R.; Hursel, R.; Westerterp-Plantenga, M.S. Long-term green tea extract supplementation does not affect fat absorption, resting energy expenditure, and body composition in adults. *J. Nutr.* **2015**, *145*, 864–870. [CrossRef] [PubMed]

12. Bell, Z.W.; Canale, R.E.; Bloomer, R.J. A dual investigation of the effect of dietary supplementation with licorice flavonoid oil on anthropometric and biochemical markers of health and adiposity. *Lipids Health Dis.* **2011**, *10*, 29. [CrossRef] [PubMed]

13. Dallas, C.; Gerbi, A.; Elbez, Y.; Caillard, P.; Zamaria, N.; Cloarec, M. Clinical study to assess the efficacy and safety of a citrus polyphenolic extract of red orange, grapefruit, and orange (Sinetrol-XPur) on weight management and metabolic parameters in healthy overweight individuals. *Phytother. Res.* **2014**, *28*, 212–218. [CrossRef] [PubMed]

14. Most, J.; Goossens, G.H.; Jocken, J.W.E.; Blaak, E.E. Short-term supplementation with a specific combination of dietary polyphenols increases energy expenditure and alters substrate metabolism in overweight subjects. *Int. J. Obes.* **2014**, *38*, 698–706. [CrossRef] [PubMed]

15. Barth, S.W.; Koch, T.C.L.; Watzl, B.; Dietrich, H.; Will, F.; Bub, A. Moderate effects of apple juice consumption on obesity-related markers in obese men: Impact of diet-gene interaction on body fat content. *Eur. J. Nutr.* **2012**, *51*, 841–850. [CrossRef] [PubMed]

16. Cases, J.; Romain, C.; Dallas, C.; Gerbi, A.; Cloarec, M. Regular consumption of Fiit-ns, a polyphenol extract from fruit and vegetables frequently consumed within the Mediterranean diet, improves metabolic ageing of obese volunteers: A randomized, double-blind, parallel trial. *Int. J. Food Sci. Nutr.* **2015**, *66*, 120–125. [CrossRef] [PubMed]

17. Almoosawi, S.; Fyfe, L.; Ho, C.; Al-Dujaili, E. The effect of polyphenol-rich dark chocolate on fasting capillary whole blood glucose, total cholesterol, blood pressure and glucocorticoids in healthy overweight and obese subjects. *Br. J. Nutr.* **2010**, *103*, 842–850. [CrossRef] [PubMed]

18. Medina-Remón, A.; Tresserra-Rimbau, A.; Pons, A.; Tur, J.A.; Martorell, M.; Ros, E.; Buil-Cosiales, P.; Sacanella, E.; Covas, M.I.; Corella, D.; et al. Effects of total dietary polyphenols on plasma nitric oxide and blood pressure in a high cardiovascular risk cohort. The PREDIMED randomized trial. *Nutr. Metab. Cardiovasc. Dis.* **2015**, *25*, 60–67. [CrossRef] [PubMed]

19. Medina-Remón, A.; Barrionuevo-González, A.; Zamora-Ros, R.; Andres-Lacueva, C.; Estruch, R.; Martínez-González, M.A.; Diez-Espino, J.; Lamuela-Raventos, R.M. Rapid Folin-Ciocalteu method using microtiter 96-well plate cartridges for solid phase extraction to assess urinary total phenolic compounds, as a biomarker of total polyphenols intake. *Anal. Chim. Acta* **2009**, *634*, 54–60. [CrossRef] [PubMed]

20. Zamora-Ros, R.; Rabassa, M.; Cherubini, A.; Urpi-Sarda, M.; Llorach, R.; Bandinelli, S.; Ferrucci, L.; Andres-Lacueva, C. Comparison of 24-h volume and creatinine-corrected total urinary polyphenol as a biomarker of total dietary polyphenols in the Invecchiare InCHIANTI study. *Anal. Chim. Acta* **2011**, *704*, 110–115. [CrossRef] [PubMed]

21. Urpi-Sarda, M.; Andres-Lacueva, C.; Rabassa, M.; Ruggiero, C.; Zamora-Ros, R.; Bandinelli, S.; Ferrucci, L.; Cherubini, A. The relationship between urinary total polyphenols and the frailty phenotype in a community-dwelling older population: The InCHIANTI study. *J. Gerontol. A Biol. Sci. Med. Sci.* **2015**, *70*, 1141–1147. [CrossRef] [PubMed]

22. Martínez-González, M.Á.; Corella, D.; Salas-Salvadó, J.; Ros, E.; Covas, M.I.; Fiol, M.; Wärnberg, J.; Arós, F.; Ruíz-Gutiérrez, V.; Lamuela-Raventós, R.M.; et al. Cohort profile: Design and methods of the PREDIMED study. *Int. J. Epidemiol.* **2012**, *41*, 377–385. [CrossRef] [PubMed]

23. Fernández-Ballart, J.D.; Piñol, J.L.; Zazpe, I.; Corella, D.; Carrasco, P.; Toledo, E.; Perez-Bauer, M.; Martínez-González, M.A.; Salas-Salvadó, J.; Martín-Moreno, J.M. Relative validity of a semi-quantitative food-frequency questionnaire in an elderly Mediterranean population of Spain. *Br. J. Nutr.* **2010**, *103*, 1808–1816. [CrossRef] [PubMed]

24. Martínez-González, M.A.; Fernández-Jarne, E.; Serrano-Martínez, M.; Wright, M.; Gomez-Gracia, E. Development of a short dietary intake questionnaire for the quantitative estimation of adherence to a cardioprotective Mediterranean diet. *Eur. J. Clin. Nutr.* **2004**, *58*, 1550–1552. [CrossRef] [PubMed]

25. Elosua, R.; Marrugat, J.; Molina, L.; Pons, S.; Pujol, E. Validation of the Minnesota Leisure Time Physical Activity Questionnaire in Spanish men. *Am. J. Epidemiol.* **1994**, *139*, 1197–1209. [CrossRef] [PubMed]

26. Willett, W.C.; Howe, R. Adjustment for total energy intake in epidemiologic studies. *Am. J. Clin. Nutr.* **1997**, *65*, 1220–1228.

27. Toledo, E.; Hu, F.B.; Estruch, R.; Buil-Cosiales, P.; Corella, D.; Salas-Salvadó, J.; Covas, M.I.; Arós, F.; Gómez-Gracia, E.; Fiol, M.; et al. Effect of the Mediterranean diet on blood pressure in the PREDIMED trial: Results from a randomized controlled trial. *BMC Med.* **2013**, *11*, 207. [CrossRef] [PubMed]

28. Martínez-González, M.A.; García-Arellano, A.; Toledo, E.; Salas-Salvadó, J.; Buil-Cosiales, P.; Corella, D.; Covas, M.I.; Schröder, H.; Arós, F.; Gómez-Gracia, E.; et al. A 14-item mediterranean diet assessment tool and obesity indexes among high-risk subjects: The PREDIMED trial. *PLoS ONE* **2012**, *7*, e43134. [CrossRef] [PubMed]

29. Razquin, C.; Martinez, J.; Martinez-Gonzalez, M.; Mitjavila, M.T.; Estruch, R.; Marti, A. A 3 years follow-up of a Mediterranean diet rich in virgin olive oil is associated with high plasma antioxidant capacity and reduced body weight gain. *Eur. J. Clin. Nutr.* **2009**, *63*, 1387–1393. [CrossRef] [PubMed]

30. Estruch, R.; Martínez-González, M.; Corella, D.; Basora-Gallisá, J.; Ruiz-Gutiérrez, V.; Covas, M.I.; Fiol, M.; Gómez-Gracia, E.; López-Sabater, M.C.; Escoda, R.; et al. Effects of dietary fibre intake on risk factors for cardiovascular disease in subjects at high risk. *J. Epidemiol. Community Health* **2009**, *63*, 582–588. [CrossRef] [PubMed]

31. Ibarrola-Jurado, N.; Bulló, M.; Guasch-Ferré, M.; Ros, E.; Martínez-González, M.A.; Corella, D.; Fiol, M.; Wärnberg, J.; Estruch, R.; Román, P.; et al. Cross-Sectional Assessment of Nut Consumption and Obesity, Metabolic Syndrome and Other Cardiometabolic Risk Factors: The PREDIMED Study. *PLoS ONE* **2013**, *8*, e57367. [CrossRef] [PubMed]

32. Bautista-Castaño, I.; Sánchez-Villegas, A.; Estruch, R.; Martínez-González, M.A.; Corella, D.; Salas-Salvadó, J.; Covas, M.I.; Schroder, H.; Alvarez-Pérez, J.; Quilez, J.; et al. Changes in bread consumption and 4-year changes in adiposity in Spanish subjects at high cardiovascular risk. *Br. J. Nutr.* **2013**, *110*, 337–346. [CrossRef] [PubMed]

33. Schröder, H. Protective mechanisms of the Mediterranean diet in obesity and type 2 diabetes. *J. Nutr. Biochem.* **2007**, *18*, 149–160. [CrossRef] [PubMed]

34. Estruch, R.; Martínez-González, M.A.; Corella, D.; Salas-Salvadó, J.; Fitó, M.; Chiva-Blanch, G.; Fiol, M.; Gómez-Gracia, E.; Arós, F.; Lapetra, J.; et al. Effect of a high-fat Mediterranean diet on bodyweight and waist circumference: A prespecified secondary outcomes analysis of the PREDIMED randomised controlled trial. *Lancet Diabetes Endocrinol.* **2016**, *4*, 666–676. [CrossRef]

35. Álvarez-Pérez, J.; Sánchez-Villegas, A.; Díaz-Benítez, E.M.; Ruano-Rodríguez, C.; Corella, D.; Martínez-González, M.Á.; Estruch, R.; Salas-Salvadó, J.; Serra-Majem, L. PREDIMED study investigators. Influence of a Mediterranean dietary pattern on body fat distribution: Results of the PREDIMED-canarias intervention randomized trial. *J. Am. Coll. Nutr.* **2016**, *35*, 568–580. [CrossRef] [PubMed]

36. Hughes, L.A.E.; Arts, I.C.W.; Ambergen, T.; Brants, H.A.M.; Dagnelie, P.C.; Goldbohm, R.A.; Van Den Brandt, P.A.; Weijenberg, M.P. Higher dietary flavone, flavonol, and catechin intakes are associated with less of an increase in BMI over time in women: A longitudinal analysis from The Netherlands Cohort Study. *Am. J. Clin. Nutr.* **2008**, *88*, 1341–1352. [PubMed]

37. Wang, H.; Wen, Y.; Du, Y.; Yan, X.; Guo, H.; Rycroft, J.A.; Boon, N.; Kovacs, E.M.R.; Mela, D.J. Effects of catechin enriched green tea on body composition. *Obesity* **2010**, *18*, 773–779. [CrossRef] [PubMed]

38. Nagao, T.; Komine, Y.; Soga, S.; Meguro, S.; Hase, T.; Tanaka, Y.; Tokimitsu, I. Ingestion of a tea rich in catechins leads to a reduction in body fat and malondialdehyde-modified LDL in men. *Am. J. Clin. Nutr.* **2005**, *81*, 122–129. [PubMed]

39. Maki, K.C.; Reeves, M.S.; Farmer, M.; Yasunaga, K.; Matsuo, N.; Katsuragi, Y.; Komikado, M.; Tokimitsu, I.; Wilder, D.; Jones, F.; et al. Green tea catechin consumption enhances exercise-induced abdominal fat loss in overweight and obese adults. *J. Nutr.* **2009**, *139*, 264–270. [CrossRef] [PubMed]

40. Stendell-Hollis, N.R.; Thomson, C.A.; Thompson, P.A.; Bea, J.W.; Cussler, E.C.; Hakim, I.A. Green tea improves metabolic biomarkers, not weight or body composition: A pilot study in overweight breast cancer survivors. *J. Hum. Nutr. Diet.* **2010**, *23*, 590–600. [CrossRef] [PubMed]

41. Mahler, A.; Steiniger, J.; Bock, M.; Klug, L.; Parreidt, N.; Lorenz, M.; Zimmermann, B.F.; Krannich, A.; Paul, F.; Boschmann, M. Metabolic response to epigallocatechin-3-gallate in relapsing-remitting multiple sclerosis: A randomized clinical trial. *Am. J. Clin. Nutr.* **2015**, *101*, 487–495. [CrossRef] [PubMed]

42. Poulsen Morten, M.; Vestergaard Poul, F.; Clasen Berthil, F.; Radko, Y.; Christensen Lars, P.; Stodkilde-Jorgensen, H.; Moller, N.; Jessen, N.; Pedersen, S.B.; Jorgensen, J.O.L. High-dose resveratrol supplementation in obese men: An investigator-initiated, randomized, placebo-controlled clinical trial of substrate metabolism, insulin sensitivity, and body composition. *Diabetes* **2013**, *62*, 1186–1195. [CrossRef] [PubMed]

43. Timmers, S.; Konings, E.; Bilet, L.; Houtkooper, R.H.; Van De Weijer, T.; Goossens, G.H.; Hoeks, J.; Van Der Krieken, S.; Ryu, D.; Kersten, S.; et al. Calorie restriction-like effects of 30 days of resveratrol supplementation on energy metabolism and metabolic profile in obese humans. *Cell Metab.* **2011**, *14*, 612–622. [CrossRef] [PubMed]

44. Yoshino, J.; Conte, C.; Fontana, L.; Mittendorfer, B.; Imai, S.; Schechtman, K.B.; Gu, C.; Kunz, I.; Rossi Fanelli, F.; Patterson, B.W.; et al. Resveratrol supplementation does not improve metabolic function in nonobese women with normal glucose tolerance. *Cell Metab.* **2012**, *16*, 658–664. [CrossRef] [PubMed]

45. Romaguera, D.; Norat, T.; Mouw, T.; May, A.M.; Bamia, C.; Slimani, N.; Travier, N.; Besson, H.; Luan, J.; Wareham, N.; et al. Adherence to the Mediterranean diet is associated with lower abdominal adiposity in European men and women. *J. Nutr.* **2009**, *139*, 1728–1737. [CrossRef] [PubMed]

46. Esposito, K.; Kastorini, C.-M.; Panagiotakos, D.B.; Giugliano, D. Mediterranean diet and weight loss: Meta-analysis of randomized controlled trials. *Metab. Syndr. Relat. Disord.* **2011**, *9*, 1–12. [CrossRef] [PubMed]

47. Mendez, M.; Popkin, B.M.; Jakszyn, P.; Berenguer, A.; Tormo, M.J.; Sanchéz, M.J.; Quirós, J.R.; Pera, G.; Navarro, C.; Martinez, C.; et al. Adherence to a Mediterranean diet is associated with reduced 3-year incidence of obesity. *J. Nutr.* **2006**, *136*, 2934–2938. [PubMed]

48. Beunza, J.-J.; Toledo, E.; Hu, F.B.; Bes-Rastrollo, M.; Serrano-Martínez, M.; Sánchez-Villegas, A.; Martínez, J.A.; Martínez-González, M.A. Adherence to the Mediterranean diet, long-term weight change, and incident overweight or obesity: The Seguimiento Universidad de Navarra (SUN) cohort. *Am. J. Clin. Nutr.* **2010**, *92*, 1484–1493. [CrossRef] [PubMed]

49. Lee, C.M.Y.; Huxley, R.R.; Wildman, R.P.; Woodward, M. Indices of abdominal obesity are better discriminators of cardiovascular risk factors than BMI: A meta-analysis. *J. Clin. Epidemiol.* **2008**, *61*, 646–653. [CrossRef] [PubMed]

50. Eguaras, S.; Toledo, E.; Buil-Cosiales, P.; Salas-Salvadó, J.; Corella, D.; Gutierrez-Bedmar, M.; Santos-Lozano, J.M.; Arós, F.; Fiol, M.; Fitó, M.; et al. Does the Mediterranean diet counteract the adverse effects of abdominal adiposity? *Nutr. Metab. Cardiovasc. Dis.* **2015**, *256*, 569–574. [CrossRef] [PubMed]

51. Panagiotakos, D.B.; Chrysohoou, C.; Pitsavos, C.; Stefanadis, C. Association between the prevalence of obesity and adherence to the Mediterranean diet: The ATTICA study. *Nutrition* **2006**, *22*, 449–456. [CrossRef] [PubMed]

52. Schröder, H.; Mendez, M.A.; Ribas-Barba, L.; Covas, M.I.; Serra-Majem, L. Mediterranean diet and waist circumference in a representative national sample of young Spaniards. *Int. J. Pediatr. Obes.* **2010**, *5*, 516–519. [CrossRef] [PubMed]

53. Nagao, T.; Hase, T.; Tokimitsu, I. A green tea extract high in catechins reduces body fat and cardiovascular risks. *Obesity* **2007**, *15*, 1473–1483. [CrossRef] [PubMed]

54. Cai, L.; Han, X.; Qi, Z.; Li, Z.; Zhang, Y.; Wang, P.; Liu, A. Prevalence of overweight and obesity and weight loss practice among Beijing adults, 2011. *PLoS ONE* **2014**, *9*, e98744. [CrossRef] [PubMed]

55. Wang, Y.; Beydoun, M.A. The obesity epidemic in the United States-Gender, age, socioeconomic, racial/ethnic, and geographic characteristics: A systematic review and meta-regression analysis. *Epidemiol. Rev.* **2007**, *29*, 6–28. [CrossRef] [PubMed]

56. Williams, R.L.; Wood, L.G.; Collins, C.E.; Callister, R. Effectiveness of weight loss interventions - is there a difference between men and women: A systematic review. *Obes. Rev.* **2015**, *16*, 171–186. [CrossRef] [PubMed]

57. Gross, G.; Jacobs, D.M.; Peters, S.; Possemiers, S.; Van Duynhoven, J.; Vaughan, E.E.; Van De Wiele, T. In vitro bioconversion of polyphenols from black tea and red wine/grape juice by human intestinal microbiota displays strong interindividual variability. *J. Agric. Food Chem.* **2010**, *58*, 10236–10246. [CrossRef] [PubMed]

58. Stevens, J.; Katz, E.G.; Huxley, R.R. Associations between gender, age and waist circumference. *Eur. J. Clin. Nutr.* **2010**, *64*, 6–15. [CrossRef] [PubMed]

59. Jo, J.; Gavrilova, O.; Pack, S.; Jou, W.; Mullen, S.; Sumner, A.E.; Cushman, S.W.; Periwal, V. Hypertrophy and/or hyperplasia: Dynamics of adipose tissue growth. *PLoS Comput. Biol.* **2009**, *5*, e1000324. [CrossRef] [PubMed]

60. Carpéné, C.; Gomez-Zorita, S.; Deleruyelle, S.; Carpéné, M.A. Novel strategies for preventing diabetes and obesity complications with natural polyphenols. *Curr. Med. Chem.* **2015**, *22*, 150–164. [CrossRef] [PubMed]

61. Szkudelska, K.; Szkudelski, T. Resveratrol, obesity and diabetes. *Eur. J. Pharmacol.* **2010**, *635*, 1–8. [CrossRef] [PubMed]

62. Tsuda, T. Dietary anthocyanin-rich plants: Biochemical basis and recent progress in health benefits studies. *Mol. Nutr. Food Res.* **2012**, *56*, 159–170. [CrossRef] [PubMed]

63. Wright, O.R.L.; Netzel, G.A.; Sakzewski, A.R. A randomized, double-blind, placebo-controlled trial of the effect of dried purple carrot on body mass, lipids, blood pressure, body composition, and inflammatory markers in overweight and obese adults: The QUENCH Trial. *Can. J. Physiol. Pharmacol.* **2013**, *91*, 480–488. [CrossRef] [PubMed]

64. Zhu, Y.; Xia, M.; Yang, Y.; Liu, F.; Li, Z.; Hao, Y.; Mi, M.; Jin, T.; Ling, W. Purified anthocyanin supplementation improves endothelial function via NO-cGMP activation in hypercholesterolemic individuals. *Clin. Chem.* **2011**, *57*, 1524–1533. [CrossRef] [PubMed]

65. Yao, L.H.; Jiang, Y.M.; Shi, J.; Tomás-Barberán, F.A.; Datta, N.; Singanusong, R.; Chen, S.S. Flavonoids in food and their health benefits. *Plant Foods Hum. Nutr.* **2004**, *59*, 113–122. [CrossRef] [PubMed]

66. Tresserra-Rimbau, A.; Medina-Remón, A.; Pérez-Jiménez, J.; Martínez-González, M.A.; Covas, M.I.; Corella, D.; Salas-Salvadó, J.; Gómez-Gracia, E.; Lapetra, J.; Arós, F.; et al. Dietary intake and major food sources of polyphenols in a Spanish population at high cardiovascular risk: The PREDIMED study. *Nutr. Metab. Cardiovasc. Dis.* **2013**, *23*, 953–959. [CrossRef] [PubMed]

67. Andersen, C.; Rayalam, S.; Della-Fera, M.A.; Baile, C.A. Phytochemicals and adipogenesis. *BioFactors* **2010**, *36*, 415–422. [CrossRef] [PubMed]

68. Galleano, M.; Calabro, V.; Prince, P.D.; Litterio, M.C.; Piotrkowski, B.; Vazquez-Prieto, M.A.; Miatello, R.M.; Oteiza, P.I.; Fraga, C.G. Flavonoids and metabolic syndrome. *Ann. N. Y. Acad. Sci.* **2012**, *1259*, 87–94. [CrossRef] [PubMed]

69. Kobayashi, M.; Kawano, T.; Ukawa, Y.; Sagesaka, Y.M.; Fukuhara, I. Green tea beverages enriched with catechins with a galloyl moiety reduce body fat in moderately obese adults: A randomized double-blind placebo-controlled trial. *Food Funct. R. Soc. Chem.* **2016**, *7*, 498–507. [CrossRef] [PubMed]

70. Brüll, V.; Burak, C.; Stoffel-Wagner, B.; Wolffram, S.; Nickenig, G.; Müller, C.; Langguth, P.; Alteheld, B.; Fimmers, R.; Naaf, S.; et al. Effects of a quercetin-rich onion skin extract on 24 h ambulatory blood pressure and endothelial function in overweight-to-obese patients with (pre-)hypertension: A randomised double-blinded placebo-controlled cross-over trial. *Br. J. Nutr.* **2015**, *114*, 1263–1277. [CrossRef] [PubMed]

71. Tresserra-Rimbau, A.; Guasch-Ferre, M.; Salas-Salvado, J.; Toledo, E.; Corella, D.; Castaner, O.; Guo, X.; Gomez-Gracia, E.; Lapetra, J.; Aros, F.; et al. Intake of total polyphenols and some classes of polyphenols is inversely associated with diabetes in elderly people at high cardiovascular disease risk. *J. Nutr.* **2016**, *146*, 767–777. [CrossRef] [PubMed]

72. Wing, R.; Lang, W.; Wadden, T.; Safford, M.; Knowler, W.; Bertoni, A.; Hill, J.; Brancati, F.; Peters, A.; Wagenknecht, L. Benefits of modest weight loss in improving cardiovascular risk factors in overweight and obese individuals with type 2 diabetes. *Diabetes Care* **2011**, *34*, 1481–1486. [CrossRef] [PubMed]

73. Guo, X.; Tresserra-Rimbau, A.; Estruch, R.; Martínez-González, M.A.; Medina-Remón, A.; Castañer, O.; Corella, D.; Salas-Salvadó, J.; Lamuela-Raventós, R.M. Effects of polyphenol, measured by a biomarker of total polyphenols in urine, on cardiovascular risk factors after a long-term follow-up in the PREDIMED study. *Oxid. Med. Cell. Longev.* **2016**, *2016*, 2572606. [CrossRef] [PubMed]

74. Nagasako-Akazome, Y.; Kanda, T.; Ohtake, Y.; Shimasaki, H.; Kobayashi, T. Apple polyphenols influence cholesterol metabolism in healthy subjects with relatively high body mass index. *J. Oleo Sci.* **2007**, *56*, 417–428. [CrossRef] [PubMed]

75. Klein, S.; Allison, D.; Heymsfield, S.; Kelley, D.; Leibel, R.; Nonas, C.; Kahn, R.E.A.; Leibe, R. Waist circumference and cardiometabolic risk: A consensus statement from Shaping America's Health: Association for weight management and obesity prevention. *Am. J. Clin. Nutr.* **2007**, *85*, 1197–1202. [PubMed]

76. Hervert-Hernández, D.; Goñi, I. Contribution of beverages to the intake of polyphenols and antioxidant capacity in obese women from rural Mexico. *Public Health Nutr.* **2012**, *15*, 6–12. [CrossRef] [PubMed]

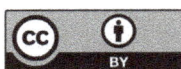

*nutrients*

MDPI

*Article*

# A Critical Review on Polyphenols and Health Benefits of Black Soybeans

**Kumar Ganesan and Baojun Xu ***

Food Science and Technology Program, Beijing Normal University-Hong Kong Baptist University United International College, Zhuhai 519085, China; kumarganesan@uic.edu.hk
* Correspondence: baojunxu@uic.edu.hk; Tel.: +86-756-3620-636; Fax: +86-756-3620-882

Received: 4 April 2017; Accepted: 28 April 2017; Published: 4 May 2017

**Abstract:** Polyphenols are plant secondary metabolites containing antioxidant properties, which help to protect chronic diseases from free radical damage. Dietary polyphenols are the subject of enhancing scientific interest due to their possible beneficial effects on human health. In the last two decades, there has been more interest in the potential health benefits of dietary polyphenols as antioxidant. Black soybeans (*Glycine max* L. Merr) are merely a black variety of soybean containing a variety of phytochemicals. These phytochemicals in black soybean (BSB) are potentially effective in human health, including cancer, diabetes, cardiovascular diseases, cerebrovascular diseases, and neurodegenerative diseases. Taking into account exploratory study, the present review aims to provide up-to-date data on health benefit of BSB, which helps to explore their therapeutic values for future clinical settings. All data of in vitro and in vivo studies of BSB and its impact on human health were collected from a library database and electronic search (Science Direct, PubMed, and Google Scholar). The different pharmacological information was gathered and orchestrated in a suitable spot on the paper.

**Keywords:** polyphenols; black soybean; antioxidants; human diseases; health benefits

---

## 1. Polyphenols

Polyphenols are phytochemicals, found largely in fruits, vegetables, tea, coffee, chocolates, legumes, cereals, and beverages. There are over 8000 polyphenols identified in nature and their main functions are as antioxidant. They protect our body from free radical damage and defense against UV radiation or aggression by pathogens. In the last two decades, there has been more interest in the potential health benefits of dietary polyphenols as antioxidant. The average 100 grams fresh weight of fruits (grapes, apple, pear, cherries, and berries) contain up to 300 mg of polyphenols. Typically, a cup of tea or coffee or a glass of red wine contains more than 100 mg of polyphenols. In addition, cereals, vegetables, dry legumes and chocolate also contribute to the polyphenolic intake and thereby protect our body from chronic diseases [1]. Dietary polyphenols are the subject of enhancing scientific interest due to their possible beneficial effects on human health. They are usually provided to the food as color, flavor, bitter, and astringent, and maintain stability from oxidation. Several epidemiological studies and associated meta-analyses strongly showed that the consumption of these polyphenols offered better protection against chronic diseases such as cancers, cardiovascular diseases, cerebrovascular diseases, diabetes, ageing and neurodegenerative diseases [2–5].

### 1.1. Types of Polyphenols

Polyphenols are divided into four different categories based on the presence of number of phenolic groups and structural elements [6]. Food usually contains complex polyphenols, predominantly found in the outer layers of the plants [1].

1. Flavonoids: Have a potential effect on radical scavenging and inflammatory reactions. They are predominantly found in fruits, vegetables, legumes, red wine, and green tea. They are further divided into a number of subgroups namely, flavones, flavonols, flavanones, isoflavones, anthocyanidins, chalcones, and catechins.
2. Stilbenes: Found in product of graphs, red wine, and peanuts. Resveratrol is the most well-known compound among the group.
3. Lignans: Found in seeds like flax, linseed, legumes, cereals, grains, fruits, algae, and certain vegetables.
4. Phenolic acids: Found in coffee, tea, cinnamon, blueberries, kiwis, plums, apples, and cherries and have two subgroups, namely hydroxybenzoic acids, and hydroxycinnamic acids.

*1.2. Role of Polyphenols in Plants and Humans*

In the plant, polyphenols protect from UV radiation, pathogens, oxidative stress, and harsh climatic conditions [1]. In the human body, polyphenols are antioxidants, and have diverse biological properties such as anti-diabetic [7,8], anticancer [9,10], anti-inflammatory [11,12], cardioprotective [13], osteoprotective [14,15], neuroprotective [16,17], antiasthmatic [18], antihypertensive [19], antiageing [20], antiseptic [21], cerebrovascular protection [22], cholesterol lowering [23], hepatoprotective [24], antifungal [25], antibacterial [26] and antiviral properties [27] (Figure 1).

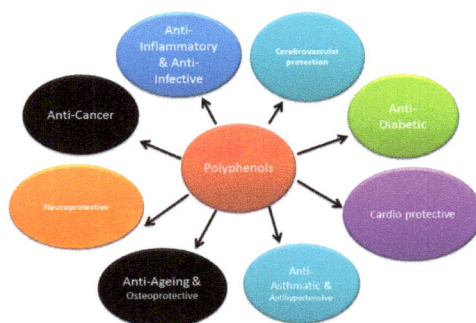

**Figure 1.** Role of polyphenols in humans.

## 2. Black Soybeans

Soybeans contain various colors of seed coat including black, yellow, green, and brown. It is due to the presence of anthocyanins, chlorophyll, and other pigments. Black soybeans (BSB) have been widely consumed as food and as material for Oriental medicine for hundreds of years in Asia. The black pigmentation is due to accumulation of anthocyanins in the epidermis palisade layer of the seed coat [28]. Different anthocyanins in BSB have been identified, including cyanidin-3-glucoside, delphinidin-3-glucoside, and pelargonidin-3-Glucoside [29]. BSB is an excellent dietary source for disease prevention and health promotion.

In the last two decades, isoflavones and proteins are the primary health beneficial components in BSB that have received attention [30–32]. Nevertheless, there are insufficient data to explain the health benefits exclusive to BSB. They have potentially active phytochemicals such as isoflavones, sterols, phytic acid, saponins, and phenolics, which are potentially effective for human health and prevention of various chronic diseases [32]. Research showed that BSB has the greatest antioxidant properties compared to other colored soybeans [33,34]. The characteristic antioxidant potential is due the presence of phenolics, which is mainly distributed in the seed coat [35,36]. In the seed coat, around 20 phenolic compounds, predominantly six anthocyanins, are greatly (13–50 times) distributed in several BSB varieties [32], which helps to reduce the risk of chronic diseases such as metabolic disorders and cancers [37–40]. These varieties have the potential to be used in functional foods and food colorant development. The predominant quantity of anthocyanins provides a black color to the seed coat and showed to have potent antioxidant properties, which is mainly responsible for health-promoting effects of BSB. In addition to the anthocyanins, BSB contain other phenolics such as tannins, isoflavones and phenolic acids [34,35].

*Nutritional Importance of BSB*

BSB has a high content of protein (32–43.6%). In addition to protein, BSB contains carbohydrates (31.7–31.85%), lipids (15.5–24.7%), water (5.6–11.5%), minerals (calcium, phosphorous, magnesium, potassium, sodium, selenium, etc.) and vitamins (Vitamin E, B complex, etc.) [41,42]. The BSB lipid composition consists of 86% unsaturated fatty acids, especially linoleic (6.48–11.6%), linolenic (0.72–2.16%) and oleic acids (3.15–8.82%), making it beneficial to human health [43]. Soybean is characterized by the most digestible proteins, lysine and methionine. However, it is limited by sulfur amino acids and tryptophan.

## 3. Anthocyanins Rich BSB

Anthocyanins are water-soluble natural pigments that belong to flavonoids, a larger subgroup of polyphenols, and widely distributed in BSB and shown to provide numerous health benefits. Major anthocyanins have been isolated and identified from the seed coat of BSB such as cyanidin 3-*O*-β-D-glucoside, delphinidin-3-*O*-β-D-glucoside, pelargonidin-3-*O*-glucoside, and petunidin 3-*O*-β-D-glucoside [29,44]. The minor anthocyanins such as catechincyanidin-3-*O*-glucoside, delphinidin-3-*O*-galactoside, cyanidin-3-*O*-galactoside, and peonidin-3-*O*-glucoside have also been isolated and identified based on the fragmentation patterns of high-performance liquid chromatography–diode array detector–electrospray ionization/mass spectrometry analysis [45,46]. 5,7,3′,4′-Tetrahydroxyflav-2-en-3-ol 3-*O*-β-D-glucoside have also been isolated from immature BSB [47]. The structure of anthocyanins-rich BSB is depicted in Figure 2.

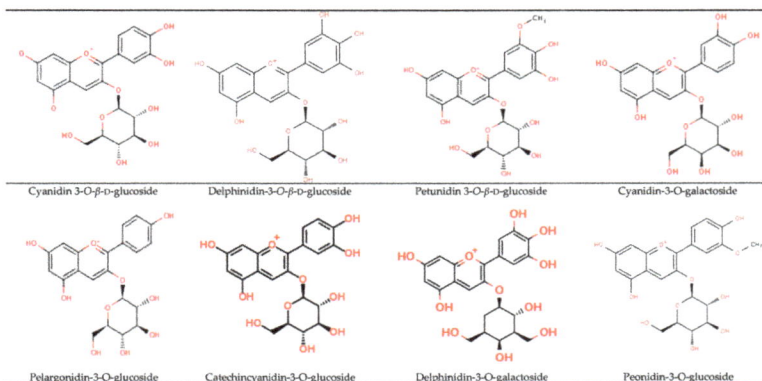

**Figure 2.** Anthocynins isolated from back soybean [45–47].

## 4. Health Benefits of Anthocyanins Rich BSB

Anthocyanins rich BSB has potential health benefit as complementary medicine and utilized in various formulation implied for antioxidant, anti-inflammatory, nephroprotective, antidiabetic, anticancer, anti-infertility, anti-obesity, anti-arthritic, neuroprotective, antihyperlipidemic, anti-cataract and wound healing properties. Detailed information on dose range, route of administration, the model used, negative controls, and other pharmacological results based on the experimental research study in vivo and in vitro, according to the appropriate title depicted, are presented in Table 1.

Some of the health benefits of anthocyanins rich BSB are listed below.

**Table 1.** Summary of in vivo and in vitro studies of health benefit potentials of Anthocyninsrich BSB.

| Model | Anthocyanin Rich BSB | Dose and Route of Administration | Negative Control | Investigation | Results | Reference |
|---|---|---|---|---|---|---|
| Mouse | Anthocyanin | 24 mg/kg/day PO | Lipopolysaccharide | Assay of phospho-c-JNK1, IL-1β, TNF-α, transcription factor NF-κB, GFAP, Iba-1, Bax, cytosolic cytochrome C, cleaved caspase-3 and PARP-1 | Neuroprotective activity | [48] |
| Obesity human | Anthocyanin-rich BSB testa extracts | 2.5 g/day PO | Obesity human | Assay of TG,LDL-C, non-HDL-C, TC/HDL-C and LDL-C/HDL-C | Anti-obesity | [49] |
| Mouse | Anthocyanin-rich BSB seed coat | 60 mg/kg/PO | Collagen induced arthritis | Assay of histological inflammation, cartilage scores, oxidative stress markers, pro-inflammatory cytokines and NF-κB signaling | Anti-arthritic activity | [50] |
| Apc (Min/+) mice | Anthocyanin-rich BSB seed coat | 0.2% or 0.5% /kg/PO | - | Assay of Number of intestinal tumors, and cellular expression of β-catenin | Anti-cancer activity | [51] |
| Apc(Min) mouse | Cyanidin-3-glucoside | 0.03%, 0.1% or 0.3% | - | Assay of Plasma, urine and intestinal mucosaanthocyaninswere determined by HPLC, UV spectrophotometry and tandem MS | Anti-cancer activity | [52] |
| Human hepatoma (HepG2) cells | BSB seed coats | 67 µg/mL | Hydrogen peroxide | Assay of ERK, intracellular total protein phosphatase activity | Anti-cancer activity | [53] |
| Human brain neuroblastoma SK-N-SH cells | Cyanidin-3-O-glucoside, Delphinidin-3-O-glucoside, and petunidin-3-O-glucoside | 67 µg/mL | Hydrogen peroxide | Assay of cell viability, ROS, expression of heme oxygenase (HO)-1, MAP kinase, ASK1-JNK/p38 pathways by MTT assay, DCF-DA assay, RT-PCR, and Western blotting | Anti-cancer activity | [54] |
| Humanhepatoma (HepG2) cells and ICR mice | BSB seed coats extracts | 25 µg/mL | Benzo[a]pyrene | Assay of cytochrome P4501A1 expression, Nrf2 to antioxidant response elements | Anti-cancer activity | [55] |
| Ratpheochromocytoma (PC12 cell line) | non-anthocyanin fraction | 3, 6, 12, and 25 µg/mL | Amyloid β peptide | Assay of cellular oxidative stress by using DCF-DA, MTT, LDH, MDA level, acetylcholinesterase activity | Anti-amnesic effect | [56] |
| Human lens epithelial cell line (HLE-B3) | BSB seed coats extracts | 0, 50, 100 and 200 µg/mL | Hydrogen peroxide | Assay of apoptosis by Annexin V assay and APO-BrdU TUNEL assay; Western blot and immunostaining of apoptosis-related molecules; Bcl2, Bax, p53 and caspase-3. | Anti- cataract effect | [57] |

**Table 1.** *Cont.*

| Model | Anthocyanin Rich BSB | Dose and Route of Administration | Negative Control | Investigation | Results | Reference |
|---|---|---|---|---|---|---|
| Rat primary cortical neuron cells | BSB (cv. Cheongja 3, Glycine max (L.) MERR,) seed coat | 50 mg/mL | Glutamate | Assay of LDH, MTT, Intracellular ROS and immunofluorescence | Neuroprotective effect | [58] |
| 3T3-L1 cells db/db mice | Anthocyanin cyanidin-3-glucoside | 60 mg/kg/PO | - | Assay of PPARγ and C/EBPα gene expressions, TNF-α, PGC-1α, SIRT1 and UCP-3 | Antiobesity and antidiabetic effects | [59] |
| 3T3-L1 cells *db/db* mice | Anthocyanin cyanidin-3-glucoside | 12.5 and 50 µg/mL | - | Assay of MTT, expression of the peroxisome proliferator-activated receptor γ and measurement of lipolysis | Antiobesity and antidiabetic effects | [60] |
| Wistar albino rats | Anthocyanin cyanidin-3-glucoside | Anthocyanins (24 mg/kg) along with and vitC (100 mg/kg) | 10% (v/v) ethanol | Assay of MTT, expression of GABAB1 receptor,Bax/Bcl-2 ratio, release of cytochrome C and activation of caspase-3 and caspase-9 | Neuroprotective effect | [61] |
| Wistar albino rats | Anthocyanin cyanidin-3-glucoside | Anthocyanins (24 mg/kg) along with and vitamin c (100 mg/kg) | 10% (v/v) ethanol | Assay of GABAB1 receptor, cellular levels of proapoptotic proteins such as Bax, activated caspase-3, and cleaved poly (ADP-ribose) polymerase 1 (PARP-1) intracellular free Ca (2+) level and CaMKII | Neuroprotective effect | [62] |
| Wistar albino rats | Anthocyanin cyanidin-3-glucoside | Anthocyanins (24 mg/kg) along with and vitamin c (100 mg/kg) | 10% (v/v) ethanol | Assay of expression of glutamate receptors, intracellular signaling molecules, and various synaptic, inflammatory, and apoptotic markers | Neuroprotective effect | [63] |
| Mouse hippocampal cell line (HT22) and primary prenatal rat hippocampal neurons | Anthocyanin cyanidin-3-glucoside | 12.5 and 50 µg/mL | Kainic acid | intracellular $Ca^{2+}$ level, ROS, AMPK, Bcl-2, cytochrome-c, and caspase-3 | Antioxidant activity | [64] |
| Human | BSB seed coat | 60 mg/kg/PO | STZ | Assay of glycemic control and lipid metabolism parameters | Anti-hyperlipidemic effect | [37] |
| in vitro (prostate cancer-DU-145 cells) and in vivo (in athymic nude mouse xenograft model) | Anthocyanin | 8 mg/kg | - | Assay of MTT, p53, Bax, Bcl, androgen receptor (AR), and prostate specific antigen | Anti-cancer activity | [65] |
| HT22 cell lines and adult wister male rats | Anthocyanin | 0.2 mg/kg | Amyloid beta 1-42 | Assay of MTT, mitochondrial membrane potential, intracellular free $Ca^{2+}$ and apoptotic cells (fluoro-jade B and TUNEL),Western blot analyses were performed | Neuroprotective effect | [66] |

**Table 1.** *Cont.*

| Model | Anthocyanin Rich BSB | Dose and Route of Administration | Negative Control | Investigation | Results | Reference |
|---|---|---|---|---|---|---|
| Wistar albino rats | Anthocyanin | 50 mg/kg/PO | Human fibrin and thrombin solutions | Assay of Masson trichrome and transforming growth factor | Anti-inflammatory and antifibrosis effects | [67] |
| In vitro | BSB seed coat | 388 mg/100 g | - | Assay of DPPH and ABTS+ | Antioxidant properties | [68] |
| Wistar albino rats and rat pheochromocytoma PC12 cell line | Non-anthocyanins | 10, 20 mg/kg/PO | $H_2O_2$ and trimethyltin | Assay of MTT, LDH, AChE in vitro inhibition, Y-maze test, Passive avoidance test and MDA levels | Beneficial for neurodegenerative disorders | [69] |
| Sprague-Dawley rats | BSB | 10, 20 mg/kg PO | ciprofloxacin, | Assay of prostate tissue, urine culture, and histological analysis | Anti-inflammatory and antimicrobial effects | [70] |
| In vitro | Black soybean tea | 10, 20 mg/kg PO | - | Assay of DPPH, ferrous ion chelating ability and reducing power | Antioxidant activity | [71] |
| In vitro | *Aspergillus awamori*-fermented BSB | 10, 20 mg/kg PO | - | Assay of DPPH, ferrous ion chelating ability and reducing power | Antioxidant activity | [72] |
| In vitro | 20 soybean hybrids | 10, 20 mg/kg PO | - | Assay of DPPH | Antioxidant activity | [73] |
| In vitro | BSB hybrids | 10, 20 mg/kg PO | - | Assay of DPPH, ferric reducing antioxidant power, oxygen radical absorbance capacity | Antioxidant activity | [34] |
| In vitro | BSB hybrids | 10, 20 mg/kg PO | - | Assay of total phenolic content, total flavonoid content, condensed tannin content, monomeric anthocyanin content, DPPH free radical scavenging activity, ferric reducing antioxidant power, and oxygen radical absorbing capacity | Antioxidant activity | [74] |
| In vitro | 30 BSB hybrids | 10, 20 mg/kg PO | - | Assay of total phenolic content, total flavonoid content, condensed tannin content, monomeric anthocyanin content, DPPH free radical scavenging activity, ferric reducing antioxidant power, and oxygen radical absorbing capacity | Antioxidant activity | [75] |
| Male Sprague-Dawley rats | Anthocyanins | 6 mg/kg and 24 mg/kg PO | - | Assay of body weight and daily food intake, neuropeptide Y, GABAB1 receptor, protein kinase A-α, and phosphorylated cAMP-response element binding protein | Hypolipidemic and anti-obesity effects | [76] |
| Wistar albino rats | BSB seed coats | 0.037%/PO | High fat diet—16% lard oil | Assay of body weight, adipose tissue weight, and serum lipids | Anti-obesity effect | [77] |

**Table 1.** *Cont.*

| Model | Anthocyanin Rich BSB | Dose and Route of Administration | Negative Control | Investigation | Results | Reference |
|---|---|---|---|---|---|---|
| C57BL/6 mice | *Monascus pilosus*-fermented BSB | 0.5 and 1.0 g/kg/PO | High fat diet—16% lard oil | Assay of blood glucose, TC, leptin and measurement of epididymal, retroperitoneal, and perirenal fat pads | Anti-obesity effect | [78] |
| Male KK-$A^g$ diabetic mice and L6 myotubes | BSB seed coat extract | 22.0 g of BE/kg diet/PO | - | Assay of blood glucose, insulin, AMP-activated protein kinase, glucose transporter 4 | Anti-diabetic effects | [79] |
| Gastric adenocarcinoma, ATCC CRL 1739 | Anthocyanin | 50 µg/mL | - | Assay of cell viability, ROS, Western blot analyses, RT-PCR were performed to assess gene and protein expression | Anti-oxidative, antibacterial and anti-inflammatory effects | [80] |
| Immortalized epidermal keratinocyte cell line (HaCaT) and human neonatal dermal fibroblasts | Anthocyanin | 50 µg/mL | $H_2O_2$ | Assay of tissue VEGF, TSP1, CD31, NF-κB, and phosphorylation of IκBα | Wound healing properties | [81] |
| Human dermal fibroblasts and keratinocytes cell lines | BSB seed coat extracts | 100 µg/mL | - | Assay of TNF-alpha, NF-kB, p65, VEGF in in fibroblasts and keratinocytes | Anti-inflammatory effects | [82] |
| Wistar albino rats | BSB seed coat extracts | 50 and 100 mg/kg/PO | - | Assay of TNF-alpha, ICAM, NF-kB,cyclooxygenase-2, VEGF in in fibroblasts and keratinocytes | Anti-inflammatory properties against ischemia-reperfusion injury | [83] |
| Bovine aortic endothelial cells and male Sprague-Dawley rats | Anthocyanin BSB seed coat | 25, 50 and 100 mg/kg/PO | LAD occlusion and reperfusion | Assay of MTT, Luciferase, TNF-alpha, ICAM, NF-kB, cyclooxygenase-2, vascular endothelial growth factor | Cardioprotective effect | [84] |
| Murine BV2 microglial cells | Anthocyanin BSB seed coat | 100 µg/mL | Lipopolysaccharides | Assay of NO, prostaglandin E(2), and pro-inflammatory cytokines, including TNF-α IL-1β, NO synthase, cyclooxygenase-2, NF-κB, ERK, c-JNK, p38 MAP kinase, and Akt. | Anti-inflammatory and potent neurodegenerative diseases | [85] |
| U2OS cells | Anthocyanin BSB seed coat | 200 µg/mL | - | Assay of extracellular signal-regulated kinase 1/2, p38 mitogen-activated protein kinase, c-Jun N-terminal kinase, protein kinase B and adenosyl mono-phosphate-dependent protein kinase | Anticancer effects | [86] |

**Table 1.** *Cont.*

| Model | Anthocyanin Rich BSB | Dose and Route of Administration | Negative Control | Investigation | Results | Reference |
|---|---|---|---|---|---|---|
| Wistar albino rats | Anthocyanin | 40 or 80 mg/kg PO | Varicocele-induced rats | Histological examination and semen analysis | Anti-infertility effects | [87] |
| Wistar albino rats | Anthocyanin | 40, 80, and 160 mg/kg PO | benign prostatic hyperplasia-induced rats | Assay of apoptosis in the prostates by the TUNEL assay | Anti-infertility effects | [88] |
| Wistar albino rats | Anthocyanin BSB seed coat | 50 mg/kg PO | N-methyl-N-nitrosourea | Electro-retinographic recordings and morphological analyses | Anti-blindness | [89] |
| Detroit 551 cells | fermented BSB broth | 200 µg/mL | - | Assay of DPPH radical scavenging effect, reducing power and ferrous ion chelating effect. | Antioxidant effect | [90] |
| Human U87 glioma cells | Anthocyanin BSB seed coat | 100 µg/mL | - | Assay of autophagy; Atg5 expression | Anti- stroke effect | [91] |
| Wistar albino rats | citric acid fermented of BSB | 10 mL/kg | Ferricnitrilotriacetate | Assay of antioxidative enzymes including catalase, glutathione peroxidase, glutathione reductase, glutathione S-transferase, glucose-6-phosphate dehydrogenase, quinone reductase, serum creatinine and urea nitrogen | Anti- renal tubular oxidative damage | [92] |
| In vitro | BSB fermented with either *Bacillus subtilis* BCRC 14715 or *Bacillus* sp. CN11 | 2, 4, 6 mL | - | Assay of ACE inhibitory activity and the reducing power of the fermented BSB | Antioxidant activity | [93] |
| In vitro | solid fermentation of steamed BSB | 100 µg/mL | 4-nitroquinoline-N-oxide and Benzo[a]pyrene | Assay of mutagenicity | Mutagenicity and antimutagenicity effects | [94] |
| In vitro | BSB with *Bacillus subtilis* BCRC 14715 | 100 µg/mL | water, 80% methanol, 80% ethanol, 80% acetone | Assay of DPPH radical-scavenging effect, and $Fe^{2+}$-chelating activity | Antioxidant activity | [95] |
| Wistar albino rats and In vitro | Anthocyanin BSB seed coat | 100 µg/mL | UVB-induced apoptotic cell death | Assay of caspase-3, Bax, NF-κB, cylooxygenase-2 | Anti-skin cancer | [96,97] |
| In vitro | Hot water extracts of BSB | 100 µg/mL | Human adenovirus type 1 and coxsackievirus B1 | WST assay and in vitro antiviral assay | Antiviral activity | [98] |

ABTS—2,2'-azino-bis(3-ethylbenzothiazoline-6-sulphonic acid; AChE—acetyl choline esterase; ASK—1-Apoptosis signal-regulating kinase 1; BSB—Black soybeans; cAMP—cyclic adenosine mono phosphate; CD—cluster of differentiation; DCF—DA-dichlorofluorescein diacetate; DNA—Deoxy ribonucleic acid; DPPH—2,2-diphenyl-1-picrylhydrazyl; ERK—extracellular signal-regulated kinases; GABA—γ-aminobutyric acid; GFAP—Glial fibrillary acidic protein; HDL—C-high density lipoprotein cholesterol; HO—heme oxygenase; HPLC—high performance liquid chromatography; ICAM—intracellular adhesion molecule-1; IL—Interleukin; JNK—Jun N-terminal Kinase; LDH—lactate dehydrogenase; LDL-C—LDL-cholesterol; MAP kinase—mitogen-activated protein kinase; MDA—melondialdehyde; MS—mass spectroscopy; MTT—3-(4,5-dimethylthiazol-2-yl)-2,5-diphenyltetrazolium bromide; NF$_κ$B—nuclear factor kappa B; NO—nitric oxide; NRF-1—Nuclear factor erythroid 2-related factor 1; PARP—Poly (ADP-ribose) polymerase; PPAR—peroxisome proliferator-activated receptors; ROS—reactive oxygen species; RT-PCR—reverse transcriptase-polymerase chain reaction; TC—total cholesterol; TG—Triglycerides; TNF—tumor necrosis factor; TSP1—thrombospondin; VCAM—vascular cell adhesion molecule-1; VEGF—Vascular endothelial growth factor; PO—per oral.

*4.1. Enhance Bone Stability*

BSB has high content of proteins and fibers. It has an enormous amount of minerals such as calcium, phosphorous magnesium, iron, manganese, copper, and zinc, which contribute to maintain and stabilize the bone and its strength [99,100]. The study showed that the consumption of BSB has a definite protective effect on bone loss in postmenopausal osteoporosis study model and thereby BSB inhibits bone turnover and prevent bone resorption. This study confirmed that the intake of BSB can be used to prevent bone loss in estrogen deficiency animal studies [101]. In addition, the observational and acute clinical trial studies also suggested that the isoflavone-genistein reduces bone loss and enhances bone mineral density in osteopenic postmenopausal women [102].

*4.2. Reduce Blood Pressure*

Owing to the beneficial health effects on the human cardiovascular system, BSB has been a focus of intensive research. BSB contains a low concentration of sodium, which helps to maintain blood pressure at a normal range. A recent epidemiological study also showed that the anthocyanins rich BSB reduce the risk of cardiovascular diseases and maintain the blood pressure in the affected individuals [38,103]. In addition, BSB has potent inhibitory activity on collagen-induced platelet aggregation and reduce cardiovascular risk, and thereby improves blood circulation [104]. BSB has enormous quantities of fiber, potassium, folic acid, pyridoxal phosphate, and phytonutrients (quercetin and saponins) and lack of cholesterol, which supports to reduce cardiovascular complications. The fiber in BSB helps to lower total cholesterol (TC), LDL-cholesterol (LDL-C) in the blood and liver that reduce the risk of heart disease. It inhibits oxidative stress in postmenopausal women by increasing antioxidant activity and improving lipid profiles [105].

*4.3. Reduce Cardiovascular Complications*

The consumption of BSB may reduce the risk of coronary heart diseases. Recent researches have shown that BSB inhibit the effect of low density lipoprotein oxidation, inhibit TNF-alpha-induced vascular cell adhesion molecule-1 (VCAM), intracellular adhesion molecule-1 (ICAM), and cyclooxygenase-2 levels [83]. Further, anthocyanins protected myocardial injury from ischemia-reperfusion in rats [83]. Thus, anthocyanins from BSB seed coat benefit for pathological conditions like coronary heart diseases [84].

*4.4. In Managing Diabetes*

BSB is known to be rich in anthocyanins, and they have been consumed since ancient times for their beneficial effects on health. It has been reported that BSB seed coat may ameliorate obesity and insulin resistance [79]. BSB has more fibers, which have a vital role to reduce the blood sugar. Notably, one cup of BSB contributes around 15 g of fibers [106]. In addition, the BSB seed coat extract contains polyphenol-rich food material consisting of 9.2% cyanidin 3-glucoside, 6.2% catechins, 39.8% procyanidins, and others. These compounds remarkably prevent obesity and diabetes by enhancing energy expenditure and suppressing inflammation [107,108].

*4.5. Cancer Prevention*

Several studies showed that anthocyanins rich BSB have been shown to inhibit cancer cell growth by suppressing oxidative stress and inflammatory responses. Anthocyanin-rich BSB seed coat extract possibly reduces the development of tumors in various organs such as intestines [51], breast [109], prostate [65,110], stomach [80], ovary [111], endometrium [112], and liver [113]. In addition to the anthocyanins, saponins also prevent cancer cells from proliferation and spreading throughout the body [114]. BSB is high in folic acid, which plays a vital role in DNA synthesis and repair, thus BSB prevents the formation of cancer cells from DNA mutations [115].

*4.6. Reduce Body Weight*

BSB contain high quantity of fibers, which enhance satiety and decrease appetite, making an individual feel full for longer time, and thereby reduce the overall calorie intake [116]. Many studies have suggested that the consumption of anthocyanins rich BSB reduces the risk of adipogenic activity, obesity [40,117], fatty acid content in subcutaneous [118] and overall mortality while promoting a healthy complexion, visceral fat, increased energy, and overall reduce the body weight [49].

*4.7. Antimicrobial Actions*

Anthocyanins rich BSB may have antibacterial, anti-fungal, and anti-viral properties. The extract from BSB produced significant growth reductions of food borne pathogens such as *Escherichia coli*, *Salmonella typhimurium* and *Campylobacter jejuni* in broth-cultures as well as on chicken skin [119]. A previous study also showed an isolated monomeric protein (molecular mass of 25 kDa), containing N-terminal sequence, which resembles a segment of chitin synthase. The protein, named glysojanin, demonstrated a potent antifungal activity against *Fusarium oxysporum* and *Mycosphaerella arachidicola* and antiviral potential against HIV-1, human adenovirus type 1 and coxsackievirus B1 [98,120].

## 5. Conclusions

Black soybeans have popularly been utilized as a food and medicinal material for a long time with low price. Anthocyanins have antioxidant effect and can be useful for the treatment of diabetes, cardiovascular disorders, cancers, etc. Although the exact mechanism by which anthocyanins prevent the expression of adhesion molecules remains to be elucidated, they can be used as good materials to modulate or prevent such chronic diseases. In any case, more support for such properties/dynamic constituents has been acquired from cellular and molecular studies, while clinical studies are as yet inadequate. Since animal research does not generally interpret human circumstances, additional clinical studies are justified for comprehending the full interpretation of the effects of Anthocyanins in BSB for human disease prevention. Subsequently, futures far-reaching clinical studies are required to warrant the therapeutic convenience of anthocyanins in BSB. Furthermore, highlighting the synergistic multi-component effects of BSB on biological functions would be a recommendation for further studies, as well as studies of the mechanism of action and new biomarkers to prove the effectiveness of BSB bioactive compounds in preventing and treating several symptoms and/or pathologies.

**Acknowledgments:** The work was jointly supported by two grants UIC 201624 and UIC 201627 from Beijing Normal University-Hong Kong Baptist University United International College, Zhuhai, Guangdong, China.

**Author Contributions:** B.X. and K.G. conceived and designed the review; K.G. wrote the paper; B.X. critically read and improved the manuscript.

**Conflicts of Interest:** The authors declare no conflict of interest.

## References

1. Pandey, K.B.; Rizvi, S.I. Plant polyphenols as dietary antioxidants in human health and disease. *Oxid. Med. Cell. Longev.* **2009**, *2*, 270–278. [CrossRef] [PubMed]
2. He, X.; Sun, L.M. Dietary intake of flavonoid subclasses and risk of colorectal cancer: Evidence from population studies. *Oncotarget* **2016**, *7*, 26617–26627. [CrossRef] [PubMed]
3. Grosso, G.; Godos, J.; Lamuela-Raventos, R.; Ray, S.; Micek, A.; Pajak, A.; Sciacca, S.; D'Orazio, N.; Del Rio, D.; Galvano, F. A comprehensive meta-analysis on dietary flavonoid and lignan intake and cancer risk: Level of evidence and limitations. *Mol. Nutr. Food Res.* **2017**. [CrossRef] [PubMed]
4. Liu, Y.J.; Zhan, J.; Liu, X.L.; Wang, Y.; Ji, J.; He, Q.Q. Dietary flavonoids intake and risk of type 2 diabetes: A meta-analysis of prospective cohort studies. *Clin. Nutr.* **2014**, *33*, 59–63. [CrossRef] [PubMed]
5. Liu, X.M.; Liu, Y.J.; Huang, Y.; Yu, H.J.; Yuan, S.; Tang, B.W.; Wang, P.G.; He, Q.Q. Dietary total flavonoids intake and risk of mortality from all causes and cardiovascular disease in the general population: A systematic review and meta-analysis of cohort studies. *Mol. Nutr. Food Res.* **2017**. [CrossRef] [PubMed]

6.  Manach, C.; Scalbert, A.; Morand, C.; Rémésy, C.; Jiménez, L. Polyphenols: Food sources and bioavailability. *Am. J. Clin. Nutr.* **2004**, *79*, 727–747. [PubMed]

7.  Omodanisi, E.I.; Aboua, Y.G.; Oguntibeju, O.O. Assessment of the anti-hyperglycaemic, anti-inflammatory and antioxidant activities of the methanol extract of *Moringa oleifera* in diabetes-induced nephrotoxic male wistar rats. *Molecules* **2017**, *22*, 439. [CrossRef] [PubMed]

8.  Venkata, K.C.; Bagchi, D.; Bishayee, A. A small plant with big benefits: Fenugreek (*Trigonella foenum*-graecum Linn.) for disease prevention and health promotion. *Mol. Nutr. Food Res* **2017**. [CrossRef]

9.  Odongo, G.A.; Schlotz, N.; Herz, C.; Hanschen, F.S.; Baldermann, S.; Neugart, S.; Trierweiler, B.; Frommherz, L.; Franz, C.M.; Ngwene, B.; et al. The role of plant processing for the cancer preventive potential of Ethiopian kale (*Brassica carinata*). *Food Nutr. Res.* **2017**, *61*, 1271527. [CrossRef] [PubMed]

10. Luo, J.; Wei, Z.; Zhang, S.; Peng, X.; Huang, Y.; Zhang, Y.; Lu, J. Phenolic fractions from muscadine grape "Noble" Pomace can inhibit breast cancer cell MDA-MB-231 Better than those from European grape "Cabernet Sauvignon" and induces-phase arrest and apoptosis. *Food Sci.* **2017**. [CrossRef] [PubMed]

11. Franceschelli, S.; Pesce, M.; Ferrone, A.; Gatta, D.M.; Patruno, A.; Lutiis, M.A.; Quiles, J.L.; Grilli, A.; Felaco, M.; Speranza, L. Biological effect of licochalcone C on the regulation of PI3K/Akt/eNOS and NF-κB/iNOS/NO Signaling pathways in H9c2 cells in response to LPS stimulation. *Int. J. Mol. Sci.* **2017**, *18*, 690. [CrossRef] [PubMed]

12. Sajid, M.; Khan, M.R.; Shah, S.A.; Majid, M.; Ismail, H.; Maryam, S.; Batool, R.; Younis, T. Investigations on anti-inflammatory and analgesic activities of *Alnus nitida* Spach (Endl). stem bark in sprague dawley rats. *J. Ethnopharmacol.* **2017**, *198*, 407–416. [CrossRef] [PubMed]

13. Rodríguez, P.R.; Figueiredo-González, M.; González-Barreiro, C.; Simal-Gándara, J.; Salvador, M.D.; Cancho-Grande, B.; Fregapane, G. State of the art on functional virgin olive oils enriched with bioactive compounds and their properties. *Int. J. Mol. Sci.* **2017**, *18*, 668.

14. Léotoing, L.; Wauquier, F.; Davicco, M.J.; Lebecque, P.; Gaudout, D.; Rey, S.; Vitrac, X.; Massenat, L.; Rashidi, S.; Wittrant, Y.; et al. The phenolic acids of *Agen prunes* (dried plums) or Agen prune juice concentrates do not account for the protective action on bone in a rat model of postmenopausal osteoporosis. *Nutr. Res.* **2016**, *36*, 161–173. [CrossRef] [PubMed]

15. An, J.; Hao, D.; Zhang, Q.; Chen, B.; Zhang, R.; Wang, Y.; Yang, H. Natural products for treatment of bone-erosive diseases: The effects and mechanisms on inhibiting osteoclastogenesis and bone resorption. *Int. Immunopharmacol.* **2016**, *36*, 118–131. [CrossRef] [PubMed]

16. Ben Mansour, R.; Wided, M.K.; Cluzet, S.; Krisa, S.; Richard, T.; Ksouri, R. LC-MS identification and preparative HPLC isolation of *Frankenia pulverulenta* phenolics with antioxidant and neuroprotective capacities in PC12 cell line. *Pharm. Biol.* **2017**, *55*, 880–887. [CrossRef] [PubMed]

17. Sarrías, A.G.; Núñez-Sánchez, M.Á.; Tomás-Barberán, F.A.; Espín, J.C. Neurorotective effects of bioavailable polyphenol-derived metabolites against oxidative stress-induced cytotoxicity in human neuroblastoma SH-SY5Y Cells. *J. Agric. Food Chem.* **2017**, *65*, 752–758. [CrossRef] [PubMed]

18. Shaw, O.M.; Hurst, R.D.; Harper, J.L. Boysenberry ingestion supports fibrolytic macrophages with the capacity to ameliorate chronic lung remodeling. *Am. J. Physiol. Lung Cell. Mol. Physiol.* **2016**, *311*, L628–L638. [CrossRef] [PubMed]

19. Gómez, C.I.G.; González-Laredo, R.F.; Gallegos-Infante, J.A.; Pérez, M.D.; Moreno-Jiménez, M.R.; Flores-Rueda, A.G.; Rocha-Guzmán, N.E. Antioxidant and angiotensin-converting enzyme inhibitory activity of *Eucalyptus camaldulensis* and *Litsea glaucescens* infusions fermented with kombucha consortium. *Food Technol. Biotechnol.* **2016**, *54*, 367–374.

20. Nobile, V.; Michelotti, A.; Cestone, E.; Caturla, N.; Castillo, J.; Benavente-García, O.; Pérez-Sánchez, A.; Micol, V. Skin photoprotective and antiageing effects of a combination of rosemary (*Rosmarinus officinalis*) and grapefruit (*Citrus paradisi*) polyphenols. *Food Nutr. Res.* **2016**. [CrossRef] [PubMed]

21. Le Sage, F.; Meilhac, O.; Gonthier, M.P. Anti-inflammatory and antioxidant effects of polyphenols extracted from *Antirhea borbonica* medicinal plant on adipocytes exposed to *Porphyromonas gingivalis* and *Escherichia coli* lipopolysaccharides. *Pharmacol. Res.* **2017**, *119*, 303–312. [CrossRef] [PubMed]

22. Forte, M.; Conti, V.; Damato, A.; Ambrosio, M.; Puca, A.A.; Sciarretta, S.; Frati, G.; Vecchione, C.; Carrizzo, A. Targeting nitric oxide with natural derived compounds as a therapeutic strategy in vascular diseases. *Oxid. Med. Cell. Longev.* **2016**, *2016*, 7364138. [CrossRef] [PubMed]

23. Tenore, G.C.; Caruso, D.; Buonomo, G.; D'Avino, M.; Campiglia, P.; Marinelli, L.; Novellino, E. A healthy balance of plasma cholesterol by a novel Annurca apple-based nutraceutical formulation: Results of a randomized trial. *J. Med. Food* **2017**, *20*, 288–300. [CrossRef] [PubMed]
24. Jia, M.; Ren, D.; Nie, Y.; Yang, X. Beneficial effects of apple peel polyphenols on vascular endothelial dysfunction and liver injury in high choline-fed mice. *Food Funct.* **2017**, *8*, 1282–1292. [CrossRef] [PubMed]
25. Ayub, M.A.; Hussain, A.I.; Hanif, M.A.; Chatha, S.A.; Kamal, G.M.; Shahid, M.; Janneh, O. Variation in phenolic profile, β-carotene and flavonoid contents, biological activities of two Tagetes species from Pakistani flora. *Chem. Biodivers.* **2017**. [CrossRef] [PubMed]
26. Miyamoto, T.; Zhang, X.; Ueyama, Y.; Apisada, K.; Nakayama, M.; Suzuki, Y.; Ozawa, T.; Mitani, A.; Shigemune, N.; Shimatani, K.; et al. Development of novel monoclonal antibodies directed against catechins for investigation of antibacterial mechanism of catechins. *J. Microbiol. Methods* **2017**, *137*, 6–13. [CrossRef] [PubMed]
27. Alam, P.; Parvez, M.K.; Arbab, A.H.; Al-Dosari, M.S. Quantitative analysis of rutin, quercetin, naringenin, and gallic acid by validated RP- and NP-HPTLC methods for quality control of anti-HBV active extract of *Guiera senegalensis*. *Pharm Biol.* **2017**, *55*, 1317–1323. [CrossRef] [PubMed]
28. Kim, J.M.; Kim, J.S.; Yoo, H.; Choung, M.G.; Sung, M.K. Effects of black soybean [*Glycine max* (L.) Merr.] seed coats and its anthocyanidins on colonic inflammation and cell proliferation in vitro and in vivo. *J. Agric. Food Chem.* **2008**, *56*, 8427–8433. [CrossRef] [PubMed]
29. Choung, M.G.; Baek, I.Y.; Kang, S.T.; Han, W.Y.; Shin, D.C.; Moon, H.P.; Kang, K.H. Isolation and determination of anthocyanins in seed coats of black soybean (*Glycine max* (L.) Merr.). *J. Agric. Food Chem.* **2001**, *49*, 5848–5851. [CrossRef] [PubMed]
30. Omoni, A.O.; Aluko, R.E. Soybean foods and their benefits: Potential mechanisms of action. *Nutr. Rev.* **2005**, *63*, 272–283. [CrossRef] [PubMed]
31. Xiao, C.W. Health effects of soy protein and isoflavones in humans. *J. Nutr.* **2008**, *138*, 1244S–1249S. [PubMed]
32. Zhang, R.F.; Zhang, F.X.; Zhang, M.W.; Wei, Z.C.; Yang, C.Y.; Zhang, Y.; Tang, X.J.; Deng, Y.Y.; Chi, J.W. Phenolic composition and antioxidant activity in seed coats of 60 Chinese black soybean (*Glycine max* L. Merr.) varieties. *J. Agric. Food Chem.* **2011**, *59*, 5935–5944. [CrossRef] [PubMed]
33. Takahashi, R.; Ohmori, R.; Kiyose, C.; Momiyama, Y.; Ohsuzu, F.; Kondo, K. Antioxidant activities of black and yellow soybeans against low density lipoprotein oxidation. *J. Agric. Food Chem.* **2005**, *53*, 4578–4582. [CrossRef] [PubMed]
34. Xu, B.; Chang, S.K. Antioxidant capacity of seed coat, dehulled bean, and whole black soybeans in relation to their distributions of total phenolics, phenolic acids, anthocyanins, and isoflavones. *J. Agric. Food Chem.* **2008**, *56*, 8365–8373. [CrossRef] [PubMed]
35. Kim, J.A.; Jung, W.S.; Chun, S.C.; Yu, C.Y.; Ma, K.H.; Gwag, J.G.; Chung, I.M. A correlation between the level of phenolic compounds and the antioxidant capacity in cooked-with-rice and vegetable soybean (*Glycine max* L.) varieties. *Eur. Food Res. Technol.* **2006**, *224*, 259–270. [CrossRef]
36. Slavin, M.; Kenworthy, W.; Yu, L.L. Antioxidant properties, phytochemical composition, and antiproliferative activity of Maryland grown soybeans with colored seed coats. *J. Agric. Food Chem.* **2009**, *57*, 11174–11185. [CrossRef] [PubMed]
37. Kusunoki, M.; Sato, D.; Tsutsumi, K.; Tsutsui, H.; Nakamura, T.; Oshida, Y. Black soybean extract improves lipid profiles in fenofibrate-treated type 2 diabetics with postprandial hyperlipidemia. *J. Med Food.* **2015**, *18*, 615–618. [CrossRef] [PubMed]
38. Zou, P. Traditional Chinese medicine, food therapy, and hypertension control: A narrative review of Chinese literature. *Am. J. Chin. Med.* **2016**, *44*, 1579–1594. [CrossRef] [PubMed]
39. Tan, Y.; Chang, S.K.; Zhang, Y. Innovative soaking and grinding methods and cooking affect the retention of isoflavones, antioxidant and antiproliferative properties in soymilk prepared from black soybean. *J. Food Sci.* **2016**, *81*, H1016–H1023. [CrossRef] [PubMed]
40. Matsukawa, T.; Villareal, M.O.; Motojima, H.; Isoda, H. Increasing cAMP levels of preadipocytes by cyanidin-3-glucoside treatment induces the formation of beige phenotypes in 3T3-L1 adipocytes. *J. Nutr. Biochem.* **2017**, *40*, 77–85. [CrossRef] [PubMed]
41. Ensminger, M.E.; Oldfield, J.E.; Heinemann, W.W. *Feeds and Nutrition*; The Ensminger Publishing Company: Clovis, CA, USA, 1990.

42. Fetriyuna, F. The potential of darmo black soybean varieties as an alternative of a promising food for future. *Int. J. Adv. Sci. Eng. Inf. Technol.* **2015**, *5*, 44–46. [CrossRef]

43. National Research Council (NRC). *Nutrient Requirements of Swine*, 10th ed.; National Academy Press: Washington, DC, USA, 1998.

44. Katsuzaki, H.; Hibasami, H.; Ohwaki, S.; Ishikawa, K.; Imai, K.; Date, K.; Kimura, Y.; Komiya, T. Cyanidin-3-*O*-beta-D-glucoside isolated from skin of black *Glycine max* and other anthocyanins isolated from skin of red grape induce apoptosis in human lymphoid leukemia Molt 4B cells. *Oncol. Rep.* **2003**, *10*, 297–300. [PubMed]

45. Lee, J.H.; Kang, N.S.; Shin, S.-O.; Shin, S.-H.; Lim, S.-G.; Suh, D.-Y.; Baek, I.-Y.; Park, K.-Y.; Ha, T.J. Characterisation of anthocyanins in the black soybean (*Glycine max* L.) by HPLC-DAD-ESI/MS analysis. *Food Chem.* **2009**, *112*, 226–231. [CrossRef]

46. Koh, K.; Youn, J.E.; Kim, H.S. Identification of anthocyanins in black soybean (*Glycine max* (L.) Merr.) varieties. *J. Food Sci. Technol.* **2014**, *51*, 377–381. [CrossRef] [PubMed]

47. Fukami, H.; Yano, Y.; Iwashita, T. Isolation of a reduced form of cyanidin 3-*O*-β-D-glucoside from immature black soybean (*Glycine max* (L.) Merr.) and its reducing properties. *J. Oleo Sci.* **2013**, *62*, 623–629. [CrossRef] [PubMed]

48. Khan, M.S.; Ali, T.; Kim, M.W.; Jo, M.H.; Jo, M.G.; Badshah, H.; Kim, M.O. Anthocyanins protect against LPS-induced oxidative stress-mediated neuroinflammation and neurodegeneration in the adult mouse cortex. *Neurochem. Int.* **2016**, *100*, 1–10. [CrossRef] [PubMed]

49. Lee, M.; Sorn, S.R.; Park, Y.; Park, H.K. Anthocyanin rich-black soybean testa improved visceral fat and plasma lipid profiles in overweight/obese Korean adults: A randomized controlled trial. *J. Med. Food* **2016**, *19*, 995–1003. [CrossRef] [PubMed]

50. Min, H.K.; Kim, S.M.; Baek, S.Y.; Woo, J.W.; Park, J.S.; Cho, M.L.; Lee, J.; Kwok, S.K.; Kim, S.W.; Park, S.H. Anthocyanin extracted from black soybean seed coats prevents autoimmune arthritis by suppressing the development of Th17 Cells and synthesis of proinflammatory cytokines by such cells, via inhibition of NF-κB. *PLoS ONE* **2015**, *10*, e0138201. [CrossRef] [PubMed]

51. Park, M.Y.; Kim, J.M.; Kim, J.S.; Choung, M.G.; Sung, M.K. Chemopreventive action of anthocyanin-rich black soybean fraction in APC (Min/+) intestinal polyposis Model. *J. Cancer Prev.* **2015**, *20*, 193–201. [CrossRef] [PubMed]

52. Cooke, D.; Schwarz, M.; Boocock, D.; Winterhalter, P.; Steward, W.P.; Gescher, A.J.; Marczylo, T.H. Effect of cyanidin-3-glucoside and an anthocyanin mixture from bilberry on adenoma development in the ApcMin mouse model of intestinal carcinogenesis–relationship with tissue anthocyanin levels. *Int. J. Cancer* **2006**, *119*, 2213–2220. [CrossRef] [PubMed]

53. Hashimoto, N.; Oki, T.; Sasaki, K.; Suda, I.; Okuno, S. Black soybean seed coat extract prevents hydrogen peroxide-mediated cell death via extracellular signal-related kinase signalling in HepG2 cells. *J. Nutr. Sci. Vitaminol.* **2015**, *61*, 275–279. [CrossRef] [PubMed]

54. Kim, S.M.; Chung, M.J.; Ha, T.J.; Choi, H.N.; Jang, S.J.; Kim, S.O.; Chun, M.H.; Do, S.I.; Choo, Y.K.; Park, Y.I. Neuroprotective effects of black soybean anthocyanins via inactivation of ASK1-JNK/p38 pathways and mobilization of cellular sialic acids. *Life Sci.* **2012**, *90*, 874–882. [CrossRef] [PubMed]

55. Zhang, T.; Jiang, S.; He, C.; Kimura, Y.; Yamashita, Y.; Ashida, H. Black soybean seed coat polyphenols prevent B(a)P-induced DNA damage through modulating drug-metabolizing enzymes in HepG2 cells and ICR mice. *Mutat. Res.* **2013**, *752*, 34–41. [CrossRef] [PubMed]

56. Jeong, J.H.; Kim, H.J.; Park, S.K.; Jin, D.E.; Kwon, O.J.; Kim, H.J.; Heo, H.J. An investigation into the ameliorating effect of black soybean extract on learning and memory impairment with assessment of neuroprotective effects. *BMC Complement. Altern. Med.* **2014**, *14*, 482. [CrossRef] [PubMed]

57. Mok, J.W.; Chang, D.J.; Joo, C.K. Antiapoptotic effects of anthocyanin from the seed coat of black soybean against oxidative damage of human lens epithelial cell induced by $H_2O_2$. *Curr. Eye Res.* **2014**, *39*, 1090–1098. [CrossRef] [PubMed]

58. Bhuiyan, M.I.; Kim, J.Y.; Ha, T.J.; Kim, S.Y.; Cho, K.O. Anthocyanins extracted from black soybean seed coat protect primary cortical neurons against in vitro ischemia. *Biol. Pharm. Bull.* **2012**, *35*, 999–1008. [CrossRef] [PubMed]

59. Matsukawa, T.; Inaguma, T.; Han, J.; Villareal, M.O.; Isoda, H. Cyanidin-3-glucoside derived from black soybeans ameliorate type 2 diabetes through the induction of differentiation of preadipocytes into smaller and insulin-sensitive adipocytes. *J. Nutr. Biochem.* **2015**, *26*, 860–867. [CrossRef] [PubMed]

60. Kim, H.K.; Kim, J.N.; Han, S.N.; Nam, J.H.; Na, H.N.; Ha, T.J. Black soybean anthocyanins inhibit adipocyte differentiation in 3T3-L1 cells. *Nutr. Res.* **2012**, *32*, 770–777. [CrossRef] [PubMed]

61. Badshah, H.; Kim, T.H.; Kim, M.O. Protective effects of anthocyanins against amyloid beta-induced neurotoxicity in vivo and in vitro. *Neurochem. Int.* **2015**, *80*, 51–59. [CrossRef] [PubMed]

62. Ali Shah, S.; Ullah, I.; Lee, H.Y.; Kim, M.O. Anthocyanins protect against ethanol-induced neuronal apoptosis via GABAB1 receptors intracellular signaling in prenatal rat hippocampal neurons. *Mol. Neurobiol.* **2013**, *48*, 257–269. [CrossRef] [PubMed]

63. Shah, S.A.; Yoon, G.H.; Kim, M.O. Protection of the developing brain with anthocyanins against ethanol-induced oxidative stress and neurodegeneration. *Mol. Neurobiol.* **2015**, *51*, 1278–1291. [CrossRef] [PubMed]

64. Ullah, I.; Park, H.Y.; Kim, M.O. Anthocyanins protect against kainic acid-induced excitotoxicity and apoptosis via ROS-activated AMPK pathway in hippocampal neurons. *CNS Neurosci. Ther.* **2014**, *20*, 327–338. [CrossRef] [PubMed]

65. Ha, U.S.; Bae, W.J.; Kim, S.J.; Yoon, B.I.; Hong, S.H.; Lee, J.Y.; Hwang, T.K.; Hwang, S.Y.; Wang, Z.; Kim, S.W. Anthocyanin induces apoptosis of DU-145 cells in vitro and inhibits xenograft growth of prostate cancer. *Yonsei Med. J.* **2015**, *56*, 16–23. [CrossRef] [PubMed]

66. Badshah, H.; Ali, T.; Ahmad, A.; Kim, M.J.; Abid, N.B.; Shah, S.A.; Yoon, G.H.; Lee, H.Y.; Kim, M.O. Co-treatment with anthocyanins and vitamin-C ameliorates ethanol-induced neurodegeneration via modulation of gabab receptor signaling in the adult rat brain. *CNS Neurol. Disord. Drug Target.* **2015**, *14*, 791–803. [CrossRef]

67. Sohn, D.W.; Bae, W.J.; Kim, H.S.; Kim, S.W.; Kim, S.W. The anti-inflammatory and antifibrosis effects of anthocyanin extracted from black soybean on a Peyronie disease rat model. *Urology* **2014**, *84*, 1112–1116. [CrossRef] [PubMed]

68. De Moraes Filho, M.L.; Hirozawa, S.S.; Prudencio, S.H.; Ida, E.I.; Garcia, S. Petit suisse from black soybean: Bioactive compounds and antioxidant properties during development process. *Int. J. Food Sci. Nutr.* **2014**, *65*, 470–475. [CrossRef] [PubMed]

69. Jeong, J.H.; Jo, Y.N.; Kim, H.J.; Jin, D.E.; Kim, D.O.; Heo, H.J. Black soybean extract protects against TMT-induced cognitive defects in mice. *J. Med. Food* **2014**, *17*, 83–91. [CrossRef] [PubMed]

70. Yoon, B.I.; Bae, W.J.; Choi, Y.S.; Kim, S.J.; Ha, U.S.; Hong, S.H.; Sohn, D.W.; Kim, S.W. The anti-inflammatory and antimicrobial effects of anthocyanin extracted from black soybean on chronic bacterial prostatitis rat model. *Chin. J. Integr. Med.* **2013**. [CrossRef] [PubMed]

71. Hsu, C.K.; Lin, W.H.; Yang, H.W. Influence of preheating on antioxidant activity of the water extract from black soybean and color and sensory properties of black soybean decoction. *J. Sci. Food Agric.* **2013**, *93*, 3883–3890. [CrossRef] [PubMed]

72. Lin, Y.C.; Chou, C.C. Effect of heat treatment on total phenolic and anthocyanin contents as well as antioxidant activity of the extract from *Aspergillus awamori*-fermented black soybeans, a healthy food ingredient. *Int. J. Food Sci. Nutr.* **2009**, *60*, 627–636. [CrossRef] [PubMed]

73. Malenčić, D.; Maksimović, Z.; Popović, M.; Miladinović, J. Polyphenol contents and antioxidant activity of soybean seed extracts. *Bioresour. Technol.* **2008**, *99*, 688–691. [CrossRef] [PubMed]

74. Xu, B.; Chang, S.K. Total phenolics, phenolic acids, isoflavones, and anthocyanins and antioxidant properties of yellow and black soybeans as affected by thermal processing. *J. Agric. Food Chem.* **2008**, *56*, 7165–7175. [CrossRef] [PubMed]

75. Xu, B.; Chang, S.K. Characterization of phenolic substances and antioxidant properties of food soybeans grown in the North Dakota-Minnesota region. *J. Agric. Food Chem.* **2008**, *56*, 9102–9113. [CrossRef] [PubMed]

76. Badshah, H.; Ullah, I.; Kim, S.E.; Kim, T.H.; Lee, H.Y.; Kim, M.O. Anthocyanins attenuate body weight gain via modulating neuropeptide Y and GABAB1 receptor in rats hypothalamus. *Neuropeptides* **2013**, *47*, 347–353. [CrossRef] [PubMed]

77. Kwon, S.H.; Ahn, I.S.; Kim, S.O.; Kong, C.S.; Chung, H.Y.; Do, M.S.; Park, K.Y. Anti-obesity and hypolipidemic effects of black soybean anthocyanins. *J. Med. Food* **2007**, *10*, 552–556. [CrossRef] [PubMed]

78. Oh, H.G.; Kang, Y.R.; Lee, H.Y.; Kim, J.H.; Shin, E.H.; Lee, B.G.; Park, S.H.; Moon, D.I.; Kim, O.J.; Lee, I.A.; et al. Ameliorative effects of *Monascus pilosus*-fermented black soybean (*Glycine max* L. Merrill) on high-fat diet-induced obesity. *J. Med. Food* **2014**, *17*, 972–978. [CrossRef] [PubMed]

79. Kurimoto, Y.; Shibayama, Y.; Inoue, S.; Soga, M.; Takikawa, M.; Ito, C.; Nanba, F.; Yoshida, T.; Yamashita, Y.; Ashida, H.; et al. Black soybean seed coat extract ameliorates hyperglycemia and insulin sensitivity via the activation of AMP-activated protein kinase in diabetic mice. *J. Agric. Food Chem.* **2013**, *61*, 5558–5564. [CrossRef] [PubMed]

80. Kim, J.M.; Kim, K.M.; Park, E.H.; Seo, J.H.; Song, J.Y.; Shin, S.C.; Kang, H.L.; Lee, W.K.; Cho, M.J.; Rhee, K.H.; et al. Anthocyanins from black soybean inhibit Helicobacter pylori-induced inflammation in human gastric epithelial AGS cells. *Microbiol. Immunol.* **2013**, *57*, 366–373. [CrossRef] [PubMed]

81. Xu, L.; Choi, T.H.; Kim, S.; Kim, S.H.; Chang, H.W.; Choe, M.; Kwon, S.Y.; Hur, J.A.; Shin, S.C.; Chung, J.I.; et al. Anthocyanins from black soybean seed coat enhance wound healing. *Ann. Plast. Surg.* **2013**, *71*, 415–420. [CrossRef] [PubMed]

82. Nizamutdinova, I.T.; Kim, Y.M.; Chung, J.I.; Shin, S.C.; Jeong, Y.K.; Seo, H.G.; Lee, J.H.; Chang, K.C.; Kim, H.J. Anthocyanins from black soybean seed coats stimulate wound healing in fibroblasts and keratinocytes and prevent inflammation in endothelial cells. *Food Chem. Toxicol.* **2009**, *47*, 2806–2812. [CrossRef] [PubMed]

83. Kim, H.J.; Xu, L.; Chang, K.C.; Shin, S.C.; Chung, J.I.; Kang, D.; Kim, S.H.; Hur, J.A.; Choi, T.H.; Kim, S.; et al. Anti-inflammatory effects of anthocyanins from black soybean seed coat on the keratinocytes and ischemia-reperfusion injury in rat skin flaps. *Microsurgery* **2012**, *32*, 563–570. [CrossRef] [PubMed]

84. Kim, H.J.; Tsoy, I.; Park, J.M.; Chung, J.I.; Shin, S.C.; Chang, K.C. Anthocyanins from soybean seed coat inhibit the expression of TNF-alpha-induced genes associated with ischemia/reperfusion in endothelial cell by NF-kappaB-dependent pathway and reduce rat myocardial damages incurred by ischemia and reperfusion in vivo. *FEBS Lett.* **2006**, *580*, 1391–1397. [CrossRef] [PubMed]

85. Jeong, J.W.; Lee, W.S.; Shin, S.C.; Kim, G.Y.; Choi, B.T.; Choi, Y.H. Anthocyanins down-regulate lipopolysaccharide-induced inflammatory responses in BV2 microglial cells by suppressing the NF-κB and Akt/MAPKs signaling pathways. *Int. J. Mol. Sci.* **2013**, *14*, 1502–1515. [CrossRef] [PubMed]

86. Choe, Y.J.; Ha, T.J.; Ko, K.W.; Lee, S.Y.; Shin, S.J.; Kim, H.S. Anthocyanins in the black soybean (*Glycine max* L.) protect U2OS cells from apoptosis by inducing autophagy via the activation of adenosyl monophosphate-dependent protein kinase. *Oncol. Rep.* **2012**, *28*, 2049–2056. [PubMed]

87. Jang, H.; Kim, S.J.; Yuk, S.M.; Han, D.S.; Ha, U.S.; Hong, S.H.; Lee, J.Y.; Hwang, T.K.; Hwang, S.Y.; Kim, S.W. Effects of anthocyanin extracted from black soybean seed coat on spermatogenesis in a rat varicocele-induced model. *Reprod. Fertil. Dev.* **2012**, *24*, 649–655. [CrossRef] [PubMed]

88. Jang, H.; Ha, U.S.; Kim, S.J.; Yoon, B.I.; Han, D.S.; Yuk, S.M.; Kim, S.W. Anthocyanin extracted from black soybean reduces prostate weight and promotes apoptosis in the prostatic hyperplasia-induced rat model. *J. Agric. Food Chem.* **2010**, *58*, 12686–12691. [CrossRef] [PubMed]

89. Paik, S.S.; Jeong, E.; Jung, S.W.; Ha, T.J.; Kang, S.; Sim, S.; Jeon, J.H.; Chun, M.H.; Kim, I.B. Anthocyanins from the seed coat of black soybean reduce retinal degeneration induced by N-methyl-N-nitrosourea. *Exp. Eye Res.* **2012**, *97*, 55–62. [CrossRef] [PubMed]

90. Lin, C.C.; Wu, P.S.; Liang, D.W.; Kwan, C.C.; Chen, Y.S. Quality, antioxidative ability, and cell proliferation-enhancing activity of fermented black soybean broths with various supplemental culture medium. *J. Food Sci.* **2012**, *77*, C95–C101. [CrossRef] [PubMed]

91. Kim, Y.K.; Yoon, H.H.; Lee, Y.D.; Youn, D.Y.; Ha, T.J.; Kim, H.S.; Lee, J.H. Anthocyanin extracts from black soybean (*Glycine max* L.) protect human glial cells against oxygen-glucose deprivation by promoting autophagy. *Biomol. Ther. (Seoul)* **2012**, *20*, 68–74. [CrossRef] [PubMed]

92. Okazaki, Y.; Iqbal, M.; Kawakami, N.; Yamamoto, Y.; Toyokuni, S.; Okada, S. A beverage containing fermented black soybean ameliorates ferric nitrilotriacetate-induced renal oxidative damage in rats. *J. Clin. Biochem. Nutr.* **2010**, *47*, 198–207. [CrossRef] [PubMed]

93. Juan, M.Y.; Wu, C.H.; Chou, C.C. Fermentation with *Bacillus* spp. as a bioprocess to enhance anthocyanin content, the angiotensin converting enzyme inhibitory effect, and the reducing activity of black soybeans. *Food Microbiol.* **2010**, *27*, 918–923. [CrossRef] [PubMed]

94. Hung, Y.H.; Huang, H.Y.; Chou, C.C. Mutagenic and antimutagenic effects of methanol extracts of unfermented and fermented black soybeans. *Int. J. Food Microbiol.* **2007**, *118*, 62–68. [CrossRef] [PubMed]

95. Juan, M.Y.; Chou, C.C. Enhancement of antioxidant activity, total phenolic and flavonoid content of black soybeans by solid state fermentation with *Bacillus subtilis* BCRC 14715. *Food Microbiol.* **2010**, *27*, 586–591. [CrossRef] [PubMed]

96. Tsoyi, K.; Park, H.B.; Kim, Y.M.; Chung, J.I.; Shin, S.C.; Lee, W.S.; Seo, H.G.; Lee, J.H.; Chang, K.C.; Kim, H.J. Anthocyanins from black soybean seed coats inhibit UVB-induced inflammatory cylooxygenase-2 gene expression and PGE2 production through regulation of the nuclear factor-kappaB and phosphatidylinositol 3-kinase/Akt pathway. *J. Agric. Food Chem.* **2008**, *56*, 8969–8974. [CrossRef] [PubMed]

97. Tsoyi, K.; Park, H.B.; Kim, Y.M.; Chung, J.I.; Shin, S.C.; Shim, H.J.; Lee, W.S.; Seo, H.G.; Lee, J.H.; Chang, K.C.; et al. Protective effect of anthocyanins from black soybean seed coats on UVB-induced apoptotic cell death in vitro and in vivo. *J. Agric. Food Chem.* **2008**, *56*, 10600–10605. [CrossRef] [PubMed]

98. Yamai, M.; Tsumura, K.; Kimura, M.; Fukuda, S.; Murakami, T.; Kimura, Y. Antiviral activity of a hot water extract of black soybean against a human respiratory illness virus. *Biosci. Biotechnol. Biochem.* **2003**, *67*, 1071–1079. [CrossRef] [PubMed]

99. Ho, S.C.; Woo, J.; Lam, S.; Chen, Y.; Sham, A.; Lau, J. Soy protein consumption and bone mass in early postmenopausal Chinese women. *Osteoporosis Int.* **2003**, *14*, 835–842. [CrossRef] [PubMed]

100. Hirata, H.; Kitamura, K.; Saito, T.; Kobayashi, R.; Iwasaki, M.; Yoshihara, A.; Watanabe, Y.; Oshiki, R.; Nishiwaki, T.; Nakamura, K. Association between dietary intake and bone mineral density in Japanese postmenopausal women: The Yokogoshi cohort study. *Tohoku J. Exp. Med.* **2016**, *239*, 95–101. [CrossRef] [PubMed]

101. Byun, J.S.; Lee, S.S. Effect of soybeans and sword beans on bone metabolism in a rat model of osteoporosis. *Ann. Nutr. Metab.* **2010**, *56*, 106–112. [CrossRef] [PubMed]

102. Marini, H.; Minutoli, L.; Polito, F.; Bitto, A.; Altavilla, D.; Atteritano, M.; Gaudio, A.; Mazzaferro, S.; Frisina, A.; Frisina, N.; et al. Effects of the phytoestrogen genistein on bone metabolism in osteopenic postmenopausal women: A randomized trial. *Ann. Intern. Med.* **2007**, *146*, 839–847. [CrossRef] [PubMed]

103. Hooper, L.; Kroon, P.A.; Rimm, E.B.; Cohn, J.S.; Harvey, I.; Le Cornu, K.A.; Ryder, J.J.; Hall, W.L.; Cassidy, A. Flavonoids, flavonoid-rich foods, and cardiovascular risk: a meta-analysis of randomized controlled trials. *Am. J. Clin. Nutr.* **2008**, *88*, 38–50. [PubMed]

104. Kim, K.; Lim, K.M.; Kim, C.W.; Shin, H.J.; Seo, D.B.; Lee, S.J.; Noh, J.Y.; Bae, O.N.; Shin, S.; Chung, J.H. Black soybean extract can attenuate thrombosis through inhibition of collagen-induced platelet activation. *J. Nutr. Biochem.* **2011**, *22*, 964–970. [CrossRef] [PubMed]

105. Byun, J.S.; Han, Y.S.; Lee, S.S. The effects of yellow soybean, black soybean, and sword bean on lipid levels and oxidative stress in ovariectomized rats. *Int. J. Vitam. Nutr. Res.* **2010**, *80*, 97–106. [CrossRef] [PubMed]

106. Ríos, J.L.; Francini, F.; Schinella, G.R. Natural Products for the Treatment of Type 2 Diabetes Mellitus. *Planta Med.* **2015**, *81*, 975–994. [CrossRef] [PubMed]

107. Kwak, J.H.; Lee, J.H.; Ahn, C.W.; Park, S.H.; Shim, S.T.; Song, Y.D.; Han, E.N.; Lee, K.H.; Chae, J.S. Black soy peptide supplementation improves glucose control in subjects with prediabetes and newly diagnosed type 2 diabetes mellitus. *J. Med. Food* **2010**, *3*, 1307–1312. [CrossRef] [PubMed]

108. Kanamoto, Y.; Yamashita, Y.; Nanba, F.; Yoshida, T.; Tsuda, T.; Fukuda, I.; Nakamura-Tsuruta, S.; Ashida, H. A black soybean seed coat extract prevents obesity and glucose intolerance by up-regulating uncoupling proteins and down-regulating inflammatory cytokines in high-fat diet-fed mice. *J. Agric. Food Chem.* **2011**, *59*, 8985–8993. [CrossRef] [PubMed]

109. Wu, Y.Y.; Liu, H.Y.; Huang, T.C.; Chen, J.H.; Chang, P.Y.; Ho, C.L.; Chao, T.Y. A phase II double-blinded study to evaluate the efficacy of EW02 in reducing chemotherapy-induced neutropenia in breast cancer. *Oncol. Lett.* **2015**, *10*, 1793–1798. [CrossRef] [PubMed]

110. Chia, J.S.; Du, J.L.; Wu, M.S.; Hsu, W.B.; Chiang, C.P.; Sun, A.; Lu, J.J.; Wang, W.B. Fermentation product of soybean, black bean, and green bean mixture induces apoptosis in a wide variety of cancer cells. *Integr. Cancer Ther.* **2013**, *12*, 248–256. [CrossRef] [PubMed]

111. Xu, B.; Chang, S.K. Comparative study on antiproliferation properties and cellular antioxidant activities of commonly consumed food legumes against nine human cancer cell lines. *Food Chem.* **2012**, *134*, 1287–1296. [CrossRef] [PubMed]

112. Horn-Ross, P.L.; John, E.M.; Canchola, A.J.; Stewart, S.L.; Lee, M.M. Phytoestrogen intake and endometrial cancer risk. *J. Natl. Cancer Inst.* **2003**, *95*, 1158–1164. [CrossRef] [PubMed]

113. Ye, X.J.; Ng, T.B. Antitumor and HIV-1 reverse transcriptase inhibitory activities of a hemagglutinin and a protease inhibitor from mini-black soybean. *Evid. Based Complement. Altern. Med.* **2011**, *2011*, 851396. [CrossRef] [PubMed]

114. Xu, B.; Chang, S.K. Reduction of antiproliferative capacities, cell-based antioxidant capacities and phytochemical contents of common beans and soybeans upon thermal processing. *Food Chem.* **2011**, *129*, 974–981. [CrossRef] [PubMed]

115. Azaïs, H.; Frochot, C.; Grabarz, A.; Khodja Bach, S.; Colombeau, L.; Delhem, N.; Mordon, S.; Collinet, P. Specific folic-acid targeted photosensitizer. The first step toward intraperitoneal photodynamic therapy for epithelial ovarian cancer. *Gynecol. Obstet. Fertil. Senol.* **2017**, *45*, 190–196. [PubMed]

116. Giusti, F.; Caprioli, G.; Ricciutelli, M.; Vittori, S.; Sagratini, G. Determination of fourteen polyphenols in pulses by high performance liquid chromatography-diode array detection (HPLC-DAD) and correlation study with antioxidant activity and colour. *Food Chem.* **2017**, *221*, 689–697. [CrossRef] [PubMed]

117. Jeon, Y.; Lee, M.; Cheon, Y.P. A testa extract of black soybean (*Glycine max* (L.) Merr.) suppresses adipogenic activity of adipose-derived stem cells. *Dev. Reprod.* **2015**, *19*, 235–242. [CrossRef] [PubMed]

118. Sato, D.; Kusunoki, M.; Seino, N.; Nishina, A.; Feng, Z.; Tsutsumi, K.; Nakamura, T. Black soybean extract reduces fatty acid contents in subcutaneous, but not in visceral adipose triglyceride in high-fat fed rats. *Int. J. Food Sci. Nutr.* **2015**, *66*, 539–545. [CrossRef] [PubMed]

119. Abutheraa, R.; Hettiarachchy, N.; Kumar-Phillips, G.; Horax, R.; Chen, P.; Morawicki, R.; Kwon, Y.M. Antimicrobial activities of phenolic extracts derived from seed coats of selected soybean varieties. *J. Food Sci.* **2017**, *82*, 731–737. [CrossRef] [PubMed]

120. Ngai, P.H.; Ng, T.B. Purification of glysojanin, an antifungal protein, from the black soybean *Glycine soja*. *Biochem. Cell Biol.* **2003**, *81*, 387–394. [CrossRef] [PubMed]

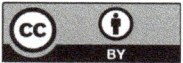

![nutrients logo] *nutrients*

MDPI

*Article*

# The Effect of Isomaltulose Together with Green Tea on Glycemic Response and Antioxidant Capacity: A Single-Blind, Crossover Study in Healthy Subjects

Passakorn Suraphad, Phim On Suklaew, Sathaporn Ngamukote, Sirichai Adisakwattana and Kittana Mäkynen *

Department of Nutrition and Dietetics, Faculty of Allied Health Sciences, Chulalongkorn University, Bangkok 10330, Thailand; tostimulus@hotmail.com (P.S.); red_flower_bow@hotmail.com (P.O.S.); amppam10@gmail.com (S.N.); Sirichai.a@chula.ac.th (S.A.)
* Correspondence: Kittana.m@chula.ac.th; Tel.: +662-218-1099

Received: 7 April 2017; Accepted: 3 May 2017; Published: 6 May 2017

**Abstract:** Isomaltulose, a naturally-occurring isomer of sucrose, is commonly used as an alternative sweetener in foods and beverages. The goal of this study was to determine the effect of isomaltulose together with green tea on postprandial plasma glucose and insulin concentration, as well as antioxidant capacity in healthy subjects. In a randomized, single-blind, crossover study, 15 healthy subjects (eight women and seven men; ages $23.5 \pm 0.7$ years; with body mass index of $22.6 \pm 0.4$ kg/m$^2$) consumed five beverages: (1) 50 g sucrose in 400 mL water; (2) 50 g isomaltulose in 400 mL of water; (3) 400 mL of green tea; (4) 50 g sucrose in 400 mL of green tea; and (5) 50 g isomaltulose in 400 mL of green tea. Incremental area under postprandial plasma glucose, insulin, ferric reducing ability of plasma (FRAP) and malondialdehyde (MDA) concentration were determined during 120 min of administration. Following the consumption of isomaltulose, the incremental 2-h area under the curve ($AUC_{0-2\,h}$) indicated a higher reduction of postprandial glucose (43.4%) and insulin concentration (42.0%) than the consumption of sucrose. The addition of green tea to isomaltulose produced a greater suppression of postprandial plasma glucose (20.9%) and insulin concentration (37.7%). In accordance with antioxidant capacity, consumption of sucrose (40.0%) and isomaltulose (28.7%) caused the reduction of green tea-induced postprandial increases in FRAP. A reduction in postprandial MDA after drinking green tea was attenuated when consumed with sucrose (34.7%) and isomaltulose (17.2%). In conclusion, green tea could enhance the reduction of postprandial glucose and insulin concentration when consumed with isomaltulose. In comparison with sucrose, isomaltulose demonstrated less alteration of plasma antioxidant capacity after being consumed with green tea.

**Keywords:** isomaltulose; green tea; sucrose; glycemic response; antioxidant capacity

---

## 1. Introduction

There has been a marked increase in the consumption of sugar-sweetened beverages across the globe [1,2]. Recent evidence has been able to substantiate the relationship between the consumption of sugar-sweetened beverages and the risks of type 2 diabetes, obesity and cardiovascular diseases [3]. A number of randomized clinical trials have reported that the consumption of sweetened beverages increased body weight and fat mass after 10 weeks [4]. There has been increasing concern regarding the health effects of being overweight and obesity in adults, and this has, therefore, led to a rising demand for low-energy food products. Low-glycemic sweeteners commonly offer an alternative approach to using caloric sugars as substitutes for sucrose and high fructose corn syrup in foods and beverages [5–7].

Isomaltulose (6-*O*-D-glucopyranosyl-D-fructose), one type of low-glycemic sweetener, is a naturally-occurring disaccharide found in honey, sugarcane and molasses [8]. Like sucrose, it is digested by α-glucosidase in the small intestine and contributes the same caloric value of approximately 4 kcal/g [9,10]. However, the rates of isomaltulose digestion and absorption are much slower than sucrose [11,12]. Furthermore, the consumption of isomaltulose was found to be safe without gastrointestinal side effects [8]. Clinical studies provided more convincing evidence in support of isomaltulose for controlling postprandial glucose profile in humans [12–14]. Therefore, isomaltulose has been applied most recently in ready-to-drink products, such as sports drinks, instant drinks and milk-based drinks [10,15].

Green tea (*Camellia sinensis*), one of the most popular beverages in the world, is a rich source of polyphenols, specifically, epicatechin (EC), epicatechin gallate (ECG) and epigallocatechin gallate (EGCG) [16]. Evidence from cohort studies showed an association between higher intake of tea-derived polyphenols, such as flavan-3-ols [17,18] and, more specifically, catechins and theaflavins [19], and lower risk of impaired glucose metabolism. However, no correlation was found for other polyphenol groups [20]. Several studies have shown the beneficial effects of green tea, including anti-hyperglycemic, anti-oxidative, anti-carcinogenic, anti-inflammatory and hypocholesterolemic activity [21–23]. For example, catechin-rich green tea improves postprandial glucose concentration and plasma antioxidant capacity in human subjects [24,25]. In a clinical trial, consumption of 1.5 g green tea extracts in 500 mL water (total polyphenols with approximately 500 mg gallic acid equivalent) with 75 g glucose decreased postprandial plasma glucose concentration in healthy subjects [26]. In a randomized crossover design, consumption of 50 g of white bread with a green tea beverage (5 g green tea in 200 mL) significantly decreased the postprandial plasma glucose level in healthy subjects [27]. Furthermore, sucrose-loading (2.0 g/kg body weight) with green tea extract (0.5 g/kg body weight) significantly decreased plasma glucose level in rats [28]. According to the literature, the plasma lowering effect of green tea was evidently supported by clinical studies in human subjects who consumed green tea with calorie sugars. However, there have not been any reports examining whether consumption of isomaltulose and green tea alters plasma glucose concentration and antioxidant status. Therefore, the aim of the current study was to investigate the effect of isomaltulose together with green tea on postprandial plasma glucose and insulin concentration and antioxidant capacity in healthy subjects.

## 2. Materials and Methods

### 2.1. Preparation of Green Tea Beverages

Instant green tea leaf products were purchased from the local market. The content of the total amount of polyphenolic compounds was determined using the Folin–Ciocalteu method, according to the ISO 14502-1 method [29]. The phytochemical analysis of catechins was determined by using high-performance liquid chromatograph (HPLC), according to the ISO 14502-2 method [30]. The polyphenol content of the instant green tea was 12.30 g/100 g (dry weight basis). The phytochemical components were 2.16 g (−)-epigallocatechin, 1.85 g (−)-epigallocatechin gallate, 0.7 g (−)-epicatechin, 0.57 g (−)-gallocatechin, 0.56 g (+)-catechin, 0.46 g (−)-epicatechin gallate, 0.16 g (−)-gallocatechin gallate and 0.01 g (−)-catechin gallate in a 100-g dry weight basis. In the experiment, instant green tea leaves in a bag (4 g) were infused with boiling water (400 mL, a serving portion) at 95 °C for 5 min. Sugars (50 g sucrose or 50 g isomaltulose) were added into the green tea beverage (400 mL).

### 2.2. Subjects

The sample size was calculated according to Torronen et al., considering the postprandial of glycemic response as the main variable [31]. A statistical power of 90% and an expected difference of 95% in the baseline values were adopted to form a total sample of at least 14 individuals. A total of eighteen subjects (aged 18–35 years old) were recruited from the local community through poster advertisement and flyers. The subjects were screened in terms of anthropometry (BMI ranged

18.5–22.9 kg/m$^2$, % body fat <20% in men and <30% in women and waist circumference ≤90 cm in men and ≤80 cm in women), blood pressure <140/90 mmHg and blood chemistry (fasting plasma glucose level ≤100 mg/dL, total cholesterol <200 mg/dL, LDL-cholesterol <150 mg/dL, triglyceride <150 mg/dL, blood creatinine level ranging from 0.7–1.4 mg/dL and alanine aminotransferase (ALT) <40 IU/L). Participants were also excluded if they met the criteria for any evidence of physical illness, smoking, heavy drinking, history of chronic diseases, allergy, gastrointestinal pathologies (e.g., short bowel syndrome) and current use of drugs and food supplements. The study protocol was approved by the Ethics Review Committee for Research Involving Human Research Subjects, Health Science Group, Chulalongkorn University (No. 135/56). All subjects provided their written informed consent to participate in this study.

### 2.3. Study Design

The study was designed as a randomized, single-blinded, five-visit crossover study with a two-week washout period. At each experimental visit, after a 12-hour overnight fast, the subjects consumed the following beverage: (1) 50 g sucrose in 400 mL of water; (2) 50 g isomaltulose in 400 mL of water; (3) 400 mL of green tea; (4) 50 g sucrose in 400 mL of green tea; or (5) 50 g isomaltulose in 400 mL of green tea; within 5 min from the starting time. Blood samples were collected before and after 15, 30, 45, 60, 90 and 120 min of administration. During the experimental period, the subjects were instructed to avoid phenolic-rich foods (e.g., tea, coffee, fruit juices, berries, fruit, chocolate, etc.), high-antioxidant diets, alcoholic beverages and excessive exercise within a week before each visit. In addition, the subjects were asked to provide their food records and physical activity questionnaire at every visit.

### 2.4. Blood Collection

Blood samples were collected into tubes containing anticoagulants from an intravenous catheter inserted into a forearm vein. Blood samples were centrifuged at 3000 rpm for 15 min at 4 °C. Plasma samples were kept in a microtube and stored at −20 °C until analysis. Plasma glucose and insulin were analyzed using a glucose oxidase method (enzymatic colorimetric kits, GLUCOSE liquicolor, Human GmbH, Wiesbaden, Wiesbaden, Germany) and insulin human ELISA kit (BQ kits, San Diego, CA, USA), respectively.

### 2.5. The Ferric Reducing Ability of Plasma

The ferric reducing ability of plasma was performed according to a previous study with slight modification [32]. In brief, the FRAP reagent was freshly prepared and warmed at 37 °C by mixing the following solution: (1) 0.3 M sodium acetate buffer solution (pH 3.6); (2) 10 mM 2,4,6-tripyridyl-1-5-triazine (TPTZ) in 40 mM HCl solution; and (3) 20 mM FeCl$_3$ solution at the ratio of 10:1:1 (*v/v/v*), respectively. Plasma (10 µL) was incubated with 90 µL of FRAP reagent in a microplate for 30 min at room temperature in the dark. After that, the mixture measured the level of absorbance at the wavelength 595 nm with a spectrophotometer. The FRAP values were calculated by using a calibration standard curve of FeSO$_4$ (0–2000 µM).

### 2.6. Lipid Peroxidation

Plasma malondialdehyde (MDA) was quantified using a method based on the formation of thiobarbituric acid reactive substances (TBARS) and determined using fluorescence detection following a previous method with slight modification [33]. The plasma sample (60 µL) was incubated with 30 µL of 10% sodium dodecyl sulfate and 1.2 mL of TBA reagent (530 mg thiobarbituric acid in a mixed solution containing 50 mL of 20% acetic acid and 50 mL of 1 M NaOH). The mixtures were incubated in a heat block at 97 °C for 1 h. Following incubation, the mixtures were immediately removed from the heat block and placed in −20 °C for 10 min to stop the reaction. Next, the mixtures were centrifuged at 13,000 rpm for 10 min at 4 °C, and then, the supernatant was loaded into the microplate. The absorbance was measured using a fluorescence reader (Perkin Elmer®, Turku, Finland) at an excitation wavelength of 530 nm and an emission wavelength of 550 nm.

### 2.7. Statistical Analysis

For each test, the incremental data of plasma glucose, insulin, FRAP and MDA after consumption were analyzed using a repeated measurement ANOVA, followed by Duncan's test at a significance level of $p < 0.05$. The incremental area under curves (iAUCs) were calculated according to the trapezoidal method. A one-way analysis of variance (ANOVA) followed by Duncan's test for multiple comparison tests were performed to assess the differences between treatments ($p < 0.05$).

## 3. Results

### 3.1. Subjects

Twenty-two subjects were recruited for this study according to the flowchart (Figure 1). Four subjects were excluded from the study following the basic inclusion and exclusion criteria of the study. The eighteen remaining subjects were randomly assigned into five groups. Three subjects withdrew after the first week due to reasons unrelated to the study. Fifteen subjects completed the study, including eight women and seven men. The baselines characteristics of the fifteen subjects are shown in Table 1. Furthermore, all subjects were instructed to maintain unchanged their lifestyles or physical behavior during the experimental period.

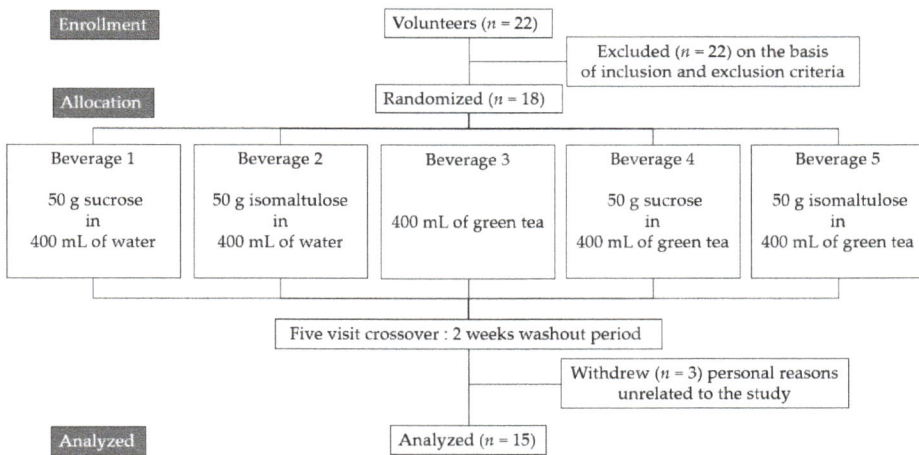

**Figure 1.** Flowchart for a randomized, single-blinded, five-visit crossover study.

### 3.2. Glycemic Response

The incremental postprandial plasma glucose and insulin concentrations after the consumption of beverages are shown in Figure 2. Consumption of isomaltulose was found to significantly lower plasma glucose concentrations at 15, 30, 45 and 60 min and insulin concentrations at 15, 30 and 45 min as compared to the consumption of sucrose. The results showed that consumption of sucrose together with green tea significantly suppressed plasma glucose concentrations at 15, 30, 45, 60 and 90 min and insulin concentration at 30 and 45 min. In addition, the ingestion of green tea-containing isomaltulose caused a higher reduction of plasma glucose concentration (15 and 30 min) and insulin concentration (30 and 45 min) than isomaltulose alone.

**Table 1.** Baseline characteristics of fifteen subjects (8 women and 7 men).

| Parameters | Mean ± SEM |
|---|---|
| Age (years) | 23.5 ± 0.7 |
| Weight (kg) | 21.0 ± 0.4 |
| BMI (kg/m$^2$) | 22.6 ± 1.4 |
| % Body fat | |
| Women | 22.6 ± 1.4 |
| Men | 13.6 ± 1.1 |
| Waist circumference (cm) | |
| Women | 69.9 ± 2.4 |
| Men | 80.0 ± 2.2 |
| Systolic blood pressure (mmHg) | 115.3 ± 1.9 |
| Diastolic blood pressure (mmHg) | 71.9 ± 2.3 |
| Fasting glucose (mg/dL) | 81.5 ± 2.3 |
| Total cholesterol (mg/dL) | 186.5 ± 3.2 |
| LDL-cholesterol (mg/dL) | 119.0 ± 5.2 |
| Triglyceride (mg/dL) | 76.5 ± 6.3 |
| Creatinine (mg/dL) | 0.9 ± 0.1 |
| Alanine aminotransferase or ALT (U/L) | 10.7 ± 1.3 |

Postprandial iAUCs for glucose (43.3%) and insulin (42.0%) were largely reduced following the ingestion of isomaltulose compared to sucrose, respectively (Figure 3). Consumption of green tea-containing sucrose solution had lower iAUCs for glucose (43.4%) and insulin (32.1%) when compared to the sucrose solution. In addition, green tea-containing isomaltulose significantly reduced the iAUCs of glucose (20.9%) and insulin concentration (37.7%) when compared to isomaltulose.

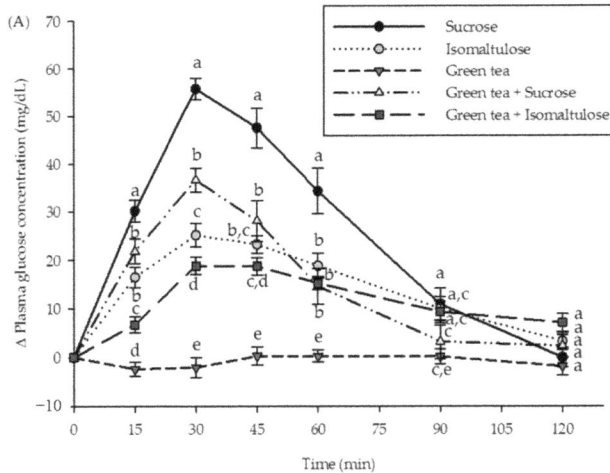

**Figure 2.** *Cont.*

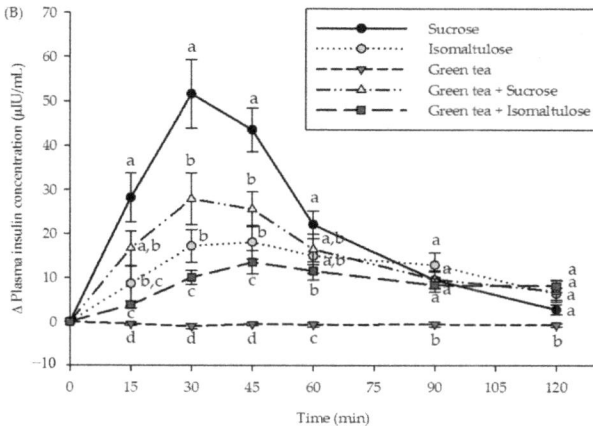

**Figure 2.** The incremental postprandial plasma (**A**) glucose concentration and (**B**) insulin concentration in healthy subjects after consumption of sucrose, isomaltulose, green tea, green tea plus sucrose and green tea plus isomaltulose ($n = 15$). Data are expressed as means $\pm$ SEM. Values not sharing the same superscript were significantly different between test groups in each time point ($p < 0.05$).

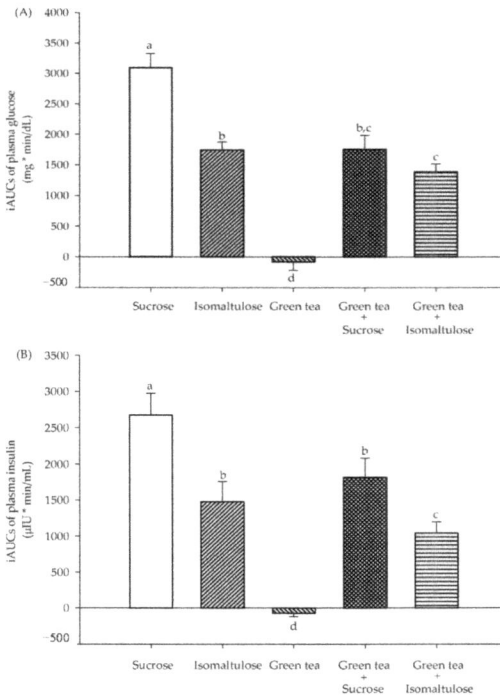

**Figure 3.** The incremental area under the curves (iAUCs) of plasma (**A**) glucose and (**B**) insulin concentration in healthy subjects after consumption of sucrose, isomaltulose, green tea, green tea plus sucrose and green tea plus isomaltulose ($n = 15$). Data are expressed as means $\pm$ SEM. Values not sharing the same superscript were significantly different between test groups ($p < 0.05$).

## 3.3. Antioxidant Capacities

The incremental postprandial plasma FRAP and MDA concentrations of treatments are shown in Figure 4. Both sucrose and isomaltulose showed a slight decrease in postprandial plasma FRAP level. Consumption of green tea increased the plasma FRAP level during the experimental period; whereas the addition of sucrose to the solution caused a reduction in plasma FRAP level at 15, 30 and 90 min. In contrast, consumption of isomaltulose together with green tea maintained an increase in the postprandial plasma FRAP level during the study. The findings also demonstrated that sucrose and isomaltulose slightly reduced postprandial plasma MDA concentration during 2 h of consumption. In comparison with sucrose and isomaltulose, consumption of green tea resulted in a higher reduction of plasma MDA concentration. This effect declined with the combination of green tea with sucrose at 15 min and 30 min. In the meantime, replacing sucrose with isomaltulose slightly suppressed green tea-induced reduction of plasma MDA concentration at 15 min and 30 min.

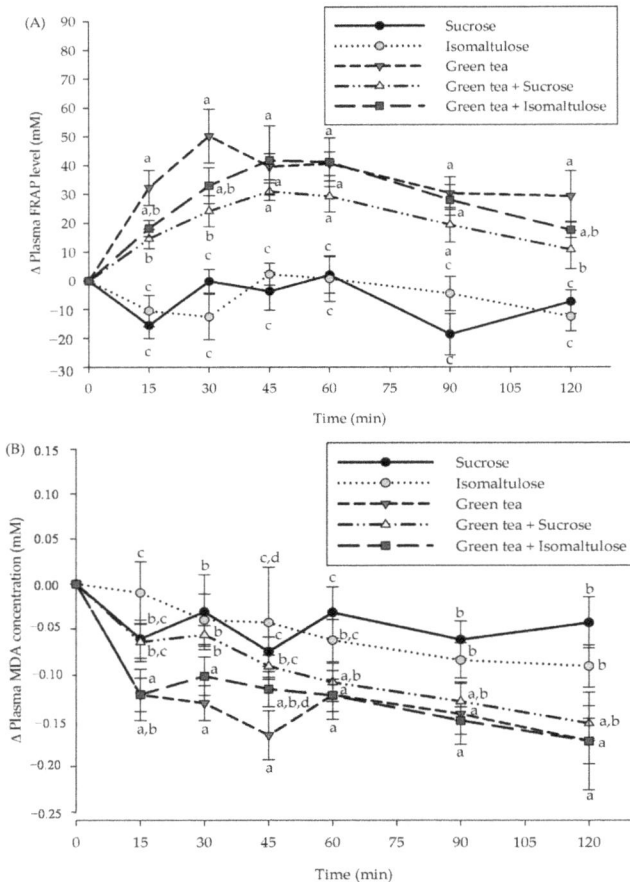

**Figure 4.** The incremental postprandial plasma (**A**) FRAP level and (**B**) malondialdehyde (MDA) concentration in healthy subjects after consumption of sucrose, isomaltulose, green tea, green tea plus sucrose and green tea plus isomaltulose ($n$ = 15). Data are expressed as means ± SEM. Values not sharing the same superscript were significantly different between test groups in each time point ($p < 0.05$).

The iAUCs of plasma FRAP and MDA concentrations are shown in Figure 5. Ingestion of green tea demonstrated the highest iAUC of plasma FRAP among all treatments. However, the iAUCs of plasma FRAP were significantly reduced with the consumption of green tea together with sucrose (40.4%) and isomaltulose (28.6%), respectively. At the same time, sucrose and isomaltulose attenuated green tea-induced reduction of iAUCs of plasma MDA by 34.7% and 17.2%, respectively.

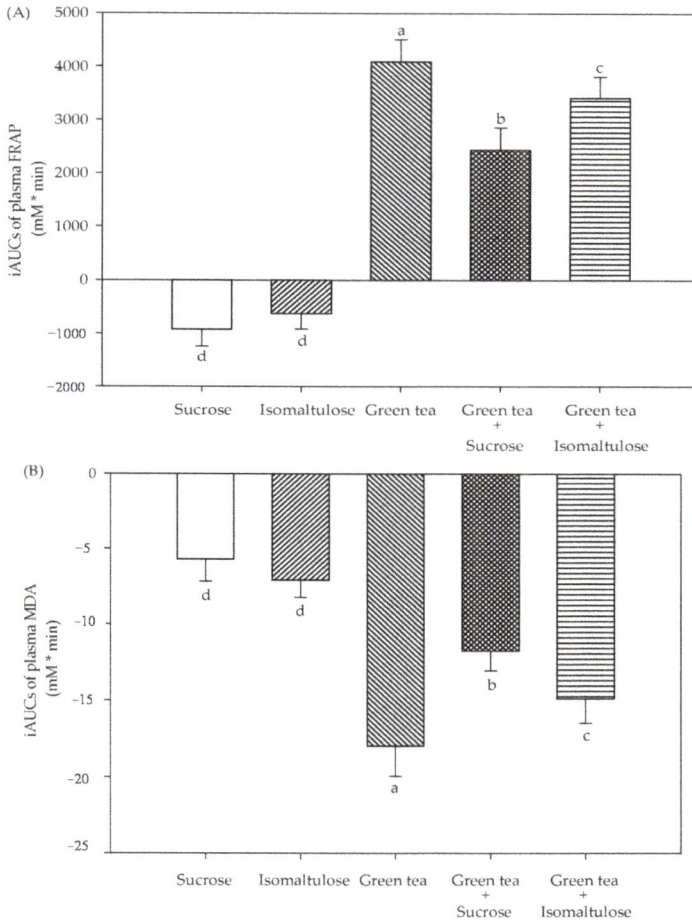

**Figure 5.** The incremental area under the curves (iAUCs) of plasma (**A**) FRAP and (**B**) MDA concentration in healthy subjects after consumption of sucrose, isomaltulose, green tea, green tea plus sucrose and green tea plus isomaltulose (*n* = 15). Data are expressed as means ± SEM. Values not sharing the same superscript were significantly different between test groups (*p* < 0.05).

## 4. Discussion

Previous studies have shown the antihyperglycemic activity of tea in healthy subjects [26,34]. Flavonoids, including catechin and its derivatives, exert effects on the reduction of postprandial glucose concentration in postmenopausal women [25]. Our findings are consistent with previous studies that the consumption of green tea together with sucrose reduces postprandial glucose and insulin concentration. The possible mechanisms of flavonoid-enriched green tea for reducing postprandial glucose include the inhibition of α-glucosidase activity, intestinal sodium-glucose co-transporter-1 (SGLT-1) and glucose transport-2 (GLUT-2) [35–37]. Furthermore, the flavins and catechins preferentially inhibited maltase rather than sucrose [38]. A recent study also revealed that epicatechin gallate competitively inhibited the glucose uptake through SGLT-1 [35]. In this connection, the postprandial glucose-lowering effects of flavonoid-enriched green might be associated with the inhibitory activity against the α-glucosidase and intestinal glucose transporter. Consistent with previous studies, replacing sucrose with isomaltulose markedly reduced postprandial plasma glucose and insulin concentrations in healthy and overweight subjects [13,39]. For example, consumption of 140 g cookies and 250 mL of liquid containing 50 g isomaltulose was found to be more effective at reducing postprandial plasma glucose and insulin concentration than sucrose in overweight subjects [39]. The suppression of hyperglycemia might be due to the slow digestion and absorption rate of isomaltulose in the small intestine [11,12]. When the subjects received isomaltulose plus green tea, a magnitude reduction of postprandial glucose and insulin concentration was achieved during the experimental period as compared to isomaltulose. The significant effect was mainly observed at 15 and 30 min. In addition to the isomerization of sucrose, isomaltulose can be slowly digested by α-glucosidase (isomaltulase). Its digestive products (glucose and fructose) are absorbed into the enterocytes by SGLT-1 and GLUT5, respectively. Finally, GLUT2 in enterocytes also aids in the transport of glucose and fructose into the blood circulation. In light of this, the inhibition of α-glucosidase activity could explain the interaction between tea catechins and isomaltulose in the gastrointestinal tract. It is possible that tea catechins might suppress the digestion of isomaltulose by inhibiting isomaltulase and/or slower absorption of the liberated glucose and fructose. Impaired digestion and/or absorption results in the reduced peak of postprandial glucose and insulin concentration.

The consumption of antioxidant-containing foods has been implicated to play a possible role in the prevention of chronic and age-related diseases [40]. Antioxidants reduce free radical-induced damage to protein, lipid and DNA, thus leading to the prevention of oxidative injury [41]. An increase in plasma FRAP level reflects the dietary intake of antioxidants and indicates the level of antioxidants in blood circulation [32]. Malondialdehyde (MDA) is commonly used as a marker of lipid peroxidation. In blood circulation, the accumulation of MDA contributes to modifying the structure of low-density lipoprotein (LDL), one of the main initiators of atherogenesis [42]. In the present study, the consumption of green tea increased plasma FRAP level concomitant with the reduction of plasma MDA concentration. Similar findings have been reported in other human studies. In a crossover study with 10 healthy subjects, green tea resulted in a 4% increase in FRAP after 40 min of consumption [43]. A greater increase in plasma FRAP was observed between 30 and 60 min after healthy volunteers drank green tea (2 g tea solids in 300 mL water) [44]. The decrease in plasma MDA concentration was seen after the consumption of green tea [45,46]. This is in accordance with previous studies in that the consumption of green tea resulted in a significant rise in plasma antioxidant activity associated with an increase in the concentration of plasma catechins [40]. Several studies support that tea catechins demonstrated antioxidant activity by scavenging free radicals and chelating redox-active transition metal ions [21,23,47]. Previous studies provided the FRAP value of tea catechins, and the order was as follows: ECG > EGCG ≈ GCG > GC ≈ EGC > C ≈ EC [48]. Furthermore, tea catechins prevented lipid peroxidation both in in vitro and in vivo models [22,23,49]. The acute rise of plasma FRAP, together with the reduction of the plasma MDA concentration, may be related in part to the presence of tea catechins. When sucrose was added to green tea, an increase in plasma FRAP level and a reduction of plasma MDA concentration were attenuated. In contrast to sucrose, isomaltulose did not impact the alteration of plasma FRAP and MDA concentration. The mechanisms by which sucrose interferes with plasma FRAP and MDA concentrations remain unclear. It is possible that sucrose remaining within the intestinal lumen may serve to interfere with the absorption of catechin and its derivatives in association with the reduction of the plasma FRAP level. A model of (−)-epicatechin gallate (ECG) absorption in the enterocyte has been recently proposed. ECG is actively absorbed across the apical membrane by monocarboxylate transporter-1 (MCT-1) [50]. Moreover, the uptake of ECG was sodium independent and pH gradient dependent. The interaction between sucrose and MCT-1 could occur in the gut; this phenomenon may be of major importance in achieving a significant reduction of the tea catechins' uptake into blood circulation. Additional experiments are required to determine the effect of sucrose and isomaltulose regarding the absorption of tea catechins in intestinal cell models. Several studies provide a correlation between the intake of the dietary total antioxidant capacity and the incidence of chronic diseases and mortality. Cohort studies investigated the inverse associations between dietary total antioxidant capacity (TAC) and stroke and myocardial infraction [51], reporting that a diet high in TAC, as measured by the Trolox equivalent antioxidant capacity (TEAC) and FRAP, has been inversely associated with pancreatic cancer risk [52]. Additionally, FRAP dietary equivalent intake was inversely associated with mortality from cancer and cardiovascular diseases [53]. The sustained elevation of total antioxidant status has been associated with the lower incidence of cardiovascular diseases (CVDs) in populations who regularly consumed red wine [54]. Consumption of green tea together with sucrose should be raised as a concern. Although drinking green tea together with sucrose suppressed a rise in postprandial plasma glucose concentration, it also caused the lower antioxidant capacity of plasma. This evidence may be a limitation regarding the inability to reach the sustained level of total antioxidant capacity for chronic disease prevention. The beneficial effects of green tea can sustain plasma antioxidant capacity concomitant with the suppression of postprandial glucose when consumed with isomaltulose. A limitation of this study is the small number of subjects enrolled. As the participants were healthy, there is a lack of an outcome associated with the alteration of antioxidant status after the intake of green tea together with sucrose or isomaltulose.

## 5. Conclusions

The consumption of green tea enhances the reduction of postprandial glucose and insulin concentration when the subjects consumed it with isomaltulose. Replacing sucrose with isomaltulose in green tea improves the plasma antioxidant capacity, as measured by the level of FRAP and the concentration of MDA. The evaluation of the long-term effects of green tea and isomaltulose deserves further attention.

**Acknowledgments:** We acknowledge the financial support of the 90th Anniversary of Chulalongkorn University Fund (Ratchadaphiseksomphot Endowment Fund). This research was supported by the Grant for International Research Integration: Chula Research Scholar, Ratchadaphiseksomphot Endowment Fund.

**Author Contributions:** P.S. and P.O.S. were responsible for the experiments, the acquisition of data, the analysis and the interpretation of the data. S.N. performed the interpretation of the data. K.M. and S.A. made substantial contributions to the conception and design, drafted the manuscript and revised it critically for important intellectual content. All authors conducted the drafting of the manuscript and agreed on the final approval of the version to be published.

**Conflicts of Interest:** The authors declare no conflict of interest.

## References

1. Ng, S.W.; Ni Mhurchu, C.; Jebb, S.A.; Popkin, B.M. Patterns and trends of beverage consumption among children and adults in Great Britain, 1986–2009. *Br. J. Nutr.* **2012**, *108*, 536–551. [CrossRef] [PubMed]
2. Kumar, G.S.; Pan, L.; Park, S.; Lee-Kwan, S.H.; Onufrak, S.; Blanck, H.M. Sugar-sweetened beverage consumption among adults 18 states, 2012. *Morb. Mortal. Wkly. Rep.* **2014**, *63*, 686–690.
3. Hu, F.B.; Malik, V.S. Sugar-sweetened beverages and risk of obesity and type 2 diabetes: Epidemiologic evidence. *Physiol. Behav.* **2010**, *100*, 47–54. [CrossRef] [PubMed]
4. Raben, A.; Vasilaras, T.H.; Moller, A.C.; Astrup, A. Sucrose compared with artificial sweeteners: Different effects on ad libitum food intake and body weight after 10 week of supplementation in overweight subjects. *Am. J. Clin. Nutr.* **2002**, *76*, 721–729. [PubMed]
5. Moraes, P.C.B.T.; Bolini, H.M.A. Different sweeteners in beverages prepared with instant and roasted ground coffee: Ideal and equivalent sweetness. *J. Sens. Stud.* **2010**, *25*, 215–225. [CrossRef]
6. Rubio-Arraez, S.; Capella, J.V.; Castelló, M.L.; Ortolá, M.D. Physicochemical characteristics of citrus jelly with non cariogenic and functional sweeteners. *J. Food Sci. Technol.* **2016**, *53*, 3642–3650. [CrossRef] [PubMed]

7.  Sylvetsky, A.C.; Rother, K.I. Trends in the consumption of low-calorie sweeteners. *Physiol. Behav.* **2016**, *2164*, 446–450. [CrossRef] [PubMed]
8.  Lina, B.A.; Jonker, D.; Kozianowski, G. Isomaltulose (Palatinose): A review of biological and toxicological studies. *Food Chem. Toxicol.* **2002**, *40*, 1375–1381. [CrossRef]
9.  Okuno, M.; Kim, M.K.; Mizu, M.; Mori, M.; Mori, H.; Yamori, Y. Palatinose-blended sugar compared with sucrose: Different effects on insulin sensitivity after 12 weeks supplementation in sedentary adults. *Int. J. Food Sci. Nutr.* **2010**, *61*, 643–651. [CrossRef] [PubMed]
10. Mu, W.; Li, W.; Wang, X.; Zhang, T.; Jiang, B. Current studies on sucrose isomerase and biological isomaltulose production using sucrose isomerase. *Appl. Microbiol. Biotechnol.* **2014**, *98*, 6569–6582. [CrossRef] [PubMed]
11. Holub, I.; Gostner, A.; Theis, S.; Nosek, L.; Kudlich, T.; Melcher, R.; Scheppach, W. Novel findings on the metabolic effects of the low glycaemic carbohydrate isomaltulose (Palatinose). *Br. J. Nutr.* **2010**, *103*, 1730–1737. [CrossRef] [PubMed]
12. Tonouchi, H.; Yamaji, T.; Uchida, M.; Koganei, M.; Sasayama, A.; Kaneko, T.; Urita, Y.; Okuno, M.; Suzuki, K.; Kashimura, J.; et al. Studies on absorption and metabolism of palatinose (isomaltulose) in rats. *Br. J. Nutr.* **2011**, *105*, 10–14. [CrossRef] [PubMed]
13. Arai, H.; Mizuno, A.; Sakuma, M.; Fukaya, M.; Matsuo, K.; Muto, K.; Sasaki, H.; Matsuura, M.; Okumura, H.; Yamamoto, H.; et al. Effects of a palatinose-based liquid diet (Inslow) on glycemic control and the second-meal effect in healthy men. *Metabolism* **2007**, *56*, 115–121. [CrossRef] [PubMed]
14. Sridonpai, P.; Komindr, S.; Kriengsinyos, W. Impact of isomaltulose and sucrose based breakfasts on postprandial substrate oxidation and glycemic/insulinemic changes in type-2 diabetes mellitus subjects. *J. Med. Assoc. Thai* **2016**, *99*, 282–289. [PubMed]
15. Dye, L.; Gilsenan, M.B.; Quadt, F.; Martens, V.E.; Bot, A.; Lasikiewicz, N.; Camidge, D.; Croden, F.; Lawton, C. Manipulation of glycemic response with isomaltulose in a milk-based drink does not affect cognitive performance in healthy adults. *Mol. Nutr. Food Res.* **2010**, *54*, 506–515. [CrossRef] [PubMed]
16. Wang, Y.; Ho, C.T. Polyphenolic chemistry of tea and coffee: A century of progress. *J. Agric. Food Chem.* **2009**, *57*, 8109–8114. [CrossRef] [PubMed]
17. Wedick, N.M.; Pan, A.; Cassidy, A.; Rimm, E.B.; Sampson, L.; Rosner, B.; Willett, W; Hu, F.B.; Sun, Q.; van Dam, R.M. Dietary flavonoid intakes and risk of type 2 diabetes in US men and women. *Am. J. Clin. Nutr.* **2012**, *95*, 925–933. [CrossRef] [PubMed]
18. Grosso, G.; Stepaniak, U.; Micek, A.; Stefler, D.; Bobak, M.; Pająk, A. Dietary polyphenols are inversely associated with metabolic syndrome in Polish adults of the HAPIEE study. *Eur. J. Nutr.* **2016**. [CrossRef] [PubMed]
19. Zamora-Ros, R.; Forouhi, N.G.; Sharp, S.J.; González, C.A.; Buijsse, B.; Guevara, M.; van der Schouw, Y.T.; Amiano, P.; Boeing, H.; Bredsdorff, L.; et al. The association between dietary flavonoid and lignan intakes and incident type 2 diabetes in European populations: The EPIC-InterAct study. *Diabetes Care* **2013**, *36*, 3961–3970. [CrossRef] [PubMed]
20. Tresserra-Rimbau, A.; Guasch-Ferré, M.; Salas-Salvadó, J.; Toledo, E.; Corella, D.; Castañer, O.; Guo, X.; Gómez-Gracia, E.; Lapetra, J.; Arós, F.; et al. PREDIMED study investigators. Intake of total polyphenols and some classes of polyphenols is inversely associated with diabetes in elderly people at high cardiovascular disease risk. *J. Nutr.* **2016**, *146*, 767–777. [CrossRef] [PubMed]
21. Frei, B.; Higdon, J.V. Antioxidant activity of tea polyphenols in vivo: Evidence from animal studies. *J. Nutr.* **2003**, *133*, 3275S–3284S. [PubMed]
22. Basu, A.; Sanchez, K.; Leyva, M.J.; Wu, M.; Betts, N.M.; Aston, C.E.; Lyons, T.J. Green tea supplementation affects body weight, lipids, and lipid peroxidation in obese subjects with metabolic syndrome. *J. Am. Coll. Nutr.* **2010**, *29*, 31–40. [CrossRef] [PubMed]
23. Chacko, S.M.; Thambi, P.T.; Kuttan, R.; Nishigaki, I. Beneficial effects of green tea: A literature review. *Chin. Med.* **2010**, *5*, 13. [CrossRef] [PubMed]
24. Koutelidakis, A.E.; Rallidis, L.; Koniari, K.; Panagiotakos, D.; Komaitis, M.; Zampelas, A.; Anastasiou-Nana, M.; Kapsokefalou, M. Effect of green tea on postprandial antioxidant capacity, serum lipids, C-reactive protein and glucose levels in patients with coronary artery disease. *Eur. J. Nutr.* **2014**, *53*, 479–486. [CrossRef] [PubMed]

25. Takahashi, M.; Miyashita, M.; Suzuki, K.; Bae, S.R.; Kim, H.K.; Wakisaka, T.; Matsui, Y.; Takeshita, M.; Yasunaga, K. Acute ingestion of catechin-rich green tea improves postprandial glucose status and increases serum thioredoxin concentrations in postmenopausal women. *Br. J. Nutr.* **2014**, *112*, 1542–1550. [CrossRef] [PubMed]

26. Tsuneki, H.; Ishizuka, M.; Terasawa, M.; Wu, J.B.; Sasaoka, T.; Kimura, I. Effect of green tea on blood glucose levels and serum proteomic patterns in diabetic (db/db) mice and on glucose metabolism in healthy humans. *BMC Pharmacol.* **2004**, *4*, 18. [CrossRef] [PubMed]

27. Azzeh, F.S. Synergistic effect of green tea, cinnamon and ginger combination on enhancing postprandial blood glucose. *Pak. J. Biol. Sci.* **2013**, *16*, 74–79. [CrossRef] [PubMed]

28. Oh, J.; Jo, S.H.; Kim, J.S.; Ha, K.S.; Lee, J.Y.; Choi, H.Y.; Yu, S.Y.; Kwon, Y.I.; Kim, Y.C. Selected tea and tea pomace extracts inhibit intestinal α-glucosidase activity in vitro and postprandial hyperglycemia in Vivo. *Int. J. Mol. Sci.* **2015**, *16*, 8811–8825. [CrossRef] [PubMed]

29. International Organization for Standardization (ISO). *ISO 14502-1: 2005. Determination of Substances Characteristic of Green and Black Tea. Part 1: Content of Total Polyphenols in Tea. Colorimetric Method Using Folin-Ciocalteu Reagent*; ISO: Geneva, Switzerland, 2005.

30. International Organization for Standardization (ISO). *ISO 14502-2: 2005. Determination of Substances Characteristic of Green and Black Tea. Part 2: Content of Catechins in Green Tea. Method Using High-Performance Liquid Chromatography*; ISO: Geneva, Switzerland, 2005.

31. Torronen, R.; Sarkkinen, E.; Tapola, N.; Hautaniemi, E.; Kilpi, K.; Niskanen, L. Berries modify the postprandial plasma glucose response to sucrose in healthy subjects. *Br. J. Nutr.* **2010**, *103*, 1094–1097. [CrossRef] [PubMed]

32. Benzie, I.F.; Strain, J.J. The ferric reducing ability of plasma (FRAP) as a measure of "antioxidant power": The FRAP assay. *Anal. Biochem.* **1996**, *239*, 70–76. [CrossRef] [PubMed]

33. Richard, M.J.; Portal, B.; Meo, J.; Coudray, C.; Hadjian, A.; Favier, A. Malondialdehyde kit evaluated for determining plasma and lipoprotein fractions that react with thiobarbituric acid. *Clin. Chem.* **1992**, *38*, 704–709. [PubMed]

34. Bryans, J.A.; Judd, P.A.; Ellis, P.R. The effect of consuming instant black tea on postprandial plasma glucose and insulin concentrations in healthy humans. *J. Am. Coll. Nutr.* **2007**, *26*, 471–477. [CrossRef] [PubMed]

35. Shimizu, M.; Kobayashi, Y.; Suzuki, M.; Satsu, H.; Miyamoto, Y. Regulation of intestinal glucose transport by tea catechins. *Biofactors* **2000**, *13*, 61–65. [CrossRef] [PubMed]

36. Kwon, O.; Eck, P.; Chen, S.; Corpe, C.P.; Lee, J.H.; Kruhlak, M.; Levine, M. Inhibition of the intestinal glucose transporter GLUT2 by flavonoids. *FASEB J.* **2007**, *21*, 366–377. [CrossRef] [PubMed]

37. Farrell, T.L.; Ellam, S.L.; Forrelli, T.; Williamson, G. Attenuation of glucose transport across Caco-2 cell monolayers by a polyphenol-rich herbal extract: Interactions with SGLT1 and GLUT2 transporters. *Biofactors* **2013**, *39*, 448–456. [CrossRef] [PubMed]

38. Matsui, T.; Tanaka, T.; Tamura, S.; Toshima, A.; Tamaya, K.; Miyata, Y.; Tanaka, K.; Matsumoto, K. Alpha-Glucosidase inhibitory profile of catechins and theaflavins. *J. Agric. Food Chem.* **2007**, *55*, 99–105. [CrossRef] [PubMed]

39. Konig, D.; Theis, S.; Kozianowski, G.; Berg, A. Postprandial substrate use in overweight subjects with the metabolic syndrome after isomaltulose (Palatinose) ingestion. *Nutrition* **2012**, *28*, 651–656. [CrossRef] [PubMed]

40. Pandey, K.B.; Rizvi, S.I. Plant polyphenols as dietary antioxidants in human health and disease. *Oxid. Med. Cell. Longev.* **2009**, *2*, 270–278. [CrossRef] [PubMed]

41. Lobo, V.; Patil, A.; Phatak, A.; Chandra, N. Free radicals, antioxidants and functional foods: Impact on human health. *Pharmacogn. Rev.* **2010**, *4*, 118–126. [CrossRef] [PubMed]

42. Kotani, K.; Tashiro, J.; Yamazaki, K.; Nakamura, Y.; Miyazaki, A.; Bujo, H.; Saito, Y.; Kanno, T.; Maekawa, M. Investigation of MDA-LDL (malondialdehyde-modified low-density lipoprotein) as a prognostic marker for coronary artery disease in patients with type 2 diabetes mellitus. *Clin. Chim. Acta* **2015**, *450*, 145–150. [CrossRef] [PubMed]

43. Benzie, I.F.; Szeto, Y.T.; Strain, J.J.; Tomlinson, B. Consumption of green tea causes rapid increase in plasma antioxidant power in humans. *Nutr. Cancer* **1999**, *34*, 83–87. [CrossRef] [PubMed]

44. Leenen, R.; Roodenburg, A.J.; Tijburg, L.B.; Wiseman, S.A. A single dose of tea with or without milk increases plasma antioxidant activity in humans. *Eur. J. Clin. Nutr.* **2000**, *54*, 87–92. [CrossRef] [PubMed]

45. Freese, R.; Basu, S.; Hietanen, E.; Nair, J.; Nakachi, K.; Bartsch, H.; Mutanen, M. Green tea extract decreases plasma malondialdehyde concentration but does not affect other indicators of oxidative stress, nitric oxide production, or hemostatic factors during a high-linoleic acid diet in healthy females. *Eur. J. Nutr.* **1999**, *38*, 149–157. [CrossRef] [PubMed]

46. Nakagawa, K.; Ninomiya, M.; Okubo, T.; Aoi, N.; Juneja, L.R.; Kim, M.; Yamanaka, K.; Miyazawa, T. Tea catechin supplementation increases antioxidant capacity and prevents phospholipid hydroperoxidation in plasma of humans. *J. Agric. Food Chem.* **1999**, *47*, 3967–3973. [CrossRef] [PubMed]

47. Zeng, L.; Luo, L.; Li, H.; Liu, R. Phytochemical profiles and antioxidant activity of 27 cultivars of tea. *Int. J. Food Sci. Nutr.* **2016**, 1–13. [CrossRef] [PubMed]

48. Lee, L.S.; Kim, S.H.; Kim, Y.B.; Kim, Y.C. Quantitative analysis of major constituents in green tea with different plucking periods and their antioxidant activity. *Molecules* **2014**, *19*, 9173–9186. [CrossRef] [PubMed]

49. Ostrowska, J.; Skrzydlewska, E. The comparison of effect of catechins and green tea extract on oxidative modification of LDL in vitro. *Adv. Med. Sci.* **2006**, *51*, 298–303. [PubMed]

50. Vaidyanathan, J.B.; Walle, T. Cellular uptake and efflux of the tea flavonoid (−)epicatechin-3-gallate in the human intestinal cell line Caco-2. *J. Pharmacol. Exp. Ther.* **2003**, *307*, 745–752. [CrossRef] [PubMed]

51. Rautiainen, S.; Larsson, S.; Virtamo, J.; Wolk, A. Total antioxidant capacity of diet and risk of stroke: A population-based prospective cohort of women. *Stroke* **2012**, *43*, 335–340. [CrossRef] [PubMed]

52. Lucas, A.L.; Bosetti, C.; Boffetta, P.; Negri, E.; Tavani, A.; Serafini, M.; Polesel, J.; Serraino, D.; La Vecchia, C.; Rossi, M. Dietary total antioxidant capacity and pancreatic cancer risk: An Italian case-control study. *Br. J. Cancer* **2016**, *115*, 102–107. [CrossRef] [PubMed]

53. Bastide, N.; Dartois, L.; Dyevre, V.; Dossus, L.; Fagherazzi, G.; Serafini, M.; Boutron-Ruault, M.C. Dietary antioxidant capacity and all-cause and cause-specific mortality in the E3N/EPIC cohort study. *Eur. J. Nutr.* **2016**, *56*, 1233–1243. [CrossRef] [PubMed]

54. Micallef, M.; Lexis, L.; Lewandowski, P. Red wine consumption increases antioxidant status and decreases oxidative stress in the circulation of both young and old humans. *Nutr. J.* **2007**, *6*, 27. [CrossRef] [PubMed]

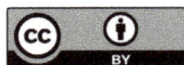

*nutrients*

MDPI

*Article*

# The Neuroprotective Effects of Phenolic Acids: Molecular Mechanism of Action

Dominik Szwajgier, Kamila Borowiec * and Katarzyna Pustelniak

Department of Biotechnology, Human Nutrition and the Science of Food Commodities, University of Life Sciences in Lublin, Lublin 20704, Poland; dszwajgier@hotmail.com (D.S.); kasia.pustus@wp.pl (K.P.)
* Correspondence: kam.borowiec@gmail.com; Tel./Fax: +48-81-462-33-53

Received: 23 March 2017; Accepted: 4 May 2017; Published: 10 May 2017

**Abstract:** The neuroprotective role of phenolic acids from food has previously been reported by many authors. In this review, the role of phenolic acids in ameliorating depression, ischemia/reperfusion injury, neuroinflammation, apoptosis, glutamate-induced toxicity, epilepsy, imbalance after traumatic brain injury, hyperinsulinemia-induced memory impairment, hearing and vision disturbances, Parkinson's disease, Huntington's disease, anti-amyotrophic lateral sclerosis, Chagas disease and other less distributed diseases is discussed. This review covers the in vitro, ex vivo and in vivo studies concerning the prevention and treatment of neurological disorders (on the biochemical and gene expression levels) by phenolic acids.

**Keywords:** cinnamic acids; benzoic acids; polyphenols; neuroprotection; neuroinflammation; central nervous system; neuron; glial cell; neurological disorder

## 1. Introduction

Phenolic acids are one of the main classes of polyphenols. They are abundantly present in foods such as berries [1], nuts [2], coffee and tea [3] and whole grains [4]. Importantly, a recent meta-analysis showed that phenolic acid-rich foods decrease the risk of depression [5,6]. Figure 1 presents the chemical structures of phenolic acids discussed in this work. Previously, authors focused mainly on the antioxidant and antiradical activities of phenolic acids. However, in recent years, the interest in protecting neurons and glial cells by phenolic acids has considerably increased, and a great number of works elaborating the neuroprotective role of phenolic acids has been published. Changes in the central nervous system, as well as in the peripheral parts of the nervous system, including sense organs, affect the patient's behavior and quality of life. Recently, we published a review paper on the anti-Alzheimer and cognition-enhancing role of phenolic acids originating from food [7]. In the following (Table 1), we present a review collating original papers concerning many other and previously omitted aspects of the neuroprotective role of phenolic acids originating from food. The presented review serves as assistance for quick access to the most prominent neuroprotective actions of phenolic acids.

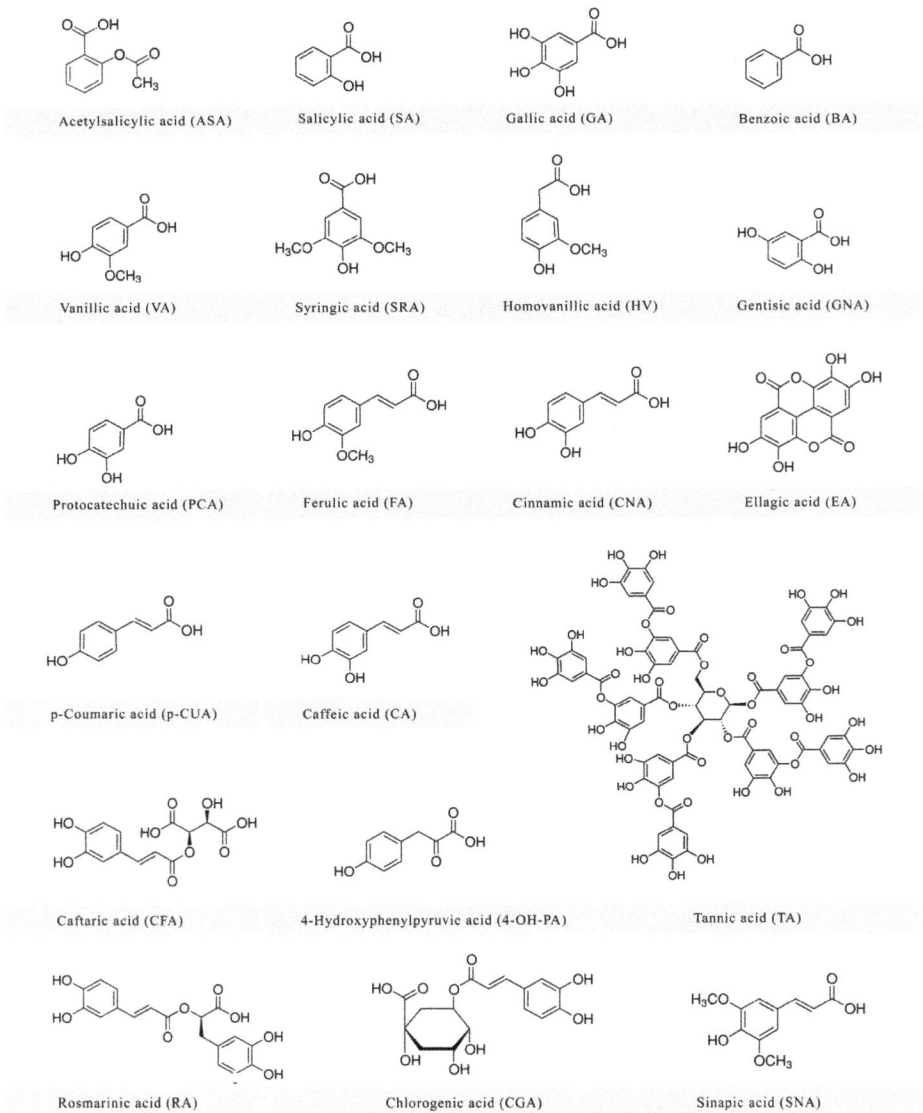

**Figure 1.** Chemical structures of phenolic acids discussed in this work.

## 2. Neuroprotective Activities of Phenolic Acids

**Table 1.** Summary of the neuroprotective activities of phenolic acids.

| Ferulic Acid | *Antidepressant-like Effect:* |
|---|---|
| | • reduction of the immobility in TST and FST; increased MAO levels in the hippocampus and frontal cortex, serotonin and norepinephrine levels in the hypothalamus; inhibition of MAO-A activity in the hippocampus and frontal cortex in mice (ferulic acid at 0.01, 0.1, 1 and 10 mg/kg/day, p.o.) [8] or 20 and 40 mg/kg b.w., p.o.) [9]; |
| | • improvement of TST and FST scores without affecting locomotor activity; amelioration of SOD, CAT in the blood and cerebral cortex, amelioration of GPx in the cerebral cortex; decrease of thiobarbituric acid-reactive substances' levels in the blood, hippocampus and cerebral cortex in mice [10]; |
| | • reversion of the TST and FST scores, significant alleviation of CUMS-induced depressive-like behaviors in sucrose preference test and FST, significant upregulation of the BDNF, postsynaptic density protein (PSD95) and synapsin I levels in the prefrontal cortex and hippocampus in male *Imprinting Control Region* mice (ferulic acid intravenously injected, 100 mg/kg b.w.) [11]. |
| | *Protection from Ischemia/Reperfusion Injury:* |
| | • promotion of EPO synthesis (increased EPO expression) in the hippocampus and the peripheral blood of male Sprague–Dawley rats after the occlusion of the right middle cerebral artery and reperfusion after 90 min [12]; |
| | • downregulation of the MEK/ERK/p90RSK signaling pathway in focal cerebral ischemic injury by the prevention of middle cerebral artery occlusion-induced injury leading to decreased phosphorylation of RAF proto-oncogene serine/threonine-protein kinase, MEK1/2 (dual specificity kinase) and ERK1/2; attenuation of the injury-induced decrease in p90RSK and BAD phosphorylation levels (ferulic acid at 100 mg/kg b.w.) [13]; |
| | • amelioration of neurological deficits and increased EPO expression in the hippocampus and the peripheral blood of male Sprague–Dawley rats (induced by focal cerebral ischemia provoked by occlusion of the right middle cerebral artery and reperfusion) [12]; |
| | • improvement of the neuroprotective activity of puerarin and astragaloside after the transient middle cerebral artery occlusion by reducing neurological deficits, decreased infarct volume and decreased expression levels of IL-1β and neuropeptide Y (single dose of ferulic acid, 43 mg/kg b.w., p.o.) [14]. |
| | *Antinociceptive Effects:* |
| | • amelioration of the descending monoaminergic system coupled with spinal β2- and 5-hydroxytryptamine 1A receptors and the downstream of δ- and mu-opioid receptors in an animal model involving CCI-induced neuropathic pain (amelioration of mechanical allodynia and thermal hyperalgesia, elevation of spinal noradrenaline and serotonin 5-hydroxytryptamine receptors, reduction of spinal MAO-A levels) (treatment with ferulic acid at 20, 40 and 80 mg/kg b.w., p.o.) [15]. |
| | *PD:* |
| | • attenuation of CCI-induced neuropathic pain (in the left sciatic nerve) in rats due to increased antioxidant and anti-inflammatory activity; decreased nociceptive thresholds, thermal hyperalgesia, mechanical hyperalgesia, tactile allodynia; reduced biochemical markers: total protein, NO, lipid peroxidase, IL-1β, and IL-6 (10, 20 or 30 mg/kg b.w., p.o.) [16]; dose-dependent amelioration of 1-methyl-4-phenyl-1,2,3,6-tetrahydropyridine-induced loss of nigrostriatal dopaminergic neurons, the decrease of the Bax/Bcl2 ratio, reduction of pro-apoptotic protein Bax levels and increased expression of anti-apoptotic protein Bcl2 in PD C57Bl/6 mice model (ferulic acid was given via injections for 7 days, at a dose of 20, 40 and 80 mg/kg/kg) [17]; |
| | • antioxidant and anti-inflammatory activities; rescue of dopamine neurons in substantia nigra pars compacta area and nerve terminals in the striatum; restored SOD, CAT, glutamate levels; prevented lipid oxidation; reduced the levels of ionized calcium-binding adapter molecule (Iba-1), GFAP hyperactivity, pro-inflammatory cytokines; and reduced COX-2 and iNOS activities in the studies using the rotenone-induced rat model of PD (chronic administration of ferulic acid for 4 weeks at a dose of 50 mg/kg b.w.) [18]. |
| | *Inflammation:* |
| | • inhibition of the LPS-induced microglial inflammation (without cytotoxicity) by partial targeting of ERK signaling and attenuation of ERK; significant inhibition of the production of TNF-α, IL-6, IL-1β and NO; and reduction of mRNA and protein levels of COX-2 and iNOS [19]; |
| | • dose-dependent prevention from LPS-induced upregulation of 3′5′-cyclic nucleotide phosphodiesterase 4B, reversion of the LPS-induced downregulation of CREB and pCREB (stimulation the cAMP/CREB signaling pathway) in PC12 cells [20]. |

**Table 1.** *Cont.*

| | |
|---|---|
| | *TBI:* |
| | • attenuation of oxidative stress caused by TBI; restriction of $H_2O_2$-induced DNA fragmentation; downregulation of ROS caused by reduced mRNA gene expression; attenuation of inflammation and apoptosis; upregulation of *BDNF* gene expression; downregulation of iNOS, endothelial NOS, neuronal NOS, COX-2, IL-1β, TNF-α, SOD, as well as apoptosis-related genes (Fas-associated protein with death domain, Casp-9 and BCL-2) in Neuro-2a cells in vitro [21]. |
| | *Anti-allergic Effect:* |
| | • restoration of Th1/Th2 balance by modulation of dendritic cell function; reduction of ovalbumin-specific immunoglobulin E and elevation of the immunoglobulin G2 antibody serum levels; inhibition of the production of eotaxin, Th2 cytokines (IL-4, IL-5 and IL-13) and proinflammatory cytokines; elevated production of Th1, interferon-γ in bronchoalveolar lavage fluid and the culture supernatant of spleen cells; reduced expression of proinflammatory cytokines IL-1β, IL-6 and TNF-α; increased expression of Notch ligand Delta-like 4 (DII4), MHX class II and CD40 protein; T-cell proliferation and Th1 cell polarization in dendritic cell cultures in an asthmatic mouse model with ovalbumin-induced Th2-mediated allergic asthma (animals were orally fed with ferulic acid at 25, 50 and 100 mg/kg b.w.) [22]. |
| | *Anti-apoptotic Activity:* |
| | • inhibition of the p38 MAPK pathway and apoptosis by increasing the cell viability, preventing membrane damage and increasing the SOD activity; reduced intracellular free $Ca^{2+}$ ion levels, lipid peroxidation, Casp-3 and COX-2 activation; reduced PGE2 production; increased scavenging of ROS in hypoxia-stressed PC12 cells [23]; |
| | • protection against 2′-azobis(2-amidinopropane) dihydrochloride-induced oxidative stress leading to the cell survival by elevating CAT and SOD activities, mitochondrial membrane potential, reduced MDA levels, reduced LDH release from PC12 cells, and accumulation of intracellular $Ca^{2+}$ levels in PC12 cells [24]. |
| **Caffeic Acid** | *Inflammation:* |
| | • antioxidant and anti-inflammatory activity, reduction (in a dose-dependent manner) of the cytokine levels in serum and whole brain in the LPS-induced model of inflammation in mice (caffeic acid administered orally at 30 mg/kg b.w.) [25]. |
| | *PD:* |
| | • inhibition (in a dose-dependent manner) of α-synuclein fibrillation in the presence of escitalopram [26]. |
| | *Glutamate-induced Toxicity:* |
| | • in vitro neuroprotection activity of SH-SY5Y cells by caffeic acid derivatives from *Arctium lappa* roots: 1,5-*O*-dicaffeoyl-3-*O*-(4-malic acid methyl ester)-quinic acid, 3,5-*O*-dicaffeoyl-quinic acid methyl ester, 3,4-*O*-dicaffeoyl-quinic acid methyl ester, 4,5-*O*-dicaffeoyl-quinic acid methyl ester, (2E)-1,4-dimethyl-2-[(4-hydroxyphenyl)methyl]-2-butenedioic acid, chlorogenic acid methyl ester, caffeic acid methyl ester, 3,4,3′,4′-tetrahydroxy-δ-truxinate [27]. |
| | *Anti-epileptic Activity:* |
| | • reduction of the levels of free radicals and DNA damage in the kindling CF-1 male mice model of epilepsy induced by PTZ (caffeic acid at 1, 4 or 8 mg/kg b.w., i.p.) [28]; |
| | • reduction of the latency to sleep in the diazepam-induced sleeping time test, decreased pilocarpine-induced genotoxic damage in acute seizure models in mice (caffeic acid at 4 or 8 mg/kg b.w., i.p.) [29]. |
| | *Memory Impairment in Hyperinsulinemia:* |
| | • high-fat diet-induced hyperinsulinemic rats: amelioration of glucose uptake and cell viability, improvement of memory impairment and brain glucose metabolism via significant reduction of plasma glucose and insulin levels, amelioration of the cerebral insulin and leptin signaling pathways (insulin receptor, phosphatidylinositol-3-kinase, protein kinase B, and insulin-degrading enzyme, leptin receptor and phosphorylated Janus tyrosine kinase 2 Tyr813/Janus tyrosine kinase 2 in the cortex of rats) (caffeic acid at 30 mg/kg b.w., p.o.) [30]. |
| **Caffeic Acid Phenethyl Ester** | *Antioxidant Activity:* |
| | • protection of brain tissue against ionizing radiation-induced oxidative damage by amelioration of the SOD activity in brains of male albino Sprague–Dawley rats (10 μmol ester/kg b.w./day, i.p., for 10 days after irradiation) [31]; |
| | • amelioration of the redox-balancing activity, positive modulation of the transcription-factor, stimulation of Nrf2, inhibition of NF-κB activity, as well as signal transducer and activator of transcription 3 (STAT3) [32]; |
| | • attenuation of the ifosfamide-induced central neurotoxicity in Wistar rats (after intraperitoneal injection) by attenuating the increase in MDA and protein carbonyl content in brain tissue (10 μmol ester/kg b.w., i.p.) [33,34]. |

**Table 1.** *Cont.*

| | |
|---|---|
| | *Anti-apoptotic Activity:*<br>• protection of PC12 cells from the cellular death induced by neurotoxin methyl-4-phenylpyridinium by increasing the neurite network (promotion of the formation, elongation and ramification; inhibition of the shortage of neurites); increasing the expression of neuron-typical proteins responsible for axonal growth (growth-associated protein 43) and synaptogenesis (synaptophysin and synapsin I) [35];<br>• reduction of the incidents of volatile anesthetic sevoflurane-induced neurodegeneration (neurotoxicity in neonatal rats) and apoptosis by activation of the phosphatidylinositide 3-kinase/protein kinase B signaling pathway, downregulation of the expression of Bax and BAD, upregulation of Bcl-2 and Bcl-extra-large levels and modification of the expression of MAPK levels (rat pups were administered with ester at 10, 20 or 40 mg/kg b.w. from postnatal Days 1–15) [36].<br>*Inflammation:*<br>• significant inhibition of the expressions of NOS, COX-2 and the production of NO; increased expression of heme oxygenase-1 and EPO in microglia in in vitro tests [37].<br>*Anticancer Activity:*<br>• reduction of NO, intracellular $Ca^{2+}$ levels, and CAT activity in C6 glioma cells when combined with Dasatinib (Bcr-abl tyrosine kinase inhibitor), in comparison to Dasatinib applied alone [38].<br>*Huntington Disease:*<br>• reduction of striatal damage, immunoreactivity to glial GFAP and lymphocyte common antigen (CD45) (markers of astrocyte and microglia activation); reduced behavioral deficits tested on the rotarod in the chemical model of Huntington disease (male C57BL/6 mice); reduced mortality of cultured striatal neurons of male C57BL/6 mice after the induction of the inflammation by 3NP [39]. |
| **Chlorogenic Acid** | *Reversing of the Glutamate-induced Toxicity:*<br>• inhibition of the glutamate-induced increase of intracellular $Ca^{2+}$ concentrations, as well as glutamate-induced death of primary cells isolated from mouse cortical neurons (cerebral cortex) [40].<br>*Inflammation:*<br>• attenuation of herpes simplex virus-1-induced inflammation in BV2 microglia, improving cell viability and increasing (at the mRNA and protein levels) Toll-like receptor 2, Toll-like receptor 9 and myeloid differentiation factor 88; significant inhibition of mRNA concentration, NF-κB p65 expression and TNF-α and IL-6 levels in microglia [41].<br>*Antidepressant Effect:*<br>• stimulation of axon and dendrite growth, promotion of serotonin release through enhancing synapsin I expression (via 5-hydroxytryptamine receptors) in the cells of fetal raphe neurons in vitro [42].<br>*Antioxidant Activity:*<br>• amelioration of the decrease of MDA and ROS levels in rat cortical slices after the $H_2O_2$-induced oxidative stress [43].<br>*Anti-epileptic:*<br>• reduction of the pilocarpine-induced epilepsy (seizures) in mice by reducing the lipid peroxidation and nitrite content, as well as the mRNA expressions of *N*-methyl-D-aspartate receptor, metabotropic glutamate receptor 1 and metabotropic glutamate receptor 5 (chlorogenic acid administered at 5 mg/kg b.w., p.o.) [44].<br>*Anti-apoptotic:*<br>• dose-dependent increase of cell viability, cell distribution ratio at the G2/M and S phases; promotion of cell differentiation by preventing ethanol-induced apoptosis in rat PC12 cells by enhancing the expression of growth-associated protein-43 (GAP-43); inhibition of the mitochondrial apoptotic pathway by promoting mitochondria transmembrane potential, upregulation of the expression of Bcl-2 and downregulation of the expression of Casp-3 [45]. |
| **Chlorogenic Acid and Its Metabolites** | *Reversing of the Glutamate-induced Toxicity:*<br>• protection from nitroprusside-induced NO generation (chlorogenic and caffeic acids), significant reduction of excitotoxicity (ferulic and caffeic acids), protection against $H_2O_2$-induced proteasome inhibition and caspase-dependent intrinsic apoptosis, as well as endoplasmic reticulum stress (caffeic acid) in primary cultures of rat cerebellar granule neurons [46]. |

Table 1. *Cont.*

| Rosmarinic Acid | |
|---|---|
| | *Antioxidant Activity:* |

**Antioxidant Activity:**

- induction/activation of the nuclear factor erythroid 2-related factor 2-antioxidant-responsive element (Nrf2-ARE) signaling pathway and potentiation of the Nrf2/HO-1 signaling pathway leading to the enhanced endogenous antioxidant defense (decreased superoxide production, reduced expression of 4-hydroxynonenal and upregulation of SOD) in a rat model of noise-induced superoxide production and overexpression of the lipid peroxidation marker 4-hydroxynonenal (rosmarinic acid administered at 10 mg/kg b.w., i.p.) [47];
- protection against the iron-induced neurotoxicity in neuroblastoma SK-N-SH cells [48];
- prevention of the progression of oxidative stress caused by $H_2O_2$ in C6 glial cells by increasing the cell viability and inhibiting the cellular lipid peroxidation, reduction of $H_2O_2$-induced expression of inducible iNOS and COX-2 at the transcriptional level, downregulation of iNOS and COX-2 protein expression in $H_2O_2$-induced C6 glial cells [49];
- antioxidant effect, inhibition of MAO-A and MAO-B and catechol-*O*-methyl transferase (COMT) with no cytotoxicity on polymorphonuclear rat cells [50];
- enhancing the antioxidant status, decreasing the oxidative stress, efficiently ameliorating inflammatory mechanisms by downregulation of NF-κB and pro-inflammatory cytokines after spinal cord injury in Wistar rats (rosmarinic acid administered at 10 mg/kg b.w., i.p.) [51].

**Anti-epileptic Activity:**

- increasing the latency and decreasing the percentage of seizure incidents, reducing the levels of free radicals and DNA damage in the kindling CF-1 male mice model of epilepsy induced by PTZ (rosmarinic acid at 1, 2 or 4 mg/kg b.w., i.p.) [28];
- attenuation of seizures, mitigation of the oxidative stress, augmentation of the activity of defensive systems, reduction of MDA and nitrite content and increase of CAT activity; prevention of the hippocampal neuronal loss in CA1 and CA3 regions and mossy fiber sprouting in the kainite model of temporal lobe epilepsy in rats (rosmarinic acid administered at 10 mg/kg b.w./d, i.p.) [52];
- acute anticonvulsant-like activity against seizures via increased latency to myoclonic jerks and generalized seizure durations in the C57BL/6 female mouse model with PTZ-induced epilepsy (rosmarinic acid at 3 or 30 mg/kg b.w., p.o., for 14 days) [53];
- improvement (in combination with diazepam) of the latency to first seizures, reduction of the latency to sleep in the diazepam-induced sleeping time test in a model of PTZ-induced seizures in mice, decreased pilocarpine-induced genotoxic damage in a mice acute seizure model (rosmarinic acid at 2 or 4 mg/kg b.w., i.p.) [29].

**Huntington Disease**

- improvement of the behavioral abnormalities and attenuation of the oxidative stress in 3NP-treated rats (an animal model of Huntington disease) (rosmarinic acid at 12 mg/kg b.w., nasal delivery) [54].

**Antidepressant Effect:**

- downregulation of mitogen-activated protein kinase phosphatase-1, upregulation of BDNF and modulation of dopamine and corticosterone synthesis in TST in a model of depression in mice with bupropion as a positive control (rosmarinic acid administered for 7 days at 5 and 10 mg/kg b.w./day) [55].

**Anti-tauopathy Activity:**

- counteracting the stress-induced tauopathy by efficient suppression of the elevation of P-tau and insoluble P-tau formation, reversion of the abnormal changes of chaperones and peptidyl-prolyl cis/trans isomerase (Pin1) in middle-aged mice with induced chronic restraint stress [56].

**Long-term Potentiation:**

- enhancement of baseline field excitatory postsynaptic potentials (fEPSPs) following high-frequency stimulation in CA1 synapses, increase of the expression of BDNF and ionotropic AMPA glutamate receptor 2 (GluR-2) proteins and prevention of cell death in scopolamine-exposed organotypic hippocampal slice cultures [57].

**Anticancer Activity:**

- dose-dependent suppression of cell proliferation and cytotoxic effect on glioblastoma cells without antioxidant effect (at 171.3–290.5 μmol/L), but at higher doses, a prooxidant effect was observed, leading to cell death through necrosis [58].

**Inflammation:**

- decrease of COX-2, PGE-2, IL-1β, matrix metallopeptidase 2 and NO levels in male Wistar rats that underwent CCI (rosmarinic acid at 40 mg/kg b.w., i.p., after 7 and 14 days) [59].

Table 1. *Cont.*

| | |
|---|---|
| **P-Coumaric Acid** | *Protection from Ischemia/Reperfusion Injury:*<br><br>• decrease of MDA, increase of NRF1 levels and SOD activity, reduction of ischemic fiber degeneration and Aβ protein expressions in rats' sciatic nerve segments after abdominal aorta clamping (p-coumaric acid at 100 mg phenolic acid/kg b.w.) [60];<br>• decrease of the oxidative damage, focal ischemia and neurological deficit scores in rat brains subjected to cerebral ischemia (via intraluminal monofilament occlusion model) due to the antioxidant and antiapoptotic activity (p-coumaric acid at 100 mg phenolic acid/kg b.w.) [61];<br>• decrease of MDA, hypoxia-inducible factor-1α levels and NF-κB immunopositive neuron number; increase of NRF1, SOD activity and the number of normal neurons after ischemia-reperfusion injury of the spinal cord (via infrarenal aorta cross-clamping model) in rats (p-coumaric acid at 100 mg/kg b.w.) [62].<br><br>*Anticancer Activity:*<br><br>• cytotoxic effect on neuroblastoma N2a cells by generation of ROS leading to dysfunction of mitochondrial membrane, the release of cytochrome c, decreased intracellular reduced glutathione, p53-mediated upregulated accumulation of Casp-8 messenger RNA, accumulation of microtubule-associated 1A/1B light chain 3B protein (LC3-II) leading to apoptosis and autophagy [63]. |
| **Sinapic Acid** | *PD:*<br><br>• partial amelioration of negative phenomena in the 6-OHDA-induced hemi-parkinsonian rat: Improved turning behavior, prevented loss of dopaminergic neurons in substantia nigra pars compacta, lowered iron reactivity and attenuated MDA and nitrite levels in midbrain homogenate (rats pretreated p.o. with sinapic acid at 20 mg/kg b.w.) [64]. |
| **Cinnamic Aldehyde** | *Inflammation and Cognition:*<br><br>• reduction of COX-2 protein activity and PGE2 concentrations in frontal cortex and hippocampus; reversal of selected abnormalities (exploratory behavior, central ambulation and total ambulation-anxiety behavior, rearing, grooming, immobility period) studied in open field exploratory behavior test in mid-aged rats after the exposure to CUMS (cinnamic aldehyde at 45 and 90 mg/kg b.w., p.o., for 21 days) [65]. |
| **Salicylic Acid** | *Antioxidant Activity:*<br><br>• sodium salicylate: amelioration of negative alterations in methamphetamine-induced mouse model, including scavenging of ROS, reversing of the mitochondrial dysfunction and movement abnormalities, and amelioration of the complex-I activity decrease leading to striatal dopamine depletion (sodium salicylate at 50 and 100 mg/kg b.w.) [66];<br>• ex vivo neuroprotective and antioxidant effect in primary cortex neurons isolated from Sprague–Dawley rat brains after the oxygen stress caused by paclitaxel and cisplatin [67]. |
| **Acetylsalicylic Acid** | *Inflammation and Antioxidant Activity:*<br><br>• counteracting the decrease of degenerative changes, decrease of inflammatory reactivity, and the expression of estrogen receptors (atrophy) in hippocampus caused by 2,3,7,8-tetrachlorodibenzo-p-dioxin (acetylsalicylic acid at 50 mg/kg b.w., p.o., for 21 days) [68];<br>• reduction of the neuroinflammation markers and oxidative stress markers PGE2, 15-epilipoxin A4, 8-isoprostane and leukotriene B4 concentrations in HIV-1 transgenic rat model associated with neurocognitive disorders (acetylsalicylic acid at 10 mg/kg/day in drinking water, for 42 days) [69].<br><br>*Protection from Ischemia/Reperfusion Injury:*<br><br>• reduction of the early neurological deterioration in patients with acute ischemic stroke (in combination with clopidogrel), in comparison to monotherapy (clopidogrel alone), in studies involving 690 patients aged > 40 years with minor stroke or transient ischemic attack (aspirin at 100 mg/day in combination with clopidogrel at 75 mg/day, in comparison to monotherapy with aspirin alone at 300 mg/day) [70];<br>• significant reduction of platelet aggregation and platelet-leukocyte aggregate numbers in patients after acute ischemic stroke (1124 patients, among which 270 experienced neurological deterioration), lower incidence of neurological deterioration in patients with pre-stroke concomitant treatment with phenolic acid (acid at 200 mg/day, p.o.) [71].<br><br>*Anti-amyotrophic Lateral Sclerosis (ALS) Effect:*<br><br>• consumption was independently inversely associated with ALS risk, predominately in patients older than 55 years, as observed in studies involving 729 patients with newly diagnosed ALS and 7390 sex-, age-, residence- and insurance premium-matched controls [72].<br><br>*Normalization of Brain Function:*<br><br>• moderate enhancement of rapamycin-mediated inhibition of dendritic cells' allostimulatory capacity: reduction of the number of mouse bone marrow-derived immature dendritic cells expressing CD40 protein and major histocompatibility complex class II (MHC II) molecules after the stimulation by LPS [73]. |

Table 1. *Cont.*

|  | |
|---|---|
| | *Inflammation:* |
| | • reduction of iron content in microglial cells by regulating the expression of iron transport proteins: downregulation of transferring receptor 1, upregulation of ferroportin 1 and ferritin expressions in microglial cells, partial reversion of LPS-induced disruption of cell iron balance under in vitro inflammatory conditions by decrease of ferritin, IL-6, TNF-α, hepcidin mRNA contents previously increased by LPS alone [74]. |
| | *Chagas Disease:* |
| | • protection of the esophageal myenteric neurons from the atrophy caused by *Trypanosoma cruzi* without alterations in the esophageal wall and the myenteric neurons in infected mice [75]. |
| | *TBI:* |
| | • upregulation of proteins involved in the neuroprotection of cellular pathways in Sprague–Dawley rats sustaining TBI, leading to the amelioration of previously provoked alterations in proteome and glycoproteins (acid at 30 mg/kg, i.p.) [76]. |
| | *Prevention of Hearing Loss:* |
| | • decrease of the progression of the age-related hearing loss, positive retinal microvascular changes, amelioration of the mean pure tone average hearing threshold (decibels) in the better ear in studies involving 1262 Australians aged over 70 years with normal cognitive functions after 3 years of phenolic acid consumption (enteric-coated aspirin at a dose of 100 mg, p.o.) [77]. |
| **Protocatechuic Acid** | *Antioxidant Activity:* |
| | • attenuation of the loss of neurons in zebrafish and mice treated by 6-hydroxydopamine; increased cell viability, Nrf2-related factor 2 protein expression, upregulation of the expression of antioxidant enzymes such as heme oxygenase-1, SOD, CAT; decrease of MDA, NF-κB, and iNOS levels; decrease of LDH release from cells in 6-OHDA-treated PC12 cells (protocatechuic acid in combination with chrysin) [78]; |
| | • protection of brain mitochondrial functions (glycemic control, reduction of oxidative stress markers) in the heart of streptozotocin-induced diabetic rats (protocatechuic acid at 50 and 100 mg/kg, p.o., for 12 weeks) [79]. |
| | *Cell Proliferation:* |
| | • induction of proliferation of RSC96 Schwann cells by phosphorylation of the insulin-like growth factor-I-mediated phosphatidylinositol 3 kinase/serine-threonine kinase (IGF-IR-PI3K-Akt) pathway; activation of expression of cell nuclear antigen in a dose-dependent manner; positive modulation of expressions of cell cycle proteins cyclin D1, E and A and a knockdown of PI3K by small interfering RNA and inhibition of IGF-IR [80]; |
| | • prevention of the reduction of mitochondrial membrane potential along with the increased cell viability, ameliorated mitochondrial complex I activity, reduction of the release of LDH and ROS from cells in midbrain dopaminergic neurons injured by 1-methyl-4-phenylpyridinium in Kun Ming mice [81]. |
| | *Inflammation:* |
| | • inhibition of Toll-like receptor 4-mediated NF-κB and MAPKs signaling pathways and the inhibition of the LPS-induced production of TNF-α, IL-6 IL-1β and PGE2 in LPS-induced BV2 (C57BL/6) microglia [82]. |
| | *PD:* |
| | • increase of tyrosine hydroxylase and dopamine receptor D2 and decrease of iNOS expression in striatum and midbrain of C57BL mice after the induction of PD by 1-methyl-4-phenyl-1,2,3,6-tetrahydropyridine (protocatechuic acid at a dose of 10 mg/kg in combination with Madopar at 125 mg/kg, i.p., for 7 days) [83]. |
| | *Inflammation:* |
| | • induction of the expressions of MAPK (ERK1/2, JNK and p38) followed by the activation of downstream expressions of matrix-degrading proteolytic enzymes Pas, matrix metallopeptidase 2, and matrix metallopeptidase 9 in RSC96 Schwann cells, which modified the cell migration and the regeneration of damaged peripheral nerve [84]. |
| **Gallic Acid** | *Antioxidant Activity:* |
| | • amelioration of the intracerebroventricular streptozotocin-induced oxidative damage by normalization of thiobarbituric acid-reactive substances and total thiol contents, as well as GPx, CAT and SOD activities in the rat striatum (gallic acid at 30 mg/kg, p.o., for 26 days) [85]; |
| | • amelioration of antioxidative enzymes in the development of depression (gallic acid at 0.8, 2 and 4 mg/kg b.w., p.o., for 10 days) [86]. |

**Table 1.** *Cont.*

| | |
|---|---|
| | *Traumatic Nerve Injury:*<br>• dose-dependent improvement during the peripheral nerve degeneration (amelioration of the motor coordination and sciatic nerve crush velocity) in rats with sciatic nerve crush (gallic acid at 200 mg/kg/2 mL, p.o.) [87].<br><br>*Antidepressant Effect:*<br>• amelioration of the anxiety and depression (tested in TST, elevated plus maze and novelty suppressed feeding test), reduction of the cell densities in the CA1, CA2, CA3 and DG hippocampal subdivisions after the administration of trimethyltin to Sprague–Dawley rats (gallic acid at 150 mg/kg b.w., i.p., for 14 days) [88].<br><br>*Cytotoxicity:*<br>• reversion of the cyclophosphamide-induced neurotoxicity in Wistar rats by restoration of normal levels of cerebellar and cerebral CAT, SOD, MDA, glutathione S-transferase, $H_2O_2$, GPx and nitrite levels (gallic acid at 60 and 120 mg/kg b.w., p.o., for 10 days) [89].<br><br>*Anticancer Activity:*<br>• dose-dependent cytotoxicity in DBTRG-05MG human brain glioblastoma cells by the elevation of intracellular $Ca^{2+}$ levels in cells, increase of intracellular $Ca^{2+}$ levels in combination with thapsigargin, increase of ROS production and activation of mitochondrial apoptotic pathways [90]. |
| **Tannic Acid** | *Antioxidant Activity:*<br>• increase of the concentrations of NR2A and NR2B subunits of *N*-methyl-D-aspartate receptors, elevation of the activities of antioxidant enzymes, decrease of lipid peroxidation in the brain hippocampus in Wistar rats after 16-weeks exposure of animals to $Al^{3+}$ and $Pb^{2+}$ (tannic acid at 50 mg/kg b.w./day; a nasogastric probe was used) [91];<br>• counteracting against $Pb^{2+}$-induced neurochemical perturbations in Wistar rats including the reduction of oxygen radical species levels and enzymatic oxidants; amelioration of the activity of non-enzymatic antioxidants, neurotoxicity biomarkers and histological changes (tannic acid at 50 mg/kg b.w., three times a week, for two weeks) [92].<br><br>*Protection from Ischemia/reperfusion Injury:*<br>• reduction of ROS and MDA levels, elevation of SOD and NRF1 levels in brain tissues in rats with brain ischemia after middle cerebral artery occlusion induced by ethanol given intraperitoneally (tannic acid at a dose of 10 mg/kg b.w. dissolved in 10% ethanol administered within half an hour intraperitoneally) [93];<br>• reduction of infarct size, improved neurological function, suppressed neuronal loss, downregulation of the GFAP expression, reduction of thiobarbituric acid reactive species and cytokine levels in Wistar rats after the middle cerebral artery occlusion followed by reperfusion (tannic acid at 50 mg/kg, i.p.) [94]. |
| **Homovanillic Acid** | *Antidepressant Effect:*<br>• reduction of depressive symptoms in a 4-week, double-blind, randomized, placebo-controlled study involving 22 men and 25 women, due to the improvement of the peripheral dopaminergic activity and increased (by 11.5%) homovanillic acid concentration in plasma of overweight or obese patients with depressive symptoms (after the co-supplementation with 1.4 g cocoa extract/day corresponding to 645 mg total polyphenols/day) [95];<br>• the lower number of suicide incidents in patients with schizophrenia and elevated homovanillic acid levels in cerebrospinal fluid (28-year follow-up studies) [96].<br><br>*Psychotic Disorders:*<br>• normalization of the disturbed dopaminergic activity in patients with psychotic spectrum disorders, especially schizophrenia, by partially taking over the functions in dopaminergic metabolism in the central nervous system [97]. |
| **Syringic Acid** | *Protection from Ischemia/reperfusion Injury:*<br>• elevation of SOD activity, NRF-1 levels; reduced MDA, Casp-3 and Casp-9 levels leading to the reduced oxidative stress and neuronal degeneration in Sprague–Dawley rat brain tissues after cerebral ischemia caused by artery occlusion (syringic acid at 10 mg/kg b.w., i.p.) [98];<br>• reduction of the oxidative stress and neuronal degeneration by reduction of the number of apoptotic neurons, beclin-1 protein and Casp-3-immunopositive neurons in spinal cords of Sprague–Dawley rats with spinal cord ischemia (infrarenal aortic cross-clamping model) (syringic acid at 10 mg/kg b.w., i.p.) [99]. |

Table 1. Cont.

|  |  |
|---|---|
|  | *Vision:* <br> • prevention of retinal ganglion cells RGC-5 from $H_2O_2$-induced apoptosis through the activation of phosphatidylinositol 3-kinase/protein kinase B signaling pathway, elevated expression of the Bcl-2 regulator proteins, decrease of the expression of Bax and cleaved Casp-3 protein [100]. <br> *Protection during Oxygen Deprivation/Reperfusion Injury:* <br> • attenuation of the injury of primary hippocampal neuronal cells by the decrease of the following: LDH leakage from cells, Bax and Casp-3 expressions, the levels of intracellular MDA, ROS, and $Ca^{2+}$; inhibition of oxygen deprivation/reperfusion-induced increase in phosphorylated JNK and p-p38 expression; increased cell viability, restoring the intracellular SOD, mitochondrial membrane potential, and Bcl-2 expression [101]. |
| **Ellagic Acid** | *Anticancer Activity:* <br> • reduction of the number of human neuroblastoma SH-SY5Y cells by alterations of the mitochondrial membrane potential, activation of Casp-3, Casp-9, fragmentation of DNA, and dose- and time-dependent cell apoptosis by the mitochondrial pathway [102,103]; <br> • decrease of cell proliferation, cell viability, decrease of the proportion at G0/G1 phase of the cell cycle together with increased cell population at S phase; upregulation of Death receptor 4, Death receptor 5, and MAP kinases (JNK, ERK1/2, and p38), as well as CCAAT-enhancer-binding homologous protein (CHOP) and glucose-regulated protein 78 (GRP78) expressions leading to the severe apoptosis in U251 human glioblastoma cells [104]. <br><br> *PD:* <br> • restoration of the locomotion, reduction of the levels of neuroinflammatory biomarkers TNF-α and IL-1β in the striatum and in hippocampus of a rat model of PD induced by 6-OHDA (right medial forebrain bundle-lesioned rats) (ellagic acid at 50 mg/kg b.w./2 mL, by gavages) [105]; <br> • amelioration of the rotenone-induced locomotor impairment in zebrafish (adult zebrafish exposed to ellagic acid at 20 or 40 mg/kg b.w. in combination with curcumin at 20 or 40 mg/kg b.w., i.m., for 14 days) and *Drosophila melanogaster* (adult wild-Type flies exposed to ellagic acid at 0.05% and 0.1% in combination with curcumin at 0.05% and 0.1%, in feed for 7 days) (swimming behavior and poorer climbing capability, respectively) [106]. <br><br> *Amnesia:* <br> • reversion of the scopolamine-induced amnesia verified in the elevated plus maze and passive avoidance paradigm tests, improvement of amnesia caused by diazepam in rats (ellagic acid at 30 or 100 mg/kg b.w., i.p.) [107]. <br><br> *Inflammation:* <br> • downregulation of the p38 mitogen-activated protein kinase (p38 MAPK), amelioration of the inflammatory pain including acetic acid-induced nociception, formalin-induced nociception, and paclitaxel-induced neuropathic pain in the murine model (ellagic acid at 50 mg/kg b.w./2 mL of saline, administered as a bolus into the subcutis for 5 days) [108]. <br><br> *Protection from the Ischemic Injury:* <br> • reduction of the infarct size, weight, and volume of the brain; reduced apoptosis by reduced levels of caspases, apoptotic pathway proteins, MAPK proteins, and inflammatory mediators NF-κB (p65) and p-IK-Ba in hypoxic-ischemic brains of rat pups (ellagic acid at 10, 20 or 40 mg/kg b.w., p.o.) [109]. <br><br> *Protection during OxygenDeprivation/Reperfusion Injury:* <br> • improvement of the rats' nerve-related abilities, remedied infarct volumes and morphological changes in the brain enhanced content of nestin protein in the brain semi-darkness zone in a photothrombosis-induced model of brain injury in rats; elevation of β-catenin expression and *cyclin D1* gene expression in an oxygen-glucose deprivation and reperfusion model established in in vitro primary cultured neural stem cells [110]. |

## 3. Penetration of Brain by Phenolic Acids

Previously, it has been estimated that the daily consumption of phenolic acids is noticeable and totals ≈200 mg [111,112]. Moreover, the pharmacokinetic properties of phenolic acids are excellent. Bourne and Rice-Evans (1998) showed that the peak concentration of ferulic acid in plasma occurred 7–9 h after the consumption of tomatoes (360–640 g), with the recovery of the phenolic acid reaching 11–25% of the amount consumed [113]. Recently, a cross-sectional analysis of the consumption of polyphenols (involving 10 European countries and over half a million participants) revealed that the total amount of these secondary plant metabolites was high (744 mg/day in men and 584 mg/day in women in Greece to 1786 mg/day in men and 1626 mg/day in women in Denmark). Among polyphenols, phenolic acids represented the largest part (52.5–56.9% in women and men, respectively) in the diets of all groups, with the exception of men in the Mediterranean countries and "health-conscious" consumers in the United Kingdom (predominantly vegetarians). However, in the Mediterranean countries and in the "health-conscious" group in the U.K., phenolic acids were the second most distributed polyphenols (34–44%). Generally, hydroxycinnamic acids (ranging from 27% in women from the "health-conscious" group in the U.K. to 53% in men from non- Mediterranean countries) were the most important contributors to total polyphenols in the diet. The most important dietary source of phenolic acids in all studied European countries was coffee (58–75%), and the most distributed phenolic acids were caffeoylquinic acids (mainly 5-caffeoylquinic, 4-caffeoylquinic and 3-caffeoylquinic acid), followed by feruloylquinic, gallic, galloylquinic, 4-hydroxyphenylacetic, homovanillic, 3,4-dihydroxyphenylacetic and dihydro-p-coumaric acids [114]. Other major research papers have confirmed the high dietary intake of phenolic acids. Tresserra-Rimbau et al. (2013) calculated that the mean consumption of phenolic acids in a group of 7200 participants was $304 \pm 156$ mg/day (a parallel-group, aged 55–80 years; a validated one-year food frequency questionnaire in a multicenter, randomized, controlled five-year feeding trial). Phenolic acids were the main polyphenolics consumed (33% of all polyphenols), and 5-caffeoylquinic acid was the most abundant individual polyphenolic compound. Other phenolic acids broadly consumed were: 3-caffeoylquinic acid ($49.75 \pm 34.18$ mg/day), 4-caffeoylquinic acid ($42.60 \pm 31.79$ mg/day), ferulic acid ($14.32 \pm 14.35$ mg/day), 5-feruloylquinic acid $7.24 \pm 5.56$ (mg/day), 4-feruloylquinic acid ($6.17 \pm 4.81$ mg/day), syringic acid ($4.82 \pm 4.76$ mg/day) and verbascoside ($4.61 \pm 7.00$ mg/day) [115]. Grosso et al. (2014), in a study involving 10,477 persons aged 45–69 years (a validated 148-item food frequency questionnaire), estimated the daily intake of phenolic acids at 800 mg (521 mg/day as aglycone equivalents, 46% of total intake of polyphenols). The main phenolic acids were 5-caffeoylquinic and 4-caffeoylquinic acids (with average intake at 150 mg/day), followed by 3-caffeoylquinic acid ($128.2 \pm 111.6$ mg/day), 5-O-galloylquinic acid ($60.8 \pm 45.4$ mg/day), ferulic acid ($43.9 \pm 33.7$ mg/day), stigmastanol ferulate ($37.5 \pm 22.6$ mg/day), 5-feruloylquinic acid ($27.9 \pm 14.3$ mg/day), gallic acid $25.0 \pm 11.2$ mg/day) and 4-feruloylquinic acid ($20.4 \pm 12$ mg/day) [116].

The experimental data collated in Table 1 prove the positive role of phenolic acids in an indirect manner. The amount of phenolic acids administered to experimental animals in feed is known, but the authors did not study the content of phenolic acids in the brain. Therefore, the activity of phenolic acids in brains (on the biochemical and gene expression levels, amelioration of the enzyme activity changes) was discussed only by comparison with reference groups of animals fed with a standard diet. Although it is assumed that the transfer of polyphenols through the blood-brain barrier is limited, a considerable number of original papers confirm the presence of absorbed phenolic acid compounds in the brain. Phenolic acids can be accumulated in the brain at pharmacologically-relevant, nanomolar or micromolar concentrations, as described below. Gallic acid has been detected in trace amounts in brains (mouse model of Alzheimer's disease) after repeated administration of grape seed polyphenolic extract for 10 days (intragastric gavage of 50, 100 and 150 mg/kg b.w.) [117]. Protocatechuic acid was detected in brain micro-dialysates (at maximal concentration of $0.09 \pm 0.07$ µg/mL, $\approx 0.58 \pm 0.45$ nmol/mL) 15 min–4 h after the administration of Danshen extract (*Salvia miltiorrhiza*, intragastrically, 40 mg/kg b.w.) to adult, male Sprague-Dawley rats [118]. 3-Hydroxybenzoic, benzoic and homovanillic acids were detected (at 0.43–1.06 nmol/g, 2.53–15.63 nmol/g and 1.84–2.39 nmol/g, respectively) in extracts of freeze-dried brain tissues of male Wistar rats orally fed with the grape seed proanthocyanidin extract (125, 250, 375, 1000 mg extract/kg b.w.). The levels of phenolic acids were dependent on the dose of the extract [119]. Benzoic acid was the main phenolic acid in brains of Sprague–Dawley rats that consumed wild blueberry for four and eight weeks. Other minor phenolic acids were also detected in brains, and the sum of all detected phenolic acids was 69.0 µg/g brain (which can be estimated for nanomolar concentrations, taking into consideration the molecular masses of the various phenolic acids) [120]. In another work, 3-hydroxybenzoic and 3-(3′-hydroxyphenyl) propionic acids were accumulated at μmol concentrations in perfused brain tissues of rats fed for 11 days with grape seed polyphenol extract. Both phenolic acids were shown to accumulate in brains in a dose-dependent manner. Treatment with 250 mg extract/kg b.w./day increased brain contents of 3-hydroxybenzoic and 3-hydroxyphenylpropionic acid 3.2-fold and 7.7-fold, respectively (in comparison to controls). Furthermore, hydroxybenzoic, 4-hydroxybenzoic, 3-hydroxyphenylacetic, 3,4-dihydroxyphenylacetic and 3-hydroxyphenylpropionic acids were detected in brains, but no detectable changes in the content of these phenolic acids were observed after the treatment with various doses of the extract [121]. Ferulic acid was detected in brains (2.6 μg/g of tissue, ≈13.39 nmol/mL) after the oral administration to rats (521 μmol acid/kg b.w.), and the concentration of this acid in brains was decreased only by 50% 60 min after the consumption [122]. Other works confirm the penetration of brain by ferulic acid [123], caffeic acid and caffeic acid phenethyl ester [124] and rosmarinic acid [125]. Ferulic, caffeic, rosmarinic acids and caffeic acid phenethyl ester can also protect blood-brain barrier and brain structures [126–129]. Chlorogenic acid was detected in the cerebrospinal fluid of rats that were fed with chlorogenic acid-enriched *Eucommia ulmoides* bark extract (200 and 400 mg extract/kg b.w./day, for seven days). The levels of phenolic acid were ≈0.42–0.56 ng/mL (≈0.0011–0.0015 nmol/mL) (1 h and 1.5 h after consumption, respectively) [42]. Moreover, degradation of absorbed, more complex polyphenols from foods yielding simple phenolic acids can be observed, thus increasing the levels of bioavailable phenolic acids in the brain. For example, cyanidin 3-*O*-glucopyranoside is degraded in vivo in SH-SY5Y bone marrow neuroblastoma cells, yielding protocatechuic acid [130]. Taking the above results into consideration, it can be claimed that phenolic acids can effectively accumulate in brain achieving the levels required for the pharmacological effect.

A very interesting aspect of the neuroprotective activity of phenolic acids in biological systems is the activity rather at low and not at high concentrations, as was explicitly stated by some authors. Caffeic acid dimethyl ether, when used at lower concentrations (15–50 μmol/L), was more efficient than applied at a higher dose (at 50–100 μmol/L) for the elevation of the expression of heme oxygenase-1 in cultivated astrocytes, leading to the increased concentrations of reduced glutathione in cultured cells [131]. Similarly, ferulic acid ethyl ester effectively induced heme oxygenase-1 protein expression in cultivated astrocytes at low (5 μmol/L), but not at high concentrations (15 μmol/L), along with the maximal expression of mRNA coding for heme oxygenase-1 [132].

## 4. Concluding Remarks

This review was designed as a compact, comprehensive, content-rich compendium of the latest reports on the role of phenolic acids in improving neurological dysfunctions by direct positive influence on neural and glial cells. Especially, the years 2014–2016 were very fruitful in terms of the very in-depth knowledge about biochemical parameters, new specific markers and gene expression modifications caused by phenolic acids, involved in the proper functioning of neural and glial cells.

In summary, it can be stated that due to a wide distribution in natural sources, a considerable daily intake, relatively high stability in foods, as well as high intestinal absorption (in comparison to more complex polyphenols) and efficient brain absorption, phenolic acids may be considered as promising compounds for the future combination therapy of neurological disorders.

**Acknowledgments:** This scientific work was supported by the Ministry of Science and Higher Education of the Republic of Poland (Scientific Grant No. 2339/B/P01/2010/38) and the University of Life Sciences in Lublin, which is financed by the Polish Government.

**Author Contributions:** All authors contributed to the gathering of source articles and writing of this paper.

**Conflicts of Interest:** The authors declare no conflict of interest.

# Abbreviations

| | |
|---|---|
| 3NP | 3-Nitropropionic acid |
| 6-OHDA | 6-Hydroxydopamine |
| BAD | Bcl-2-associated death promoter |
| Bax | Bcl-2-like protein 4 |
| BCL | B-cell lymphoma |
| BCL-2 | B-cell lymphoma 2 |
| Bcr-Abl | fusion between break point cluster (Bcr) gene and the Abelson (Abl) tyrosine kinase gene |
| BDNF | Brain-derived neurotrophic factor |
| b.w. | Body weight |
| Casp-3 | Caspase-3 |
| Casp-8 | Caspase-8 |
| Casp-9 | Caspase-9 |
| CAT | Catalase |
| CCI | Chronic constriction injury |
| CD40 | Cluster of differentiation 40 |
| COX-2 | Cyclooxygenase-2 |
| CREB | cAMP response element-binding protein |
| CUMS | Chronic unexpected mild stress |
| EPO | Erythropoietin |
| ERK | Extracellular signal-regulated kinase, protein-serine/threonine kinase |
| ERK1 | Extracellular signal-regulated kinase 1, protein-serine/threonine kinase 1 |
| ERK2 | Extracellular signal-regulated kinase 2 protein-serine/threonine kinase 2 |
| FST | Forced swimming test |
| GFAP | Glial fibrillary acidic protein |
| GPx | Glutathione peroxidase |
| i.p. | Intraperitoneally |
| IL-1$\beta$ | Interleukin 1$\beta$ |
| IL-4 | Interleukin 4 |
| IL-5 | Interleukin 5 |
| IL-6 | Interleukin 6 |
| IL-13 | Interleukin 13 |
| iNOS | Inducible nitric oxide synthase |
| JNK | c-Jun N-terminal kinase |
| LDH | Lactate dehydrogenase |
| LPS | Lipopolysaccharide |
| MAO | Monoamine oxidase |
| MDA | Malondialdehyde |
| MEK | Mitogen-activated protein kinase |
| MHX | major histocompatibility complex II molecules |
| NF-$\kappa$B | Nuclear factor-$\kappa$B |
| NO | Nitric oxide |
| NRF1 | Nuclear respiratory factor 1 |
| Nrf2 | Nuclear factor (erythroid-derived 2)-like 2 |
| Nrf2/HO-1 | Nuclear factor (erythroid-derived 2)-like 2/heme oxygenase-1 |
| p38 | MAP Kinase (MAPK), CSBP Cytokinin-Specific Binding Protein or RK |
| p90RSK | MAPK-activated protein kinase-1 (MAPKAP-K1) |
| pCREB | phosphorylated cAMP response element-binding protein |
| PD | Parkinson disease |
| PGE2 | Prostaglandin E2 |
| p.o. | Orally |
| p-p38 | phosphorylated p38 |
| PTZ | Pentylenetetrazol |
| ROS | Reactive oxygen species |
| SOD | Superoxide dismutase |
| TBI | Traumatic brain injury |
| Th1 | T helper type 1 (Th1) cells |
| Th2 | T helper type 2 (Th2) cells |
| TNF-$\alpha$ | Tumor necrosis factor-$\alpha$ |
| TST | Tail suspension test |

## References

1. Mattila, P.; Hellström, J.; Törrönen, R. Phenolic acids in berries, fruits, and beverages. *J. Agric. Food Chem.* **2006**, *54*, 7193–7199. [CrossRef] [PubMed]
2. Grosso, G.; Estruch, R. Nut consumption and age-related disease. *Maturitas* **2016**, *84*, 11–16. [CrossRef] [PubMed]
3. Crozier, A.; Jaganath, I.B.; Clifford, M.N. Dietary phenolics: Chemistry, bioavailability and effects on health. *Nat. Prod. Rep.* **2009**, *26*, 1001–1043. [CrossRef] [PubMed]
4. Van Hung, P. Phenolic compounds of cereals and their antioxidant capacity. *Crit. Rev. Food Sci. Nutr.* **2016**, *56*, 25–35. [CrossRef] [PubMed]
5. Liu, X.; Yan, Y.; Li, F.; Zhang, D. Fruit and vegetable consumption and the risk of depression: A meta-analysis. *Nutrition* **2016**, *32*, 296–302. [CrossRef] [PubMed]
6. Grosso, G.; Micek, A.; Castellano, S.; Pajak, A.; Galvano, F. Coffee, tea, caffeine and risk of depression: A systematic review and close-response meta-analysis of observational studies. *Mol. Nutr. Food Res.* **2016**, *60*, 223–234. [CrossRef] [PubMed]
7. Szwajgier, D.; Baranowska-Wójcik, E.; Borowiec, K. Phenolic acids exert anticholinesterase and cognition-improving effects. *Curr. Alzheimer Res* **2017**, in press.
8. Li, G.; Ruan, L.; Chen, R.; Wang, R.; Xie, X.; Zhang, M.; Chen, L.; Yan, Q.; Reed, M.; Chen, J.; et al. Synergistic antidepressant-like effect of ferulic acid in combination with piperine: Involvement of monoaminergic system. *Metab. Brain Dis.* **2015**, *30*, 1505–1514. [CrossRef] [PubMed]
9. Chen, J.; Lin, D.; Zhang, C.; Li, G.; Zhang, N.; Ruan, L.; Yan, Q.; Li, J.; Yu, X.; Xie, X.; et al. Antidepressant-like effects of ferulic acid: Involvement of serotonergic and norepinergic systems. *Metab. Brain Dis.* **2015**, *30*, 129–136. [CrossRef] [PubMed]
10. Lenzi, J.; Rodriguez, A.F.; Rós Ade, S.; de Castro, A.B.; de Lima, D.D.; Magro, D.D.; Zeni, A.L. Ferulic acid chronic treatment exerts antidepressant-like effect: Role of antioxidant defense system. *Metab. Brain Dis.* **2015**, *30*, 1453–1463. [CrossRef] [PubMed]
11. Liu, Y.M.; Hu, C.Y.; Shen, J.D.; Wu, S.H.; Li, Y.C.; Yi, L.T. Elevation of synaptic protein is associated with the antidepressant-like effects of ferulic acid in a chronic model of depression. *Physiol. Behav.* **2017**, *169*, 184–188. [CrossRef] [PubMed]
12. Zhang, L.; Wang, H.; Wang, T.; Jiang, N.; Yu, P.; Chong, Y.; Fu, F. Ferulic acid ameliorates nerve injury induced by cerebral ischemia in rats. *Exp. Ther. Med.* **2015**, *9*, 972–976. [CrossRef] [PubMed]
13. Koh, P.O. Ferulic acid attenuates the down-regulation of MEK/ERK/p90RSK signaling pathway in focal cerebral ischemic injury. *Neurosci. Lett.* **2015**, *588*, 18–23. [CrossRef] [PubMed]
14. Ge, L.J.; Fan, S.Y.; Yang, J.H.; Wei, Y.; Zhu, Z.H.; Lou, Y.J.; Guo, Y.; Wan, H.T.; Xie, Y.Q. Pharmacokinetic and pharmacodynamic analysis of ferulic acid-puerarin-astragaloside in combination with neuroprotective in cerebral ischemia/reperfusion injury in rats. *Asian Pac. J. Trop. Med.* **2015**, *8*, 299–304. [CrossRef]
15. Xu, Y.; Lin, D.; Yu, X.; Xie, X.; Wang, L.; Lian, L.; Fei, N.; Chen, J.; Zhu, N.; Wang, G.; et al. The antinociceptive effects of ferulic acid on neuropathic pain: Involvement of descending monoaminergic system and opioid receptors. *Oncotarget* **2016**, *7*, 20455–20468. [CrossRef] [PubMed]
16. Aswar, M.; Patil, V. Ferulic acid ameliorates chronic constriction injury induced painful neuropathy in rats. *Inflammopharmacology* **2016**, *24*, 181–188. [CrossRef] [PubMed]
17. Nagarajan, S.; Chellappan, D.R.; Chinnaswamy, P.; Thulasingam, S. Ferulic acid pretreatment mitigates MPTP-induced motor impairment and histopathological alterations in C57BI/6 mice. *Pharm. Biol.* **2015**, *53*, 1591–1601. [CrossRef] [PubMed]
18. Ojha, S.; Javed, H.; Azimullah, S.; Khair, S.B.A.; Haque, M.E. Neuroprotective potential of ferulic acid in the rotenone model of Parkinson's disease. *Drug Des. Devel. Ther.* **2015**, *9*, 5499–5510. [PubMed]
19. Wu, J.L.; Shen, M.M.; Yang, S.X.; Wang, X.; Ma, Z.C. Inhibitory effect of ferulic acid on neuroinflammation in LPS-activated microglia. *Chin. Pharm. Bull.* **2015**, *31*, 97–102.
20. Huang, H.; Hong, Q.; Tan, H.L.; Xiao, C.R.; Gao, Y. Ferulic acid prevents LPS-induced up-regulation of PDE4B and stimulates the cAMP/CREB signaling pathway in PC12 cells. *Acta Pharm. Sin.* **2016**, *37*, 1543–1554. [CrossRef] [PubMed]

21. Dong, G.C.; Kuan, C.Y.; Subramaniam, S.; Zhao, J.Y.; Sivasubramaniam, S.; Chang, H.Y.; Lin, F.H. A potent inhibition of oxidative stress induced gene expression in neural cells by sustained ferulic acid release from chitosan based hydrogel. *Mat. Sci. Eng. C* **2015**, *49*, 691–699. [CrossRef] [PubMed]
22. Lee, C.C.; Wang, C.C.; Huang, H.M.; Lin, C.L.; Leu, S.J.; Lee, Y.L. Ferulic acid induces Th1 responses by modulating the function of dendritic cells and ameliorates Th2-mediated allergic airway inflammation in mice. *Evid-Based Compl. Alt. Med.* **2015**. [CrossRef] [PubMed]
23. Lin, W.C.; Peng, Y.F.; Hou, C.W. Ferulic acid protects PC12 neurons against hypoxia by inhibiting the p-MAPKs and COX-2 pathways. *Iran. J. Basic Med. Sci.* **2015**, *18*, 478–484. [PubMed]
24. Shen, Y.; Zhang, H.; Wang, L.; Qian, H.; Qi, H.; Miao, X.; Cheng, L.; Qi, X. Protective effect of ferulic acid against 2,2′-azobis(2-amidinopropane) dihydrochloride-induced oxidative stress in PC12 cells. *Cell. Mol. Biol.* **2016**, *62*, 109–116. [PubMed]
25. Basu Mallik, S.; Mudgal, J.; Nampoothiri, M.; Hall, S.; Dukie, S.A.; Grant, G.; Rao, C.M.; Arora, D. Caffeic acid attenuates lipopolysaccharide-induced sickness behavior and neuroinflammation in mice. *Neurosci. Lett.* **2016**, *632*, 218–223. [CrossRef] [PubMed]
26. Fazili, N.A.; Naeem, A. Anti-fibrillation potency of caffeic acid against an antidepressant induced fibrillogenesis of human α-synuclein: Implications for Parkinson's disease. *Biochimie* **2015**, *108*, 178–185. [CrossRef] [PubMed]
27. Baj, J.P.; Hu, X.L.; Jiang, X.W.; Tian, X.; Zhao, Q.C. Caffeic acids from roots of Arctium lappa and their neuroprotective activity. *Chin. Trad. Herb. Drugs* **2015**, *46*, 163–168.
28. Coelho, V.R.; Vieira, C.G.; de Souza, L.P.; Moysés, F.; Basso, C.; Picada, J.N.; Pereira, P. Antiepileptogenic, antioxidant and genotoxic evaluation of rosmarinic acid and its metabolite caffeic acid in mice. *Life Sci.* **2015**, *122*, 65–71. [CrossRef] [PubMed]
29. Coelho, V.R.; Vieira, C.G.; de Souza, L.P.; da Silva, L.L.; Pflüger, P.; Regner, G.G.; Papke, D.K.; Picada, J.N.; Pereira, P. Behavioral and genotoxic evaluation of rosmarinic and caffeic acid in acute seizure models induced by pentylenetetrazole and pilocarpine in mice. *Naunyn-Schmiedeberg's Arch. Pharmacol.* **2016**, *389*, 1195–1203. [CrossRef] [PubMed]
30. Chang, W.C.; Kuo, P.L.; Chen, C.W.; Wu, J.S.B.; Shen, S.C. Caffeic acid improves memory impairment and brain glucose metabolism via ameliorating cerebral insulin and leptin signaling pathways in high-fat diet–induced hyperinsulinemic rats. *Food Res. Int.* **2015**, *77*, 24–33. [CrossRef]
31. Alkis, H.E.; Kuzhan, A.; Dirier, A.; Tarakcioglu, M.; Demir, E.; Saricicek, E.; Demir, T.; Ahlatci, A.; Demirci, A.; Cinar, K.; Taysi, S. Neuroprotective effects of propolis and caffeic acid phenethyl ester (CAPE) on the radiation-injured brain tissue (Neuroprotective effects of propolis and CAPE). *Int. J. Radiat. Res.* **2015**, *13*, 297–303.
32. Khan, M.; Baarine, M.; Singh, I. Therapeutic potential of caffeic acid phenethyl ester in neurodegenerative diseases. In *Caffeic Acid: Biological Properties, Structure and Health Effects*; Nova Science Publishers: New York, NY, USA, 2015.
33. Ginis, Z.; Ozturk, G.; Albayrak, A.; Kurt, S.N.; Albayrak, M.; Fadillioglu, E. Protective effects of caffeic acid phenethyl ester on ifosfamide-induced central neurotoxicity in rats. *Toxicol. Ind. Health.* **2016**, *32*, 337–343. [CrossRef] [PubMed]
34. Akyol, S.; Erdemli, H.K.; Amautou, F.; Akyol, O. In vitro and in vivo neuroprotective effect of caffeic acid phenethyl ester. *J. Intercult. Ethnopharmacol.* **2015**, *4*, 192–193. [CrossRef] [PubMed]
35. Santos, N.A.G.D.; Martins, N.M.; Silva, R.D.B.; Ferreira, R.S.; Sisti, F.M.; dos Santos, A.C. Caffeic acid phenethyl ester (CAPE) protects PC12 cells from MPP+ toxicity by inducing the expression of neuron-typical proteins. *Neurotoxicology* **2014**, *45*, 131–138. [CrossRef] [PubMed]
36. Wang, L.Y.; Tang, Z.J.; Han, Y.Z. Neuroprotective effects of caffeic acid phenethyl ester against sevoflurane-induced neuronal degeneration in the hippocampus of neonatal rats involve MAPK and PI3K/Akt signaling pathways. *Mol. Med. Rep.* **2016**, *14*, 3403–3412. [CrossRef] [PubMed]
37. Tsai, C.F.; Kuo, Y.H.; Yeh, W.L.; Wu, C.Y.; Lin, H.Y.; Lai, S.W.; Liu, Y.S.; Wu, L.H.; Lu, J.K.; Lu, D.Y. Regulatory effects of caffeiccidphenethyl ester on neuroinflammation in microglial cells. *Int. J. Mol. Sci.* **2015**, *16*, 5572–5589. [CrossRef] [PubMed]
38. Balkhi, H.M.; Gul, T.; Haq, E. Anti-neoplastic and calcium modulatory action of caffeic acid phenethyl ester and desatinib in C6 glial cells: A therapeutic perspective. *CNS Neurol. Disord. Drug Targets* **2016**, *15*, 54–63. [CrossRef] [PubMed]

39. Bak, J.; Kim, H.J.; Kim, S.Y.; Choi, Y.S. Neuroprotective effect of caffeic acid phenethyl ester in 3-nitropropionic acid-induced striatal neurotoxicity. *Korean J. Physiol. Pharmacol.* **2016**, *20*, 279–286. [CrossRef] [PubMed]

40. Mikami, Y.; Yamazawa, T. Chlorogenic, a polyphenol in coffee, protects neurons against glutamate neurotoxicity. *Life Sci.* **2015**, *139*, 69–74. [CrossRef] [PubMed]

41. Guo, Y.J.; Luo, T.; Wu, F.; Mei, Y.W.; Peng, J.; Liu, H.; Li, H.R.; Zhang, S.L.; Dong, J.H.; Fang, Y.; et al. Involvement of TLR2 and TLR9 in the anti-inflammatory effects of chlorogenic acid in HSV-1-infected microglia. *Life Sci.* **2015**, *127*, 12–18. [CrossRef] [PubMed]

42. Wu, J.M.; Chen, H.X.; Li, H.; Tang, Y.; Yang, L.; Cao, S.S.; Qin, D.L. Antidepressant potential of chlorogenic acid-enriched extract from Eucommia ulmoides Oliver bark with neuron protection and promotion of serotonin release through enhancing synapsin I expression. *Molecules* **2016**, *21*. [CrossRef] [PubMed]

43. Gul, Z.; Demircan, C.; Bagdas, D.; Buyukuysal, R.L. Protective effects of chlorogenic acid and its metabolites on hydrogen peroxide-induced alterations in rat brain slices: a comparative study with resveratrol. *Neurochem. Res.* **2016**, *41*, 2075–2085. [CrossRef] [PubMed]

44. Aseervatham, G.S.B.; Suryakala, U.; Doulethunisha; Sundaram, S.; Bose, P.C.; Sivasudha, T. Expression pattern of NMDA receptors reveals antiepileptic potential of apigenin 8-Cglucoside and chlorogenic acid in pilocarpine induced epileptic mice. *Biomed. Pharmacother.* **2016**, *82*, 54–64. [CrossRef] [PubMed]

45. Fang, S.Q.; Wang, J.X.; Wei, J.X.; Shu, Y.H.; Xiao, L.; Lu, X.M. Beneficial effects of chlorogenic acid on alcohol-induced damage in PC12 cells. *Biomed. Pharmacother.* **2016**, *79*, 254–262. [CrossRef] [PubMed]

46. Taram, F.; Winter, A.N.; Linseman, D.A. Neuroprotection comparison of chlorogenic acid and its metabolites against mechanistically distinct cell death-inducing agents in cultured cerebellar granule neurons. *Brain Res.* **2016**, *1648*, 69–80. [CrossRef] [PubMed]

47. Fetoni, A.R.; Paciello, F.; Rolesi, R.; Eramo, S.L.; Mancuso, C.; Troiani, D.; Paludetti, G. Rosmarinic acid up-regulates the noise-activated Nrf2/HO-1 pathway and protects against noise-induced injury in rat cochlea. *Free Radic. Biol. Med.* **2015**, *85*, 269–281. [CrossRef] [PubMed]

48. Qu, L.; Xu, H.M.; Jiang, H.; Hie, J.X. Protective effects of rosmarinic acid against iron-induced neurotoxicity in SK-N-SH cells. *Am. J. Hematol.* **2015**, *91*, E95.

49. Lee, A.Y.; Wu, T.T.; Hwang, B.R.; Lee, J.; Lee, M.H.; Lee, S.; Cho, E.J. The neuro-protective effect of the methanolic extract of Perillafrutescens var. japonica and rosmarinic acid against $H_2O_2$-induced oxidative stress in C6 glial cells. *Biomol. Ther.* **2016**, *24*, 338–345. [CrossRef] [PubMed]

50. Andrade, J.M.D.; Passos, C.D.; Kieling Rubio, M.A.; Mendonça, J.N.; Lopes, N.P.; Henriques, A.T. Combining in vitro and in silico approaches to evaluate the multifunctional profile of rosmarinic acid from Blechnum brasiliense on targets related to neurodegeneration. *Chem. Biol. Interact.* **2016**, *254*, 135–145. [CrossRef] [PubMed]

51. Shang, A.J.; Yang, Y.; Wang, H.Y.; Tao, B.Z.; Wang, J.; Wang, Z.F.; Zhou, D.B. Spinal cord injury effectively ameliorated by neuroprotective effects of rosmarinic acid. *Nutr. Neurosci.* **2017**, *20*, 172–179. [CrossRef] [PubMed]

52. Khamse, S.; Sadr, S.S.; Roghani, M.; Hasanzadeh, G.; Mohammadian, M. Rosmarinic acid exerts a neuroprotective effect in the kainite rat model of temporat lobe epilepsy: Underlying mechanisms. *Pharm. Biol.* **2015**, *53*, 1818–1825. [CrossRef] [PubMed]

53. Grigoletto, J.; de Oliveira, C.V.; Grauncke, A.C.; de Souza, T.L.; Souto, N.S.; de Freitas, M.L.; Furian, A.F.; Santos, A.R.S.; Oliveira, M.S. Rosmarinic acid is anticonvulsant against seizures induced by pentylenetetrazol and pilocarpine in mice. *Epilepsy Behav.* **2016**, *62*, 27–34. [CrossRef] [PubMed]

54. Bhatt, R.; Singh, D.; Prakash, A.; Mishra, N. Development, characterization and nasal delivery of rosmarinic acid-loaded solid lipid nanoparticles for the effective management of Huntingtons disease. *Drug Deliv.* **2015**, *22*, 931–939. [CrossRef] [PubMed]

55. Kondo, S.; El Omri, A.; Han, J.; Isoda, H. Antidepressant-like effects of rosmarinic acid through mitogen-activated protein kinase phosphatase-1 and brain-derived neurotrophic factor modulation. *J. Funct. Food.* **2015**, *14*, 758–766. [CrossRef]

56. Shan, Y.; Wang, D.D.; Xu, Y.X.; Wang, C.; Cao, L.; Liu, Y.S.; Zhu, C.Q. Aging as a precipitating factor in chronic restraint stress-induced tau aggregation pathology, and the protective effects of rosmarinic acid. *J. Alzheimers Dis.* **2016**, *49*, 829–844. [CrossRef] [PubMed]

57. Hwang, E.S.; Kim, H.B.; Choi, G.Y.; Lee, S.; Lee, S.O.; Kim, S.; Park, J.H. Acute rosmarinic acid treatment enhances long-term potentiation, BDNF and GluR-2 protein expression, and cell survival rate against scopolamine challenge in rat organotypic hippocampal slice cultures. *Biochem. Biophs. Res. Commun.* **2016**, *475*, 44–50. [CrossRef] [PubMed]

58. Ramanauskiene, K.; Raudonis, R.; Majiene, D. Rosmarinic acid and Melissa officinalis extracts differently affect glioblastoma cells. *Oxid. Med. Cell. Longev.* **2016**. [CrossRef] [PubMed]

59. Ghasemzadeh Rahbardar, M.; Amin, B.; Mehri, S.; Mirnajafi-Zadeh, S.J.; Hosseinzadeh, H. Anti-inflammatory effects of ethanolic extract of Rosmarinus officinalis L. and rosmarinic acid in a rat model of neuropathic pain. *Biomed. Pharmacother.* **2016**, *86*, 441–449. [CrossRef] [PubMed]

60. Güven, M.; Yuksel, Y.; Sehitoglu, M.H.; Tokmak, M.; Aras, A.B.; Akman, T.; Golge, U.H.; Goksel, F.; Karavelioglu, E.; Cosar, M. The effect of coumaric acid on ischemia-reperfusion injury of sciatic nerve in rats. *Inflammation* **2015**, *38*, 2124–2132. [CrossRef] [PubMed]

61. Güven, M.; Aras, A.B.; Akman, T.; Sen, H.M.; Ozkan, A.; Salis, O.; Sehitoglu, I.; Kalkan, Y.; Silan, C.; Deniz, M.; et al. Neuroprotective effect of p-coumaric acid in rat model of embolic cerebral ischemia. *Iran. J. Basic Med. Sci.* **2015**, *18*, 356–363. [PubMed]

62. Güven, M.; Sehitoglu, M.H.; Yuksel, Y.; Tomkak, M.; Aras, A.B.; Akman, T.; Golge, U.H.; Karavelioglu, E.; Bal, E.; Cosar, M. The neuroprotective effect of p-coumaric acid on spinal cord ischemia/reperfusion injury in rats. *Inflammation* **2015**, *38*, 1986–1995. [CrossRef] [PubMed]

63. Shailasree, S.; Venkataramana, M.; Niranjana, S.R. Cytotoxic effect of p-coumaric acid on neuroblastoma, N2a cell via generation of reactive oxygen species leading to dysfunction of mitochondria inducing apoptosis and autophagy. *Mol. Neurobiol.* **2015**, *51*, 119–130. [CrossRef] [PubMed]

64. Zare, K.; Eidi, A.; Roghani, M.; Haeri-Rohani, A. The neuroprotective potential of sinapic acid in the 6-hydroxydopamine-induced hem-parkinsonian rat. *Metab. Brain Dis.* **2015**, *30*, 205–213. [CrossRef] [PubMed]

65. Yao, Y.; Huang, H.Y.; Yang, Y.X.; Guo, J.Y. Cinnamic aldehyde treatment alleviates chronic unexpected stress-induced depressive-like behaviors via targeting cyclooxygenase-2 in mid-aged rats. *J. Ethnopharmacol.* **2015**, *162*, 97–103. [CrossRef] [PubMed]

66. Thrash-Williams, B.; Karuppagounder, S.S.; Bhattacharya, D.; Ahuja, M.; Suppiramaniam, V.; Dhanasekaran, M. Methamphetamine-induced dopaminergic toxicity prevented owing to the neuroprotective effects of salicylic acid. *Life Sci.* **2016**, *1*, 24–29. [CrossRef] [PubMed]

67. Cetin, D.; Hacimuftuoglu, A.; Tatar, A.; Turkez, H.; Togar, B. The in vitro protective effect of salicylic acid against paclitaxel and cisplatin-induced neurotoxicity. *Cytotechnology* **2016**, *68*, 1361–1367. [CrossRef] [PubMed]

68. Rosińczuk, J.; Dymarek, R.; Całkosiński, I. Histopathological, ultrastructural, and immunohistochemical assessment of hippocampus structures of rats exposed to TCDD and high doses of tocopherol and acetylsalicylic acid. *Biomed. Res. Int.* **2015**. [CrossRef] [PubMed]

69. Blanchard, H.C.; Taha, A.Y.; Rapoport, S.I.; Yuan, Z.X. Low-dose aspirin (acetylsalicylate) prevents increases in brain PGE2, 15-epi-lipoxin A4 and 8-isoprostane in 9 month-old HIV-1 transgenic rats, a model for HIV-1 associated neurocognitive disorders. *Prostag. Leukot. Ess.* **2015**, *96*, 25–30. [CrossRef] [PubMed]

70. He, F.; Xia, C.; Zhang, J.H.; Li, X.Q.; Zhou, Z.H.; Li, F.P.; Li, W.; Lv, Y.; Chen, H.S. Clopidogrel plus aspirin versus aspirin alone for preventing early neurological deterioration in patients with acute ischemic stroke. *J. Clin. Neurosci.* **2015**, *22*, 83–86. [CrossRef] [PubMed]

71. Yi, X.; Han, Z.; Wang, C.; Zhou, Q.; Lin, J. Statin and aspirin pretreatment are associated with lower neurological deterioration and platelet activity in patients with acute ischemic stroke. *J. Stroke Cerebrovasc. Dis.* **2017**, *26*, 352–359. [CrossRef] [PubMed]

72. Tsai, C.P.; Lin, F.C.; Lee, J.K.W.; Lee, C.T.C. Aspirin use associated with amyotrophic lateral sclerosis: A total population-based case control study. *J. Epidemiol.* **2015**, *25*, 172–177. [CrossRef] [PubMed]

73. Roehrich, M.E.; Wyss, J.C.; Kumar, R.; Pascual, M.; Golshayan, D.; Vssalli, G. Additive effects of rapamycin and aspirin on dendritic cell allostimulatory capacity. *Immunopharm. Immunot.* **2015**, *37*, 434–441. [CrossRef] [PubMed]

74. Xu, Y.X.; Du, F.; Jiang, L.R.; Gong, J.; Zhou, Y.F.; Luo, Q.Q.; Qian, Z.M.; Ke, Y. Effects of aspirin on expression of iron transport and storage proteins in BV-2 microglial cells. *Neurochem. Int.* **2015**, *91*, 72–77. [CrossRef] [PubMed]

75. Massocatto, C.L.; Moreira, N.M.; Muniz, E.; Pinge-Filho, P.; Rossi, R.M.; Araújo, E.J.; Sant'Ana, D.M. Aspirin prevents atrophy of esophageal nitrergic myenteric neurons in a mouse model of chronic Chagas disease. *Dis. Esophagus* **2016**. [CrossRef] [PubMed]

76. Abou-Abbass, H.; Bahmad, H.; Abou-El-Hassan, H.; Zhu, R.; Zhou, S.; Dong, X.; Hamade, E.; Mallah, K.; Zebian, A.; Ramadan, N.; et al. Deciphering glycomics and neuroproteomic alterations in experimental traumatic brain injury: Comparative analysis of aspirin and clopidogrel treatment. *Electrophoresis* **2016**, *37*, 1562–1576. [CrossRef]

77. Lowthian, J.A.; Britt, C.J.; Rance, G.; Lin, F.R.; Woods, R.L.; Wolfe, R.; Nelson, M.R.; Dillon, H.A.; Ward, S.; Reid, C.M.; et al. Slowing the progression of age-related hearing loss: Rationale and study design of the ASPIRIN in HEARING, retinal vessels imaging and neurocognition in older generations (ASPREE-HEARING) trial. *Contemp. Clin. Trials* **2016**, *46*, 60–66. [PubMed]

78. Zhang, Z.; Li, G.; Szeto, S.S.; Chong, C.M.; Quan, Q.; Huang, C.; Cui, W.; Guo, B.; Wang, Y.; Han, Y.; et al. Examining the neuroprotective effects of protocatechuic acid and chrysin on in vitro and in vivo models of Parkinson disease. *Free Radic. Biol. Med.* **2015**, *84*, 331–343. [CrossRef] [PubMed]

79. Semaming, Y.; Sripetchwandee, J.; Sa-nguanmoo, P.; Pintana, H.; Pannangpetch, P.; Chattipakorn, N.; Chattipakorn, S.C. Protocatechuic acid protects brain mitochondrial function in streptozotocin-induced diabetic rats. *Appl. Physiol. Nutr. Metab.* **2015**, *40*, 1078–1081. [CrossRef]

80. Ju, D.T.; Liao, H.E.; Shibu, M.A.; Ho, T.J.; Padma, V.V.; Tsai, F.J.; Chung, L.C.; Day, C.H.; Lin, C.C.; Huang, C.Y. Nerve regeneration potential of protocatechuic acid in RSC96 Schwann cells by induction of cellular proliferation and migration through IGF-IR-PI3K-Akt signaling. *Chin. J. Physiol.* **2015**, *58*, 412–419. [CrossRef] [PubMed]

81. Ning, Q.-Q.; Liu, S.; Li, Y.-C.; Li, L.; Yu, Y.; Zhao, W.-X.; Zhang, X.-L. Protective effect of protocatechuic acid on midbrain dopaminergic neurons injured by 1-methyl-4-phenylpyridinium. *Chin. Trad. Herb. Drugs* **2016**, *47*, 2497–2501.

82. Wang, H.Y.; Wang, H.; Wang, J.H.; Wang, Q.; Ma, Q.F.; Chen, Y.Y. Protocatechuic acid inhibits inflammatory responses in LPS-stimulated BV2 microglia via NF-κB and MAPKs signaling pathways. *Neurochem. Res.* **2015**, *40*, 1655–1660. [CrossRef] [PubMed]

83. Yin, X.; Su, X.Y.; Wang, X.H.; Su, J.L.; Lian, Y.; Zhang, X.L. Effects of protocatechuic acid on expression of D2DR, iNOS, and TH in striatum and midbrain of Parkinson's disease model mice. *Chin. Trad. Herb. Drugs* **2015**, *46*, 866–870.

84. Ju, D.T.; Kuo, W.W.; Ho, T.J. Protocatechuic acid from Alpinia oxyphylla induces Schwann cell migration via ERK1/2, JNK and p38 activation. *Am. J. Chin. Med.* **2015**, *43*, 653–665. [CrossRef] [PubMed]

85. Naghizadeh, B.; Mansouri, M.T. Protective effects of gallic acid against streptozotocin-induced oxidative damage in rat striatum. *Drug Res.* **2015**, *65*, 515–520. [CrossRef] [PubMed]

86. Pemminati, S. Effect of gallic acid on antioxidative enzymes activities in depression. *Indian J. Psychiat.* **2015**, *57*, S125.

87. Hajimoradi, M.; Fazilati, M.; Gharib-Naseri, M.K.; Sarkaki, A. Gallic acid and exercise training improve motor function, nerve conduction velocity but not pain sense reflex after experimental sciatic nerve crush in male rats. *Avicenna J. Phytomed.* **2015**, *5*, 288–297. [PubMed]

88. Moghadas, M.; Edalatmanesh, M.A.; Robati, R. Histopathological analysis from gallic acid administration on hippocampal cell density, depression, and anxiety related behaviors in a trimethyltin intoxication model. *Cell. J.* **2016**, *17*, 659–667. [PubMed]

89. Oyagbemi, A.A.; Omobowale, T.O.; Saba, A.B.; Olowu, E.R.; Dada, R.O.; Akinrinde, A.S. Gallic acid ameliorates cyclophosphamide-induced neurotoxicity in Wistar rats through free radical scavenging activity and improvement in antioxidant defense system. *J. Diet. Suppl.* **2016**, *13*, 402–419. [CrossRef] [PubMed]

90. Hsu, S.S.; Chou, C.T.; Liao, W.C.; Shieh, P.; Kuo, D.H.; Kuo, C.C.; Jan, C.R.; Liang, W.Z. The effect of gallic acid on cytotoxicity, $Ca^{2+}$ homeostasis and ROS production in DBTRG-05MG human glioblastoma cells and CTX TNA2 rat astrocytes. *Chem. Biol. Interact.* **2016**, *252*, 61–73. [CrossRef] [PubMed]

91. Tüzmen, M.N.; Yücel, N.C.; Kalburcu, T.; Demiryas, N. Effects of curcumin and tannic acid on the aluminum-and lead-induced oxidative neurotoxicity and alterations in NMDA receptors. *Toxicol. Mech. Method.* **2015**, *25*, 120–127. [CrossRef] [PubMed]

92. Ashafaq, M.; Tabassum, H.; Vishnoi, S.; Salman, M.; Raisuddin, S.; Parvez, S. Tannic acid alleviates lead acetate-induced neurochemical perturbations in rat brain. *Neurosci. Lett.* **2016**, *617*, 94–100. [CrossRef] [PubMed]

93. Sen, H.M.; Ozkan, A.; Güven, M.; Akman, T.; Aras, A.B.; Sehitoglu, I.; Alacam, H.; Silan, C.; Cosar, M.; Ozisik Karaman, H.I. Effects of tannic acid on the ischemic brain tissue of rats. *Inflammation* **2015**, *38*, 1624–1630. [CrossRef] [PubMed]

94. Ashafaq, M.; Tabassum, H.; Parvez, S. Modulation of behavioral deficits and neurodegeneration by tannic acid in experimental stroke challenged Wistar rats. *Mol. Neurobiol.* **2016**. [CrossRef] [PubMed]

95. Ibero-Baraibar, I.; Perez-Cornago, A.; Ramirez, M.J.; Martinez, J.A.; Zulet, M.A. An increase in plasma homovanillic acid with cocoa extract consumption is associated with the alleviation of depressive symptoms in overweight or obese adults on an energy restricted diet in a randomized controlled trial. *J. Nutr.* **2016**, *146*, 897S–904S. [CrossRef] [PubMed]

96. Neider, D.; Lindstrom, L.H.; Boden, R. Risk factors for suicide among patients with schizophrenia: A cohort study focused on cerebrospinal fluid levels of homovanillic acid and 5-hydroxyindoleacetic acid. *Neuropsych. Dis. Treat.* **2016**, *12*, 1711–1714. [CrossRef] [PubMed]

97. Van de Kerkhof, N.W.A.; Fekkes, D.; van der Heijden, F.M.M.A.; Egger, J.I.M.; Verhoeven, W.M.A. Relationship between plasma homovanillic acid and outcome in patients with psychosis spectrum disorders. *Neuropsychobiology* **2015**, *71*, 212–217. [CrossRef] [PubMed]

98. Güven, M.; Aras, A.B.; Topaloğlu, N.; Özkan, A.; Şen, H.M.; Kalkan, Y.; Okuyucu, A.; Akbal, A.; Gökmen, F.; Coşar, M. The protective effect of syringic acid on ischemia injury in rat brain. *Turk. J. Med. Sci.* **2015**, *45*, 233–240. [CrossRef] [PubMed]

99. Tokmak, M.; Yuksel, Y.; Sehitoglu, M.H.; Güven, M.; Akman, T.; Aras, A.B.; Cosar, M.; Abbed, K.M. The neuroprotective effect of syringic acid on spinal cord ischemia/reperfusion injury in rats. *Inflammation* **2015**, *38*, 1969–1978. [CrossRef] [PubMed]

100. Song, M.; Du, Z.; Lu, G.; Li, P.; Wang, L. Syringic acid protects retinal ganglion cells against $H_2O_2$-induced apoptosis through the activation of Pl3K/Akt signaling pathway. *Cell. Mol. Biol.* **2016**, *62*, 50–54. [PubMed]

101. Cao, Y.; Zhang, L.; Sun, S.; Yi, Z.; Jiang, X.; Jia, D. Neuroprotective effects of syringic acid against OGD/R-induced injury in cultured hippocampal neuronal cells. *Int. J. Mol. Med.* **2016**, *38*, 567–573. [CrossRef] [PubMed]

102. Alfredsson, C.F.; Ding, M.; Liang, Q.-L.; Sundström, B.E.; Nånberg, E. Ellagic acid induces a dose-and time-dependent depolarization of mitochondria and activation of caspase-9 and -3 in human neuroblastoma cells. *Biomed. Pharmacother.* **2014**, *68*, 129–135. [CrossRef] [PubMed]

103. Alfredsson, C.F.; Rendel, F.; Liang, Q.L.; Sundström, B.E.; Nånberg, E. Altered sensitivity to ellagic acid in neuroblastoma cells undergoing differentiation with 12-O-tetradecynoylphorbol-13-acetate and all-trans retinoic acid. *Biomed. Pharmacother.* **2015**, *76*, 39–45. [CrossRef] [PubMed]

104. Wang, D.; Chen, Q.; Liu, B.; Li, Y.; Tan, Y.; Yang, B. Ellagic acid inhibits proliferation and induces apoptosis in human glioblastoma cells. *Acta Cir. Bras.* **2016**, *31*, 143–149. [CrossRef] [PubMed]

105. Farbood, Y.; Sarkaki, A.; Dolatshahi, M.; Mansouri, S.M.T.; Khodadadi, A. Ellagic acid protects the brain against 6-hydroxydopamine induced neuroinflammation in a rat model of Parkinson's disease. *Basic Clin. Neurosci.* **2015**, *6*, 15–22.

106. Khatri, D.; Juvekar, A. Abrogation of locomotor impairment in a rotenone-induced Drosophila melanogaster and zebrafish model of Parkinson's disease by ellagic acid and curcumin. *Int. J. Nutr. Pharm. Neurol. Dis.* **2016**, *6*, 90–96.

107. Mansouri, M.T.; Farbood, Y.; Naghizadeh, B.; Shabani, S.; Mirshekar, M.A.; Sarkaki, A. Beneficial effects of ellagic acid against animal models of scopolamine- and diazepam-induced cognitive impairments. *Pharm. Biol.* **2016**, *54*, 1947–1953. [CrossRef] [PubMed]

108. Liu, H.P.; Ren, T.W.; Yan, W.J.; Liu, J.; Liu, R.B. Ellagic acid alleviates inflammatory pain and paclitaxel-induced neuropathic pain in murine models. *Int. J. Clin. Exp. Med.* **2016**, *9*, 12514–12520.

109. Chen, S.Y.; Zheng, K.; Wang, Z.Q. Neuroprotective effects of ellagic acid on neonatal hypoxic brain injury via inhibition of inflammatory mediators and down-regulation of JNK/p38 MAPK activation. *Trop. J. Pharm. Res.* **2016**, *15*, 241–251. [CrossRef]

110. Liu, Q.S.; Li, S.R.; Li, K.; Li, X.; Yin, X.; Pang, Z. Ellagic acid improves endogenous neural stem cells proliferation and neurorestoration through Wnt/β-catenin signaling in vivo and in vitro. *Mol. Nutr. Food Res.* **2017**, *61*. [CrossRef] [PubMed]

111. Herrmann, K. Occurrence and content of hydroxycinnamic and hydroxybenzoic acid compounds in foods. *Crit. Rev. Sci. Food Nutr.* **1989**, *28*, 315–347. [CrossRef] [PubMed]

112. Scalbert, A.; Williamson, G. Dietary intake and bioavailability of polyphenols. *J. Nutr.* **2000**, *130*, 2073S–2085S. [PubMed]

113. Bourne, L.C.; Rice-Evans, C. Bioavailablility of ferulic acid. *Biochem. Biophys. Res. Commun.* **1998**, *253*, 222–227. [CrossRef] [PubMed]

114. Zamora-Ros, R.; Knaze, V.; Rothwell, J.A.; Hémon, B.; Moskal, A.; Overvad, K.; Tjønneland, A.; Kyrø, C.; Fagherazzi, G.; Boutron-Ruault, M.C.; et al. Dietary polyphenol intake in Europe: The European prospective investigation into cancer and nutrition (EPIC) study. *Eur. J. Nutr.* **2016**, *55*, 1359–1375. [CrossRef] [PubMed]

115. Tresserra-Rimbau, A.; Medina-Remón, A.; Pérez-Jiménez, J.; Martínez-González, M.A.; Covas, M.I.; Corella, D.; Salas-Salvadó, J.; Gómez-Gracia, E.; Lapetra, J.; Arós, F.; et al. Dietary intake and major food sources of polyphenols in a Spanish population at high cardiovascular risk: The PREDIMED study. *Nutr. Metab. Cardiovasc. Dis.* **2013**, *23*, 953–959. [CrossRef] [PubMed]

116. Grosso, G.; Stepaniak, U.; Topor-Mądry, R.; Szafraniec, K.; Pająk, A. Estimated dietary intake and major food sources of polyphenols in the Polish arm of the HAPIEE study. *Nutrition* **2014**, *30*, 1398–1403. [CrossRef] [PubMed]

117. Ferruzzi, M.G.; Lobo, J.K.; Janle, E.M.; Cooper, B.; Simon, J.E.; Wu, Q.L.; Welch, C.; Ho, L.; Weaver, C.; Pasinetti, G.M. Bioavailability of gallic acid and catechins from grape seed polyphenol extract is improved by repeated dosing in rats: implications for treatment in Alzheimer's disease. *J. Alzheimers Dis.* **2009**, *18*, 113–124. [CrossRef] [PubMed]

118. Zhang, Y.J.; Wu, L.; Zhang, Q.L.; Li, J.; Yin, F.X.; Yuan, Y. Pharmacokinetics of phenolic compounds of Danshen extract in rat blood and brain by microdialysis sampling. *J. Ethnopharmacol.* **2011**, *136*, 129–136. [CrossRef] [PubMed]

119. Margalef, M.; Pons, Z.; Bravo, F.I.; Muguerza, B.; Arola-Arnal, A. Tissue distribution of rat flavanol metabolites at different doses. *J. Nutr. Biochem.* **2015**, *26*, 987–995. [CrossRef] [PubMed]

120. Del Bo, C.; Ciapellano, S.; Klimis-Zacas, D.; Martini, D.; Gardana, C.; Riso, P.; Porrini, M. Anthocyanin absorption, metabolism, and distribution from a wild blueberry-enriched diet (Vaccinium angustifolium) is affected by diet duration in the Sprague-Dawley rat. *J. Agric. Food Chem.* **2010**, *58*, 2491–2497. [PubMed]

121. Wang, D.; Ho, L.; Faith, J.; Ono, K.; Janle, E.M.; Lachcik, P.J.; Cooper, B.R.; Jannasch, A.H.; D'Arcy, B.R.; Williams, B.A.; et al. Role of intestinal microbiota in the generation of polyphenol derived phenolic acid mediated attenuation of Alzheimer's disease β-amyloid oligomerization. *Mol. Nutr. Food. Res.* **2015**, *59*, 1025–1040. [CrossRef] [PubMed]

122. Chang, M.X.; Xu, L.Y.; Tao, J.S.; Feng, Y. Metabolism and pharmacokinetics of ferulic acid in rats. *China J. Chin. Mater. Medica* **1993**, *18*, 300–2319.

123. Wu, K.; Wang, Z.Z.; Liu, D.; Qi, X.R. Pharmacokinetics, brain distribution, release and blood-brain barrier transport of Shunaoxin pills. *J. Ethnopharmacol.* **2014**, *151*, 1133–1140. [CrossRef] [PubMed]

124. Pinheiro Fernandes, F.D.; Fontenele Menezes, A.P.; de Sousa Neves, J.C.; Fonteles, A.A.; da Silva, A.T.; de Araújo, R.P.; Santos do Carmo, M.R.; de Souza, C.M.; de Andrade, G.M. Caffeic acid protects mice from memory deficits induced by focal cerebral ischemia. *Behav. Pharmacol.* **2014**, *25*, 637–647. [CrossRef] [PubMed]

125. Ritschel, W.A.; Starzacher, A.; Sabouni, A.; Hussain, A.S.; Koch, H.P. Percutaneous absorption of rosmarinic acid in the rat. *Method. Find. Exp. Clin. Pharmacol.* **1989**, *11*, 345–352.

126. Yan, J.J.; Cho, J.Y.; Kim, H.S.; Kim, K.L.; Jung, J.S.; Huh, S.O.; Suh, H.W.; Kim, Y.H.; Song, D.K. Protection against b-amyloid peptide toxicity in vivo with long-term administration of ferulic acid. *Br. J. Pharmacol.* **2001**, *133*, 89–96. [CrossRef] [PubMed]

127. Zhao, J.; Pati, S.; Redell, J.B.; Zhang, M.; Moore, A.N.; Dash, P.K. Caffeic acid phenethyl ester protects blood-brain barrier integrity and reduces contusion volume in rodent models of traumatic brain injury. *J. Neurotraum.* **2012**, *29*, 1209–1218. [CrossRef] [PubMed]

128. Vauzour, D.; Vafeiadou, K.; Corona, G.; Pollard, S.E.; Tzounis, X.; Spencer, J.P. Champagne wine polyphenols protect primary cortical neurons against peroxynitrite-induced injury. *J. Agric. Food Chem.* **2007**, *55*, 2854–2860. [CrossRef] [PubMed]

129. Luan, H.; Kan, Z.; Xu, Y.; Lv, C.; Jiang, W. Rosmarinic acid protects against experimental diabetes with cerebral ischemia: relation to inflammation response. *J. Neuroinflamm.* **2013**, *10*. [CrossRef] [PubMed]

130. Tarozzi, A.; Morroni, F.; Hrelia, S.; Angeloni, C.; Marchesi, A.; Cantelli-Forti, G.; Hrelia, P. Neuroprotective effects of anthocyanins and their in vivo metabolites in SH-SY5Y cells. *Neurosci. Lett.* **2007**, *424*, 36–40. [CrossRef] [PubMed]

131. Scapagnini, G.; Foresti, R.; Calabrese, V.; Giuffrida Stella, A.M.; Green, C.J.; Motterlini, R. Caffeic acid phenethyl ester and curcumin: A novel class of heme oxygenase-1 inducers. *Mol. Pharmacol.* **2002**, *3*, 554–561. [CrossRef]

132. Scapagnini, G.; Butterfield, D.A.; Colombrita, C.; Sultana, R.; Pascale, A.; Calabrese, V. Ethyl ferulate, a lipophilic polyphenol, induces HO-1 and protects rat neurons against oxidative stress. *Antioxid. Redox Signal.* **2004**, *6*, 811–818. [CrossRef] [PubMed]

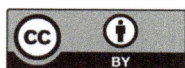

*nutrients*

MDPI

Article

# NAFLD and Atherosclerosis Are Prevented by a Natural Dietary Supplement Containing Curcumin, Silymarin, Guggul, Chlorogenic Acid and Inulin in Mice Fed a High-Fat Diet

Antonella Amato [1,*], Gaetano-Felice Caldara [1], Domenico Nuzzo [2], Sara Baldassano [1], Pasquale Picone [2], Manfredi Rizzo [3], Flavia Mulè [1,†] and Marta Di Carlo [2,*,†]

[1] Biological, Chemical and Pharmaceutical Sciences and Technologies (STEBICEF), University of Palermo, Palermo 90128, Italy; gaetanofelice.caldara@unipa.it (G.-F.C.); sara.baldassano@unipa.it (S.B.); flavia.mule@unipa.it (F.M.)

[2] Institute of Biomedicine and Molecular Immunology "Alberto Monroy" (IBIM), Consiglio Nazionale delle Ricerche (CNR), 90146 Palermo, Italy; domenico.nuzzo@ibim.cnr.it (D.N.); pasquale.picone@ibim.cnr.it (P.P.)

[3] Biomedical Department of Internal Medicine and Medical Specialties, University of Palermo, Palermo 90127, Italy; manfredi.rizzo@unipa.it

* Correspondence: antonella.amato@unipa.it (A.A.); marta.di.carlo@ibim.cnr.it (M.D.C.); Tel.: +39-091-2399-7506 (A.A.); +39-091-6809538 (M.D.C.)

† These authors contribute equally to this work.

Received: 11 April 2017; Accepted: 9 May 2017; Published: 13 May 2017

**Abstract:** Non-alcoholic fatty liver disease (NAFLD) confers an increased risk of cardiovascular diseases. NAFDL is associated with atherogenic dyslipidemia, inflammation and renin-angiotensin system (RAS) imbalance, which in turn lead to atherosclerotic lesions. In the present study, the impact of a natural dietary supplement (NDS) containing *Curcuma longa*, silymarin, guggul, chlorogenic acid and inulin on NAFLD and atherosclerosis was evaluated, and the mechanism of action was examined. C57BL/6 mice were fed an HFD for 16 weeks; half of the mice were simultaneously treated with a daily oral administration (os) of the NDS. NAFLD and atherogenic lesions in aorta and carotid artery (histological analysis), hepatic expression of genes involved in the NAFLD (PCR array), hepatic angiotensinogen (AGT) and $AT_1R$ mRNA expression (real-time PCR) and plasma angiotensin (ANG)-II levels (ELISA) were evaluated. In the NDS group, steatosis, aortic lesions or carotid artery thickening was not observed. PCR array showed upregulation of some genes involved in lipid metabolism and anti-inflammatory activity (Cpt2, Ifng) and downregulation of some genes involved in pro-inflammatory response and in free fatty acid up-take (Fabp5, Socs3). Hepatic AGT, $AT_1R$ mRNA and ANG II plasma levels were significantly lower with respect to the untreated-group. Furthermore, NDS inhibited the dyslipidemia observed in the untreated animals. Altogether, these results suggest that NDS prevents NAFLD and atherogenesis by modulating the expression of different genes involved in NAFLD and avoiding RAS imbalance.

**Keywords:** non-alcoholic fatty liver disease; atherogenic lesions; diet-induced obesity; natural dietary supplement; renin-angiotensin system imbalance; Profiler PCR array

## 1. Introduction

Non-alcoholic fatty liver disease (NAFLD) is the most frequent hepatic disorder in developed countries and may lead to steatohepatitis, cirrhosis and liver cancer. NAFLD is also considered the hepatic component of metabolic syndrome (MetS) because it is associated with atherogenic dyslipidemia, obesity and type 2 diabetes (T2DM) [1]. The precise mechanism of the onset and progression of NAFLD remains unclear although increased fatty acid syntheses, oxidative stress and inflammation may play a fundamental role [2].

Emerging evidence suggests that angiotensin (ANG) II, a pro-oxidant cytokine, synthesized mainly from the hepatic precursor angiotensinogen (AGT), may have a relevant importance in the pathogenesis of NAFLD by generating reactive oxygen species and regulating the production of pro-inflammatory mediators [3]. Patients with NAFLD present elevated ANG II levels [4,5], and animals with liver steatosis show increased hepatic expression of AGT, AGT II and ANG II type 1 receptor (AT$_1$R) [6,7]. The renin-angiotensin system (RAS) and its primary mediator ANG II have also a direct influence on the progression of the atherosclerotic process via effects on endothelial function, inflammation, fibrinolytic balance and plaque stability [8]. Increasing clinical evidence supports a strong association between NAFLD and cardiovascular diseases (CVD), which represents the principal cause of death in NAFLD patients, more so than liver-related complications [9,10]. Patients with NAFLD have an altered flow-mediated vasodilatation and increased carotid-artery intimal medial thickness, two reliable markers of subclinical atherosclerosis [11]. Therefore, the involvement of AGT II in NAFLD pathogenesis and in atherosclerotic plaque formation may provide one of the possible links between NAFLD and accelerated atherogenesis. Accordingly, the use of RAS blockers seems to be potentially useful as a therapeutic approach against NAFLD [12] and atherosclerosis [13]. To date, there is no single approved pharmacologic therapy to treat metabolic dysfunctions occurring in obesity, such as NAFLD and related atherosclerosis. The backbone of therapy currently includes lifestyle management to induce weight loss and therapeutic treatment to reduce cardiovascular risk or hyperglycemia [14]. Recently, natural herbs have been the focus of many researches both because of their safety and efficacy and because their potential bio-active ingredients could help to prevent or treat obesity and the related metabolic disorders [15]. The natural dietary supplement (NDS) used in this study contains extracts from *Cynara scolymus* (chlorogenic acid), *Silybum marianum* (silymarin), *Taraxacum officinale* (inulin), *Curcuma Longa* (curcuma) and *Commiphora mukul* (guggul), plant extracts that exert protective actions mainly towards the liver. Recent evidence has shown that the treatment with the NDS exerts beneficial effects in patients with MetS, reducing anthropometric parameters and total cholesterol levels, but the mechanism of action is still unknown [16].

This study aims to investigate whether the treatment with this NDS is able to prevent the development of NAFLD and related atherosclerotic lesions in aorta and carotid artery in a mouse model of diet-induced obesity (DIO). In order to investigate the mechanism of action of the natural supplement, its ability to modulate the expression of some RAS components (AGT and AT$_1$R mRNA in liver and circulating concentration of AGT II) or of genes involved in NAFLD was examined. In addition, the impact of the NDS treatment in the plasma lipid profile was also analyzed.

## 2. Materials and Methods

### 2.1. Animals

The procedures were performed in accordance with the conventional guidelines for animal experimentation (Italian D.L. (Legislative Decree) No. 116 of 27 January 1992 and subsequent variations) and the recommendations of the European Economic Community (86/609/ECC).

Male C57BL/6J (B6) mice, purchased from Harlan Laboratories (San Pietro al Natisone Udine, Italy) at 4 weeks of age, were housed in a room with controlled temperature and dark-light cycles, with free access to water and food. After acclimatization (1 week), the animals were weighed and divided into two groups, both fed a high-fat diet (HFD) (PF4051/D, Mucedola, Milan, Italy) composed of 60% of energy as fat, 20% protein and 20% carbohydrates, for 16 weeks.

It has been shown that these animals, consequent to an HFD, develop obesity, hyperglycemia [17], hepatic steatosis [18], atherosclerosis [19] and neurodegeneration [20].

One group served as a control of obesity-related dysfunctions (*n* = 6, untreated group), and the other one (*n* = 6, treated group) received, simultaneously to the HFD, a daily administration of NDS

(0.9 mg/mouse) for 16 weeks. The dose given to the DIO mice was extrapolated from the human dosage (1.6 g/day) and calculated on the basis of the average body weight (40 mg).

The NDS used in this study is, in Italy, commercialized under the name Kèpar® and was provided by Rikrea® S.r.l. (Modica-RG, Italy). The main constituents of the NDS are plant-derived polyphenolic compounds that are well known for their antioxidant and anti-inflammatory properties. In particular, NDS consists of extract from five plant sources, and each extract was obtained from a different part of the plant (Table 1).

**Table 1.** Ingredients of the natural dietary supplement (NDS) formulation.

| Herbal Components | Part Used | Quantity/100 g |
|---|---|---|
| *Cynara scolymus*, e.s. tit. 2.5% chlorogenic acid | Leaf | 35 g (extract) 0.87 g (Chlor. acid) |
| *Silybum marianum*, e.s. tit. 80% silymarin | Seed | 8 g (extract) 6.4 g (silymarin) |
| *Taraxacum officinale* e.s. tit. 2% inulin | Root | 10 g (extract) 0.2 g (inulin) |
| *Curcuma Longa* e.s. tit. 95% curcumin | Rhizome | 10 g (powder) 9.5 g (curcumin) |
| *Commiphora mukul* Guggul e.s. tit. 10% guggulipids | Resin | 15 g (extract) 1.5 g (guggulipids) |

e.s. tit.: Dry extract titrated; Chlor. acid: Chlorogenic acid.

The tablets of the NDS (Kèpar, Batch No. SL0010) were ground by pestle and 9 mg of powder dissolved in 200 μL of water and used as stock solution. The daily dose was freshly made up, by diluting 1:10 the stock solution (0.9 mg/mouse in 20 μL), and was administered by oral gavaging. The administrated dose contained: 0.09 mg of *Curcuma*, 0.057 mg of silymarin, 0.0135 mg of guggul lipids, 0.008 of chlorogenic acid and 0.002 mg of inulin. During the 16 weeks of the treatment, changes in body weight and food-intake, determined by measuring the difference between the pre-weighed chow and the weight of chow at intervals of 24 h [21], were periodically monitored and compared between the two groups of animals. After 16 weeks of treatment, mice were sacrificed, and blood, liver, aorta and carotid artery were immediately collected for subsequent analysis.

*2.2. Histological Analysis*

Aorta, carotid arteries and liver specimens excised from each hepatic lobe were fixed in 4% formalin for 24 h. After this treatment, the tissues were dehydrated in alcohol and embedded in paraffin wax. Paraffin histological sections (5 μm thick) were stained with hematoxylin and eosin and observed using an automated Leica DM5000 B microscope (Leica, Milan, Italy) connected to a high-resolution camera, Leica DC300 F (Leica, Milan, Italy). According to the Non-alcoholic Steatohepatitis Clinical Research Network (NASH CRN) scoring system, steatosis was determined by analyzing the morphology and percentage of lipid vesicles in hepatocytes [22].

*2.3. Atherogenic Index (AIS)*

The atherogenic index serum (AIS), which is the measure of the atherosclerotic lesion extent based on serum lipids [23], was determined in all groups. The atherogenic index serum is calculated using the formula AIS = total cholesterol (TC)/HDL [24].

*2.4. Biochemical Analysis*

Lipid profile was measured in mice fasted for 6 h with free access to water. After this time, the mice were euthanized, and the blood was drawn by cardiac puncture and immediately transferred into chilled tubes containing a final concentration of 1 mg/mL EDTA. Then, the samples were centrifuged at 825 g for 10 min, and the obtained plasma was stored at −80 °C until analysis. Plasma triglyceride, cholesterol, low density lipoprotein (LDL), high density lipoprotein (HDL) levels and AST- and ALT-serum concentrations were measured using the ILAB 600 Analyzer (Instrumentation Laboratory, Bedford, Massachusetts).

## 2.5. Quantitative Real-Time qPCR

Total RNA from livers of treated and untreated obese mice were extracted using the RNEasy Mini Kit (Qiagen, Milan, Italy). Two nanograms of RNA were used to synthesize the first strand cDNA using the RT First-Strand kit (Qiagen, Milan, Italy). Synthesized cDNAs were amplified using RT2 SYBR Green/ROX qPCR Mastermix (Qiagen, Milan, Italy) and StepOne Real-Time instrument (Applied Biosystem, Foster City, CA, USA).

Gene expression analysis was performed using sequence primers for mice AGT, $AT_1R$ and β-actin (SigmaLife Sciences, Milan, Italy). The primers were as follows: AGT forward 5'-GTA CAG ACA GCA CCC TAC TT-3', reverse 5'-TTG TTG AAG AGG CAC TGC AC-3'; $AT_1R$ forward 5'-GAC CAA CTC AAC CCA GAA AAGC-3', reverse 5'-CCT TTG TCG AAC CAC CACTA-3'; β-actin forward 5'-CGG GAT CCC CGC CCT AGG CAC CAG GGT-3', reverse 5'-GGA ATT CGG CTG GGG TGT TGA AGG TCT CAAA-3'. Each PCR reaction was amplified in triplicate, and levels of expression were calculated after normalization to β-actin. On the basis of the Ct value (threshold cycle; the number of reaction cycles after which fluorescence exceeds the defined threshold) of the examined gene and of the internal control gene, the relative expression level of RNA was calculated according to the $2^{-\Delta\Delta Ct}$ approximation method.

## 2.6. $RT^2$ Profiler PCR Array

Synthesized cDNAs from NDS-treated and NSD-untreated livers were added to 96-well reaction plates of the Mouse Fatty Liver PCR Array (PAMM-157Z, SABiosciences, Qiagen, Milan, Italy) according to the manufacturer's instructions. The array profiles the expression of 84 key genes involved in the mechanisms of non-alcoholic fatty liver disease (NAFLD) and hepatic insulin resistance. The reaction was performed by using a StepOne Real-Time instrument (Applied Biosystem, Foster City, CA, USA). Analysis was performed using the spreadsheet provided by Qiagen Company, Milan, Italy.

## 2.7. Measurement of Circulating Levels of Angiotensin II

Quantification of plasma AGT II was carried out by the ELISA kit for mice (Enzo Life Sciences, Inc. Farmingdale NY, USA) according to the manufacturer's instructions. The experimental detection limit of the analysis was 3.9 pg/mL.

## 2.8. Statistical Analyses

Results are shown as means ± the standard error of the mean (S.E.M.). The letter n indicates the number of animals. Statistical analyses were performed using Prism Version 6.0 Software (Graph Pad Software, Inc., San Diego, CA, USA). The comparison between the groups was performed by ANOVA followed by Bonferroni's post-test. A $p$-value $\leq 0.05$ was considered statistically significant.

## 3. Results

### 3.1. The Natural Dietary Supplement Prevents the Development of NAFLD

At the end of the treatment, the untreated mice had greater mass gain compared to the animals treated with NDS (Figure 1A), although no difference in the food intake was observed (Figure 1B). Furthermore, the liver weight (Figure 1C) and ratio liver weight/body weight (Figure 1D) was higher than the treated group. In the untreated mice, steatosis affected the liver gross appearance.

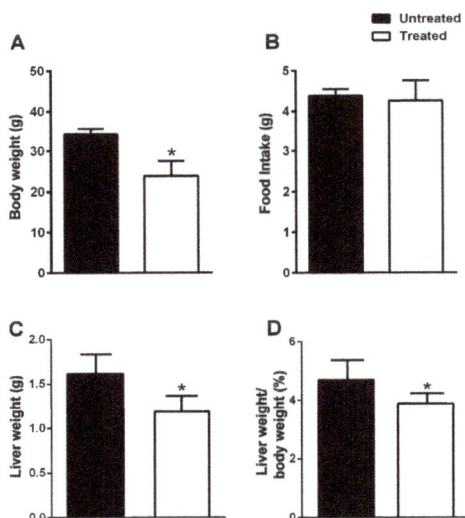

**Figure 1.** NDS reduces food intake, body and liver weight in HFD mice. Effects of the NDS treatment (0.9 mg/mouse) on body weight (**A**), food intake (**B**), liver weight (**C**) and the ratio of liver weight/body weight (**D**), in mice fed a high-fat diet (HFD). Data are the means ± S.E.M. (*n* = 6/group). * $p \leq 0.05$.

In particular, the organ appeared enlarged with rounded edges. Moreover, it was pale-yellowish color, friable with a greasy texture attributable to the fat accumulation in the hepatic parenchyma (Figure 2A). Histologically, the liver exhibited micro- and macro-vesicular steatosis (Grade I: >5%–33%) in the perivenular area (Zone 3) and transition area (Zone 2) (Figure 2C) with focal infiltration of polymorphonuclear cells (Figure 2E). The hepatocytes showed a typical foamy aspect; numerous small vacuoles coalesced and created cleared space displacing the nucleus to the periphery of the cells (Figure 2E). On the contrary, in the NDS-treated mice, the liver gross anatomy was not affected by fat accumulation (Figure 2B), and the histological analysis did not reveal the presence of steatosis (Grade 0: <5%), but only the presence of small inclusions of lipids within hepatocytes (Figure 2D–F). Moreover, in agreement with the liver maintaining the lobular architecture, plasma AST and ALT were significantly lower in treated mice than in the untreated ones (Figure 2G).

In addition, NDS-treated mice showed decreased triglycerides, cholesterol and LDL and increased HDL plasma levels in comparison with untreated animals (Figure 3).

### 3.2. The Natural Dietary Supplement Modulates the Expression of Genes Involved in NAFLD

To compare differences in the profile gene expression involved in NAFLD between the treated and the untreated groups, we analyzed hepatic expression levels of 84 genes by PCR array analysis. The position of the genes is signified in Table S1. In the hepatic tissue of treated mice, the expression levels of 23 genes were affected (Table S1). Among these, nine were up- or down-regulated by more than two-fold in comparison with the untreated animals (Figure 4A–C). In particular, NDS treatment upregulates genes involved in lipid metabolism and anti-inflammatory mediators (Cpt2, Ifng), whereas it downregulates genes involved in FFA up-take and in pro-inflammatory activity (Fabp5, Socs3).

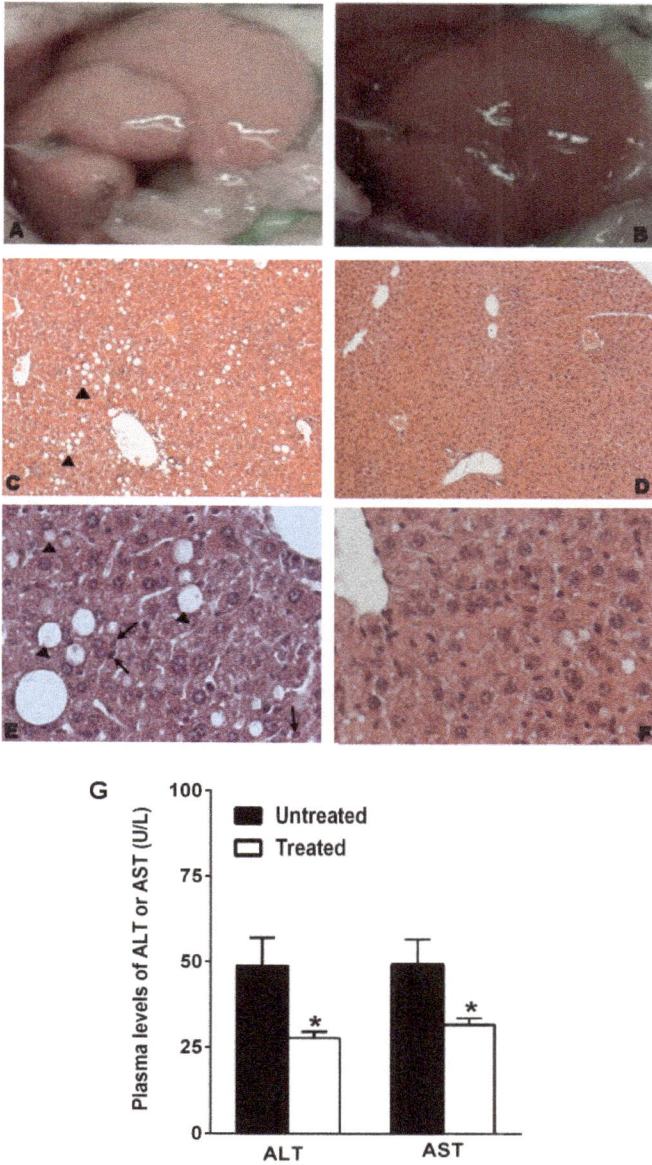

**Figure 2.** NDS prevents NAFLD development in diet-induced obesity (DIO) animals. Representative images of gross anatomy and histological cross-sections of liver from NDS-treated and untreated high-fat diet (HFD) mice. Liver morphologies of untreated HFD mice (**A**) and NDS-treated HFD mice (**B**). Cross-sections from untreated HFD mice (**C,E**) show micro- and macro-vesicular steatosis (black arrowhead) with polymorphonuclear cell infiltration (black arrow). Histological cross-sections from NDS-treated HFD mice (**D,F**) show normal hepatocytes and maintaining of the lobular architecture. Hematoxylin and eosin stain. Original magnification: (C,D) = ×200, (E,F) = ×400. (**G**) Plasma levels of AST and ALT. Data are the mean values ± S.E.M. ($n$ = 6/group). * $p \leq 0.05$.

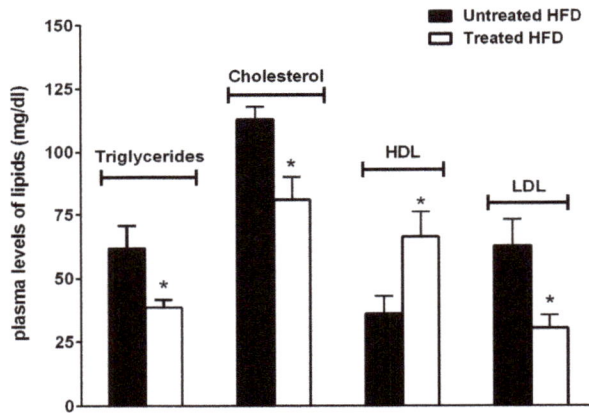

**Figure 3.** NDS prevents altered the plasma lipid profile. Effects of NDS treatment (0.9 mg/mouse) on plasma lipid concentrations. Data are the mean values ± S.E.M. ($n$ = 6/group).* $p \leq 0.05$.

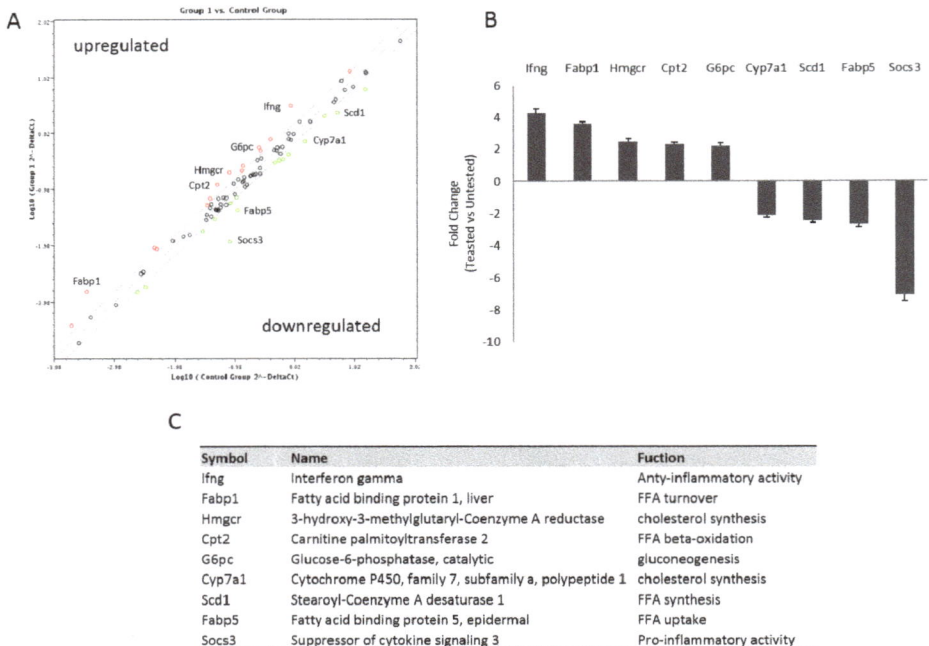

| Symbol | Name | Fuction |
|--------|------|---------|
| Ifng | Interferon gamma | Anty-inflammatory activity |
| Fabp1 | Fatty acid binding protein 1, liver | FFA turnover |
| Hmgcr | 3-hydroxy-3-methylglutaryl-Coenzyme A reductase | cholesterol synthesis |
| Cpt2 | Carnitine palmitoyltransferase 2 | FFA beta-oxidation |
| G6pc | Glucose-6-phosphatase, catalytic | gluconeogenesis |
| Cyp7a1 | Cytochrome P450, family 7, subfamily a, polypeptide 1 | cholesterol synthesis |
| Scd1 | Stearoyl-Coenzyme A desaturase 1 | FFA synthesis |
| Fabp5 | Fatty acid binding protein 5, epidermal | FFA uptake |
| Socs3 | Suppressor of cytokine signaling 3 | Pro-inflammatory activity |

**Figure 4.** NDS reduces the expression of genes involved in NAFLD pathogenesis. Livers of untreated and treated high-fat diet (HFD) mice were used to perform the RNA for the PCR array analysis. (**A**) Scatter plot of relative expression levels for each gene in mice samples (treated vs. untreated). The figure depicts a log transformation plot of the relative expression level of each gene ($2^{-\Delta Ct}$) between untreated (x-axis) and treated mice (y-axis). The grey lines indicate a two-fold change in gene expression threshold. Red rings indicate upregulated genes; green rings indicate downregulated genes. (**B**) Histogram of some up- and down-regulated genes with a greater than two-fold expression change. (**C**) Table of the names and functions of the quantitative real-time PCR of the chosen genes.

### 3.3. The Natural Dietary Supplement Prevents Atherosclerosis Development

Untreated mice showed atherosclerotic lesions with features of the earliest stages of the disease. In fact, the observed lesions did not develop beyond the fatty-streak presence. The lesions of aorta were confined to the aortic root and were characterized predominantly by lipid-laden areas in the tunica media, between smooth muscle cells and elastic lamina (Figure 5A,B). Carotid arteries showed an increased thickening of the intima characterized by hyperplasia and the presence of myocytes proliferating from the tunica media (Figure 5E,F). On the contrary, in NDS-treated mice, neither lesions in aortic root (Figure 5C,D), nor carotid intimal hyperplasia and alterations in the tunica media or adventitia (Figure 5G,H) were observed.

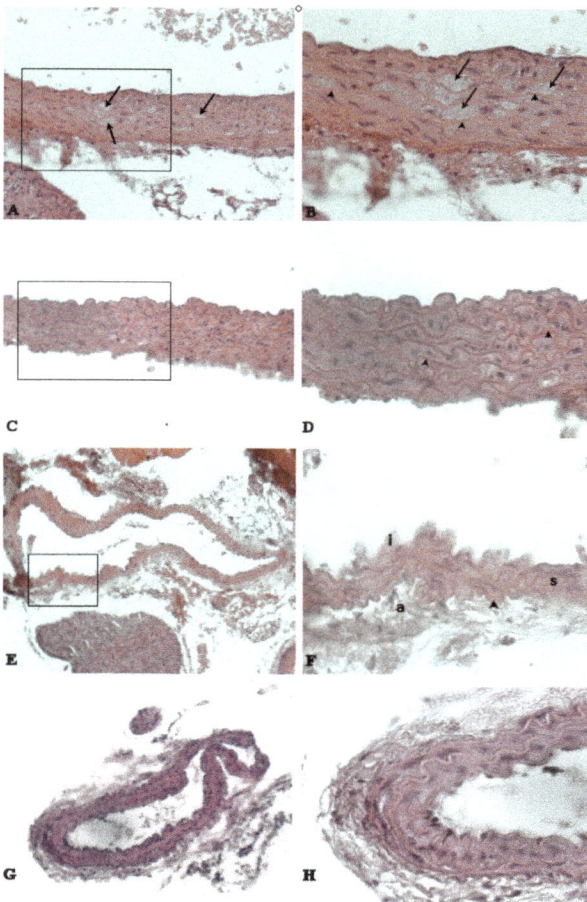

**Figure 5.** NDS prevents the development of atherosclerotic lesions. Representative images of histological cross-sections of aortic arch and carotid artery in high-fat diet (HFD) mice. The black arrow (**A,B**) denotes the prominent fatty streak between elastic laminae (arrowhead) in the aortic root wall of untreated vs. treated (**C,D**) HFD mice. Carotid artery shows a hyperplasia of the intima (i) in untreated HFD mice (**E,F**). On the contrary, no alterations of carotid artery are detected in treated HFD mice (**G,H**). a = tunica adventitia. s = smooth muscle cells. Hematoxylin and eosin stain. Original magnification: (**A,C**) = ×400; (**B,D,F**) and (**H**) = ×600; (**E,G**) = ×200.

According to these data, the AIS was significantly higher in untreated HFD-fed mice in comparison with the treated obese mice (Figure 6).

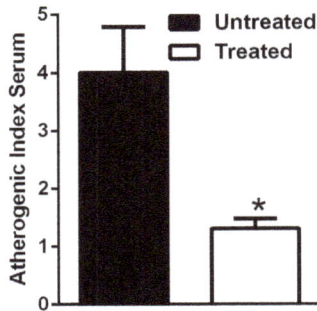

**Figure 6.** Atherogenic index serum (AIS) in HFD mice is reduced by NDS. Effects of NDS treatment (0.9 mg/mouse) on AIS of high-fat diet (HFD)-fed mice. Data are the mean values ± S.E.M. ($n$ = 6/group). * $p \leq 0.05$.

### 3.4. The Natural Dietary Supplement Reduces RAS Component Expression

To investigate whether variations in the levels of the RAS system are specifically involved in the preventive effects of the natural supplement, we analyzed the hepatic mRNA levels of AGT and AT1R by quantitative real-time PCR and circulating ANG II concentration by ELISA assay. In NDS-treated mice, hepatic AGT and AT1R mRNA expression and plasma ANG II levels were significantly lower in comparison with untreated mice (Figure 7A,B).

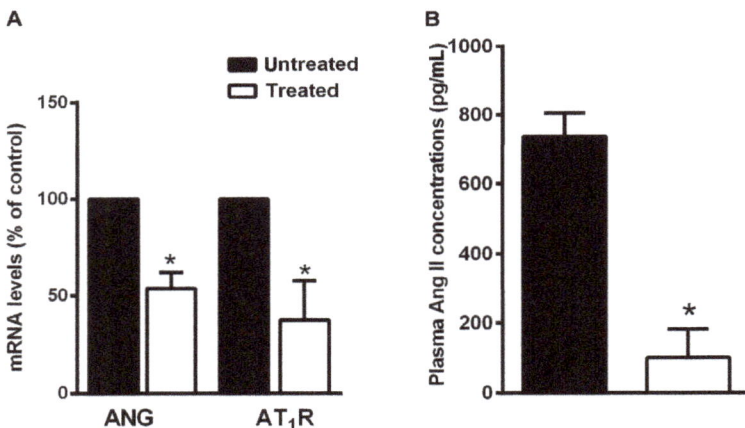

**Figure 7.** NDS reduces RAS component expression. (**A**) Expression levels of AGT and AT1R mRNAs in liver of treated high-fat diet (HFD) mice and the untreated HFD group, by real-time RT-PCR analysis. Data are the mean values ± S.E.M. ($n$ = 3/group). * $p \leq 0.05$. (**B**) Effects of NDS treatment (0.9 mg/mouse) on circulating levels of angiotensin II in HFD mice, by ELISA. Data are the mean values ± S.E.M. ($n$ = 6/group). * $p \leq 0.05$.

## 4. Discussion

The present study shows that the natural supplement, here utilized, is able to prevent the development of NAFLD and atherogenic lesions in HFD obese mice. Such a preventive role is determined by its ability to reduce the expression of the RAS components (AGT, AT1R and AGT II) and modulate positively the expression of genes involved in NAFLD. The NDS also improves the lipid profile, a typical obesity-related dysfunction.

In recent years, there has been an increasing interest in the use of plant extracts as potential therapeutic agents. A mixture of natural products is used in various therapeutic areas obtaining a number of interesting outcomes due to their synergistic effects [25]. The natural dietary supplement used in this work, known as Képar, is used in the Italian market to treat liver discomfort, caused by gallstones, cirrhosis and toxic agents. It is composed of several plant extracts (*Curcuma*, silymarin, guggul, chlorogenic acid and inulin) that exert, at least individually, beneficial effects on different components of MetS. Curcumin improves insulin resistance and dyslipidemia [26]; silymarin exerts anti-inflammatory effects in animal models of NAFLD [27]; guggul lipids have been successfully used in obesity and hypercholesterolemia [28]; and chlorogenic acid, as well as inulin, may improve lipidic and glycidic metabolism [29,30]. In the present study, we have demonstrated that the diet natural supplement is able to prevent body weight gain, hepatic fat accumulation, atherosclerotic lesions development and dysregulation of lipidic metabolism. In fact, NDS-treated HFD mice showed a body weight significantly lower than the untreated HFD animals, without any differences in the food intake. This suggests that NDS prevents body mass gain by an independent mechanism from central control of the feeding behavior.

It is interesting to note that our study represents the first experimental evidence for a preventive role of the natural supplement against obesity-associated steatosis development. In fact, the liver of treated obese mice did not show hepatomegaly or other histomorphological alterations; on the contrary, the untreated group liver showed the presence of moderate micro- and macro-vesicular steatosis in Zone 3, a zonal distribution highly associated with the severity of steatosis [31]. The positive impact of NDS treatment, besides liver morphology, was also observed on the hepatic function, as suggested by the reduced ALT and AST plasma levels in treated-obese animals compared to the untreated group. In addition, the results showed that plasma triglycerides and LDL were lower and HDL higher in treated HFD animals in comparison to the untreated mice, demonstrating that NDS exerts beneficial effects on lipid metabolism and, consequently, on cardiovascular functions [32].

In order to examine the mechanism by which NDS prevents NAFLD, we also analyzed and compared the hepatic expression of genes involved in NAFLD pathogenesis in treated vs. untreated animals. For the first time, it was demonstrated that NDS is able to modulate different signaling pathways involved in de novo hepatic lipogenesis, lipid oxidation and inflammatory responses. In fact, in NDS-treated liver, genes involved in fatty acid turnover (such as Fabp1 and Cpt2) and anti-inflammatory activity (Ifng) were upregulated, while genes involved in FFA uptake (Fabp5), lipogenesis (Scd1) and inflammation (Socs3) were downregulated. The increased level of Cpt-2 and Fabp-1 provides an explanation of the reduced hepatic lipid depots observed in the NDS-treated liver. Cpt-2 is involved in beta-oxidation and Fabp-1 in the rapid removal of fatty acid in the oxidative organelles [33]. Downregulation of Fabp5 and Scd1 also contributes to preventing hepatic lipid accumulation, as Fabp5 leads to the fatty acid uptake [34] and Scd1 converts saturated FA to monounsaturated FA, the major substrates necessary for the synthesis of other lipids [35]. On the other hand, Scd1 knockout mice result in being resistant to the development of obesity and hepatic steatosis [36], and the fatty livers of ob/ob mice show increased Scd1 expression [37].

Microarray analysis also showed that the treatment with the natural supplement is able to modulate the expression of factors involved in the inflammatory process. In particular, the liver of treated HFD mice showed upregulation of Ifng, a protective mediator against the liver inflammatory process [38], and a very strong downregulation of Socs3, usually overexpressed in inflamed steatotic liver [39], providing a molecular basis for the protective role of the NDS in the HFD liver.

It is well known that NAFLD shares many risk factors with cardiovascular diseases, implying a close relationship between NAFLD and adverse cardiovascular events, such as hypertension and atherosclerosis [9]. Accordingly, we analyzed the impact of NDS treatment on the development of atherogenic lesions in our animal models. Our results showed that no atherosclerotic lesions were present in the vessels of NDS-treated obese mice. On the contrary, early hallmarks of atherosclerosis were highlighted in the untreated-HFD group. In fact, in agreement with Whitman's report [40], we observed "fatty streak-type" lesions in the aortic root, representative of foam cells, which are lipid-laden macrophages. We also observed carotid artery intimal-medial wall thickening. Additionally, AIS, a measure of the atherosclerotic lesion extent based on serum lipid concentration [23,24], was significantly lower in NDS-treated animals compared with untreated mice, suggesting a preventive action of the natural supplement on atherogenesis development. Therefore, the improvement of the lipid profile could explain the absence of lesions in the NDS-treated animals. Different mechanisms explain the increased risk of cardiovascular events in patients with NAFLD. In fact, besides the proatherogenic lipid profile, the disease is associated with an increased production of pro-inflammatory cytokines [41,42] and RAS imbalance. Patients with NAFLD present elevated circulating levels of ANG II and over-activation of intrahepatic RAS [4,5]. Our results showed that in the liver of NDS-treated obese mice, angiotensinogen and $AT_1R$ mRNA were significantly decreased, as well as the circulating levels of ANG II, suggesting that the treatment with the natural supplement protects from NAFLD and atherogenesis by preventing RAS imbalance.

## 5. Conclusions

In conclusion, the natural dietary supplement (Kèpar) is effective in protecting against the development of NAFLD and atherosclerotic lesions in obesity conditions. The NDS prevents liver fat accumulation, development of atherosclerotic lesions and improves hyperlipidemia. These beneficial effects seem to be mediated by the ability of the natural supplement to modulate the expression of different genes involved in NAFLD and to prevent the imbalance of RAS components.

**Supplementary Materials:** The following are available online at http://www.mdpi.com/2072-6643/9/5/492/s1: Table S1: List of the 84 genes involved in the NAFLD pathogenesis pathway in the array used.

**Acknowledgments:** This work was supported by a grant from Rikrea© (Agreement STEBICEF-Rikrea, N.3252, 11-07-2014). The Rikrea fund covered publication charges. The authors thank Pierluigi Rosa for his contribution to the idea of study.

**Author Contributions:** A.A. conceived of the idea, designed the study, performed some of the experiments, analyzed and interpreted the data critically and wrote the manuscript. G.F.C. performed histological analysis. S.B. contributed to data analyses. D.N. and P.P. performed real-time PCR and microarray analysis. M.R. contributed to a critical revision of the manuscript. F.M. and M.D.C. contributed to supervising the study, writing and reviewing the manuscript.

**Conflicts of Interest:** The authors declare no conflict of interest. The funding sponsors had no role in the design of the study; in the collection, analyses or interpretation of data; in the writing of the manuscript; nor in the decision to publish the results.

## References

1. Lim, S.; Oh, T.J.; Koh, K.K. Mechanistic link between nonalcoholic fatty liver disease and cardiometabolic disorders. *Int. J. Cardiol.* **2015**, *201*, 408–414. [CrossRef] [PubMed]

2. Harrison, S.A.; Day, C.P. Benefits of lifestyle modification in NAFLD. *Gut* **2007**, *56*, 1760–1769. [CrossRef] [PubMed]

3. Paschos, P.; Tziomalos, K. Nonalcoholic fatty liver disease and the renin-angiotensin system: Implications for treatment. *World J. Hepatol.* **2012**, *4*, 327–331. [CrossRef] [PubMed]

4. Xu, Y.Z.; Zhang, X.; Wang, L.; Zhang, F.; Qiu, Q.; Liu, M.L.; Zhang, G.R.; Wu, X.L. An increased circulating angiotensin II concentration is associated with hypoadiponectinemia and postprandial hyperglycemia in men with nonalcoholic fatty liver disease. *Intern. Med.* **2013**, *52*, 855–861. [CrossRef] [PubMed]

5. Moreira de Macêdo, S.; Guimarães, T.A.; Feltenberger, J.D.; Sousa Santos, S.H. The role of renin-angiotensin system modulation on treatment and prevention of liver diseases. *Peptides* **2014**, *62*, 189–196. [CrossRef] [PubMed]

6.  Kurita, S.; Takamura, T.; Ota, T.; Matsuzawa-Nagata, N.; Kita, Y.; Uno, M.; Nabemoto, S.; Ishikura, K.; Misu, H.; Ando, H.; et al. Olmesartan ameliorates a dietary rat model of non-alcoholic steatohepatitis through its pleiotropic effects. *Eur. J. Pharmacol.* **2008**, *588*, 316–324. [CrossRef] [PubMed]

7.  Wei, Y.; Rector, R.S.; Thyfault, J.P.; Ibdah, J.A. Nonalcoholic fatty liver disease and mitochondrial dysfunction. *World J. Gastroenterol.* **2008**, *14*, 193–199. [CrossRef] [PubMed]

8.  Husain, K.; Hernandez, W.; Ansari, R.A.; Ferder, L. Inflammation, oxidative stress and renin angiotensin system in atherosclerosis. *World J. Biol. Chem.* **2015**, *6*, 209–217. [CrossRef] [PubMed]

9.  Fargion, S.; Porzio, M.; Fracanzani, A.L. Nonalcoholic fatty liver disease and vascular disease: State-of-the-art. *World J. Gastroenterol.* **2014**, *20*, 13306–13324. [CrossRef] [PubMed]

10. Stepanova, M.; Younossi, Z.M. Independent association between nonalcoholic fatty liver disease and cardiovascular disease in the US population. *Clin. Gastroenterol. Hepatol.* **2012**, *10*, 646–650. [CrossRef] [PubMed]

11. Targher, G.; Day, C.P.; Bonora, E. Risk of cardiovascular disease in patients with Nonalcoholic Fatty Liver Disease. *N. Engl. J. Med.* **2010**, *363*, 1341–1350. [CrossRef] [PubMed]

12. Frantz, E.D.; Penna-de-Carvalho, A.; Batista Tde, M.; Aguila, M.B.; Mandarim-de-Lacerda, C.A. Comparative effects of the renin-angiotensin system blockers on nonalcoholic fatty liver disease and insulin resistance in C57BL/6 mice. *Metab. Syndr. Relat. Disord.* **2014**, *12*, 191–201. [CrossRef] [PubMed]

13. Fraga-Silva, R.A.; Savergnini, S.Q.; Montecucco, F.; Nencioni, A.; Caffa, I.; Soncini, D.; Costa-Fraga, F.P.; De Sousa, F.B.; Sinisterra, R.D.; Capettini, L.A.; et al. Treatment with Angiotensin-(1-7) reduces inflammation in carotid atherosclerotic plaques. *Thromb. Haemost.* **2014**, *111*, 736–747. [CrossRef] [PubMed]

14. Malhotra, N.; Beaton, M.D. Management of non-alcoholic fatty liver disease in 2015. *World J. Hepatol.* **2015**, *7*, 2962–2967. [CrossRef] [PubMed]

15. Kim, S.B.; Kang, O.H.; Lee, Y.S.; Han, S.H.; Ahn, Y.S.; Cha, S.W.; Seo, Y.S.; Kong, R.; Kwon, D.Y. Hepatoprotective effect and synergism of bisdemethoycurcumin against MCD Diet-Induced Nonalcoholic Fatty Liver Disease in mice. *PLoS ONE* **2016**, *11*. [CrossRef] [PubMed]

16. Patti, A.M.; Al-Rasadi, K.; Katsiki, N.; Banerjee, Y.; Nikolic, D.; Vanella, L.; Giglio, R.V.; Giannone, V.A.; Montalto, G.; Rizzo, M. Effect of a Natural Supplement Containing Curcuma Longa, Guggul, and Chlorogenic Acid in Patients With Metabolic Syndrome. *Angiology* **2015**, *66*, 856–861. [CrossRef] [PubMed]

17. Baldassano, S.; Amato, A.; Cappello, F.; Rappa, F.; Mulè, F. Glucagon-like peptide-2 and mouse intestinal adaptation to a high-fat diet. *J. Endocrinol.* **2013**, *217*, 11–20. [CrossRef] [PubMed]

18. Baldassano, S.; Amato, A.; Rappa, F.; Cappello, F.; Mulè, F. Influence of endogenous glucagon like peptide-2 on lipid disorders in mice fed a high fat diet. *Endoc. Res.* **2016**, *23*, 1–8. [CrossRef] [PubMed]

19. Jawień, J.; Nastałek, P.; Korbut, R. Mouse models of experimental atherosclerosis. *J. Physiol. Pharmacol.* **2004**, *55*, 503–517. [PubMed]

20. Nuzzo, D.; Picone, P.; Baldassano, S.; Caruana, L.; Messina, E.; Marino Gammazza, A.; Cappello, F.; Mulè, F.; Di Carlo, M. Insulin Resistance as Common Molecular Denominator Linking Obesity to Alzheimer's Disease. *Curr. Alzheimer Res.* **2015**, *12*, 723–735. [CrossRef] [PubMed]

21. Amato, A.; Baldassano, S.; Caldara, G.; Mulè, F. Neuronostatin: Peripheral site of action in mouse stomach. *Peptides* **2015**, *64*, 8–13. [CrossRef] [PubMed]

22. Liang, W.; Menke, A.L.; Driessen, A.; Koek, G.H.; Lindeman, J.H.; Stoop, R.; Havekes, L.M.; Kleemann, R.; van den Hoek, A.M. Establishment of a general NAFLD scoring system for rodent models and comparison to human liver pathology. *PLoS ONE* **2014**, *9*. [CrossRef] [PubMed]

23. Frediani Brant, N.M.; Mourão Gasparotto, F.; de Oliveira Araújo, V.; Christian Maraschin, J.; Lima Ribeiro Rde, C.; Botelho Lourenço, E.L.; Cardozo Junior, E.L.; Gasparotto Junior, A. Cardiovascular protective effects of Casearia sylvestris Swartz in Swiss and C57BL/6 LDLr-null mice undergoing high fat diet. *J. Ethnopharmacol.* **2014**, *154*, 419–427. [CrossRef] [PubMed]

24. Balzan, S.; Hernandes, A.; Reichert, C.L.; Donaduzzi, C.; Pires, V.A.; Gasparotto, A., Jr.; Cardozo, E.L., Jr. Lipid-lowering effects of standardized extracts of Ilex paraguariensis in high-fat-diet rats. *Fitoterapia* **2013**, *86*, 115–122. [CrossRef] [PubMed]

25. Gibbons, S. An overview of plant extracts as potential therapeutics. *Expert. Opin. Ther. Pat.* **2003**, *13*, 489–497. [CrossRef]

26. Sahebkar, A. Why it is necessary to translate curcumin into clinical practice for the prevention and treatment of metabolic syndrome? *Biofactors* **2013**, *39*, 197–208. [CrossRef] [PubMed]

27. Salamone, F.; Galvano, F.; Cappello, F.; Mangiameli, A.; Barbagallo, I.; Li Volti, G. Silibinin modulates lipid homeostasis and inhibits nuclear factor kappa B activation in experimental nonalcoholic steatohepatitis. *Transl. Res* **2012**, *159*, 477–486. [CrossRef] [PubMed]

28. Nohr, L.A.; Rasmussen, L.B.; Straand, J. Resin from the mukul myrrh tree, guggul, can it be used for treating hypercholesterolemia? A randomized, controlled study. Complement. *Ther. Med.* **2009**, *17*, 16–22. [CrossRef]

29. Mubarak, A.; Hodgson, J.M.; Considine, M.J.; Croft, K.D.; Matthews, V.B. Correction to Supplementation of a high-fat diet with chlorogenic acid is associated with insulin resistance and hepatic lipid accumulation in mice. *J. Agric. Food Chem.* **2013**, *61*, 4371–4378. [CrossRef] [PubMed]

30. Russo, F.; Riezzo, G.; Chiloiro, M.; De Michele, G.; Chimienti, G.; Marconi, E.; D'Attoma, B.; Linsalata, M.; Clemente, C. Metabolic effects of a diet with inulin-enriched pasta in healthy young volunteers. *Curr. Pharm. Des.* **2010**, *16*, 825–831. [CrossRef] [PubMed]

31. Chalasani, N.; Wilson, L.; Kleiner, D.E.; Cummings, O.W.; Brunt, E.M. Relationship of steatosis grade and zonal location to histological features of steatohepatitis in adult patients with non-alcoholic fatty liver disease. *J. Hepatol.* **2008**, *48*, 829–834. [CrossRef] [PubMed]

32. Corey, K.E.; Chalasani, N. Management of dyslipidemia as a cardiovascular risk factor in individuals with nonalcoholic fatty liver disease. *Clin. Gastroenterol. Hepatol.* **2014**, *12*, 1077–1084. [CrossRef] [PubMed]

33. Atshaves, B.P.; Martin, G.G.; Hostetler, H.A.; McIntosh, A.L.; Kier, A.B.; Schroeder, F. Liver fatty acid-binding protein and obesity. *J. Nutr. Biochem.* **2010**, *21*, 1015–1032. [CrossRef] [PubMed]

34. Westerbacka, J.; Kolak, M.; Kiviluoto, T.; Arkkila, P.; Sirén, J.; Hamsten, A.; Fisher, R.M.; Yki-Järvinen, H. Genes involved in fatty acid partitioning and binding, lipolysis, monocyte/macrophage recruitment, and inflammation are overexpressed in the human fatty liver of insulin-resistant subjects. *Diabetes* **2007**, *56*, 2759–2765. [CrossRef] [PubMed]

35. Kotronen, A.; Seppänen-Laakso, T.; Westerbacka, J.; Kiviluoto, T.; Arola, J.; Ruskeepää, A.L.; Oresic, M.; Yki-Järvinen, H. Hepatic stearoyl-CoA desaturase (SCD)-1 activity and diacylglycerol but not ceramide concentrations are increased in the nonalcoholic human fatty liver. *Diabetes* **2009**, *58*, 203–208. [CrossRef] [PubMed]

36. Miyazaki, M.; Dobrzyn, A.; Sampath, H.; Lee, S.H.; Man, W.C.; Chu, K.; Peters, J.M.; Gonzalez, F.J.; Ntambi, J.M. Reduced adiposity and liver steatosis by stearoyl-CoA desaturase deficiency are independent of peroxisome proliferator-activated receptor-alpha. *J. Biol. Chem.* **2004**, *279*, 35017–35024. [CrossRef] [PubMed]

37. Cohen, P.; Miyazaki, M.; Socci, N.D.; Hagge-Greenberg, A.; Liedtke, W.; Soukas, A.A.; Sharma, R.; Hudgins, L.C.; Ntambi, J.M.; Friedman, J.M. Role for stearoyl-CoA desaturase-1 in leptin-mediated weight loss. *Science* **2002**, *297*, 240–243. [CrossRef] [PubMed]

38. Kandhi, R.; Bobbala, D.; Yeganeh, M.; Mayhue, M.; Menendez, A.; Ilangumaran, S. Negative regulation of the hepatic fibrogenic response by suppressor of cytokine signaling 1. *Cytokine* **2016**, *82*, 58–69. [CrossRef] [PubMed]

39. Klein, T.; Fujii, M.; Sandel, J.; Shibazaki, Y.; Wakamatsu, K.; Mark, M.; Yoneyama, H. Linagliptin alleviates hepatic steatosis and inflammation in a mouse model of non-alcoholic steatohepatitis. *Med. Mol. Morphol.* **2014**, *47*, 137–149. [CrossRef] [PubMed]

40. Whitman, S.C. A practical approach to using mice in atherosclerosis research. *Clin. Biochem. Rev.* **2004**, *25*, 81–93. [PubMed]

41. Villanova, N.; Moscatiello, S.; Ramilli, S.; Bugianesi, E.; Magalotti, D.; Vanni, E.; Zoli, M.; Marchesini, G. Endothelial dysfunction and cardiovascular risk profile in nonalcoholic fatty liver disease. *Hepatology* **2005**, *42*, 473–480. [CrossRef] [PubMed]

42. Wieckowska, A.; Papouchado, B.G.; Li, Z.; Lopez, R.; Zein, N.N.; Feldstein, A.E. Increased hepatic and circulating interleukin-6 levels in human nonalcoholic steatohepatitis. *Am. J. Gastroenterol.* **2008**, *103*, 1372–1379. [CrossRef] [PubMed]

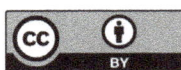

nutrients

MDPI

*Review*

# Nutraceutical Value of Citrus Flavanones and Their Implications in Cardiovascular Disease

**Lara Testai [1,2,\*] and Vincenzo Calderone [1,2]**

[1] Department of Farmacia, University of Pisa, via Bonanno, 6 56120 Pisa, Italy; vincenzo.calderone@unipi.it
[2] Interdepartmental Center of Nutrafood, University of Pisa, via Del Borghetto, 80 56124 Pisa, Italy
\* Correspondence: lara.testai@unipi.it

Received: 29 March 2017; Accepted: 10 May 2017; Published: 16 May 2017

**Abstract:** Background- Cardiovascular diseases, including myocardial infarction, dyslipidaemia and coronary artery pathology, are a major cause of illness and death in Western countries. Therefore, identifying effective therapeutic approaches and their cellular signalling pathways is a challenging goal for medicine. In this regard, several epidemiological studies demonstrate a relationship between the intake of flavonoid-rich foods and the reduction of cardiovascular risk factors and mortality. In particular, flavonoids present in citrus fruits, such as oranges, bergamots, lemons and grapefruit (95% from flavanones), are emerging for their considerable nutraceutical value. Methods- In this review an examination of literature was performed while considering both epidemiological, clinical and pre-clinical evidence supporting the beneficial role of the flavanone class. We evaluated studies in which citrus fruit juices or single flavanone administration and cardiovascular risk factors were analysed; to identify these studies, an electronic search was conducted in PUBMED for papers fulfilling these criteria and written in English. Results- In addition to epidemiological evidence and clinical studies demonstrating that fruits in the *Citrus* genus significantly reduce the incidence of cardiovascular disease risk, pre-clinical investigations highlight cellular and subcellular targets that are responsible for these beneficial effects. There has been special attention on evaluating intracellular pathways involved in direct cardiovascular and cardiometabolic effects mediated by naringenin, hesperetin and eriodictyol or their glycosylated derivatives. Conclusions- Although some mechanisms of action remain unclear and bioavailability problems remain to be solved, the current evidence supports the use of a nutraceutical approach with citrus fruits to prevent and cure several aspects of cardiovascular disease.

**Keywords:** citrus flavonoids; cardiovascular benefit; nutraceutical value

## 1. Introduction

Cardiovascular diseases are a main cause of illness and death in Western countries, and cardiovascular drugs are the most commonly used medications. Therefore, cardiovascular diseases remain a therapeutic and sanitary issue, affecting the largest number of patients in the world. To alleviate the social and economic burden of cardiovascular diseases, recommendations have been proposed for health and lifestyle interventions targeting multiple risk factors. Prevention of risk factors is considered a primary approach for containing cardiovascular diseases [1].

The availability of nutraceuticals with a positive impact on cardiac function to reduce the incidence and lethality of cardiovascular diseases is a challenging topic [2,3].

In this regard, flavonoids are important constituents endowed with beneficial properties that humans can obtain through food, particularly through consuming fruit and vegetables. Some of these are characteristic of specific foods (i.e., genistein and daidzein), whereas others are widespread in several foods (i.e., quercetin and apigenin). Generally, flavonoids are distinct based on structural characteristics in the following six sub-classes: flavonols, flavones, isoflavones, flavanones, anthocyanins and flavanols (catechins and proanthocyanidins) [4].

In particular, the flavanone class is abundant in fruits and fruit juices of the *Citrus* genus; approximately 95% of flavonoids are represented by this sub-class [5], and these foods are the main source of flavanones. However, they are not unique because there are high levels in other foods, such as in tomatoes [6].

Citrus flavanones are glycosylated in vegetables; of note, a disaccaridic moiety is linked to the 7 position of aglycone and the aglycone type is characteristic of the fruit. Therefore, the same aglycone can be combined with several glycosides to give different flavanones; for example, the most representative flavanones in grapefruit are narirutin and naringin, those in orange fruit are hesperidin and narirutin, and that in lemon is eriocitrin.

Of note, narirutin and naringin have the same aglycone, naringenin, and hesperidin is the glycoside of hesperetin, while eriocitrin contains the aglycone eriodictyol (Figure 1) [7].

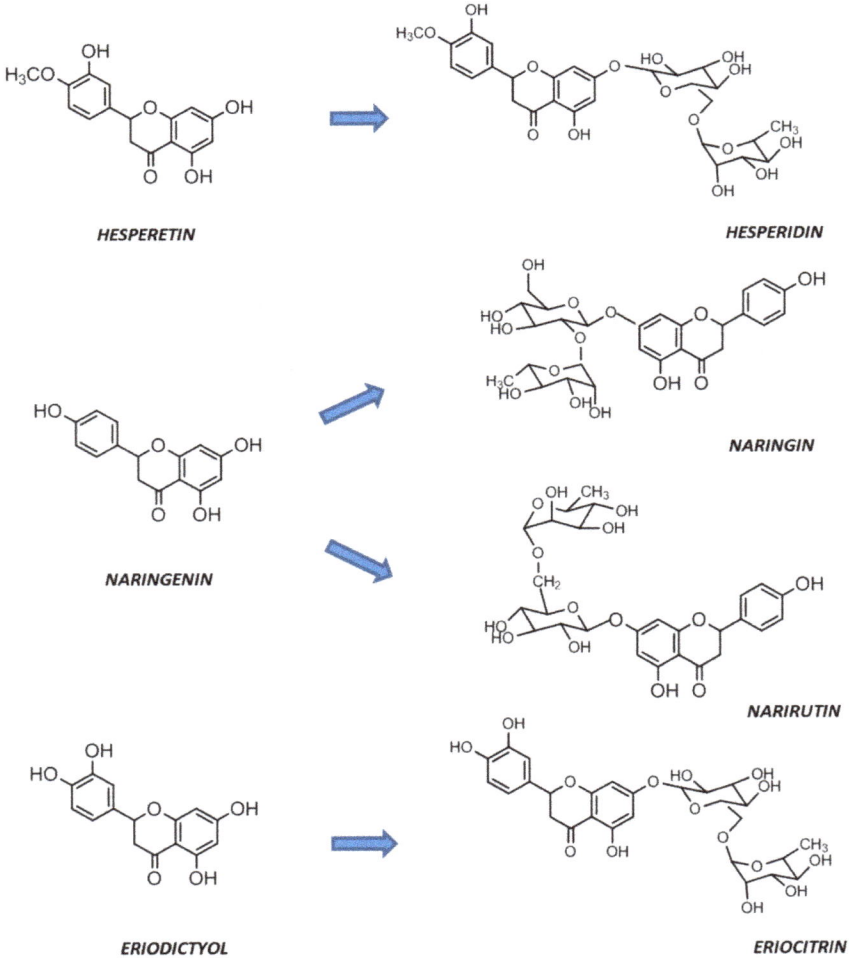

**Figure 1.** Chemical structures of citrus flavanones.

These flavanones are not evenly distributed in the fruit; they are particularly present in the albedo and in the membranes separating cloves rather than in the pulp. Peterson and his colleagues report flavanone levels in the orange range between 35 and 147 mg/100 g, and naringin and narirutin in grapefruit are present in a range between 44 and 106 mg/100 g [5].

Because the albedo and membranous parts are usually discarded to prepare fruit juices, the actual level of flavanones is lower. Indeed, as reported by Tomas-Barbean and Clifford, the levels of hesperidin and narirutin in orange juice are between 13 and 77 mg/100 mg. Ross et al. quantified naringenin in grapefruit juice in the range of 17–76 mg/100 mL [8,9].

In Europe, orange or its fruit juice is the most commonly consumed citrus fruit; therefore, it is the principal fruit source of citrus flavanones [10]. Moreover, *O*-glycoside flavanones are present in all cultivars of orange, both red or pigmented and blond or non-pigmented; nevertheless, the number of flavanones is higher in red cultivars in which a high level of anthocyanins is also present, representing a peculiar feature [11].

## 2. Cardiovascular Benefits of Citrus Flavanones—Epidemiological, Clinical and Pre-Clinical Evidence

Epidemiological evidence and clinical and pre-clinical studies suggest that flavanones present in the *Citrus* genus positively influence cardio-metabolic parameters, preventing cardiovascular disease [12–15].

In particular, a recent epidemiological study performed a Nurses' Health Study on approximately 70,000 women, highlighting an inverse correlation between flavanone intake and cerebral ischaemia risk, which is significant when considering women who consume high levels of flavanones (>63 mg/day) versus low levels (<13.7 mg/day) [16].

Another prospective study was performed in Finland on approximately 10,000 men and women, considering the correlation between the cardiovascular risk and flavonoid intake, revealing a 20% reduction in cerebrovascular diseases in those who consumed the highest levels of flavanones (4.7–26.8 mg aglycone/day) [17].

Similar results have been obtained in a Japanese cohort study conducted at JICHI Medical School. In Japan, citrus fruits represent 30% of the annual consumption of fruit and, in enrolled individuals, the incidence of cardiovascular diseases was evaluated during a period of approximately 11 years, confirming the inverse correlation between these [18].

Moreover, Wang and colleagues published a systematic review and meta-analysis of prospective cohort studies, which demonstrated that flavonoid consumption, especially of flavanones, was associated with a decreased risk of cardiovascular disease ($p$ = 0.002) [19]

Very recently, a meta-analysis of three randomized clinical trials, including 233 patients, demonstrated a correlation between grapefruit intake and a reduction in blood pressure. Although grapefruit intake does not significantly reduce body weight, it was responsible for a small, but significant, reduction in the systolic blood pressure and waist circumference in overweight and obese adults. The authors speculated that such beneficial effects can be related to naringin considering its great abundance in grapefruit [20].

Cassidy et al. reported approximately three prospective studies (Nurses's Health Studies) in middle-aged and older US women and men in which the association between habitual intake of several flavonoid sub-classes and risk of incident hypertension was examined. This analysis confirmed that habitual flavonoid intake (principally from the consumption of flavanones present in grapefruits, oranges and citrus juices) is correlated with a reduced incidence of hypertension [21].

Another recognized cardiovascular risk factor is metabolic syndrome, a condition characterized by impaired glucose metabolism, dyslipidaemia, elevated blood pressure and abdominal obesity. Grosso et al. published a cohort study in 2016 on another 10,000 Polish subjects, demonstrating an interesting inverse association between polyphenols and metabolic syndrome, which is particularly evident in individuals with the biggest intake of these [22].

Therefore, evidence gathered thus far supports a preventive role of citrus fruits in addressing the main risk factors of cardiovascular diseases, including overweight, hypertension and hyperglycaemia; a deeper examination of specific cardio-vascular and cardio-metabolic parameters influenced by such a flavonoid sub-class has been performed below.

A schematic table of the epidemiological and clinical evidence supporting the cardiovascular benefits obtained with citrus flavanones is reported in Table 1.

**Table 1.** Epidemiological evidence, clinical trials or meta-analysis in which beneficial effects of citrus flavanones or citrus fruits have been studied.

| Type and Duration of Study | Number of Subjects Enrolled | Dietary Intervention | Outcomes | Reference |
|---|---|---|---|---|
| Epidemiological study "Nurses's Healthy Study" | 70,000 women | Flavonoid intake (>63 mg/day) | Reduction of cerebral ischaemia risk | [16] |
| Finnish prospective study | 10,000 men and women | Flavanone intake (4.7–26.8 mg aglycone/day) | Significant reduction of cerebrovascular diseases (20%) | [17] |
| Japanese cohort study | 12,500 men and women | Habitual citrus fruit consumption | Significant reduction of cardiovascular disease incidence (30%) | [18] |
| Meta-analysis of three prospective cohort studies | 250 participants | Naringenin contained in grapefruit | Significant reduction of pressure parameters | [19] |
| Prospective studies | 8821 middle-aged and older men and women | Habitual citrus fruits consumed | Reduction of hypertension incidence | [21] |
| Cohort clinical trial | 10,000 Polish subjects | Habitual consumption of flavonoids, among which flavanones | Reduction of incidence of metabolic syndrome | [22] |
| Clinical trial of 5 weeks | 12 mild hypertension (stage I) subjects | Sweetie fruits (containing 25% naringin and 30% narirutin) | Significant reduction of diastolic pressure parameters | [23] |
| Clinical trial of 4 weeks | 24 overweight subjects | Hesperidin (292 mg, corresponding to levels in 500 mL of orange juice) | Pressure parameter reduction (4 mmHg), amelioration of post-prandial microvascular reactivity | [24] |
| Controlled clinical trials of 3 weeks | 28 subjects with metabolic syndrome | Capsules of hesperidin (500 mg/day) | Reduction of sE-selectin expression, cholesterol and ApoB level reduction, enhancement of NO levels | [25,26] |
| Clinical trials of 6 months | 52 post-menopausal women | Intake of grapefruit juice (containing 105 mg of naringenin) | Improvement of arterial stiffness | [27] |
| French prospective cohort study | 59 middle-aged women | Habitual intake of flavonoids, among which flavanones | Improvement of vascular function and slowing down of atherosclerotic progression | [28] |
| Clinical trials of 2 months | 30 healthy subjects + 30 hypercholesterolemic subjects | Capsules of naringin (400 mg/day) | Reduction of LDL-C, cholesterol and ApoB levels. Increase of HDL-C levels and detoxifying enzymes. | [29] |
| Clinical trial of 4 or 6 months | 20 healthy subjects and 33 subjects with metabolic syndrome | Intake of 300 mL of fruit juice (containing 95% of citrus flavonoids) | No variations of glucidic parameters, improvement of lipidic panel | [30] |
| Clinical trial of 4 weeks treatment | 25 hyperchoesterolemic subjects | Intake of 200 mL of blond orange juice (three times a day) | ApoA levels reduction | [31] |

Table 1. *Cont.*

| Type and Duration of Study | Number of Subjects Enrolled | Dietary Intervention | Outcomes | Reference |
|---|---|---|---|---|
| Prospective study with 6-month treatment | 80 patients with mild hypercholesterolaemia | Intake of Bergavit® (bergamot extract containing 150 mg/day of flavonoids) | Improvement of lipidic panel and reduction of cholesterol levels | [32] |
| Randomized controlled study of 4 weeks of treatment | 204 healthy and with moderate hypercholesterolaemia subjects (men and women) | Intake of capsules containing naringin+hesperidin (500 mg and 800 mg/day respectively) | No improvement of lipidic panel | [33] |
| Clinical trial of 4 weeks of treatment | 24 overweight subjects | Hesperidin (292 mg/day) | No improvement of lipidic panel | [34] |

*2.1. Effects on Cardiovascular Parameters*

2.1.1. Reduction of Endothelial Dysfunction and Improvement of Vascular Function

The paradigm between hypertension and endothelial dysfunction has been widely demonstrated, as well as that between the reduction of endothelial integrity and atherosclerotic processes. Indeed, the vascular endothelium is a very active organ responsible for regulating vascular tone through the effects of locally synthesized mediators, especially nitric oxide (NO), endothelial NO synthase (eNOS), and superoxide, and its depletion is both a sign and cause of endothelial dysfunction resulting from reduced activity of eNOS and amplified production of reactive oxygen species. Then, the integrity and reactivity of endothelium must be ensured to prevent the progression of cardiovascular disease [35].

Clinical trials in the literature indicate a clear correlation between citrus flavanone intake, vasodilatation and reduction of endothelial dysfunction. In particular, Reshef and colleagues described a study on patients with mild hypertension (stage I) treated with sweetie fruit, which is a hybrid between grapefruit and pomelo that contains a high level of flavonoids from the *Citrus* genus (25% of naringin and 30% of narirutin). Two types of sweetie juices were obtained, one with a low flavonoid level (166 mg/L naringin and 64 mg/L narirutin) and one with a high flavonoid level (677 mg/L of naringin and 212 mg/L narirutin). After 5 weeks, a significant reduction in the diastolic pressure value was observed in the high flavonoid group ($p = 0.04$) [23]. In agreement with this study, a study on 4 weeks of treatment with 292 mg of hesperidin (corresponding to the levels present in 500 mL of orange juice) showed a reduction in the diastolic pressure by 4 mmHg in moderately overweight men ($p = 0.02$). Moreover, the intake of hesperidin supplement improved the post-prandial reactivity of the microvascular endothelium ($p < 0.05$), demonstrating that hesperidin can positively influence endothelial function. Based on these results, the authors encourage the consumption of citrus foods [24].

A further confirmation of these observations was demonstrated in a clinical trial performed on 25 patients with metabolic syndrome. After 3 weeks of treatment with 500 mg daily of capsules containing 98% of pure hesperidin, the expression of E-selectin, a biomarker of endothelial dysfunction, was significantly reduced. This clinical effect was accompanied by an improvement in endogenous NO production, inspiring the hypothesis that the vascular protection could be mediated by enhancement of endothelial function [25,26].

Of note, a primary risk factor for cardiovascular diseases in aged women is the post-menopausal condition, which is mainly due to dysfunction of the endothelium. Morand's group reported a clinical trial enrolling 52 women after menopause who were asked to consume a bottle (340 mL) of a concentrated blond grapefruit juice (containing 105 mg of naringenin) or a iso-caloric and iso-energetic drink daily. After 6 months of treatment, volunteers consuming grapefruit juice had a significant change in their anthropometric parameters and vascular function, with improvement in arterial stiffness that was independent of blood pressure changes [36]. A positive impact of flavonoids on hypertension has also been shown in a prospective cohort on French middle-aged women [28]. In agreement with several previously described studies, improvement in vascular function and slowing of atherosclerosis progression have been reported in normotensive subjects (healthy volunteers and patients with type 2 diabetes or coronary artery disease) [37,38] and in overweight men [39].

### 2.1.2. Lipid Level Reduction

Elevated levels of low-density lipoprotein cholesterol (LDL-C) and its deposition in the macrophages of arterial walls contribute to the main cause of atherosclerosis progression, which is a gateway for cardiovascular complications, including heart attacks, ischaemic stroke and coronary diseases [40]. Several large randomized clinical trials with statin-based and non-statin based therapies have demonstrated that a reduction in LDL-C levels reduced the cardiovascular risks [41].

Interestingly, naringenin promotes a decrease in LDL-C and triglycerides as well as inhibiting glucose uptake. On the other hand, it increases high-density lipoprotein (HDL-C) and ameliorates anti-oxidant defences, downregulating atherosclerosis-related genes [42].

Several pre-clinical studies have demonstrated the role of flavanones in atherosclerosis progression. In particular, a 0.1% naringin or 0.05% naringenin supplement given to rabbits with high cholesterol levels significantly decreased the expression levels of vascular cell adhesion molecule-1 (VCAM-1) and monocyte chemotactic protein-1 (MCP-1) after 8 weeks; at the same time, the hepatic cholesterol acyltransferase (ACAT) activity, the basis for reducing atherosclerotic plaques, appeared to decrease [43,44]. Similarly, another research group demonstrated that mice given high cholesterol levels plus naringin (0.02%, corresponding to a half grapefruit) had a significant reduction (41%) of atherosclerotic plaque compared to the high cholesterol level-alone group [45].

In terms of clinical evidence, the administration of capsules containing 400 mg/day of naringenin for two months promoted a drop in the LDL-C, cholesterol and ApoB levels and an increase in HDL-C levels in hypercholesterolemic, but not control, subjects, and there was an improvement in detoxifying enzymes [29].

Moreover, patients with metabolic syndrome given a supplement of hesperidin (500 mg/day) for 3 weeks had reduced cholesterol and ApoB levels [25]. In agreement, in a 2012 clinical study performed in Spain on patients with a diagnosis of metabolic syndrome, the glycaemic profile was unchanged after 4 and 6 months of citrus fruit juice treatment (300 mL daily), but the lipid profile improved, as observed by decrease in the cholesterol, LDL-C, and C-reactive peptide (a well-known inflammatory marker) levels ($p < 0.05$) [30].

Of the citrus fruits, bergamot fruit is worth noting because it is considered a promising nutraceutical approach for controlling hypercholesterolaemia. *Citrus bergamia* administered to rats with hyperlipidaemia (1 mL/rat/day) showed hepatic protection and a significant reduction in the cholesterol, triglycerides and LDL-C levels (−29%, −46% and −52%, respectively) with an approximately 28% increase in the HDL-C levels. These effects are the basis for anti-atherogenic activity and are responsible for cardiovascular disease prevention [46]. Additionally, the authors reported that bergamot can increase the excretion of sterols and bile acids. The mechanisms through which bergamot has beneficial effects are not completely clear, though it cannot only be due to citrus flavanones (naringenin, hesperetin and eriodictyol) [47]. Indeed, Di Donna et al. reported the presence of 3-hydroxy-3-methyl-glutaryl flavanones with a behaviour similar to simvastatin in a model of hypercholesterolaemic rats, speculating that these statin-like compounds could potentiate the hypocholesterolaemic effects [48].

However, beyond these encouraging data, a more nebulous scenario appears based on consideration for the citrus flavanone effects on hypercholesterolaemic patients. On the one hand, a study enrolling 25 volunteers with high LDL-C and cholesterol levels demonstrated that 4 weeks of feed with 600 mL/day of blond orange juice significantly reduced the plasma levels of oxidative stress markers and apo A levels [31]. In agreement, a recent 6-month prospective study showed that bergamia extract (containing 150 mg of flavonoids with 16% neoericitrin, 47% neohesperidin and 37% naringin) reduced the plasma levels of lipids and improved the lipoproteic profile in moderate hypercholesterolemic patients. Of note, such an ipolipidaemic effect was more evident in the group with higher cholesterol levels [32].

On the other hand, a clinical study with 500 mg of naringin plus 800 mg of hesperidin did not show a significant improvement in the lipid profile in moderate hypercholesterolaemia patients. Of note, the citrus flavanone doses in the study correspond to the 95th percentile of daily consumption in Western populations and were finalized to minimize the chance of not detecting a LDL-C lowering effect. This outcome suggests that citrus flavonoids have no effect on LDL-C in people, at least not when consumed in a capsule format [33]. Similar results have been reported in overweight patients consuming 292 mg of hesperidin and 47.5 mg of narirutin for 4 weeks [24]. A possible explanation for this discrepancy, according to some authors, could be caused by high inter-individual variability in the pharmacokinetic parameters beyond by the type formulation. Although pre-clinical results are clearer and encouraging, further clinical studies need to be performed.

## 3. Putative Mechanisms of Action Responsible for the Cardiovascular Benefits of Citrus Flavanones

### 3.1. Anti-Oxidant and Anti-Inflammatory Action

Oxidative stress and inflammation are pathologic processes that contribute to atherosclerotic progression and the evolution of cardiovascular diseases. In healthy subjects, citrus flavanones do not have significant anti-oxidant effects, suggesting that their anti-oxidant potency is negligible in normal conditions. In hypercholesterolaemic subjects, Jung et al. demonstrated that naringin, administered for 8 weeks at a dose of 400 mg/day, significantly increased the SOD and catalase levels [29]. This result suggests that flavanones of the *Citrus* genus could have an important impact on the improvement of endogenous anti-oxidant defences in dyslipidaemia. Very recently, hesperidin has been demonstrated to elevate anti-oxidant defences through increasing Nrf2 expression, suggesting an anti-ageing effect of this flavonoid on senescent rat hearts [34]. Similar results emerged from an in vitro study on H9c2 cells in which naringenin significantly reduced the production of beta-galactosidase, a typical marker of senescence, after doxorubicin treatment [49].

Several in vivo studies showed that flavanones can reduce chemokines as well as inflammatory and adhesion molecules, whose expression is tightly regulated by the pro-inflammatory factor NF-kB. This anti-inflammatory action accounts for anti-atherogenesis at the endothelium, smooth muscle cell and monocyte/macrophage levels [50–52].

Five hundred milligrams of hesperidin can help reduce the plasma values of inflammatory factors and genetic expression of proteins involved in cell proliferation, chemotaxis and platelet adhesion [23]. Moreover, a very recent in vitro study on human endothelial cells, showed that hesperetin and its main metabolites inhibited TNF-$\alpha$-induced cell migration [53]. On the other hand, 5 $\mu$M naringenin decreased the production of a pro-inflammatory eicosanoid, PGE2, and reduced the expression of the COX2 enzyme, while higher concentrations (30–100 $\mu$M) inhibited NFkB activation [54–56]. A further central inflammatory target is represented by matrix metallopeptidases; MMP9 is particularly involved in atherosclerotic lesions, and one study indicated that naringenin and naringin reduced MMP9 expression, reducing smooth muscle cell migration. Such an action could be at least partly related to the suppression of NF-kB activation [57].

### 3.2. Vasodilator Activity

Vasoactive properties of the main flavonoids of the *Citrus* genus, naringenin and hesperetin, have been widely described; particularly, Rizza et al. demonstrated that hesperetin induces vasodilatation through endothelial production of nitric oxide (NO) and its derivative, glycosyl-hesperidin, which was administered for 8 weeks to spontaneously hypertensive rats, was able to reduce pressure parameters 3% in addition to improving the endothelial response [25,58–60]. Moreover, on isolated coronary arteries of rodents, hesperetin caused vasodilatation by activating voltage-operated calcium channels and potassium currents [61].

With respect to naringenin-mediated vasorelaxing effects, they are probably linked to opening a calcium-activated potassium channel (BKCa) located on the sarcolemmatic membrane of smooth muscle cells, as demonstrated by Saponara and colleagues [62,63].

Finally, a unique paper reported the vasorelaxing property of eriodictyol, a flavanone typical of lemon; nevertheless, the authors reported a concentration-dependent reduction in the vascular tone in the rat aortic rings without elucidating the mechanism of action. More recently, in vitro protective effects on endothelial cells have also been demonstrated [64,65].

### 3.3. Anti-Ischaemic Activity

Myocardial infarction represents the main and often lethal manifestation of cardiovascular risk such that agents able to prevent it are useful for containing the damage.

Several pre-clinical studies have demonstrated the cardioprotection conferred by citrus flavanones. In ex vivo and in vivo myocardial ischaemia–reperfusion (I/R) models, naringenin could confer cardioprotection, and this action seemed to be mediated through activation of BKCa channels expressed on the inner mitochondrial membrane. This channel is structurally similar to that expressed on the sarcolemma and is involved in vasodilatation that, at the mitochondrial level, plays a crucial role in I/R events. Indeed, naringenin promoted reduced mitochondrial calcium uptake and mild mitochondrial depolarization as well as restricting the probability of mitochondrial permeability transition pore (MPTP) formation and apoptotic death of myocardiocytes [66–68].

On the other hand, hesperetin can have anti-apoptotic effects on cardiomyoblasts through the mitochondrial JNK/Bax pathway [69].

### 3.4. Glucose Tolerance

A supplement for 4 or more weeks with flavanones reduces glycaemia and insulinaemia in diabetic or insulin-resistant animals fed a high fat diet; moreover, glucose tolerance was improved. The insulin-like property of naringenin has been demonstrated, and it has added to the in vitro evidence that demonstrates the ability of naringin and hesperidin to reduce the PPAR-γ expression and glucokinase activity, a key enzyme involved in the glucose use [70–72]. In this context, a poly-methoxy flavone abundant in mandarin, tangeretin, should be mentioned. In diabetic rats, tangeretin markedly reduced the plasmatic glucose levels, while it also increased the insulin secretion, enhancing complex glucose metabolism [73].

## 4. Pharmacokinetic Profile of Citrus Flavanones

A significant problem with citrus flavonoids is their low bioavailability, restricting their efficacy to the point of having to enrich the fruit juice with citrus flavanones or their analogues, which are enzymatically more stable. Usually, the peak plasma concentration is reached 6 h after consumption with a μM concentration and relative differences among several flavonoid types [74].

Their metabolism concerns conjugation at the intestinal and hepatic levels, leading to two types of metabolites, glucuronide- and sulfate-conjugated. Principal excretion occurs through urine with a peak between 6 and 12 hours after intake [75].

Another factor that could influence the bioavailability of citrus flavanones is their solubility in fruit juice, and the preparation technique, homemade or industrial, is very important. Indeed, an analytical evaluation revealed that the qualitative composition is not changed, but quantitative analysis highlights significant differences [76]. However, the matrix factor is not the most critical. The main factor responsible for the high inter-individual variability seems to be the colon bacteria microflora [77], which is essential for flavonoid metabolism. Indeed, the consumption of fruit juice guarantees intake of glycosylated flavanones, but they are pro-drugs that require bio-activation via the hydrolysis of the glycoside portion to release the aglycone that is then responsible for pharmacological activity. Of note, an innovative view to improve the bioavailability of flavonoids and, more generally, of polyphenols is represented by the evaluation of human intestinal microbiota. Indeed, it has been demonstrated that the intestinal microbiota controls the bio-activation of flavonoids and regulates their catabolism [78]. On the other hand, other authors have noted that polyphenolic components could act as prebiotics and influence the growth of intestinal bacteria [79]. Further knowledge of the role of microbiota in metabolic diseases, as well as in cardiovascular diseases, and of factors that modulate microbiota will allow us to understand the true therapeutic benefits of various diet components and suggest an appropriate diet that optimizes these beneficial effects [80].

## 5. Conclusions

In conclusion, the mechanisms responsible for the beneficial effects of citrus flavanones on the cardiovascular system are multiple and remain somewhat unclear, although, in general, the available clinical and pre-clinical studies suggest a positive correlation between their intake and a significant reduction in the cardiovascular risk factors. However, such evidence is satisfactory to confer citrus fruits with an interesting nutraceutical value in the context of the spread of cardiovascular disease in Western countries and their heavy impact on the quality of life of patients.

Indeed, to date, cardiovascular drugs represent the most commonly used category in the world, and, although there are large-scale pharmacological treatments, cardiovascular diseases are the most widespread, consuming a high level of therapeutic resources and affecting health significantly. Furthermore, their prevalence is expected to rise, particularly in Western countries, because of obesity and the ageing population.

A nutraceutical approach, such as with citrus fruits, aimed at preventing and curing several aspects of cardiovascular diseases could be very useful.

**Acknowledgments:** This work was supported by the Research Project of Ateneo-PRA2017.

**Author Contributions:** L.T. wrote the paper, V.C. organized and revised the paper.

**Conflicts of Interest:** The authors declare no conflict of interest.

## References

1. Mendis, S.; Puska, P.; Norrving, B. *Global Atlas on Cardiovascular Disease Prevention and Control*; WHO: Geneva, Switzerland, 2017.
2. Butler, J.; Tahhan, A.S.; Georgiopoulou, V.V.; Kelkar, A.; Lee, M.; Khan, B.; Peterson, E.; Fonarow, G.C.; Kalogeropoulos, A.P.; Gheorghiade, M. Trends in characteristics of cardiovascular clinical trials 2001–2012. *Am. Heart J.* **2015**, *170*, 263–272. [CrossRef] [PubMed]
3. Moran, A.E.; Forouzanfar, M.H.; Roth, G.A.; Mensah, G.A.; Ezzati, M.; Murray, C.J.; Naghavi, M. Temporal trends in ischemic heart disease mortality in 21 world regions, 1980 to 2010: The Global Burden of Disease 2010 study. *Circulation* **2014**, *129*, 1483–1492. [CrossRef] [PubMed]
4. Shashank, K.; Abhay, K.P. Chemistry and Biological Activities of Flavonoids: An Overview. *Sci. World J.* **2013**, *2013*, 1–16.
5. Peterson, J.J.; Dwyer, J.T.; Beecher, G.R.; Bhagwat, S.A.; Gabhardt, S.E.; Haytowitz, D.B.; Holden, J.M. Flavanones in oranges, tangerines (mandarins), tangors and tangelos: A compilation and review of the data from the analytical literature. *J. Food Compos. Anal.* **2006**, *19*, S66–S73. [CrossRef]
6. Bharti, S.; Rani, N.; Krishnamurthy, B.; Arya, D.S. Preclinical evidence for the pharmacological actions of naringin: A review. *Planta Med.* **2014**, *80*, 437–451. [CrossRef] [PubMed]
7. Chanet, A.; Milenkovic, D.; Manach, C.; Mazur, A.; Morand, C. Citrus flavanones: What is their role in cardiovascular protection? *J. Agric. Food Chem.* **2012**, *60*, 8809–8822. [CrossRef] [PubMed]
8. Tomas-Barberan, F.A.; Clifford, M.N. Flavanones, chalcones and dihydrochalcones. Nature, occurrence and dietary burden. *J. Sci. Food Agric.* **2000**, *80*, 1073–1080. [CrossRef]
9. Ross, S.A.; Ziska, D.S.; Zhao, K.; ElSohly, M.A. Variance of common flavonoids by brand of grapefruit juice. *Fitoterapia* **2000**, *71*, 154–161. [CrossRef]

10. Zamora-Ros, R.; Andres-Lacueva, C.; Lamuela-Raventós, R.M.; Berenguer, T.; Jakszyn, P.; Barricarte, A.; Ardanaz, E.; Amiano, P.; Dorronsoro, M.; Larrañaga, N.; et al. Estimation of dietary sources and flavonoid intake in a Spanish adult population (EPIC-Spain). *J. Am. Diet. Assoc.* **2010**, *110*, 390–398. [CrossRef] [PubMed]

11. Grosso, G.; Galvano, F.; Mistretta, A.; Marventano, S.; Nolfo, F.; Calabrese, G.; Buscemi, S.; Drago, F.; Veronesi, U.; Scuderi, A. Red orange: Experimental models and epidemiological evidence of its benefits on human health. *Oxid. Med. Cell. Longev.* **2013**, *2013*, 157240. [CrossRef] [PubMed]

12. Dauchet, L.; Amouyel, P.; Dallongeville, J. Fruit and vegetable consumption and risk of stroke: A meta-analysis of cohort studies. *Neurology* **2005**, *65*, 1193–1197. [CrossRef] [PubMed]

13. Dauchet, L.; Amouyel, P.; Hercberg, S.; Dallongeville, J. Fruit and vegetable consumption and risk of coronary heart disease: A meta-analysis of cohort studies. *J. Nutr.* **2006**, *136*, 2588–2593. [PubMed]

14. He, F.J.; Nowson, C.A.; MacGregor, G.A. Fruit and vegetable consumption and stroke: Meta-analysis of cohort studies. *Lancet* **2006**, *367*, 320–326. [CrossRef]

15. He, F.J.; Nowson, C.A.; Lucas, M.; MacGregor, G.A. Increased consumption of fruit and vegetables is related to a reduced risk of coronary heart disease: Meta-analysis of cohort studies. *J. Hum. Hypertens.* **2007**, *21*, 717–728. [CrossRef] [PubMed]

16. Cassidy, A.; Rimm, E.B.; O'Reilly, E.J.; Logroscino, G.; Kay, C.; Chiuve, S.E.; Rexrode, K.M. Dietary flavonoids and risk of stroke in women. *Stroke* **2012**, *43*, 946–951. [CrossRef] [PubMed]

17. Knekt, P.; Kumpulainen, J.; Järvinen, R.; Rissanen, H.; Heliövaara, M.; Reunanen, A.; Hakulinen, T.; Aromaa, A. Flavonoid intake and risk of chronic diseases. *Am. J. Clin. Nutr.* **2002**, *76*, 560–568. [PubMed]

18. Yamada, T.; Hayasaka, S.; Shibata, Y.; Ojima, T.; Saegusa, T.; Gotoh, T.; Ishikawa, S.; Nakamura, Y.; Kayaba, K.; Jichi Medical School Cohort Study Group. Frequency of citrus fruit intake is associated with the incidence of cardiovascular disease: The Jichi Medical School cohort study. *J. Epidemiol.* **2011**, *21*, 169–175. [CrossRef] [PubMed]

19. Wang, X.; Ouyang, Y.Y.; Liu, J.; Zhao, G. Flavonoid intake and risk of CVD: A systematic review and meta-analysis of prospective cohort studies. *Br. J. Nutr.* **2014**, *111*, 1–11. [CrossRef] [PubMed]

20. Onakpoya, I.; O'Sullivan, J.; Heneghan, C.; Thompson, M. The Effect of Grapefruits (Citrus paradisi) on Body Weight and Cardiovascular Risk Factors: A Systematic Review and Meta-analysis of Randomized Clinical Trials. *Crit. Rev. Food Sci. Nutr.* **2017**, *57*, 602–612. [CrossRef] [PubMed]

21. Cassidy, A.; O'Reilly, É.J.; Kay, C.; Sampson, L.; Franz, M.; Forman, J.P.; Curhan, G.; Rimm, E.B. Habitual intake of flavonoid subclasses and incident hypertension in adults. *Am. J. Clin. Nutr.* **2011**, *93*, 338–347. [CrossRef] [PubMed]

22. Grosso, G.; Stepaniak, U.; Micek, A.; Stefler, D.; Bobak, M.; Pająk, A. Dietary polyphenols are inversely associated with metabolic syndrome in Polish adults of the HAPIEE study. *Eur. J. Nutr.* **2016**, in press. [CrossRef] [PubMed]

23. Reshef, N.; Hayari, Y.; Goren, C.; Boaz, M.; Madar, Z.; Knobler, H. Antihypertensive effect of sweetie fruit in patients with stage I hypertension. *Am. J. Hypertens.* **2005**, *18*, 1360–1363. [CrossRef] [PubMed]

24. Morand, C.; Dubray, C.; Milenkovic, D.; Lioger, D.; Martin, J.F.; Scalbert, A.; Mazur, A. Hesperidin contributes to the vascular protective effects of orange juice: A randomized crossover study in healthy volunteers. *Am. J. Clin. Nutr.* **2011**, *93*, 73–80. [CrossRef] [PubMed]

25. Rizza, S.; Muniyappa, R.; Iantorno, M.; Kim, J.A.; Chen, H.; Pullikotil, P.; Senese, N.; Tesauro, M.; Lauro, D.; Cardillo, C.; et al. Citrus polyphenol hesperidin stimulates production of nitric oxide in endothelial cells while improving endothelial function and reducing inflammatory markers in patients with metabolic syndrome. *J. Clin. Endocrinol. Metab.* **2011**, *96*, E782–E792. [CrossRef] [PubMed]

26. Roohbakhsh, A.; Parhiz, H.; Soltani, F.; Rezaee, R.; Iranshahi, M. Molecular mechanisms behind the biological effects of hesperidin and hesperetin for the prevention of cancer and cardiovascular diseases. *Life Sci.* **2015**, *124*, 64–74. [CrossRef] [PubMed]

27. Teede, H.J.; McGrath, B.P.; DeSilva, L.; Cehun, M.; Fassoulakis, A.; Nestel, P.J. Isoflavones reduce arterial stiffness: A placebo-controlled study in men and postmenopausal women. *Arterioscler. Thromb. Vasc. Biol.* **2003**, *23*, 1066–1071. [CrossRef] [PubMed]

28. Lajous, M.; Rossignol, E.; Fagherazzi, G.; Perquier, F.; Scalbert, A.; Clavel-Chapelon, F.; Boutron-Ruault, M.C. Flavonoid intake and incident hypertension in women. *Am. J. Clin. Nutr.* **2016**, *103*, 1091–1098. [CrossRef] [PubMed]

29. Jung, U.J.; Kim, H.J.; Lee, J.S.; Lee, M.K.; Kim, H.O.; Park, E.J.; Kim, H.K.; Jeong, T.S.; Choi, M.S. Naringin supplementation lowers plasma lipids and enhances erythrocyte antioxidant enzyme activities in hypercholesterolemic subjects. *Clin. Nutr.* **2003**, *22*, 561–568. [CrossRef]

30. Mulero, J.; Bernabé, J.; Cerdá, B.; García-Viguera, C.; Moreno, D.A.; Albaladejo, M.D.; Avilés, F.; Parra, S.; Abellán, J.; Zafrilla, P. Variations on cardiovascular risk factors in metabolic syndrome after consume of a citrus-based juice. *Clin. Nutr.* **2012**, *31*, 372–377. [CrossRef] [PubMed]

31. Constans, J.; Bennetau-Pelissero, C.; Martin, J.F.; Rock, E.; Mazur, A.; Bedel, A.; Morand, C.; Bérard, A.M. Marked antioxidant effect of orange juice intake and its phytomicronutrients in a preliminary randomized cross-over trial on mild hypercholesterolemic men. *Clin. Nutr.* **2015**, *34*, 1093–1100. [CrossRef] [PubMed]

32. Toth, P.P.; Patti, A.M.; Nikolic, D.; Giglio, R.V.; Castellino, G.; Biancucci, T.; Geraci, F.; David, S.; Montalto, G.; Rizvi, A.; et al. Bergamot Reduces Plasma Lipids, Atherogenic Small Dense LDL, and Subclinical Atherosclerosis in Subjects with Moderate Hypercholesterolemia: A 6 Months Prospective Study. *Front. Pharmacol.* **2016**, *6*, 299. [CrossRef] [PubMed]

33. Demonty, I.; Lin, Y.; Zebregs, Y.E.; Vermeer, M.A.; van der Knaap, H.C.; Jäkel, M.; Trautwein, E.A. The citrus flavonoids hesperidin and naringin do not affect serum cholesterol in moderately hypercholesterolemic men and women. *J. Nutr.* **2010**, *140*, 1615–1620. [CrossRef]

34. Elavarasan, J.; Velusamy, P.; Ganesan, T.; Ramakrishnan, S.K.; Rajasekaran, D.; Periandavan, K. Hesperidin-mediated expression of Nrf2 and upregulation of antioxidant status in senescent rat heart. *J. Pharm. Pharmacol.* **2012**, *64*, 1472–1482. [CrossRef] [PubMed]

35. Bleakley, C.; Hamilton, P.K.; Pumb, R.; Harbinson, M.; McVeigh, G.E. Endothelial Function in Hypertension: Victim or Culprit? *J. Clin. Hypertens. (Greenwich)* **2015**, *17*, 651–654. [CrossRef] [PubMed]

36. Habauzit, V.; Verny, M.A.; Milenkovic, D.; Barber-Chamoux, N.; Mazur, A.; Dubray, C.; Morand, C. Flavanones protect from arterial stiffness in postmenopausal women consuming grapefruit juice for 6 mo: A randomized, controlled, crossover trial. *Am. J. Clin. Nutr.* **2015**, *102*, 66–74. [CrossRef] [PubMed]

37. Curtis, P.J.; Potter, J.; Kroon, P.A.; Wilson, P.; Dhatariya, K.; Sampson, M.; Cassidy, A. Vascular function and atherosclerosis progression after 1 y of flavonoid intake in statin-treated postmenopausal women with type 2 diabetes: A double-blind randomized controlled trial. *Am. J. Clin. Nutr.* **2013**, *97*, 936–942. [CrossRef] [PubMed]

38. Dohadwala, M.M.; Holbrook, M.; Hamburg, N.M.; Shenouda, S.M.; Chung, W.B.; Titas, M.; Kluge, M.A.; Wang, N.; Palmisano, J.; Milbury, P.E.; et al. Effects of cranberry juice consumption on vascular function in patients with coronary artery disease. *Am. J. Clin. Nutr.* **2011**, *93*, 934–940. [CrossRef] [PubMed]

39. Nestel, P.; Fujii, A.; Zhang, L. An isoflavone metabolite reduces arterial stiffness and blood pressure in overweight men and postmenopausal women. *Atherosclerosis* **2007**, *192*, 184–189. [CrossRef] [PubMed]

40. Expert Dyslipidemia Panel of the International Atherosclerosis Society Panel members, An International Atherosclerosis Society Position Paper: Global recommendations for the management of dyslipidemia–full report. *J. Clin. Lipidol.* **2014**, *8*, 29–60.

41. Naci, H.; Brugts, J.J.; Fleurence, R.; Tsoi, B.; Toor, H.; Ades, A.E. Comparative benefits of statins in the primary and secondary prevention of major coronary events and all-cause mortality: A network meta-analysis of placebo-controlled and active-comparator trials. *Eur. J. Prev. Cardiol.* **2013**, *20*, 641–657. [CrossRef] [PubMed]

42. Orhan, I.E.; Nabavi, S.F.; Daglia, M.; Tenore, G.C.; Mansouri, K.; Nabavi, S.M. Naringenin and atherosclerosis: A review of literature. *Curr. Pharm. Biotechnol.* **2015**, *16*, 245–251. [CrossRef] [PubMed]

43. Choe, S.C.; Kim, H.S.; Jeong, T.S.; Bok, S.H.; Park, Y.B. Naringin has an antiatherogenic effect with the inhibition of intercellular adhesion molecule-1 in hypercholesterolemic rabbits. *J. Cardiovasc. Pharmacol.* **2001**, *38*, 947–955. [CrossRef] [PubMed]

44. Lee, C.H.; Jeong, T.S.; Choi, Y.K.; Hyun, B.H.; Oh, G.T.; Kim, E.H.; Kim, J.R.; Han, J.I.; Bok, S.H. Anti-atherogenic effect of citrus flavonoids, naringin and naringenin, associated with hepatic ACAT and aortic VCAM-1 and MCP-1 in high cholesterol-fed rabbits. *Biochem. Biophys. Res. Commun.* **2001**, *284*, 681–688. [CrossRef] [PubMed]

45. Chanet, A.; Milenkovic, D.; Deval, C.; Potier, M.; Constans, J.; Mazur, A.; Bennetau-Pelissero, C.; Morand, C.; Bérard, A.M. Naringin, the major grapefruit flavonoid, specifically affects atherosclerosis development in diet-induced hypercholesterolemia in mice. *J. Nutr. Biochem.* **2012**, *23*, 469–477. [CrossRef] [PubMed]

46. Cappello, A.R.; Dolce, V.; Iacopetta, D.; Martello, M.; Fiorillo, M.; Curcio, R.; Muto, L.; Dhanyalayam, D. Bergamot (Citrus bergamia Risso) Flavonoids and Their Potential Benefits in Human Hyperlipidemia and Atherosclerosis: An Overview. *Mini Rev. Med. Chem.* **2016**, *16*, 619–629. [CrossRef] [PubMed]

47. Di Donna, L.; Iacopetta, D.; Cappello, A.R.; Gallucci, G.; Martello, E.; Fiorillo, M.; Dolce, V.; Sindona, G. Hypocholesterolaemic activity of 3-hydroxy-3-methyl-glutaryl flavanones enriched fraction from bergamot fruit (Citrus bergamia): "In vivo" studies. *J. Funct. Foods* **2014**, *7*, 558–568. [CrossRef]

48. Di Donna, L.; De Luca, G.; Mazzotti, F.; Napoli, A.; Salerno, R.; Taverna, D.; Sindona, G. Statin-like principles of bergamot fruit (Citrus bergamia): Isolation of 3-hydroxymethylglutaryl flavonoid glycosides. *J. Nat. Prod.* **2009**, *72*, 1352–1354. [CrossRef] [PubMed]

49. Da Pozzo, E.; Costa, B.; Cavallini, C.; Testai, L.; Martelli, A.; Calderone, V.; Martini, C. The citrus flavanone naringenin protects myocardial cells against age-associated damage. *Oxid. Med. Cell. Longev.* **2017**, in press. [CrossRef] [PubMed]

50. Yamamoto, M.; Jokura, H.; Hashizume, K.; Ominami, H.; Shibuya, Y.; Suzuki, A.; Hase, T.; Shimotoyodome, A. Hesperidin metabolite hesperetin-7-O-glucuronide, but not hesperetin-3'-O-glucuronide, exerts hypotensive, vasodilatory, and anti-inflammatory activities. *Food Funct.* **2013**, *4*, 1346–1351. [CrossRef] [PubMed]

51. Liu, Y.; Su, W.W.; Wang, S.; Li, P.B. Naringin inhibits chemokine production in an LPS-induced RAW 264.7 macrophage cell line. *Mol. Med. Rep.* **2012**, *6*, 1343–1350. [PubMed]

52. Park, H.Y.; Kim, G.Y.; Choi, Y.H. Naringenin attenuates the release of pro-inflammatory mediators from lipopolysaccharide-stimulated BV2 microglia by inactivating nuclear factor-κB and inhibiting mitogen-activated protein kinases. *Int. J. Mol. Med.* **2012**, *30*, 204–210. [PubMed]

53. Giménez-Bastida, J.A.; González-Sarrías, A.; Vallejo, F.; Espín, J.C.; Tomás-Barberán, F.A. Hesperetin and its sulfate and glucuronide metabolites inhibit TNF-α induced human aortic endothelial cell migration and decrease plasminogen activator inhibitor-1 (PAI-1) levels. *Food Funct.* **2015**, *7*, 118–126. [CrossRef] [PubMed]

54. Raso, G.M.; Meli, R.; Di Carlo, G.; Pacilio, M.; Di Carlo, R. Inhibition of inducible nitric oxide synthase and cyclooxygenase-2 expression by flavonoids in macrophage J774A.1. *Life Sci.* **2001**, *68*, 921–931. [CrossRef]

55. Tsai, S.H.; Lin-Shiau, S.Y.; Lin, J.K. Suppression of nitric oxide synthase and the down-regulation of the activation of NFkappaB in macrophages by resveratrol. *Br. J. Pharmacol.* **1999**, *126*, 673–680. [CrossRef] [PubMed]

56. Hämäläinen, M.; Nieminen, R.; Vuorela, P.; Heinonen, M.; Moilanen, E. Anti-inflammatory effects of flavonoids: Genistein, kaempferol, quercetin, and daidzein inhibit STAT-1 and NF-kappaB activations, whereas flavone, isorhamnetin, naringenin, and pelargonidin inhibit only NF-kappaB activation along with their inhibitory effect on iNOS expression and NO production in activated macrophages. *Mediat. Inflamm.* **2007**, *2007*, 45673.

57. Lee, E.J.; Kim, D.I.; Kim, W.J.; Moon, S.K. Naringin inhibits matrix metalloproteinase-9 expression and AKT phosphorylation in tumor necrosis factor-alpha-induced vascular smooth muscle cells. *Mol. Nutr. Food Res.* **2009**, *53*, 1582–1591. [CrossRef] [PubMed]

58. Yamamoto, M.; Suzuki, A.; Hase, T. Short-term effects of glucosyl hesperidin and hesperetin on blood pressure and vascular endothelial function in spontaneously hypertensive rats. *J. Nutr. Sci. Vitaminol.* **2008**, *54*, 95–98. [CrossRef] [PubMed]

59. Yamamoto, M.; Jokura, H.; Suzuki, A.; Hase, T.; Shimotoyodome, A. Effects of continuous ingestion of hesperidin and glucosyl hesperidin on vascular gene expression in spontaneously hypertensive rats. *J. Nutr. Sci. Vitaminol.* **2013**, *59*, 470–473. [CrossRef] [PubMed]

60. Yamada, M.; Tanabe, F.; Arai, N.; Mitsuzumi, H.; Miwa, Y.; Kubota, M.; Chaen, H.; Kibata, M. Bioavailability of glucosyl hesperidin in rats. *Biosci. Biotechnol. Biochem.* **2006**, *70*, 1386–1394. [CrossRef] [PubMed]

61. Liu, Y.; Niu, L.; Cui, L.; Hou, X.; Li, J.; Zhang, X.; Zhang, M. Hesperetin inhibits rat coronary constriction by inhibiting Ca(2+) influx and enhancing voltage-gated K(+) channel currents of the myocytes. *Eur. J. Pharmacol.* **2014**, *735*, 193–201. [CrossRef] [PubMed]

62. Saponara, S.; Testai, L.; Iozzi, D.; Martinotti, E.; Martelli, A.; Chericoni, S.; Sgaragli, G.; Fusi, F.; Calderone, V. (+/−)-Naringenin as large conductance Ca(2+)-activated K+ (BKCa) channel opener in vascular smooth muscle cells. *Br. J. Pharmacol.* **2006**, *149*, 1013–1021. [CrossRef] [PubMed]

63. Calderone, V.; Chericoni, S.; Martinelli, C.; Testai, L.; Nardi, A.; Morelli, I.; Breschi, M.C.; Martinotti, E. Vasorelaxing effects of flavonoids: Investigation on the possible involvement of potassium channels. *Naunyn Schmiedebergs Arch. Pharmacol.* **2004**, *370*, 290–298. [CrossRef] [PubMed]

64. Ramón Sánchez de Rojas, V.; Somoza, B.; Ortega, T.; Villar, A.M.; Tejerina, T. Vasodilatory effect in rat aorta of eriodictyol obtained from Satureja obovata. *Planta Med.* **1999**, *65*, 234–238. [CrossRef] [PubMed]

65. Lee, S.E.; Yang, H.; Son, G.W.; Park, H.R.; Park, C.S.; Jin, Y.H.; Park, Y.S. Eriodictyol Protects Endothelial Cells against Oxidative Stress-Induced Cell Death through Modulating ERK/Nrf2/ARE-Dependent Heme Oxygenase-1 Expression. *Int. J. Mol. Sci.* **2015**, *16*, 14526–14539. [CrossRef] [PubMed]

66. Testai, L.; Martelli, A.; Cristofaro, M.; Breschi, M.C.; Calderone, V. Cardioprotective effects of different flavonoids against myocardial ischaemia/reperfusion injury in Langendorff-perfused rat hearts. *J. Pharm. Pharmacol.* **2013**, *65*, 750–756. [CrossRef] [PubMed]

67. Testai, L.; Martelli, A.; Marino, A.; D'Antongiovanni, V.; Ciregia, F.; Giusti, L.; Lucacchini, A.; Chericoni, S.; Breschi, M.C.; Calderone, V. The activation of mitochondrial BK potassium channels contributes to the protective effects of naringenin against myocardial ischemia/reperfusion injury. *Biochem. Pharmacol.* **2013**, *85*, 1634–1643. [CrossRef] [PubMed]

68. Testai, L. Flavonoids and mitochondrial pharmacology: A new paradigm for cardioprotection. *Life Sci.* **2015**, *135*, 68–76. [CrossRef] [PubMed]

69. Yang, Z.; Liu, Y.; Deng, W.; Dai, J.; Li, F.; Yuan, Y.; Wu, Q.; Zhou, H.; Bian, Z.; Tang, Q. Hesperetin attenuates mitochondria-dependent apoptosis in lipopolysaccharide-induced H9C2 cardiomyocytes. *Mol. Med. Rep.* **2014**, *9*, 1941–1946. [CrossRef] [PubMed]

70. Sharma, A.K.; Bharti, S.; Ojha, S.; Bhatia, J.; Kumar, N.; Ray, R.; Kumari, S.; Arya, D.S. Up-regulation of PPARγ, heat shock protein-27 and -72 by naringin attenuates insulin resistance, β-cell dysfunction, hepatic steatosis and kidney damage in a rat model of type 2 diabetes. *Br. J. Nutr.* **2011**, *106*, 1713–1723. [CrossRef] [PubMed]

71. Cho, K.W.; Kim, Y.O.; Andrade, J.E.; Burgess, J.R.; Kim, Y.C. Dietary naringenin increases hepatic peroxisome proliferators-activated receptor α protein expression and decreases plasma triglyceride and adiposity in rats. *Eur. J. Nutr.* **2011**, *50*, 81–88. [CrossRef] [PubMed]

72. Jung, U.J.; Lee, M.K.; Park, Y.B.; Kang, M.A.; Choi, M.S. Effect of citrus flavonoids on lipid metabolism and glucose-regulating enzyme mRNA levels in type-2 diabetic mice. *Int. J. Biochem. Cell Biol.* **2006**, *38*, 1134–1145. [CrossRef] [PubMed]

73. Sundaram, R.; Shanthi, P.; Sachdanandam, P. Effect of tangeretin, a polymethoxylated flavone on glucose metabolism in streptozotocin-induced diabetic rats. *Phytomedicine* **2014**, *21*, 793–799. [CrossRef] [PubMed]

74. Manach, C.; Scalbert, A.; Morand, C.; Remesy, C.; Jimenez, L. Polyphenols: Food sources and bioavailability. *Am. J. Clin. Nutr.* **2004**, *79*, 727–747. [PubMed]

75. Urpi-Sarda, M.; Rothwell, J.; Morand, C.; Manach, C. Bioavailability of flavanones. In *Flavonoids and Related Compounds: Bioavailability and Function*; Spencer, J., Crozier, A., Eds.; CRC Press: Boca Raton, FL, USA, 2012; pp. 1–65.

76. Silveira, J.Q.; Cesar, T.B.; Manthey, J.A.; Baldwin, E.A.; Bai, J.; Raithore, S. Pharmacokinetics of flavanone glycosides after ingestion of single doses of fresh-squeezed orange juice versus commercially processed orange juice in healthy humans. *J. Agric. Food Chem.* **2014**, *62*, 12576–12584. [CrossRef] [PubMed]

77. Ozdal, T.; Sela, D.A.; Xiao, J.; Boyacioglu, D.; Chen, F.; Capanoglu, E. The Reciprocal Interactions between Polyphenols and Gut Microbiota and Effects on Bioaccessibility. *Nutrients* **2016**, *8*, 78. [CrossRef] [PubMed]

78. Rowland, I.; Gibson, G.; Heinken, A.; Scott, K.; Swann, J.; Thiele, I.; Tuohy, K. Gut microbiota functions: Metabolism of nutrients and other food components. *Eur. J. Nutr.* **2017**, in press. [CrossRef] [PubMed]

79. Shen, L.; Hong-Fang, J. Intestinal microbiota and metabolic diseases: Pharmacological implications. *Trends Pharmacol. Sci.* **2016**, *37*, 169–171. [CrossRef] [PubMed]

80. Cassidy, A.; Minihane, A.M. The role of metabolism (and the microbiome) in defining the clinical efficacy of dietary flavonoids. *Am. J. Clin. Nutr.* **2017**, *105*, 10–22. [CrossRef] [PubMed]

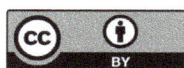

*nutrients*

MDPI

*Review*

# Effects of Polyphenols on Oxidative Stress-Mediated Injury in Cardiomyocytes

**Rosanna Mattera [1], Monica Benvenuto [1], Maria Gabriella Giganti [1], Ilaria Tresoldi [1], Francesca Romana Pluchinotta [2], Sonia Bergante [2], Guido Tettamanti [2], Laura Masuelli [3], Vittorio Manzari [1], Andrea Modesti [1,4] and Roberto Bei [1,4,\***

[1] Department of Clinical Sciences and Translational Medicine, University of Rome "Tor Vergata", 00133 Rome, Italy; rosannamatter@gmail.com (R.M.); monicab4@hotmail.it (M.B.); giganti@med.uniroma2.it (M.G.G.); ilaria3soldi@hotmail.com (I.T.); manzari@uniroma2.it (V.M.); modesti@med.uniroma2.it (A.M.)

[2] IRCCS "S. Donato" Hospital, San Donato Milanese, Piazza Edmondo Malan, 20097 Milan, Italy; FrancescaRomana.Pluchinotta@cardio.chboston.org (F.R.M.); sonia.bergante@unimi.it (S.B.); guido.tettamanti@grupposandonato.it (G.T.)

[3] Department of Experimental Medicine, University of Rome "Sapienza", 00164 Rome, Italy; laura.masuelli@uniroma1.it

[4] Center for Regenerative Medicine (CIMER), University of Rome "Tor Vergata", 00133 Rome, Italy

[*] Correspondence: bei@med.uniroma2.it; Tel.: +39-06-7259-6522

Received: 27 March 2017; Accepted: 16 May 2017; Published: 20 May 2017

**Abstract:** Cardiovascular diseases are the main cause of mortality and morbidity in the world. Hypertension, ischemia/reperfusion, diabetes and anti-cancer drugs contribute to heart failure through oxidative and nitrosative stresses which cause cardiomyocytes nuclear and mitochondrial DNA damage, denaturation of intracellular proteins, lipid peroxidation and inflammation. Oxidative or nitrosative stress-mediated injury lead to cardiomyocytes apoptosis or necrosis. The reactive oxygen (ROS) and nitrogen species (RNS) concentration is dependent on their production and on the expression and activity of anti-oxidant enzymes. Polyphenols are a large group of natural compounds ubiquitously expressed in plants, and epidemiological studies have shown associations between a diet rich in polyphenols and the prevention of various ROS-mediated human diseases. Polyphenols reduce cardiomyocytes damage, necrosis, apoptosis, infarct size and improve cardiac function by decreasing oxidative stress-induced production of ROS or RNS. These effects are achieved by the ability of polyphenols to modulate the expression and activity of anti-oxidant enzymes and several signaling pathways involved in cells survival. This report reviews current knowledge on the potential anti-oxidative effects of polyphenols to control the cardiotoxicity induced by ROS and RNS stress.

**Keywords:** polyphenols; oxidative stress; cardiovascular disease; cardiomyocytes

## 1. Introduction

Cardiovascular diseases are the main cause of mortality and morbidity in the world [1]. Hypertension, ischemia, diabetes, anti-cancer drugs contribute to heart failure through oxidative and nitrosative stresses which induce nuclear and mitochondrial DNA damage, denaturation of intracellular proteins, lipid peroxidation and inflammation in cardiomyocytes [2,3]. Oxidative or nitrosative stress-mediated injury lead to cardiomyocytes apoptosis or necrosis [2,3]. Reactive oxygen (ROS) and nitrogen species (RNS) concentration is dependent on their production and on the expression and activity of anti-oxidant enzymes [2]. ROS production is influenced by many factors, such as dysfunction of oxidative enzymes (xanthine oxidase (XO), aldehyde oxidase, nicotinamide adenine dinucleotide phosphate (NADPH) oxidase and uncoupled nitric oxide synthase (NOS)), dysregulation of mitochondria, microsomes and/or nuclei transport, neutrophil activation, arachidonic acid metabolism and auto-oxidation of catecholamines, flavins, quinones and proteins [4,5]. The main ROS and RNS are superoxide, hydrogen peroxide, hydroxyl radical, nitric oxide (NO) and peroxynitrite. The production of hydrogen peroxide regulates the expression of genes, in particular those activated by nuclear factor-kappa B (NF-κB), and the overload of $Ca^{2+}$ levels in cardiomyocytes subjected to heart failure. The nitric oxide initiates lipid peroxidation and produces, by interacting with superoxide anion, peroxynitrite which is implicated in atherosclerosis [4]. Peroxynitrites trigger lipid peroxidation, protein oxidation, nitration and activation of matrix metalloproteinases (MMPs) [6]. However, NO can also maintain inactive the oxidant enzymes (XO and NADPH oxidase) and balance the superoxide/NO ratio [6]. In addition, iron and copper are the principal metal ions that induce the production of ROS by Fenton or Haber-Weiss reactions. Iron and copper enhance the lipid peroxidation and production of free radicals, including alkyl, alkoxy, peroxy and hydroxyl radicals. Conversely, selenium is an important anti-oxidant ion which regulates the glutathione peroxidase (GSH-Px) [4].

The mitochondria are identified as a major source of ROS production in several organs with high metabolic activity, for example in the heart [7]. Enzymes that produce ROS, both in membrane (NADPH oxidase) and in matrix (tricarboxylic acid cycle, TCA) are present in the mitochondria. Under normal conditions, ROS levels are low for the intra-mitochondrial presence of anti-oxidant systems. The increase of ROS production simultaneously to the inhibition of anti-oxidant systems and/or of ETC (electron transport chain) complex increase ROS levels [7]. Furthermore, sirtuins (SIRTs), localized in the mitochondria, play an essential role in cardiovascular disease and influence energy metabolism, DNA repair and oxidative stress. Sirtuins induce the deacetylation of forkhead box O (FoxO), NF-κB, protein kinase B (Akt), p53, superoxide dismutase (SOD), and members of ETC complex I and influence fatty acid oxidation, cardiac hypertrophy, ischemia/reperfusion (I/R) injury, apoptosis, oxidative stress and autophagy in cardiomyocytes [8]. Angiotensin (Ang) II, platelet-derived growth factor (PDGF), and tumor necrosis factor (TNF)-α induce the production of ROS in the cardiac muscle through the NADPH oxidase and then cardiomyocytes apoptosis, cardiac hypertrophy, reduction of myofilament sensitivity and cardiac contractility [9].

Several enzymatic and non-enzymatic mechanisms balance the production of ROS and transform ROS into non-toxic molecules in myocardium, as in other organs [9]. An anti-oxidant enzyme is SOD, which is present in three forms, copper-zinc SOD (CuZnSOD or SOD1), manganese SOD (MnSOD or SOD2) and extracellular SOD (EC-SOD or SOD3) [8]. Other enzymes, including the catalase (CAT) and GSH-Px reduce the production of ROS. SOD converts superoxide in hydrogen peroxide, which is transformed into water and oxygen by CAT and GSH-Px. Thioredoxin and thioredoxin reductase form an additional system that blocks ROS production through protein-disulfide oxidoreductase activity. Intracellular non-enzymatic anti-oxidants are vitamins E and C, β-carotene, ubiquinone, lipoic acid, urate and glutathione [6,10]. Anti-oxidant enzymes are activated during oxidative stress and after activation of cytokines. However, these enzymes are down-regulated during the end stage of heart failure [10].

Recently, many studies identified the potential anti-oxidant effects of polyphenols in cardiac diseases. Polyphenols can reduce the cardiac damage due to ROS and RNS production [11] (Figure 1). In this review, we report the last ten years researches on the potential effects of polyphenols in modulating the cardiotoxicity induced by ROS or RNS.

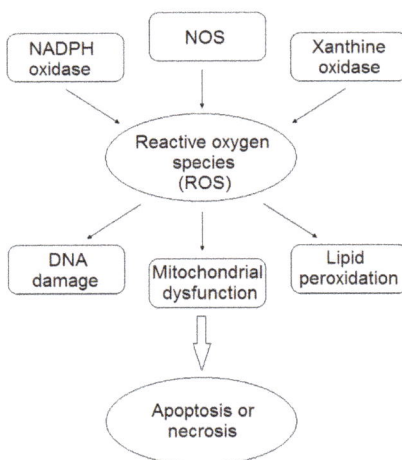

**Figure 1.** Generation of reactive oxygen species (ROS) and their cellular effects.

## 2. Polyphenols

### 2.1. Classification

Polyphenols are a large group of natural compounds found in foods and beverages of plant origin (fruits, vegetables, cereals, herbs, spices, legumes, nuts, olives, chocolate, tea, coffee, and wine) [12,13].

Polyphenols are classified in flavonoids and non-flavonoids, according to the number of phenol rings and structural elements bound to these rings. The most important classes of flavonoids found in foods are flavonols, flavones, flavan-3-ols, anthocyanins, flavanones and isoflavones. The subclasses of dihydroflavonols, flavan-3,4-diols, chalcones, dihydrochalcones, and aurones are minor components of our diet. The most important classes of non-flavonoids are phenolic acids, stilbenes and lignans [14–16] (Figure 2).

### 2.2. Polyphenols and Oxidative Stress and Epigenetic Regulation

Epidemiological studies have shown associations between a diet rich in polyphenols and the prevention of human diseases [12,17–21]. Polyphenols are natural anti-oxidants present in the human diet. This activity is related to their metal ions chelating and free radical scavenger properties. Structural features of polyphenols allow them to act as direct free radical scavengers, such as the catechol group on the B-ring, the presence of hydroxyl groups at the 3 and 5 position and the 2,3-double bond in conjugation with a 4-oxofunction of a carbonyl group in the C-ring [22]. However, polyphenols can also behave as pro-oxidants at high doses or in the presence of metal ions, leading to DNA degradation. However, there is no evidence of sistemic pro-oxidant effect of polyphenols in humans [23].

It is of note that the direct anti-oxidant activity of polyphenols appears to be ineffective in vivo, because of the low bioavailability and kinetic constraints, and it has been proposed that the beneficial effects observed are due to an indirect anti-oxidant effect rather than to their direct free radical scavenger properties. Indeed, it has been demonstrated that polyphenols possess an indirect anti-oxidant capacity by modulating genes expression and by inducing the endogenous anti-oxidant enzymatic defense system [24–26]. The indirect modality of oxidative stress protection and the health benefits exerted by polyphenols are due to the hormetic mechanism of action. Polyphenols activate adaptive cellular response pathways (hormetic pathways) that induce the expression of genes encoding for anti-oxidant enzymes, phase-2 enzymes, protein chaperones and survival-promoting proteins. Example of these pathways are the Keap1/Nrf2/ARE, the Sirtuin-FoxO and the NF-κB pathways [27,28]. In particular, it has been demonstrated that polyphenols activate the Keap1/Nrf2/ARE pathway through an oxidative mechanism. In fact, polyphenols must be metabolized into electrophilic compounds for inactivating the inhibitor Keap 1 and thus activating Nrf2, a transcription factor regulating the expression of most Phase II and some Phase III genes [26]. By transcription-mediated signalling, polyphenols exert long-lasting effects as compared to other direct anti-oxidant agents [27,29]. However, the hypothesis of activation of Phase II enzymes by polyphenols has not been proven in human yet [28,30].

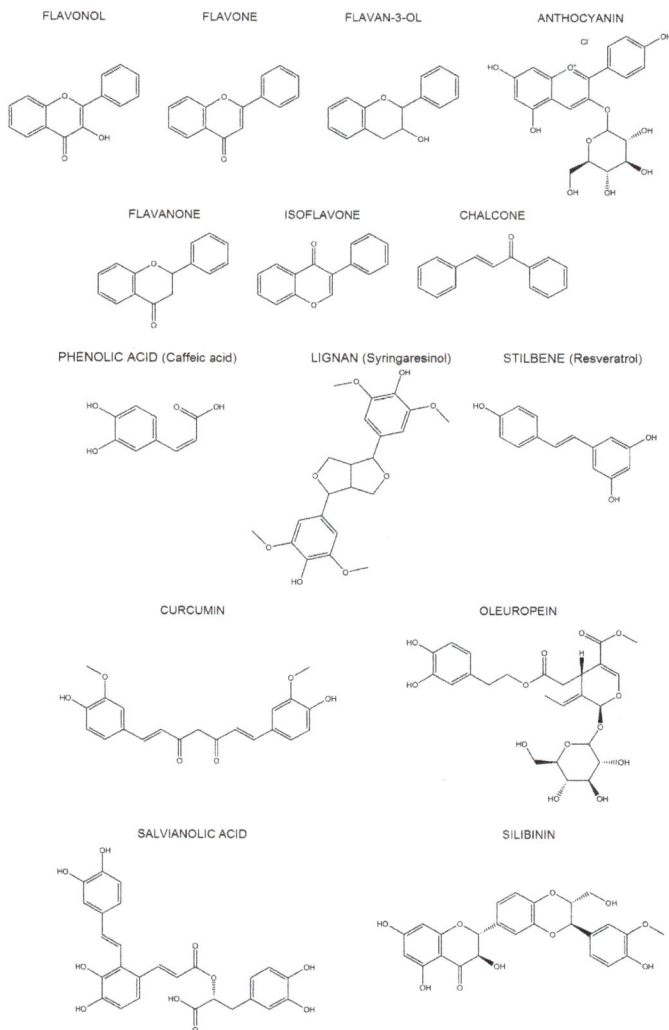

**Figure 2.** Chemical structure of polyphenols.

Several studies reported that epigenetic mechanisms are involved in the development and progression of different diseases, including cardiovascular diseases [31]. Polyphenols can reduce the risk of cardiovascular disease by interacting with signaling cascades and epigenetic factors [32]. Several evidence reported that epigenetic mechanisms are involved in hormesis-like responses [33]. Epigenetic modifications depend on the cell type and the stage of the cardiovascular disease. For example, the global DNA is hypermethylated in the early stage of atherosclerosis and hypomethylated in the atherosclerotic lesions, while the peripheral blood leucocytes show global hypermethylation of DNA. In addition, the methylation or acetylation of DNA regulatory regions up- or down-regulate the expression of genes involved in cardiovascular diseases [34]. Polyphenols can reduce DNA methylation, as well as histone modifications and can modify the expression of transcription factors by epigenetic regulation [32,34–36]. Polyphenols silence chromatin by the inhibition of DNA methyltransferases and the activation of class III histone deacetylases (commonly called sirtuins) in vascular endothelium. These effects occur in atherosclerosis and other cardiovascular diseases [36,37].

MicroRNAs (miRNAs) are non-coding RNAs which modify the transcription with no interference with DNA sequences [34]. miRNAs regulate gene transcription through the degradation or repression of mRNA. Various miRNAs are also associated with cardiovascular diseases as biomarkers [34]. For example, increased levels of miRNA-1, miRNA-133b and miRNA-499 are observed in acute myocardial infarction [38,39]. Elevated levels of miRNA-217 are associated with inhibited expression of SIRT1 in atherosclerosis [40]. However, the levels of several miRNAs can also decrease in cardiovascular diseases. In fact, miRNA-126 and miRNA-145 levels decrease in patients with coronary artery disease [41]. Polyphenols modulate the expression of several miRNAs [42]. For example, resveratrol regulates the cardiac function through the expression of miRNA-20b, miRNA-149, miRNA-133, miRNA-21, and miRNA-27 [32]. In addition, it has been reported that resveratrol exerts cardioprotective effects through the up-regulation of miRNA-21 and SIRT1 expression in ischemic rats. miRNA-21 regulates cardiac remodeling, cardiac cell growth and apoptosis [43].

In vitro studies underlying molecular mechanisms through which polyphenols affect oxidative stress-induced cardiotoxicity are reported below.

## 3. In Vitro Effects of Polyphenols Against Oxidative Stress-Induced Cardiotoxicity

### 3.1. Flavonoids

#### 3.1.1. Flavonols

Flavonols are the most common flavonoids present in plant-derived foods, wine and tea. Quercetin, kaempferol and myricetin are the main flavonols [17].

Several studies investigated the effect of flavonols against $H_2O_2$-induced cardiotoxicity. Quercetin or 3'-*O*-methyl quercetin treatment (30 µM) or rhamnetin, from berries of *Rhamnus petiolaris*, (1, 3, 5 µM) treatment of rat/H9c2 cardiomyocytes exposed to $H_2O_2$ decreased ROS production and number of death cells by up-regulating the NQO-1, HO-1, TR (thioredoxin reductase 1), and total glutathione *S*-transferase (GST) activities or by inhibiting MAPKs activation [44–46]. Conversely, 3',4'-dihydroxyflavonol (DiOHF, 10 µM) protected rat cardiomyocytes against $H_2O_2$-induced oxidative stress by increasing the phosphorylation of MAPKs and Akt and regulated the activation of the reperfusion injury survival kinase (RISK) pathways [47].

Doxorubicin (DOX)/Adriamycin is an anthracycline antibiotic used in chemotherapy and it is associated with cardiotoxicity. The treatment of H9c2 cardiomyocytes with quercetin (50, 100 µM), isorhamnetin (6.25–25 µg/mL), kaempferol (20 µM) or dihydromyricetin (50 µM, a flavonoid extracted from *Ampelopsis grossedentata*), decreased the DOX-induced apoptosis, ROS production, lipid peroxidation and NADPH oxidase activity. Isorhamnetin also increased the production of anti-oxidant enzymes and modulated MAPK activity [48–51].

Quercetin pretreatment (20 µM) of H9c2 cardiomyocytes significantly attenuated trauma-induced apoptosis, TNF-α levels, ROS production and $Ca^{2+}$ levels [52].

$PKC_\varepsilon$, a member of the PKC family of serine and threonine kinases, regulates several processes, including mitogenesis, cell survival, metastasis and transcriptional regulation. The treatment of rat cardiomyocytes with quercetin (40 µM) or kaempferol (20 µM) before anoxia/reoxygenation (A/R) mediated-injury increased $PKC_\varepsilon$, cells viability and the expression of SIRT1, decreased apoptosis and ROS generation and restored the mitochondrial membrane potential [53,54]. The incubation of sheep myocardial tissues with DiOHF ($10^{-4}$–$10^{-6}$ M) blocked ROS production after myocardial I/R injury [55].

Taxifolin (5–50 µM), a derivative of dihydroquercetin, reduced hypertrophy, ROS generation and protein synthesis induced by Ang II in neonatal rat cardiomyocytes [56].

The effects of quercetin and hydroxytyrosol, present in the leaves of olive (*Olea europaea* L.), have been evaluated in H9c2 cardiomyocytes exposed to xanthine/XO-induced oxidative stress. Both quercetin and hydroxytyrosol (0.1, 10 µg/mL) reduced the number of death cells, ROS generation and the phosphorylation of the MAPK-activated protein kinase 2 (MAPKAPK-2) after exposure to xanthine/XO [57].

### 3.1.2. Flavones

Flavones are found in plants as 7-*O*-glycosides. The most abundant flavones in foods are apigenin (parsley, celery, onion, garlic, pepper, chamomile tea) and luteolin (Thai chili, onion leaves, celery). Others flavones, less abundant in edible plants, are tangeretin, nobiletin, baicalein, wogonin and chrysin [17].

The effect of apigenin and vitexin (a flavone glycoside of apigenin isolated from the leaf of *Crataegus pinnatifida Bunge*) on A/R injury was recently assessed in H9c2 and neonatal rat cardiomyocytes. Apigenin (40 µM) or vitexin (10, 30 and 100 µM) were able to increase cells viability and to decrease ROS generation, cells apoptosis and necrosis [58,59].

Vitexin has also been shown to possess significant protective effects against myocardial I/R injury in isolated rat hearts. Hearts were perfused with vitexin (50, 100, 200 µM) for 20 min before ischemia. Treatment with vitexin inhibited I/R-induced reduction of coronary flow and decreased I/R-induced histopathological alterations of myocardium, inflammatory cytokines and it inhibited apoptosis [60]. Baicalein from the root of *Scutellaria baicalensis* was analyzed for its anti-oxidative effects in chick cardiomyocyte models during hypoxia, simulated I/R, or mitochondrial complex III inhibition with antimycin A. Baicalein (10–100 µM) was able to scavenge ROS and to decrease the number of death cells in all different models [61]. Recently, it has been proven that baicalein protected H9c2 cardiomyocytes and also human embryonic stem cells-derived cardiomyocites (hESC-CMs) against oxidative stress-induced cell injury. Baicalein (10, 30 µM) decreased ROS generation and the number of death cells and activated Nrf2 pathway [62].

Conversely, Chang et al. reported that preconditioning with baicalein (10 µM) for a brief time before I/R injury protected chick embryonic ventricular myocytes from apoptosis through mitochondrial pro-oxidant mechanisms. Thus, the authors hypothesized that the oxidant-mediated protective effects of baicalein was probably due to the modulation of mitochondrial pro-oxidant signaling as well [63]. Baicalein (1 µM) also reduced H/R-induced myocardium necrosis and apoptosis through µ- and δ-opioid but not κ-opioid receptors pathways in chick embryonic cardiomyocites [64].

### 3.1.3. Flavan-3-Ols

The flavan-3-ol subclass includes several compounds with different chemical structures that can be divided in monomers, (+)-catechin, (−)-epicatechin, (+)-gallocatechin, (−)-epigallocatechin, (−)-epicatechin-3-*O*-gallate, (−)-epigallocatechin-3-*O*-gallate (EGCG), and polymers (proanthocyanidins). They are found in fruits, berries, cereals, nuts, chocolate, red wine, and tea [17].

Several studies investigated the effects of flavan-3-ols in cardiomyocytes exposed to exogenous and endogenous oxidant stress. Pretreatment of rat cardiomyocytes exposed to $H_2O_2$ with EGCG (20, 50 µM or 50–100 mg/L) and theaflavin-3,3′ digallate (TF3, 20 µM) decreased ROS production, cellular damage and apoptosis through the inhibition of telomere dependent apoptotic pathway [65–68]. EGCG (50 µM) was also able to protect H9c2 cardiomyocytes from $H_2O_2$-induced changes in the expression of β-catenin, *N*-cadherin and the gap junction protein Cx43 and to activate caveolin-1 by modulating Akt/GSK-3β signaling [66].

Other studies investigated the cardioprotective role of flavan-3-ols in cardiomyocytes exposed to DOX. EGCG (25, 38, 50, or 100 μM) and grape seed proanthocyanidin extract (GSPE, 50 μg/mL) protected rat cardiomyocytes against DOX-induced oxidative stress by reducing apoptosis, ROS generation and the distruption of mitochondrial membrane potential, and by increasing anti-oxidant enzymes and by reversing DOX-induced intracellular $Ca^{2+}$ depletion in the sarcoplasmic reticulum [69–71]. GSPE prevented cardiotoxicity induced by DOX, without interfering with DOX anti-neoplastic activity in primary cultures of cardiomyocytes [71]. Two studies showed the role of flavan-3-ols against toxicity induced by I/R injury. EGCG (10, 100 μM), and GSPE (50 μg/mL) protected rat and chick cardiomyocytes from I/R-induced apoptosis and cellular damage [72,73]. Similarly, Hirai et al. evaluated the cardioprotective effects of EGCG and the catechin epimer (GCG) in isolated guinea-pig Langendorff hearts subjected to I/R. EGCG ($3 \times 10^{-5}$ M) or GCG ($3 \times 10^{-6}$ M) was introduced into the perfusate 4 min before ischemia and during reperfusion. EGCG and GCG improved the recovery of left ventricular end diastolic pressure (LVDP), increased the tissue levels of ATP and phosphocreatine and inhibited apoptosis [74]. Wei and Meng analyzed the effect of EGCG against bisulfite/sulfite, an agent that induces sulfur- and oxygen-based free radicals and affects voltage-gated sodium ($Na^+$) channels (VGSC), or lead in rat ventricular myocytes. EGCG (30 μg/mL) increased anti-oxidant enzymes and decreased ROS levels and lipid peroxidation in ventricular myocytes of rats exposed to sulfite or lead [75,76]. EGCG also protected $Na^+$ channels against the oxidative damage induced by sulfite [75].

An in vitro study observed the effects of flavonoids isolated from *Lindera erythrocarpa* in H9c2 cardiomyocytes exposed to BSO (buthionine-(*S*,*R*)-sulfoximine), an inducer of oxidative stress and cell death. It was found that (−)-epicatechin (3 μM), avicularin (3 μM) and quercitrin (3 μM) had the ability to inhibit BSO-induced cardiomyocytes death [77].

### 3.1.4. Anthocyanins

Anthocyanins are a subclass of more than 550 compounds. The most abundant anthocyanins are cyanidin, pelargonidin, delphinidin, peonidin, petunidin, and malvidin. They occur in two forms: the aglycone form (anthocyanidin) and the heteroside form (anthocyanin). They are found mainly in berries, cherries, red grapes, and currants [17].

Two studies evaluated the effects of malvidin, an anthocyanidine present in red wine, and cyanidin-3-*O*-glucoside (Cy3G) in isolated rat hearts after I/R. Pretreatment with malvidin ($10^{-7}$ M) or Cy3G (20 μM) increased left ventricular (LV) pressure, reduced cells apoptosis and necrosis [78,79].

Louis et al. investigated the in vitro effect of blueberry phenol fractions (BF) to prevent the pathologic damage induced by norepinephrine (NE) in adult rat cardiomyocytes. NE induced cells hypertrophy and death by activating calpains. Pretreatment with BF (6.55 μg/mL) reduced activation of calpains and apoptosis and increased activity of anti-oxidant enzymes [80].

### 3.1.5. Flavanones

Flavanones are found mainly in citrus fruits and occur as aglycones, mono- and di-glycosides. Naringenin and hesperetin are the most important aglycones; neohesperidin (hesperetin-7-*O*-neohesperidoside) and naringin (naringenin-7-*O*-neohesperidoside) are neohesperidosides, and hesperidin (hesperetin-7- *O*-rutinoside) and narirutin (naringenin-7-*O*-rutinoside) are rutinosides [17].

Naringenin (NGN) was proven to possess a cytoprotective effect against oxidative stress by up-regulating the transcription of Nrf2 and its target genes (GCL and NQO-1). Indeed NGN (50 μM) protected H9c2 cardiomyocytes from $H_2O_2$-mediated cells death, reduced lipid peroxidation and increased the activity of anti-oxidant enzymes [81].

Several studies demonstrated that naringin was able to protect H9c2 cardiomyocytes against high glucose (HG)-induced injury. Pretreatment with naringin (5 or 80 μM) increased cells viability and reduced the number of apoptotic cells, and dissipation of mitochondrial membrane potential (MMP). Naringin protected H9c2 cardiomyocytes by inhibiting ROS production and activation of MAPKs [82–84]. Naringin also confered protection against A/R-induced injury in H9c2 cardiomyocytes. Pretreatment with naringin (10, 20, 40 μg/mL) inhibited apoptosis and oxidative stress. Naringin protected H9c2 cardiomyocytes through the activation of ERK1/2, PKCδ, Akt and then the activation of Nrf2 signaling pathway [85].

Several studies analyzed the effect of naringenin-7-*O*-glucoside (NARG) extracted from Chinese traditional medicine herb *Dracocephalum Rupestre* against DOX-induced oxidative stress and apoptosis. NARG (5–40 μM) reduced DOX-induced apoptosis, necrosis, ROS generation and it up-regulated the expression of endogenous anti-oxidant enzymes in H9c2 cardiomyocytes [86–88].

Yang et al. demonstrated that hesperetin (25 μM) exerted an anti-apoptotic effect in LPS-stimulated H9c2 cardiomyocytes, through the mitochondria-dependent intrinsic apoptosis pathway [89].

### 3.1.6. Isoflavones

Isoflavones are classified as phyto-estrogens for their chemical structure. They are found in soybeans, soy products, and leguminous plants. Isoflavones are present in plant food mainly as aglycones (genistein, daidzein) and glycosides (genistin, daidzin, puerarin) [17].

Puerarin, a bioactive daidzein glucoside derived from *Radix puerariniae*, was studied for its effects on Ang II-induced cardiac hypertrophy. In vitro pretreatment of neonatal murine cardiomyocytes with puerarin (50, 100 μM) decreased NADPH oxidase activity, inhibited ROS production and the activation of oxidative stress-related signaling pathways [90].

Calycosin, an O-methylated isoflavone derived from *Astragali radix*, has been evaluated for its effects on oxidative stress-induced apoptosis in H9c2 cardiomyocytes. It has been found that pretreatment with calycosin (5, 10, 20 μM) enhanced the expression and activation of ERα/β and Akt phosphorylation and inhibited $H_2O_2$-induced cell injury and apoptosis [91].

### 3.1.7. Chalcones and Dihydrochalcones

Chalcones occur in tomatoes, licorice, shallots and bean sprouts, while dihydrochalcones are present in apples [17].

Several studies reported the important role of chalcones against I/R injury. Isolated rat hearts, pretreated with licochalcone D (1 μg/mL) or licochalcone B (0.5, 1 μg/mL) and then subjected to I/R, showed decreased apoptosis, decreased expression of pro-inflammatory cytokines, reduced cells necrosis and increased expression of anti-oxidant enzymes. The authors supposed that licochalcone D exerted these effects through the activation of Akt and the block of NF-κB/p65 and p38 MAPK pathways [92,93]. Isoliquiritigenin treatment (100 μM) of cardiomyocytes isolated from hearts with I/R, activated the AMP-activated protein kinase (AMPK) and MAPKs signaling pathways while reduced the mitochondrial potential and cardiac ROS levels [94]. It has been reported that safflor yellow A (SYA), a chalcone extracted from *Carthamus tinctorius*, and hydroxysafflor yellow A (HSYA) protected H9c2 and primary cultured neonatal rat cardiomyocytes exposed to A/R. The treatment with SYA (40, 60, 80 nM) or HSYA (20 μM) before A/R injury increased the levels of anti-oxidant enzymes and decreased cells necrosis and apoptosis through the up-regulation of HO-1 expression [95,96].

Another study investigated the in vitro effect of L6H9, a novel chalcone derivative, in the pathogenesis of diabetic cardiomyopathy (DCM). The treatment with L6H9 (10 μM) before incubation with glucose decreased the levels of pro-inflammatory cytokines, pro-apoptotic proteins and ROS in H9c2 cardiomyocytes. In addition, L6H9 increased the expression of Nrf2 and Nrf2-downstream anti-oxidant genes and inhibited fibrosis and hypertrophy [97].

Dludla et al. performed a study on the effects of a popular South African herbal tea, rooibos, produced from the leaves and stems of *Aspalathus linearis*, on diabetic cardiomyopathy (DCM). The authors evaluated the effects of an aqueous extract of fermented rooibos (FRE), containing the chalcone aspalathin and the flavonoids isoorientin, orientin, quercetin-3-*O*-robinobioside, in cardiomyocytes isolated from STZ-induced diabetic rats. Pretreatment of cardiomyocytes with FRE (1 and 10 μg/mL) protected cardiomyocytes against experimentally induced oxidative stress and ischemia [98]. Another study demonstrated that aspalathin, found in *Aspalathus linearis* (rooibos), protected H9c2 cardiomyocytes from chronic hyperglycemia-mediated apoptosis, by inhibiting the loss of mitochondrial membrane potential and ROS production and by increasing anti-oxidant enzymes [99].

### 3.2. Phenolic Acids

Phenolic acids are derivatives of benzoic acid and cinnamic acid and include the hydroxybenzoic acids (protocatechuic acid, and gallic acid) and the hydroxycinnamic acids (caffeic acid, ferulic acid, *p*-coumaric acid, and sinapic acid). The formers are found in few edible plants, while the laters are found in fruits, coffee, and cereal grains [17]. Phenolic acids were able to protect cardiomyocytes against $H_2O_2$-induced injury [100–104]. Gui-ling-gao (GLG, also known as turtle jelly) is a traditional food in Southern China and Hong Kong. Li et al. revealed nine compounds in GLG using mass spectrometry: caffeoylquinic acid, 5-*O*-caffeoylshikimic acid, astilbin, 3,4-dicaffeoylquinic acid, 4,5-dicaffeoylquinic acid, neoisoastilbin, isoastilbin, engeletin and 3,5-dicafeoyylquinic acid. GLG (1.372 mM) had the ability to scavenge free radicals and to abolish hemolysis, an index of oxidative damage. GLG increased cell survival and reduced apoptosis in H9c2 cardiomyocytes exposed to $H_2O_2$ [100]. *Castanea sativa* Mill. (CSM)-bark extract contains tannins and phenolic compounds, including ellagic acid, gallic acid, and 4 ellagitannins (vescalin, castalin, vescalagin and castalagin). Pretreatment with CSM-bark extract (50, 100 μg/mL) of neonatal rat cardiac myocytes for 24 h prior to $H_2O_2$ exposure protected cells from oxidative stress-induced injury [101]. *Phellinus linteus* is a medicinal mushroom rich of a phenolic compound, the hispidin. H9c2 cardiomyocytes treated with hispidin (30 μM) prior to $H_2O_2$ exposure, showed increased cell viability, reduced cells necrosis and ROS generation. In addition, hispidin decreased $H_2O_2$-induced apoptosis through the activation of Akt/GSK3β and MAPKs [102]. Neonatal rat cardiac myocytes (RCMs) pretreated with methyl gallate (50 μM) for 30 min prior to exposure to cobalt or $H_2O_2$, showed reduced apoptosis and ROS levels [103]. Ku et al. compared the in vitro effect of caffeic acid (CA) and pyrrolidinyl caffeamide (PLCA), a derivative of CA. HL-1, a mouse atrial cardiomyocyte cell line, was pretreated with CA and PLCA (3 μM) for 1 h before $H_2O_2$ administration. PLCA reduced the production of ROS and increased cells viability more than CA. In addition, PLCA treatment preserved the expression of anti-oxidant enzymes in cardiomyocytes [104].

Song et al. demonstrated the cytoprotective effect of ferulic acid (1, 5, or 10 μg/mL) in hepatocytes and cardiomyocytes against HG-induced injury and oxidative stress [105].

Atale et al. analyzed the effect of gallic acid-enriched methanolic *Syzygium cumini* pulp extract (MPE) on cardiotoxicity induced by malathion, an organophosphate pesticide. MPE treatment (20 μg/mL) restored the integrity of extra cellular matrix components and reduced the malathion-induced oxidative stress in H9c2 cardiomyocytes [106].

The beneficial effects of caffeic, chlorogenic and rosmarinic acids against DOX-induced toxicity were investigated in neonatal rat cardiomyocytes. Hydroxycinnamic acids (100, 200 μM) attenuated DOX-induced cell damage and the iron-dependent DOX-induced lipid peroxidation of microsomal and mitochondrial membranes [107].

Danshensu (3-(3,4-dihydroxyphenyl)-2-hydroxypropanoic acid) is the major water-soluble active component of Danshen, the dried root of the traditional Chinese herb *Salvia miltiorrhiza*, and it has been analyzed for its cardioprotective effects. Treatment with danshensu (10 μM) during reperfusion protected H9c2 cardiomyocytes from I/R-induced apoptosis [108]. Similarly, isolated rat hearts, perfused with danshensu (1, 10 μM) for 20 min and then subjected to I/R, showed reduced cells necrosis and ROS production and increased activity of anti-oxidant enzymes. These effects were achieved by the activation of Akt/ERK1/2/Nrf2 signaling pathways [109].

### 3.3. Lignans

Lignans (ecoisolariciresinol, matairesinol, medioresinol, pinoresinol, and lariciresinol) are found in high concentration in linseed and in minor concentration in algae, leguminous plants, cereals, vegetables, and fruits [17].

Two studies investigated the transduction pathways involved in the cytoprotective effect of (−) schisandrin B (Sch B), the most abundant dibenzocyclooctadiene lignan in *S. chinensis* (Turcz.) Baill, in H9c2 cardiomyocytes. The treatment of H9c2 cardiomyocytes with (−)Sch B (15 or 20 μM) activated the MAPKs, increased the nuclear expression of Nrf2 and reduced the H/R-induced apoptosis and inflammation [110,111]. Chang et al. showed that the treatment with deoxyschizandrin (DSD, 1 μM) and schisantherin A (STA, 1 μM) reduced apoptosis in cardiac cells subjected to I/R [112].

Cho et al. investigated the effect of syringaresinol in modulating HIF-1 (hypoxia inducible factor-1) during H/R injury. Syringaresinol (25 μM) protected H9c2 cardiomyocytes against H/R induced-cells damage, and reduced apoptosis. In addition, syringaresinol suppressed the expression of HIF-1 but stimulated the nuclear expression and activation of FoxO3, which decreased the expression of ROS and increased the expression of anti-oxidant enzymes [113].

Su et al. evaluated the in vitro effect of sesamin in DOX-induced citotoxicity in H9c2 cardiomyocytes. Treatment with sesamin (40 μM) increased cells viability, reduced the release of free radicals and the mitochondrial damage induced by DOX [114]. Zheng et al. demonstrated that sesamin treatment reduced the Ang II-induced apoptotic rate and ROS production in H9c2 cardiomyocytes [115].

### 3.4. Stilbenes (Resveratrol)

The main dietary source of stilbenes is resveratrol (3,5,4′-trihidroxystilbene) from red wine, grapes, berries, plums, peanuts, and pine nuts [17]. Many studies investigated the protective effects of resveratrol against $H_2O_2$-induced damage in cardiomyocytes. Resveratrol treatment (10–50 μM) protected H9c2 cardiomyocytes from $H_2O_2$-induced cell injury, apoptosis and autophagy and reduced ROS generation through activation of SIRT1 and mitochondrial biogenesis signaling pathways [116–118]. Movahed et al. also demonstrated that pretreatment with resveratrol (30 μM) prevented necrosis and the reduction of anti-oxidant enzymes activity in $H_2O_2$-exposed adult rat cardiomyocytes [119]. In addition, resveratrol treatment (50 μM) was effective in protecting rabbit ventricular myocytes against the oxidative stress-induced arrhythmogenic activity and $Ca^{2+}$ overload, through the reduction of ROS production and inhibition of $Ca^{2+}$/calmodulin-dependent protein kinases II (CaMKII) [120]. A study by Chen et al. demonstrated the protective effect of resveratrol against apoptosis induced by hypoxia in H9c2 cardiomyocytes. Resveratrol (20 μM) increased SIRT1 expression, leading to inhibition of forkhead box protein O1 (FoxO1) expression and activity [121].

Several studies showed the cardioprotective role of resveratrol in cardiomyocytes exposed to I/R injury. Pretreatment with resveratrol (20 μM) protected neonatal rat ventricular cardiomyocytes from I/R-induced oxidative injury, apoptosis, necrosis and mitochondrial dysfunction through the induction of SIRT1 which modulated MAPKs signaling [122]. Resveratrol was effective in attenuating the cardiotoxicity induced by chemotherapeutic drugs, such as DOX and arsenic trioxide, and by anti-retroviral agents, such as azidothymidine (AZT). Danz et al. observed that resveratrol (10 μM) inhibited DOX-induced ROS generation and necrosis through the activation of SIRT1 pathway in neonatal rat ventricular myocytes [123]. Similarly, Gao and colleagues reported that pretreatment with resveratrol (3μM) attenuated the mitochondrial ROS generation, apoptosis and necrosis induced by AZT in human primary cardiomyocytes [124]. Zhao et al. investigated the protective effect of resveratrol against arsenic trioxide ($As_2O_3$)-induced cardiotoxicity in H9c2 cardiomyocytes. They demonstrated that pretreatment with resveratrol (10 μM) reduced cells apoptosis and necrosis, increased cell viability and inhibited the generation of ROS and the intracellular $Ca^{2+}$ mobilization induced by $As_2O_3$ [125].

Resveratrol was also able to protect primary cultures of neonatal rat cardiomyocytes against HG-induced apoptosis through the AMPK pathway. Resveratrol (50 μM) inhibited apoptosis and

ROS production and increased the activity of anti-oxidant enzymes [126]. Das et al. demonstrated that the treatment of human and murine cardiomyocytes with resveratrol (100 μM) reduced the iron-induced oxidative stress by decreasing the levels of free radicals. The authors observed that the inhibition of oxidative stress was dependent on the increase of SIRT1 and on the reduction of FoxO1 expression [127].

Several studies investigated the in vitro effects of resveratrol derivatives. The effect of polydatin, a resveratrol glucoside, against phenylephrine induced-cardiac hypertrophy was investigated in neonatal rat cardiomyocytes. Polydatin (50 μM) induced an anti-hypertrophic effect by decreasing ROS production and by inhibiting the RhoA/ROCK signaling pathway, that play a role in mediating the development of cardiac hypertrophy and heart failure [128]. Recently, Feng et al. investigated the effect of an analog of resveratrol, bakuchiol (BAK), a monoterpene phenol isolated from the seeds of *Psoralea corylifolia* (Leguminosae), against the I/R-induced oxidative damage. Pretreatment with BAK (1 μM), administered 5 min before I/R, protected isolated rat hearts from I/R through the activation of the SIRT1 pathway. BAK improved cardiac function, reduced apoptosis and increased anti-oxidant enzymes [129].

### 3.5. Other Polyphenols

#### 3.5.1. Curcumin

Curcumin (1,7-bis-(4-hydroxy-3-methoxyphenyl)-1,6-heptadiene-3,5-dione) is another polyphenol compound and a member of the curcuminoid family. It is found in turmeric, a spice produced from the rhizome of *Curcuma longa* [17].

Several studies investigated the protective effect of curcumin against the oxidative stress in cardiomyocytes. Pretreatment of HL-1 cells with curcumin (5 μM) reduced Ang II-induced cardiomyocytes hypertrophy, oxidative stress and apoptosis [130]. Kim et al. showed that the curcumin (10 μM) pretreatment reduced the cardiotoxicity caused by TNF-α, peptidoglycan or H/R in rat cardiomyocytes [131]. Curcumin also attenuated the I/R-induced toxicity through SIRT1 pathway [132]. Xu et al. analyzed the protective role of curcumin against A/R-induced mitochondrial injuries in rat hearts. Curcumin (1 μM) restored the mitochondrial respiratory activity, inhibited the lipoperoxidation, protein carbonylation and cells apoptosis [133]. Treatment of primary cultures of neonatal rat cardiomyocytes with curcumin (10 μM) reduced the glucose-induced toxicity by decreasing the apoptotic rate and ROS production. Curcumin reduced the toxicity through the NADPH-mediated oxidative stress and PI3K/Akt pathway [134].

Several studies investigated the cardioprotective effects of curcumin derivatives. Nehra et al. evaluated the effect of nanocurcumin after hypoxia. H9c2 cardiomyocytes treated with nanocurcumin (50 μM), compared to cells treated with curcumin, showed reduced hypertrophy and apoptosis [135]. In addition, nanocurcumin (50 ng/mL) inhibited the hypertrophy, reduced necrosis and ROS generation, restored the mitochondrial membrane potential and glucose transporters and increased ATP levels in primary human ventricular cardiomyocytes (HVCM) [136]. The treatment of hearts with AID (alpha-interacting domain of the L-type $Ca^{2+}$ channel) peptide tethered nanoparticles containing 25 mg of curcumin (NP-C-AID) or resveratrol (NP-R-AID) reduced cells necrosis, ROS generation and mitochondrial membrane potential in response to I/R injury. However, only NP-C-AID reduced the oxidative stress by balancing the GSH/GSSG ratio, and the muscle damage [137]. The effects of monocarbonyl analogues of curcumin (MACs) with high stability was evaluated in I/R-induced toxicity and injuries. Among these MACs, the curcumin analogue 14p (10 μM) reduced the toxicity by blocking the oxidative stress, apoptosis and by activating the Nrf2 pathway in H9c2 cardiomyocytes [138].

#### 3.5.2. Olive Oil Polyphenols

Olive oil is a source of at least 30 phenolic compounds. The three phenolic compounds found in highest concentration in olive oil are oleuropein, hydroxytyrosol and tyrosol [139].

Bali et al. compared the effects of the ethanolic and methanolic extracts of olive leaves with the effects of oleuropein, hydroxytyrosol, and quercetin, as a positive control, in H9c2 cardiomyocytes exposed to 4-hydroxy-2-nonenal (HNE), which induced oxidative damage. H9c2 cardiomyocytes were pretreated with each compound (0.1, 10 μg/mL) and then exposed to HNE. Both extracts of olive leaves and the other compounds inhibited cells apoptosis, blocked ROS production, counteracted mitochondrial dysfunction. The ethanolic extract, that contained large amounts of oleuropein, hydroxytyrosol, verbascoside, luteolin, and quercetin, exerted a better protection against HNE-induced cardiotoxicity than the methanolic extract or each phenolic compound [140].

### 3.5.3. Salvianolic Acid

Salvianolic acid B (SalB), derived from the Chinese herb *Salvia miltiorrhiza*, was investigated against TNF-α-induced MMP-2 up-regulation and oxidative stress in human aortic smooth muscle cells (HASMCs). Pretreatment with SalB (0.1, 1, 10 μM) inhibited the TNF-α-induced increase of ROS production. In addition, the polyphenol suppressed the TNF-α-induced MMP-2 enzymatic activity [141]. SalB (5, 10 μM) was also able to protect human aortic endothelial cells (HAECs) from oxidized-low density lipoprotein (ox-LDL) induced oxidative injury via inhibition of ROS production [142].

### 3.5.4. Silymarin and Silibinin

Silymarin (SM) is a standardized extract from the seeds of *Silybum marianum L. Gaertneri*, and the main constituents are silibinin, and other flavonolignans (dehydrosilibinin, silychristin and silydianin). Silymarin (0.50 mg/mL) showed ROS radical scavenging activities. Silymarin (0.50 mg/mL) improved mitochondrial functions, reduced NO levels, protein carbonyl content and lipid peroxidation and increased anti-oxidant and Kreb's cycle enzymes in cardiac mitochondria exposed to copper-ascorbate [143].

Silibinin (50–200 μM) reduced cellular damage after $H_2O_2$-exposure in H9c2 cardiomyocytes. In addition, the treatment with silibinin (100–200 μM) inhibited MAPKs and Akt activation in phenylephrine-induced hypertrophic H9c2 cardiomyocytes [144]. Gabrielova et al. demonstrated that the treatment of rat neonatal cardiomyocytes with 2,3-dehydrosilybin (DHS) (10 μM) attenuated the H/R-induced damage by decreasing the generation of ROS and protein carbonyls [145].

### 3.6. Combination of Polyphenols and Comparative Studies

Esmaeili and Sonboli demonstrated the anti-oxidant and free radical scavenging activities of *Salvia brachyantha* extract, which contains phenolic and flavonoid compounds such as rosmarinic acid, caffeic acid, luteolin, gallic acid, rutin and catechin. The pretreatment of H9c2 cardiomyocytes with the *Salvia brachyantha* extract (50–100 μg/mL) reduced the production of ROS, increased anti-oxidant enzymes and prevented cells apoptosis induced by xanthine/XO [146].

Chen et al. analyzed the cardioprotective role of the total flavonoids from *Clinopodium chinense* (Benth.) O. Ktze (TFCC), against the adverse effects of DOX treatment in H9c2 cardiomyocytes. H9c2 cardiomyocytes treated with TFCC (25 μM) showed increased levels of anti-oxidant enzymes and decreased cells necrosis and apoptosis and ROS production. Furthermore, TFCC blocked DOX-induced over-expression of p53 and regulated the phosphorylation of MAPKs, Akt and PI3K [147].

Chang et al. evaluated and compared the oxidant scavenging capacity of five flavonoids (wogonin, baicalin, baicalein, catechin and procyanidin B2) and their protective efficacy in a chick cardiomyocytes model. Catechin and procyanidin $B_2$ showed the best scavenging capacity for DPPH (1,1-diphenyl-2-picryhydrazyl) and superoxide radicals. Only baicalein exhibited a significant hydroxyl radical scavenging potency. The cardiomyocytes were treated with three different treatment protocols during I/R. The cardiomiocytes were exposed to flavonoids (25 μM) before and during I/R (chronic treatment) or during I/R or during reperfusion phase. The administration of all flavonoids, except for wogonin, reduced apoptosis in chronic treatment. Baicalein, procyanidin $B_2$, and catechin reduced apoptosis when flavonoids were administered only during I/R. In addition, only baicalein and

*Nutrients* **2017**, *9*, 523

procyanidin $B_2$ treatment during reperfusion phase reduced cells apoptosis. Flavonoids had different radical scavenging capacities and protective effects against I/R injury depending on the timing of treatment [148].

Akhlaghi et al. analyzed the effects of several flavonoids (all at 25 μM) in H9c2 cardiomyocytes exposed to I/R injury. The pretreatment with catechin improved cells viability, while cyanidin showed a mild protection. However, only the pretreatment of H9c2 cardiomyocytes with quercetin and EGCG reduced the oxidative stress [149].

Mechanisms of action of in vitro effects of polyphenols to counteract the oxidative stress-induced cardiotoxicity are summarized in Table 1.

## 4. Bioavailability of Polyphenols: Is the Effective Polyphenols Dose Feasible In Vivo?

Although in vitro studies reported that polyphenols exert strong anti-oxidant activity, their beneficial effects in humans remains poor, because of their low bioavailability. Bioavailability is the quantity of a compound that is absorbed and metabolized within the human body after dietary intake and it is measured commonly with the maximum plasma concentration (Cmax) reached after the intake. In fact, in order to produce in vivo effects, a compound must enter the circulation and reach the tissues, in the native or metabolized form, in a sufficient dose to exert biological activity [17]. After dietary intake, polyphenols are metabolized and then the metabolites induce the physiological effects observed in in vivo models [150,151]. The doses of polyphenols employed in vitro usually range between μmol/L and mmol/L, but the concentrations of metabolites in the plasma are of only nmol/L [150]. Endogenous factors affect the bioavailability of polyphenols, such as their metabolism in the gastrointestinal tract and liver, their binding on the surfaces of blood cells and microbial flora in the oral cavity and gut, and regulatory mechanisms that prevent the toxic effects of high polyphenols levels on mitochondria or other organelles [152]. Furthermore, polyphenols are often used as aglycones or conjugates to sugar and not as their active metabolites in in vitro studies [150].

Polyphenols can interact with several substances that influence their bioavailability. For example, polyphenols can bind proteins and metal cations that modify their absorption [153]. Dietary factors can affect the bioavailability of polyphenols, such as food matrix and food preparation techniques [154]. The rate and extent of intestinal absorption and the metabolites in the plasma mainly depend on the chemical structure of polyphenols. Polyphenols show different bioavailability and it has been estimated that the plasma concentration of polyphenols and total metabolites reached after an intake of 50 mg of aglycones ranged from 0 to 4 μM. In addition, the half-lives of polyphenols in human plasma are in the range of few hours and depend on the food source [155]. However, in order to assess the real in vivo potential of polyphenols it is essential to know not only their plasma concentration, but the concentration of the active metabolites in the target tissues [155]. Thus, it would be necessary to employ the active metabolites of polyphenols in in vitro studies [151]. Accordingly, although it is very difficult, it would be important to analyze the concentration of polyphenols in a specific tissue [150]. A limited number of studies detected the concentration of polyphenols in different tissues of mice and rats, including endothelial cells and heart, after administration of the compounds. The tissue concentrations are different depending on the type of tissue and the dose administered, but tipically range from 30 to 3000 ng aglycone equivalents/g tissue [13]. Unfortunately, it is much more difficult to evaluate the tissue concentrations of polyphenols in humans and in fact the studies are very scarce [150]. Overall, a better knowledge of this issue is needed.

Despite the limit of the in vitro studies, anti-oxidative effects of polyphenols have been reported in in vivo experimental models.

Table 1. In vitro protective effects of polyphenols against the oxidative stress-induced cardiotoxicity.

| Polyphenol | Cardiac Damage Inducers | Cell Type | In Vitro Effects | Ref. |
|---|---|---|---|---|
| Quercetin | DOX $H_2O_2$ A/R Xanthine/XO | H9c2 cells | ↓ Apoptosis, ROS, LDH release<br>↓ DNA fragmentation<br>↓ Bid, p53 and NADPH oxidase<br>↓ ERK1/2, Akt, p38, JNK, TNF-α<br>↓ Phospho-ERK1/2 and –Akt<br>↑ Phospho-c-Jun and –PKC$_\varepsilon$<br>↓ AΨm loss and $Ca^{2+}$<br>↓ Phospho-MAPKAPK-2 and caspase 3 | [45,48,52,53,57] |
| 3′-O-methyl quercetin | $H_2O_2$ | H9c2 cells | ↓ Apoptosis and LDH release | [45] |
| Hydroxytyrosol | Xanthine/XO | H9c2 cells | ↑ Phospho-ERK1/2 and -Hsp-27<br>↓ Phospho-c-Jun | [57] |
| Taxifolin | Ang II | Neonatal rat cardiomyocytes | ↓ ROS and hypertrophy | [56] |
| Rhamnetin | $H_2O_2$ | H9c2 cells | ↓ Apoptosis and ROS<br>↑ CAT and MnSOD<br>↓ Phospho-Akt/GSK-3β, -ERK1/2, -p38 and -JNK | [46] |
| Isorhamnetin | DOX | H9c2 cells | ↓ Apoptosis and ROS<br>↓ LDH release and lipid peroxidation<br>↑ Anti-oxidant markers<br>↓ Bax/Bcl-2 ratio, p53, caspases 9 and 3, PARP and cytochrome *c* release<br>↓ Phospho-ERK, -p38 and -JNK | [49] |
| Dihydromyricetin | DOX | Primary myocardial H9c2 cells | ↓ Apoptosis and ROS<br>↑ GSH<br>↓ Nuclear damage, caspase 3 and 8, PARP, AΨm loss and Bax/Bcl-2 ratio | [51] |
| Kaempferol | DOX A/R | H9c2 cells Neonatal primary rat cardiomyocytes | ↓ Apoptosis and ROS<br>↓ LDH release<br>↑ SIRT1, AΨm and Bcl-2<br>↓ mPTP opening and DNA fragmentation<br>↓ Phospho-ERK1/2<br>↓ p53, cytochrome *c* release, and caspase 3 and PARP cleavage | [50,54] |
| 3′,4′-dihydroxyflavonol | I/R $H_2O_2$ | Cardiomyocytes | ↓ Superoxide<br>↑ Phospho-ERK, -MEK and -Akt | [47,55] |
| Apigenin | A/R | H9c2 cells | ↓ Apoptosis and ROS<br>↓ LDH release and cytochrome *c* release | [58] |

**Table 1.** *Cont.*

| Polyphenol | Cardiac Damage Inducers | Cell Type | In Vitro Effects | Ref. |
|---|---|---|---|---|
| Apigenin glucoside, vitexin | A/R | Neonatal rat cardiomyocytes | ↓ Apoptosis and ROS<br>↓ LDH and CK release<br>↑ Phospho-ERK1/2 | [59] |
| Baicalein | Ipoxia<br>I/R<br>DOX | Chick cardiomyocytes<br>H9c2 cells<br>hESC-CMs | ↓ Apoptosis and ROS<br>↓ LDH release<br>↑ Nrf2 pathway and HO-1<br>↑ Contractile activity | [61–64] |
| EGCG | $H_2O_2$<br>I/R<br>DOX<br>Bisulfite/sulfite<br>Lead | Neonatal and adult rat cardiomyocytes<br>H9c2 cells<br>Cultures of cardiomyocytes<br>Rat ventricular myocytes | ↓ Apoptosis and ROS<br>↓ Cellular damage and citosolic $Ca^{2+}$<br>↓ LDH release and MDA formation<br>↑ MnSOD, CAT and GSH-Px<br>↑ HO-1 and caveolin-1<br>↓ β-catenin, N-cadherin and Cx43<br>↓ p53, p21, caspase 3 and FasR<br>↓ STAT-1 activation, telomere attrition and $TRF_2$ loss | [65–70,72,75,76] |
| EGCG and TF3 | $H_2O_2$ | Neonatal rat cardiomyocytes | ↓ Cellular damage<br>↑ Akt, ERK1/2 and p38 MAPK | [65] |
| (−)-epicatechin, avicularin and quercitrin | BSO | H9c2 cells | ↓ Apoptosis and LDH release | [77] |
| Grape seed proanthocyanidin extract | I/R<br>DOX | Chick cardiomyocytes<br>Primary cultures cardiomyocytes | ↓ Apoptosis and ROS<br>↑ NO and GSH-GSSG ratio<br>↓ Δψm loss and DNA fragmentation<br>↑ Contractile activity | [71,73] |
| Malvidin | I/R | Rat cardiomyocytes | ↑ LV pressure, Akt, eNOS, ERK1/2, and phospho-GSK3β | [78] |
| Cyanidin-3-O-glucoside | I/R | Rat cardiomyocytes | ↓ Apoptosis and LDH release | [79] |
| Blueberry phenol fractions | NE | Adult rat cardiomyocytes | ↓ Apoptosis and calpains<br>↑ SOD and CAT | [80] |
| Narigenin | $H_2O_2$ | H9c2 cells | ↓ Apoptosis and lipid peroxidation<br>↑ GSH-Px, GST, CAT, Nrf2, GCL and NQO-1 | [81] |
| Naringin | High glucose | H9c2 cells | ↓ Apoptosis and ROS<br>↑ GSH-Px, SOD, CAT and Bcl-2<br>↓ Δψm loss, p53, Bax, Bad, caspase, release of cytochrome c<br>↓ ERK1/2, p38 MAPK, JNK and leptin | [82–85] |

Table 1. *Cont.*

| Polyphenol | Cardiac Damage Inducers | Cell Type | In Vitro Effects | Ref. |
|---|---|---|---|---|
| Naringenin-7-O-glucoside | DOX | H9c2 cells | ↓ Apoptosis and ROS; ↑ SOD, CAT, GSH-Px and NQO-1; ↓ CK, LDH, caspase 9 and 3 mRNA; ↑ ERK, Nrf2, HO-1 and Bcl-2 | [86–88] |
| Hesperetin | LPS | H9c2 cells | ↓ Apoptosis; ↑ Bcl-2; ↓ Bax and phopsho-JNK | [89] |
| Puerarin | Ang II | Neonatal murine cardiomyocytes | ↓ ROS; ↓ NADPH oxidase; ↓ ERK 1/2, JNK and AP-1 | [90] |
| Calycosin | $H_2O_2$ | H9c2 cells | ↓ Apoptosis; ↑ ERα/β and Akt | [91] |
| Licochalcone D | I/R | Rat cardiomyocytes | ↓ Caspase 3 and PARP; ↓ IL-6, TNF-α, CRP, LDH, CK, MDA, NO, NF-κB and p38 MAPK; ↑ SOD, GSH/GSSG ratio, eNOS and Akt | [92] |
| Isoliquiritigenin | I/R | Cardiomyocytes | ↓ ROS and mitochondrial potential; ↑ AMPK and ERK | [94] |
| Safflor yellow A | A/R | Neonatal rat cardiomyocytes | ↓ LDH, CK, MDA and Bax; ↑ SOD, CAT, GSH, GSH-Px and Bcl-2 | [95] |
| Hydroxysafflor yellow A | A/R | H9c2 cells | ↓ Apoptosis; ↑ Nrf2 | [96] |
| Chalcone derivative L6H9 | Glucose | H9c2 cells | ↓ ROS, Hypertrophy and fibrosis; ↓ Bax, caspase 9 and 3; ↓ IL-6, TNF-α, COX and NF-κB; ↑ Nrf2, HO-1, NQO-1 and GCLC | [97] |
| Aspalathin | Hyperglycemia | H9c2 cells | ↓ ROS; ↓ DNA nick and Δψm loss; ↑ GSH, SOD and Bcl-2/Bax ratio | [99] |
| GLG | $H_2O_2$ | H9c2 cells | ↓ Apoptosis, ROS and hemolysis; ↓ Caspase 3 and nuclear condensation and fragmentation | [100] |
| CSM-bark extract | $H_2O_2$ | Neonatal cardiomyocytes | ↓ Apoptosis and ROS | [101] |

**Table 1.** *Cont.*

| Polyphenol | Cardiac Damage Inducers | Cell Type | In Vitro Effects | Ref. |
|---|---|---|---|---|
| Hispidin | $H_2O_2$ | H9c2 cells | ↓ Apoptosis, ROS and LDH release<br>↓ DNA fragmentation, caspase 3 and Bax<br>↑ HO-1, CAT, Bcl-2, Akt/GSK3β and ERK 1/2 | [102] |
| Methyl gallate | $H_2O_2$ | Neonatal rat cardiomyocytes | ↓ Apoptosis and ROS<br>↓ DNA damage, caspase 3 and Δψm loss<br>↑ GSH | [103] |
| Pyrrolidinyl caffeamide | $H_2O_2$ | HL-1 cells | ↓ Apoptosis and ROS<br>↑ CAT, MnSOD, HO-1 and phospho-Akt | [104] |
| Ferulic acid | High glucose | Cardiomyocytes | ↓ Apoptosis and ROS<br>↑ GSH, Nrf2, HO-1 and Keap-1 | [105] |
| MPE | Malathion | H9c2 cells | ↓ ROS, DPPH, ABTS and NO<br>↑ Integrity of extra cellular matrix components | [106] |
| Hydroxycinnamic acids | DOX | Neonatal rat cardiomyocytes | ↓ Cellular damage and lipid peroxidation | [107] |
| Danshensu | I/R | H9c2 cells | ↓ Apoptosis, ROS, LDH release, CK, MDA and caspase 3<br>↑ SOD, CAT, GSH-Px, HO-1, Bcl-2/Bax ratio, PI3K/Akt and ERK1/2 | [108,109] |
| Sch B | I/R | H9c2 cells | ↓ Apoptosis, inflammation and ROS<br>↓ Bax/Bcl-2 ratio, NF-κB<br>↑ ERK and Nrf2 | [110,111] |
| Syringaresinol | I/R | H9c2 cells | ↓ ROS, MDA, Bax/Bcl-2 ratio, caspase 3 and HIF-1<br>↑ FoxO3 and anti-oxidant markers | [113] |
| Sesamin | DOX<br>Ang II | H9c2 cells | ↓ Apoptosis, ROS and MDA<br>↓ Caspase 3, p47phox and Δψm loss<br>↑Bcl-2, SOD and T-AOC | [114,115] |
| Resveratrol | $H_2O_2$<br>Hypoxia<br>DOX<br>AZT<br>$As_2O_3$<br>High glucose<br>Iron | H9c2 cells<br>Neonatal rat ventricular cardiomyocytes<br>Human and rat primary cardiomyocytes | ↓ Apoptosis, necrosis, autophagy, mitochondrial dysfunction and cell injury<br>↓ ROS, NADPH oxidase, LDH release, FoxO1, CaMKII<br>↓ Bax, phospho-p38 and -JNK<br>↑ SIRT1, Bcl-2, phospho-Akt and -ERK<br>↑ SOD, CAT | [116–127] |
| Polydatin | Phenylephrine | Neonatal rat cardiomyocytes | ↓ ROS and RhoA/ROCK | [128] |
| Bakuchiol | I/R | Rat cardiomyocytes | ↓ Apoptosis<br>↑ SIRT1, SDH, cytochrome *c* oxidase and SOD | [129] |

Table 1. Cont.

| Polyphenol | Cardiac Damage Inducers | Cell Type | In Vitro Effects | Ref. |
|---|---|---|---|---|
| Curcumin | TNF-α Peptidoglycan H/R I/R Glucose | Rat cardiomyocytes | ↓ Apoptosis, ROS, NADPH oxidase, MDA, lipid peroxidation and protein carbonylation ↓ Bax, cytochrome $c$ and cardiolipin release, FoxO1, TLR2 and MCP-1 ↑ Bcl-2, SDH, COX, SOD, SIRT1, Akt and phospho-GSK-3β | [131–134] |
| Nanocurcumin | Hypoxia | H9c2 cells HVCM | ↓ Apoptosis, hypertrophy and ROS ↓ HIF-1α, caspase 3 and 7, p53 translocation ↓ AMPKα, p-300 HAT, LDH, acetyl-CoA and Δψm loss ↑ c-Fos, c-Jun and ATP | [135,136] |
| Curcumin analogue 14p | I/R | H9c2 cells | ↓ Apoptosis, ROS and MDA ↑ Nrf2, SOD | [138] |
| Salvianolic acid B | TNF-α | HASMC | ↓ ROS, NADPH oxidase, MMP-2 | [141] |
| Silymarin | Copper-ascorbate | Neonatal rat cardiomyocytes | ↓ ROS, NO, protein carbonylation and lipid peroxidation ↑ mitochondrial function, GSH, GSH-Px, GR, SOD, PDH | [143] |
| Silibinin | $H_2O_2$ Phenylephrine | H9c2 cells | ↓ Apoptosis, DNA damage, ROS ↓ ERK and Akt | [144] |
| 2,3-dehydrosilybin | H/R | Neonatal rat cardiomyocytes | ↓ ROS, protein carbonylation and LDH release | [145] |
| TFCC | DOX | H9c2 cells | ↓ Apoptosis, ROS, MDA and LDH release ↓ DNA fragmentation, caspase 3, cytochrome $c$ release, Bax/Bcl-2 ratio, p53, phospho-ERK, -p38 and -JNK ↑ SOD, CAT, GSH-Px, phospho-Akt and PI3K | [147] |

Abbreviations: ↑: increase; ↓: decrease; DOX: doxorubicin; $H_2O_2$: hydrogen peroxide; A/R: anoxia/reoxygenation; XO: xanthine oxidase; ROS: reactive oxygen species; ERK: extracellular signal-regulated kinase; JNK: c-Jun N-terminal kinase; TNF-α: tumor necrosis factor-α; PKC$_ε$: Protein kinase C epsilon type; Δψm: mitochondrial membrane potential; LDH: lactate dehydrogenase; MAPKAPK-2: mitogen-activated protein kinase-activated protein kinase 2; Hsp: heat shock protein; Ang II: angiotensin II; CAT: catalase; MnSOD: manganese superoxide dismutase; GSH: glutathione; SIRT1: sirtuin 1; mPTP: mitochondrial permeability transition pore; I/R: ischemia/reperfusion; CK: creatin kinase; H/R: hypoxia/reoxygenation; hESC-CMs: human embryonic stem cells-derived cardiomyocytes; Nrf2: nuclear factor erythroid 2-related factor 2; HO-1: heme oxygenase-1; EGCG: (−)-epigallocatechin-3-gallate; MDA: malondialdehyde; GSH-Px: glutathione peroxidase; TF3: theaflavin-3,3′ digallate; BSO: buthionine-(S,R)-sulfoximine; NO: nitric oxide; GSSG: glutathione disulfide; LV: left ventricular; NE: norepinephrine; GCL: glutamate cysteine ligase; NQO-1: NAD(P)H:quinone oxidoreductase 1; LPS: lipopolysaccharide; ER: estrogen receptor; IL: interleukin; CRP: C reactive protein; eNOS: endothelial nitric oxide synthase; COX: cyclooxygenase; GCLC: glutamate cysteine ligase catalytic subunit; GLG: Gui-ling-gao; CSM: *Castanea Sativa* Mill.; MPE: gallic acid-enriched methanolic *Syzygium cumini* pulp extract; DPPH: 1,1-diphenyl-1-picrylhydrazyl; ABTS: 2,2′-azino-bis (3-ethylbenzthiazoline-6-sulfonic acid); Sch: schisandrin; HIF-1: hypoxia inducible factor-1; FoxO: Forkhead box protein O; T-AOC: total antioxidant capacity; AZT: azidothymidine; As$_2$O$_3$: arsenic trioxide; CaMKII: Ca$^{2+}$/Calmodulin-dependent protein kinases II; GR: glutathione reductase; GST: glutathione s-transferase; TLR2: Toll-like receptor 2; MCP-1: monocyte chemoattractant protein; SDH: succinate dehydrogenase; HASMC: human aortic smooth muscle cells; MMP: metalloproteinase; PDH: piruvate dehydrogenase; TFCC: *Clinopodium chinense* (Benth.) O. Ktze.

## 5. In Vivo Effects of Polyphenols Against Oxidative Stress-Induced Cardiotoxicity

### 5.1. Flavonoids

#### 5.1.1. Flavonols

Several studies showed the in vivo cardioprotective effects of flavonols against DOX-induced cardiotoxicity. The quercetin (100 or 15 mg/kg) pretreatment of mice and rats treated with DOX improved cardiac function, blocked ROS generation and lipid peroxidation and increased anti-oxidant enzymes [48,156]. Isorhamnetin (5 mg/kg, i.p.), kaempferol (10 mg/kg, i.p.) and dihydromyricetin (125–500 mg/kg) administration reduced cardiomiocytes necrosis and apoptosis, ROS production and lipid peroxidation and increased the production of anti-oxidant enzymes in in vivo models exposed to DOX [49–51].

Flavonols effects were analyzed also in rats underewent I/R injury. Rats treated with kaempferol (15 mM) recovered cardiac function, reduced infarct size and cardiomyocytes apoptosis [157].

Astragalin (kaempferol-3-*O*-glucoside) pretreatment (10 μM) showed cardioprotective effects in rats via its anti-oxidative, anti-apoptotic, and anti-inflammatory activities [158]. The in vivo effects of 3′,4′-dihydroxyflavonol (DiOHF) was investigated in sheep. The in vivo administration of DiOHF (5 mg/kg) after I/R injury reduced ROS generation, neutrophil accumulation in coronary microvessels, left ventricular diastolic pressure (LVDP) and infarct size, increased the left anterior descending (LAD) coronary artery blood flow, the total plasma nitrate and nitrite and restored the myocardial function [55]. The myocardial I/R injury was blocked by NP202, a novel pro-drug of DiOHF, through the activation of MAPKs signaling in sheep [47].

A study by Bhandary et al. investigated the preventive effects of rutin, quercetin and various isoflavones (biochanin A, daidzein, genistein) in an ex vivo model of I/R injury. They perfused rat hearts with isoflavones (10 μM), quercetin (10 μM), and rutin (50 μM) before ischemia and during the reperfusion time. Only rutin possessed the ability to attenuate cardiac I/R-associated hemodynamic alterations [159]. In addition, rutin increased anti-oxidant molecules and reduced cells necrosis and apoptosis and overall cardiac dysfunction in rats exposed to sodium fluoride-induced oxidative stress [160].

The isoproterenol injection induced cardiotoxicity in rats. The co-treatment with vincristine (25 mg/kg) and quercetin (10 mg/kg) attenuated the cardiotoxicity induced by isoproterenol [161].

Guo et al., employing a mouse model with transverse aortic constriction (TAC), demonstrated that taxifolin, a dihydroquercetin derivative decreased ROS levels, attenuated the pressure overload, blocked the cardiac remodeling, ventricular dysfunction and fibrosis [56].

#### 5.1.2. Flavones

Several studies demonstrated the in vivo cardioprotective role of flavones against I/R. In murine and rat models baicalein (30 mg/kg), apigenin (5 mg/kg) and vitexin (6, 3, 1.5 mg/kg) reduced I/R injury-induced infarct size, apoptosis, pro-inflammatory cytokines and oxidative stress [162–164]. Employing diabetic rats subjected to myocardial I/R, it has been assessed the protective effects of luteolin or breviscapine, a flavonoid extracted by *Erigeron breviscapus*. Luteolin (100 mg/kg/day intragastrically) or breviscapine (60 mg/kg orally) reduced the ROS production [165,166]. Luteolin also improved left ventricular function and cardiac tissue viability [165]. In addition, breviscapine reduced the expression of ICAM-1 in rat myocardium, the inactivation of ATPase and associated ionic disturbances [166].

The protective effect of apigenin in isolated rat heart suffered from A/R was also demonstrated. Rats intraperitoneally injected with apigenin (4 mg/kg) showed reduced cells death and infarct size [58].

### 5.1.3. Flavan-3-Ols

Several studies reported that the administration of green tea extract (GTE) (200 mg/kg or 400 mg/kg, prior to I/R injury) to rats reduced the myocardium damage, infarct size and apoptosis and increased the anti-oxidant enzymes [167,168]. The anti-oxidant properties of flavan-3-ols were also evaluated in DOX-exposed in vivo models. Oral pretreatment for 30 days with GTE (100, 200 and 400 mg/kg) or procyanidins (150 mg/kg daily) decreased the cardyomyocytes death and increased anti-oxidant enzymes in rat models exposed to DOX [169,170].

Sheng et al. reported the protective effects of EGCG in cardiac hypertrophy induced by abdominal aortic constriction in rats. They showed that EGCG (50 and 100 mg/kg) administered intragastrically to rats for 6 weeks, decreased myocardium damage and ROS generation. The highest doses of EGCG improved histological changes in the heart tissue, inhibited fibrosis and myocytes apoptosis [67]. Using the same rat model, the authors evaluated the effect of EGCG and other traditional anti-hypertrophic therapeutic agents on telomere dysfunction mediated apoptotic signal. They demonstrated that treatment for 6 weeks with EGCG (50 and 100 mg/kg) or quercetin (100 mg/kg) reduced heart weight indices and cardiac myocytes apoptosis in the hypertrophic myocardium [171].

Another investigation reported the effect of grape seed proanthocyanidins (GSP) against cadmium (Cd), a toxic heavy metal that induced oxidative stress and cardiotoxicity. In this study, GSP pretreatment (100 mg/kg) reduced Cd-induced disruption of cardiac myofibrils, cardiomyocytes necrosis and apoptosis, production of pro-inflammatory cytokines and increased the levels of anti-oxidant enzymes in rats [172]. Wang et al. demonstrated that GSP (195 mg/kg, intragastric administration) treatment prevented deoxycorticosterone (DOCA)-salt-induced cardiovascular remodeling and endothelial dysfunction in mice, in part through the involvement of oxidative stress [173].

### 5.1.4. Anthocyanins

Liu et al. reported the effects of blueberry anthocyanins-enriched extracts (BAE) on cyclophosphamide (CTX)-induced cardiac toxicity in rats. BAE (20 and 80 mg/kg daily by gavage) treatment attenuated the CTX-induced cardiac injury through its anti-inflammatory and anti-oxidant proprieties. BAE decreased mean arterial blood pressure and myocardial leukocyte infiltration, increased heart rate and improved cardiac dysfunction, and reduced LV hypertrophy and fibrosis. Rats treated with BAE showed a decrease expression of pro-inflammatory cytokines, an increase of anti-inflammatory cytokines and anti-oxidant enzymes [174].

### 5.1.5. Flavanones

Two studies reported the cardioprotective role of the flavanone glycoside hesperidin on I/R-induced arrhythmias in an in vivo rat model. Rats were administered with hesperidin (100 mg/kg, p.o. for 15 days) and then subjected to I/R. The administration of hesperidin induced antiarrhythmic effects, a reduction of inflammation, oxidative stress and cardiomyocytes apoptosis [175,176]. A similar study was conducted with naringin. Naringin was administered *per os* (40, 80 mg/kg, daily) to rats for 14 days and then I/R injury was induced by coronary artery occlusion. Naringin restored I/R injury, as demonstrated by the normalization of cardiac injury markers, by the increased activity of anti-oxidant enzymes, by the reduction of cells apoptosis, infarct size and inflammation [177].

The protective effect of hesperetin against DOX-induced oxidative stress and DNA damage was analyzed in rat heart. Rat, treated with DOX and hesperetin (50 and 100 mg/kg b.w., p.o. by gavage for 5 consecutive days in a week), showed decreased ROS production and cells apoptosis [178]. Hesperetin (30 mg/kg, p.o.) and hesperidin (200 mg/kg, p.o.) administration to murine and rat models inhibited the cardiac remodeling and fibrosis, oxidative stress and apoptosis induced by pressure overload and isoproterenol [179,180].

In addition, Elavarasan et al. also demonstrated that the anti-oxidant activity of hesperidin protected cardiac tissue of aged rats against age-related increase in oxidative stress. Hesperidin (100 mg/kg/day, p.o. for 90 days) increased the activity of anti-oxidant enzymes [181].

The cardioprotective role of hesperidin and naringin on hyperglycemia-induced oxidative damage in HFD/streptozotocin (STZ)-induced diabetic rats has been reported by Mahmoud et al. Diabetes was induced and then rats were treated with hesperidin or naringin (50 mg/kg, p.o.) daily for 4 weeks. Oral administration of hesperidin and naringin prevented diabetic complications and increased the activities of anti-oxidant enzymes in experimental diabetic rats [182].

### 5.1.6. Isoflavones

In vivo effects of calycosin-7-O-β-D-glucoside (CG) on I/R injury were investigated by Ren et al. Pretreatment of rats with CG (30 mg/kg i.v.) 30 min before the ligation of the left anterior descending (LAD) coronary artery was able to improve cardiac function, to decrease infarct size and to enhance the activity of SOD. CG alleviated I/R injury through the activation of the PI3K/Akt pathway and the inhibition of apoptosis [183].

Gang et al. investigated the in vivo effect of puerarin in Ang II-induced cardiac hypertrophy. Puerarin (100 and 200 mg/kg, gavage) reduced cardiac hypertrophy induced by Ang II in mice [90]. The effect of puerarin on severe burn-induced acute myocardial injury in rats was assessed by Liu et al. Groups of adult Wistar rats were subjected to a 30% TBSA (total body surface area) full-thickness dermal burn and resuscitated with an intraperitoneal injection of 4 mL/kg/TBSA of lactated Ringer's solution with or without puerarin (10 mg/kg). Results showed that puerarin protected cardiomyocytes from severe burn-induced ultrastructural modifications and death [184].

### 5.1.7. Chalcones and Dihydrochalcones

Zhong et al. evaluated the in vivo effects of the chalcone derivative L6H9 against STZ-induced diabetes in C57BL/6 mice. L6H9 (20 mg/kg by gavage) protected multiple organs in diabetic mice. In particular, the heart of mice treated with L6H9 did not show structural abnormalities and fibrosis. These mice showed lower levels of ROS, cytokines, and apoptosis [97].

Several studies investigated the in vivo effects of chalcones against I/R. Treatment with licochalcone C (2.0 mM) increased LVDP, levels of anti-oxidant enzymes and decreased cardiomyocytes mitochondrial injury, necrosis and apoptosis in rats [185]. Another study showed the effects of intraperitoneal injection of Cl-chalcone (50 μg/kg) and F-chalcone (100 μg/kg) in albino rats with I/R. Rat hearts treated with Cl-chalcone and F-chalcone showed limited infarct size and high levels of anti-oxidant enzymes [186]. A study reported the protective effect of rooibos extract against myocardial I/R injury. They showed that the aortic output recovery after reperfusion was improved in hearts isolated from male Wistar rats supplemented with aqueous rooibos extract for 7 weeks when compared to that supplemented with green tea (*Camellia sinensis*) extract [187].

### 5.2. Phenolic Acids

Ku et al. analyzed the response of pyrrolidinyl caffeamide (PLCA) against I/R-induced oxidative stress in rats. PCLA administration (1 mg/kg i.p.) reduced the levels of troponin and lipid peroxidation, improved cardiac functions and attenuated the myeloperoxidase (MPO) activity, a marker of neutrophil accumulation [104].

Tang et al. investigated the effect of danshensu in spontaneously hypertensive rats (SHR). Danshensu (10 mg/kg/day i.p.) decreased the HW/BW index, prevented the increase of blood pressure, and reduced arrhythmias in rats exposed to I/R [188]. In addition, danshensu possessed a cardioprotective effect against I/R injury when given to rats during reperfusion (30 and 60 mg/kg, for 3 h) [108].

The protective effects of the preparation Shenge, composed by 1:1 ratio of puerarin and danshensu, has been evaluated on acute ischemic myocardial injury in rats. Rats were subjected to LAD coronary artery occlusion and were injected intravenously with Shenge (30, 60, or 120 mg/kg b.w.) 15 min later.

Shenge was able to improve electrocardiographic changes, the size of ischemic area and anti-oxidant activities induced by the acute myocardial ischemia [189].

*5.3. Lignans*

Several studies analyzed the cardioprotective effects of Schisandrin (Sch) B against DOX-induced oxidative stress. The administration of Sch B (25, 50 and 100 mg/kg) to mice and rats reduced cardiomyocytes apoptosis and necrosis in left ventricle and the activity of MMPs induced by DOX [190,191]. The pretreatment with Sch B (100 mg/kg) significantly increased the levels of GSH redox cycling enzymes [190]. Su et al. also evaluated the in vivo effect of sesamin in DOX-induced cardiotoxicity in rats. The treatment of rats with sesamin (20 mg/kg, orally, for 10 consecutive days) reduced the DOX-induced toxicity through the normalization of the electrocardiography and the decrease of histopathological changes [114]. Daily sesamin treatment (80 or 160 mg/kg, by gavage) in SHR for 16 weeks improved LV hypertrophy and fibrosis. The treatment reduced the systolic blood pressure, enhanced cardiac total anti-oxidant capabilities and TGF-β1 expression [192].

Chen et al., employing a mice model of myocardial infarction (MI) established by a permanent ligation of the left anterior descending (LAD) coronary artery, reported that the MI mice treated with Sch B (80 mg/kg) showed increased survival rate, improved heart function and decreased infarct size [111].

Chiu et al. demonstrated that Sch B also exerted a protective role against myocardial I/R injury through the activation of ERK pathway in rats. Sch B (1.2 mmol/kg, intragastric) decreased LDH leakage and increased GSH levels [110].

The effects of magnolol, extracted from *Magnolia officinalis*, deoxyschizandrin (DSD) and schisantherin A (STA) was analyzed in rats subjected to I/R. Magnolol (10 mg/kg, i.p.), DSD (40 µmol/kg, i.v.) and STA (40 µmol/kg, i.v.) reduced infarct size, arrhythmias and improved I/R-induced myocardial dysfunctions [112,193].

*5.4. Stilbenes (Resveratrol)*

Resveratrol was able to prevent the development of oxidative stress in SHR. Treatment with resveratrol (2.5 mg/kg b.w., daily, by oral gavage for 10 weeks) reduced ROS production [119]. Dolinsky et al. reported that resveratrol (2.5 mg/kg b.w., daily, by oral gavage for 2 weeks) reduced the levels of cardiac HNE-protein adducts and the HNE adducts formation on liver kinase B1 (LKB1), leading to a reduction of left ventricular hypertrophy [194].

Zhao et al. investigated the effect of resveratrol in a mouse model of arsenic trioxide ($As_2O_3$)-induced cardiomyopathy in vivo. Pretreatment with resveratrol (3 mg/kg, i.v., on alternate days for three days 1 h before $As_2O_3$ administration) attenuated $As_2O_3$-induced structural and electrocardiographic abnormalities, increased increased anti-oxidant activity of mice treated with $As_2O_3$ [125].

Resveratrol exerted a beneficial effect in mice with diabetic cardiomyopathy induced by strepozotocin (STZ). Mice fed with a diet enriched with resveratrol (60 and 300 mg/kg/day, for 16 weeks) showed an attenuation of oxidative injury, a decreased cardiomyocytes apoptosis and an improved cardiac function. In addition, resveratrol increased the autophagic flux in diabetic mouse hearts [195].

Das et al. reported that the oral administration of resveratrol reduced the myocardial injury induced by iron. Mice treated with resveratrol decreased oxidative stress and myocardial fibrosis. These responses were achieved by the increase in SIRT1 expression and the reduction in FoxO1 expression [127].

Resveratrol and polydatin, a resveratrol glucoside, attenuated DOX-induced cardiotoxicity in rats. Resveratrol (10 or 15 mg/kg) reduced cardiac dysfunction, oxidative damage and apoptosis and increased anti-oxidant enzymes [196,197]. In addition, a synergistic effect of polydatin and vitamin C to reduce the cardiotoxicity of DOX was observed. The combined treatment (polydatin and vitamin C both 200 µmol/kg) improved electrocardiography, reduced ROS production, increased anti-oxidant activities, and improved the myocardial metabolism in rats [198].

The treatment with resveratrol (20 mg/kg, s.c. or 5, 15, 45 mg/kg/day for 10 days, by gavage) protected mice and rats against LPS and cisplatin-induced cardiotoxicity by restoring the intracellular redox status [199,200]. The anti-hypertrophic effect of polydatin or isorhapontigenin, a resveratrol analogue, was demonstrated in C57BL/6 mice subjected to transverse aortic constriction (TAC), a model of pressure-overload-induced cardiac hypertrophy in vivo. Polydatin (50 mg/kg, daily by gavage) reduced the TAC-induced cardiac hypertrophy [128].

*5.5. Other Polyphenols*

5.5.1. Curcumin

Several studies investigated the effect of curcumin in I/R. Curcumin exerts a cardioprotective effect against I/R injury through the reduction of oxidative stress and mitochondrial dysfunction. Curcumin pretreatment (200 mg/kg) reduced the loss of cardiac mechanical work, the lipid peroxidation and the levels of inflammatory markers in rats [131,201]. In addition, curcumin reduced the cardiotoxicity induced by I/R injury through the SIRT1 pathway. In fact, the in vivo pretreatment of rats with curcumin increased the levels of SIRT1, anti-oxidant enzymes and reduced the cellular damage and necrotic and apoptotic cells [132]. Li et al. showed that the administration of curcumin analogue 14p (10 mg/kg) decreased the infarct size and myocardial apoptosis to the same extent as the high dose curcumin (100 mg/kg) in a mouse model of myocardial I/R [138]. In another study, the co-treatment of rats with curcumin (60 mg/kg) and isoprenaline reduced the percentage of isoprenaline-induced apoptotic and necrotic cells and restored the levels of anti-oxidants. Curcumin decreased the opening of mPTP induced by isoprenaline without modify mitochondria [202].

Diabetic cardiomyopathies are associated with high levels of membrane-bound protein kinase C (PKC). Treatment of STZ-induced diabetic rats with curcumin (100 mg/kg/day for 8 weeks) reduced cardiomyocyte hypertrophy, oxidative stress, myocardial fibrosis and left ventricular dysfunctions [203].

Imbaby et al. analyzed the cardioprotective effects of curcumin and nebivolol against cardiotoxicity induced by DOX therapy in rats. Oral administration of curcumin (200 mg/kg) attenuated DOX-induced cardiotoxicity. The treatment increased survival rate and anti-oxidant enzymes, decreased lipid peroxidation and histological alterations [204].

5.5.2. Olive Oil Polyphenols

In several studies, Andreadou et al. demonstrated the cardioprotective effect of oleuropein against DOX. Oleuropein administration (100 or 200 mg/kg for 5 or 3 consecutive days) reduced cells damage and necrosis in rats induced by DOX [205]. In addition, the same authors investigated the effect of oleuropein in chronic DOX-induced cardiomyopathy in rats. The intraperitoneal administration of oleuropein (1000 or 2000 mg/kg for 14 days) improved heart contractility, reduced apoptosis and production of inflammatory cytokines, degenerative myocardial lesions and levels of nitro-oxidative compounds [206].

5.5.3. Silymarin and Silibinin

Several studies analyzed the effect of silymarin against the cardiotoxicity induced by anti-cancer drugs. Silymarin protected rats against DOX-induced injury. It has been observed that silymarin (50 or 100 mg/kg) reduced myocardial and renal damage and NO levels [207,208]. Silymarin treatment (25, 50 or 100 mg/kg) reduced the serum levels of necrosis markers, enhanced anti-oxidant activities and attenuated the damage of mitochondria in mice and rats exposed to cisplatin or acrolein [209,210].

The protective effect of silibinin against arsenic-induced oxidative stress has been analyzed in rats. Silibinin administration (75 mg/kg) reduced the myocardial damage, the activity of heart mitochondrial enzymes, levels of plasma and cardiac lipids, while it up-regulated the levels of anti-oxidant enzymes in hepatic tissues. Thus, silibinin attenuated the mitochondrial damage and restored the heart function [211].

### 5.6. Combination of Polyphenols

Chen et al. evaluated the cardioprotection of flavonoids extracted from *Clinopodium chinense* (Benth.) O. Ktze (TFCC) against DOX treatment in rats. TFCC (20, 40 and 80 mg/kg) treatment induced the recovery of body and heart weights, balanced the levels of cardiac enzymes, inhibited ROS production and apoptosis and up-regulated the level of anti-oxidant enzymes [147].

Table 2 summarizes molecular mechisms of in vivo effects of polyphenols against the oxidative stress-induced cardiotoxicity.

Overall, Figure 3 shows the in vitro and in vivo effects of polyphenols in cardiovascular disease.

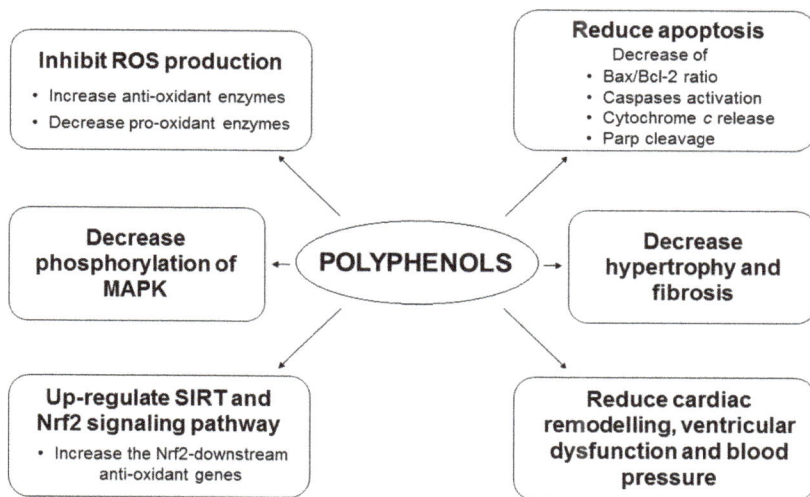

**Figure 3.** In vitro and in vivo effects of polyphenols in cardiovascular disease.

**Table 2.** In vivo protective effects of polyphenols against the oxidative stress-induced cardiotoxicity.

| Polyphenol | In Vivo Model | Protective Effects | Ref. |
|---|---|---|---|
| Quercetin | Mice treated with DOX | ↑ Cardiac function<br>↓ ROS and lipid peroxidation<br>↑ Bmi-1 and SOD expression | [48] |
| | Rats treated with DOX | ↓ Blood pressure and heart rate increase<br>↓ Cellular damage<br>↓ MMP-2 activation and apoptosis<br>↑ SOD activity | [156] |
| Vincristine and quercetin | Rats exposed to isoproterenol | ↓ CK-MB, LDH, ALT, cTnT<br>↓ Lipid peroxidation<br>↓ SOD, CAT, GR, GSH-Px activities<br>↓ Heart rate and ST-segment elevation | [161] |
| Taxifolin | Mouse model of TAC | ↓ Pressure overload, fibrosis, ROS, MDA, HNE<br>↓ Cardiac remodeling and ventricular dysfunction<br>↓ ANP, BNP, β-MHC expression<br>↓ Phospho-ERK1/2, phospho-JNK1/2, Smad2 | [56] |
| DiOHF | Sheep model of I/R injury | ↓ ROS, neutrophil accumulation, LVDP, infarct size<br>↑ Myocardial function | [55] |
| Isorhamnetin | Rats treated with DOX | ↓ Cardiac enzymes, apoptosis, ROS, lipid peroxidation<br>↑ Anti-oxidant enzymes | [49] |
| Rutin | Rats exposed to sodium fluoride | ↓ Cardiac dysfunction, cardiac serum markers<br>↓ Lipid peroxidation and DNA fragmentation<br>↑ SOD, CAT, GSH levels | [160] |
| Dihydromyricetin | Mice treated with DOX | ↑ Survival rate<br>↓ AST, CK-MB, LDH activities | [51] |
| Kaempferol | Rats treated with DOX | ↑ Body and heart weights, SOD, CAT<br>↓ LDH levels, apoptosis, mitochondrial damage | [50] |
| | Rat model of I/R injury | ↑ Cardiac function, SOD activity, GSH/GSSG ratio<br>↓ CK, LDH, MDA levels, infarct size, apoptosis | [157] |
| Astragalin | Rat model of I/R injury | ↑ Cardiac function, SOD activity, GSH/GSSG ratio<br>↓ CK, LDH, MDA levels, infarct size, apoptosis | [158] |
| Baicalein | Murine model of I/R injury | ↓ Infarct size, apoptosis, pro-inflammatory cytokines<br>↓ ROS, MDA levels<br>↑ GSH-Px | [162] |
| Apigenin | Rat model of I/R injury | ↓ Infarct size, apoptosis, CK, LDH, MDA levels<br>↑ SOD | [163] |

**Table 2.** *Cont.*

| Polyphenol | In Vivo Model | Protective Effects | Ref. |
|---|---|---|---|
| Vitexin | Rat model of I/R injury | ↑ Cardiac function, SOD activity <br> ↓ Infarct size, apoptosis, inflammatory cytokines <br> ↓ CK, LDH, MDA | [164] |
| Luteolin | Rat model of I/R injury | ↑ Cardiac function, MnSOD activity <br> ↓ LDH, MDA levels | [165] |
| Breviscapine | Rat model of I/R injury | ↓ ICAM-1, ROS, MDA <br> ↑ SOD, GSH-Px activities | [166] |
| Green Tea Exctract (GTE) | Rat model of I/R injury | ↓ Infarct size, apoptosis <br> ↑ GSH, GCL, QR | [167] |
| | Rats treated with DOX | ↓ AST, CK, LDH, lipid peroxidation <br> ↑ Cyt P450, GSH, GSH-Px, GR, GST, SOD, CAT | [169] |
| EGCG, quercetin | Rats with cardiac hypertrophy | ↓ Systolic blood pressure, heart weight indices, MDA <br> ↑ SOD, GSH-Px activities, apoptosis | [67,171] |
| GSP | Rats treated with cadmium | ↓ Cardiac damage, CK-MB, AST, ALT, ALP, LDH <br> ↓ Pro-inflammatory cytokines, apoptosis <br> ↑ GSH-Px, GR, GST, SOD, CAT, G6PD | [172] |
| Procyanidins | Rats treated with DOX | ↑ Cardiac function <br> ↓ Lipid peroxidation | [170] |
| BAE | Rats treated with CTX | ↑ Cardiac function , IL-10, SOD, GSH <br> ↓ Apoptosis, pro-inflammatory cytokines, MDA | [174] |
| Hesperidin | Rat model of I/R injury | ↑ Cardiac function <br> ↓ Apoptosis, oxidative stress | [176] |
| Naringin | Rat model of I/R injury | ↓ CK-MB, LDH, apoptosis, infarct size, inflammation <br> ↑ SOD, GSH-Px | [177] |
| Hesperetin | Rats treated with DOX | ↓ MDA, DNA damage <br> ↑ GSH | [178] |
| Hesperidin | Rats treated with isoproterenol | ↓ Lipid peroxidation <br> ↓ CK, CK-MB, LDH, AST, ALT, cTnI, cTnT <br> ↑ SOD, CAT, GSH-Px, GST, GR | [180] |
| Hesperidin, naringin | HFD/STZ-induced diabetic rats | Prevention of diabetic complications <br> ↓ MDA, NO <br> ↑ SOD, CAT, GSH-Px, GR | [182] |

**Table 2.** *Cont.*

| Polyphenol | In Vivo Model | Protective Effects | Ref. |
|---|---|---|---|
| Puerarin | Mice treated with Ang II | ↓ Cardiac hypertrophy, HW/BW, LVW/BW | [90] |
| | Rats subjected to severe burn | ↓ CK-MB, cTnT, MDA, MPO | [184] |
| Calycosin-7-O-β-D-glucoside | Rat model of I/R injury | ↑ Cardiac function, SOD activity<br>↓ Infarct size, CK, LDH, MDA, apoptosis | [183] |
| Chalcone derivative L6H9 | STZ-induced diabetic mice | ↓ Cardiac damage and fibrosis<br>↓ ROS, TNF-α, IL-6, COX2, Bax<br>↑ HO-1, NQO-1, GCLC, Bcl-2 | [97] |
| Licochalcone B | Rat model of I/R injury | ↓ Apoptosis, MDA, LDH, CK, TNF-α<br>↑ LVDP, SOD, GSH/GSSG ratio | [185] |
| Cl-chalcone, F-chalcone | Rat model of I/R injury | ↓ Infarct size, lipid peroxidation, MDA<br>↑ SOD, CAT | [186] |
| Pyrrolidinyl caffeamide (PLCA) | Rat model of I/R injury | ↓ Troponin, MDA, MPO<br>↑ Cardiac function, CAT, HO-1, MnSOD | [104] |
| Danshensu | I/R in spontaneously hypertensive rats (SHR) | ↓ Blood pressure increase, arrhythmias, HW/BW<br>↑ NO content, iNOS activity | [188] |
| | Rat model of I/R injury | ↓ Infarct size, CK-MB, cTnI | [108] |
| Shenge | Rats subjected to LAD | ↓ ST-segment elevation, infarct size<br>↓ CK-MB, LDH, MDA<br>↑ SOD activity | [189] |
| Schisandrin B (Sch B) | Rats treated with DOX | ↓ CK, CK-MB, LDH, AST, MDA, MMP<br>↓ Cardiac damage, cell death<br>↑ GSH, GSH/GSSG, GR, GST, GSH-Px, SOD | [190] |
| | Mice treated with DOX | ↓ Cardiac damage, apoptosis, DNA damage<br>↓ ROS, MDA, TNF-α, IL-1β, IL-6, MMP-2, MMP-9<br>↑ GSH, LV performance | [191] |
| | Mouse model of myocardial infarction (MI) | ↑ Survival rate, heart function, eNOS<br>↓ Infarct size, TGF-β1, TNF-α, IL-1β, Bax/Bcl-2 | [111] |
| | Rat model of I/R injury | ↑ GSH<br>↓ LDH | [110] |
| Magnolol | Rat model of I/R injury | ↓ Infarct size, apoptosis, myocardial dysfunction | [193] |

**Table 2.** *Cont.*

| Polyphenol | In Vivo Model | Protective Effects | Ref. |
|---|---|---|---|
| Sesamin | SHR rats | ↓ Cardiac fibrosis, systolic blood pressure<br>↓ HW/BW, LVW/BW, MDA, TGF-β1<br>↑ Cardiac total anti-oxidant capability | [192] |
| | Rats treated with DOX | Normalization QT intervals, QRS complexes<br>↑ SIRT1 activation, MnSOD | [114] |
| Deoxyshizandrin (DSD) + Schisantherin (STA) | Rat model of I/R injury | ↓ Infarct size, LVDP, arrhythmias, MDA<br>↑ LVSP, SOD | [112] |
| | SHR rats | ↓ $H_2O_2$, left ventricular hypertrophy<br>↑ CAT activity | [119,194] |
| Resveratrol | Mice treated with arsenic trioxide ($As_2O_3$) | ↓ QT-interval prolongation, cardiac damage, LDH<br>↑ GSH-Px, CAT, SOD | [125] |
| | Mice treated with LPS | ↑ SERCA2a, Nrf2<br>↓ MDA, HNE | [199] |
| | Rats treated with cisplatin | ↓ LDH, CK, MDA<br>↑ SOD, GSH, GSH-Px, CAT | [200] |
| | Rats treated with DOX | ↓ Cardiac dysfunction, apoptosis, MDA, CK, LDH<br>↑ SIRT1, GSH | [196,197] |
| | STZ-induced diabetic mice | ↓ Apoptosis, p62<br>↑ Cardiac function, SIRT1, autophagy | [195] |
| Polydatin + vitamin C | Rats treated with DOX | ↓ ROS, MDA, CRP, ST and QT intervals<br>↑ GSH-Px, SOD | [198] |
| Polydatin | Mice subjected to TAC | ↓ Cardiac hypertrophy | [128] |
| Curcumin | Rat model of I/R | ↓ Lipid peroxidation<br>↑ Cardiac function, SOD, CAT, GSH, GSH-Px | [201] |
| | Rats treated with isoprenaline | ↓ Apoptosis, MPO, MDA<br>↑ CAT, GSH | [202] |
| | Rat model of I/R | ↑ SIRT1, Bcl-2, SDH, COX<br>↓ Bax, CK, LDH | [132] |
| | STZ-induced diabetic rats | ↓ MDA, hypertrophy, fibrosis, ventricular dysfunction<br>↑ GSH-Px | [203] |

207

Table 2. Cont.

| Polyphenol | In Vivo Model | Protective Effects | Ref. |
|---|---|---|---|
| Curcumin + nebivolol | Rats treated with DOX | ↑ Survival rate, SOD, GSH-Px, Body and heart weights; ↓ Cardiac damage, lipid peroxidation, NO; ↓ QT and ST intervals | [204] |
| Oleuropein | Rats treated with DOX | ↓ CK, CK-MB, LDH, ALT, AST, apoptosis; ↓ MDA, protein carbonyl, nitrotyrosine, iNOS | [205,206] |
| Silymarin | Rats treated with DOX | ↓ CK, LDH, creatinine, urea, MDA; ↑ GSH | [207] |
| | Rats treated with cisplatin | ↓ LDH, CK, CK-MB, cTnI, MDA; ↑ GSH, SOD | [209] |
| | Mice treated with acrolein | ↓ Lipid peroxidation, apoptosis, MDA, cTnI, CK-MB; ↑ GSH, SOD, CAT | [210] |
| Silibinin | Rats treated with arsenic | ↑ Cardiac function, Nrf-2, HO-1; ↑ SOD, CAT, GSH-Px, GST, GR, G6PD; ↓ CK-MB, LDH, AST, ALT, ALP, HW/BW | [211] |
| Clinopodium chinense (Benth.) O. Ktze (TFCC) | Rats treated with DOX | ↑ Body and heart weights; ↓ CK, AST, LDH, MDA, apoptosis; ↑ SOD, CAT, GSH-Px | [147] |

Abbreviations: ↑: increase. ↓: decrease; DOX: doxorubicin; ROS: reactive oxygen species; SOD: superoxide dismutase; MMP: metalloproteinase; CK-MB: creatin kinase-MB; LDH: lactate dehydrogenase; ALT: alanine aminotransferase; cTn: cardiac troponin; CAT: catalase; GR: glutathione reductase; GSH-Px: glutathione peroxidase; TAC: transverse aortic constriction; MDA: malondialdehyde; HNE: 4-hydroxy-2-nonenal; ANP: atrial natriuretic peptide; BNP: brain natriuretic peptide; ERK: extracellular signal-regulated kinase; JNK: c-jun N-terminal kinase; DiOHF: 3′,4′-dihydroxyflavonol; I/R: ischemia/reperfusion; LVDP: left ventricular end diastolic pressure; GSH: glutathione; AST: aspartate aminotransferase; GSSG: glutathione disulfide; MnSOD: manganese superoxide dismutase; EGCG: (−)-epigallocatechin-3-gallate; IL: interleukin; GCL: glutamate cysteine ligase; QR: quinone reductase; Cyt: cytochrome; GST: glutathione s-transferase; GSP: grape seed proanthocyanidins; ALP: alkaline phosphatase; G6PD: glucose-6-phosphate dehydrogenase; BAE: blueberry anthocyanins-enriched extracts; CTX: cyclophosphamide; HFD/STZ: high fat diet/streptozotocin; Ang II: angiotensin II; HW/BW: heart weight/body weight ratio; LVW/BW: left ventricular weight/body weight ratio; MPO: myeloperoxidase; TNF-α: tumor necrosis factor-α; COX: cyclooxygenase; HO-1: heme oxygenase-1; NQO-1: NAD(P)H:quinone oxidoreductase 1; GCLC: glutamate cysteine ligase catalytic subunit; NO: nitric oxide; iNOS: inducible nitric oxide sinthase; LAD: left anterior descending; SHR: spontaneously hypertensive rats; SIRT1: sirtuin 1; LVSP: left ventricular systolic pressure; SERCA: sarcoplasmic reticulum Ca$^{2+}$ ATPase; Nrf2: nuclear factor erythroid 2-related factor 2; CRP: C reactive protein; SDH: succinate dehydrogenase.

## 6. Evidence from Human Studies

Although human studies are not the main focus of this review and have been reviewed elsewhere [153,212,213], a short section of results from clinical trials is reported. This section might help to understand whether in vitro and in vivo results obtained in experimental models can be mimicked in humans. Many human studies have investigated the potential effects of polyphenols, such as cocoa-, olive-, tea-, grape-contained polyphenols, in cardiovascular diseases [212]. Recently, it has been reported that resveratrol intake (10 mg resveratrol capsule, per day for 3 months) reduced LDL, platelet aggregation and improved endothelial function and vasodilation in 40 patients with coronary artery disease [214]. In another study, resveratrol (400 mg, daily, for one month) reduced the expression of ICAM-1, VCAM-1, IL-8 and mRNA of inflammatory and adhesion molecules in 44 healthy subjects. The inflammatory markers are related with atherosclerosis and oxidative stress. Thus, resveratrol intake could represents a preventive measure for the onset of atherosclerosis [215].

Zunino et al. investigated the effects of dietary grapes in a randomized, double-blind crossover study in 24 obese human subjects. The obesity is associated with a major risk of cardiovascular diseases. The authors reported that dietary grape powder supplementation (46 g, two times per day for 3 weeks) reduced the plasma concentration of LDL and increased the production of IL-1β and IL-6 in supernatants from lipopolysaccharide-activated peripheral blood mononuclear cells (PBMCs) [216]. Zern et al. observed that the grape powder supplementation (36 g, per day for 4 weeks) showed an improvement in plasma lipids, inflammatory cytokines, and oxidative stress in 24 pre- and 20 post-menopausal women. This trial suggested that grape powder can influence the expression of key risk factors for coronary heart disease in pre- and post-menopausal women [217]. Vaisman and Niv showed that red grape cell powder consumption (200 or 400 mg, per day for 12 weeks) improved the endothelial function, diastolic blood pressure and reduced oxidative stress without adverse effects in 50 subjects with pre-hypertension and mild hypertension [218]. However, several randomized placebo-controlled trials did not show differences between placebo and treated groups [212]. For example, in a double-blind, randomized crossover trial, Mellen and colleagues reported that the muscadine grape seed supplementation (1300 mg, per day for 4 weeks) did not improve endothelial function, blood pressure or did not change the plasma markers of cardiovascular risk in 50 subjects with increased cardiovascular risk [219].

Several studies reported the improvement of blood pressure after cocoa intake, in particular dark chocolate, in hypertensive subjects and with endothelial dysfunction. It has been reported that flavanol-enriched cocoa drink increased the levels of NO and NOS activity by improving the endothelial dysfunction. But some trials did not show this effects both in short treatments and in supplementation of one year with 27 g flavonoid-enriched chocolate [212].

Overall, the conclusions that may be drawn from clinical trials are much different from in vitro and in vivo studies. Indeed, results from human trials employing polyphenols showed a controversial response [212].

## 7. Limitations of the Polyphenols Studies

Overall, although in vitro studies were necessary to determine the polyphenols effective dose and their mechanism of action, they have some limitations. One of the major drawback of in vitro studies is the use of polyphenols in the aglycones form or in coniugation with sugar moieties and not the use of the active metabolites. In addition, the effective doses were much higher than the concentrations that can be reached in humans. Accordingly, the in vitro results must be carefully decoded.

The results obtained from in vivo studies also have some limitations. Indeed, the majority of the information regarding the metabolism and distribution of polyphenols in target tissues is the results of animal studies. However, the metabolism, the genome, the physiology and colonic microflora of animals are much different from those of humans. Accordingly, these results are needed to be carefully translated in humans. In addition, a variety of employed animal models does not mimic the progression of the human disease.

The controversial results obtained from human trials might reflect these drawbacks and further be amplified by the human inter-individual variability in the colonic microflora composition that might affect the absorption and the production of the polyphenol active metabolites. In addition, the number of participants in many human studies might be too low and the observation time too short for obtaining an unbeatable result.

Finally, a better knowledge of polyphenols interaction is required for understanding the polyphenols beneficial effects observed in epidemiological studies.

## 8. Conclusions

Polyphenols possess many biological activities, including anti-oxidant, anti-inflammatory, anti-microbial, anti-viral and anti-cancer properties. Several epidemiological studies have shown a relation between a diet rich in polyphenols and the prevention of various human diseases.

Cardiovascular diseases are the mainly cause of mortality and morbidity in the world. Overall, several in vitro and in vivo studies demonstrated the ability of polyphenols to counteract oxidative stress-induced cardiomyocytes damage and death. Polyphenols exert long-lasting effects compared to other direct anti-oxidant agents, because they induce a transcription-mediated signaling, thus activating endogenous anti-oxidant enzymatic defense systems.

In light of the results from in vitro, in vivo and in some clinical trials, and of the activity of polyphenols in the regulation of oxidative stress and inflammation, polyphenols could be useful for the design of novel agents for the treatment of cardiovascular diseases [213]. However, it is necessary a better understanding of the reason why not all individuals show cardiovascular benefits after administration with dietary polyphenols. This knowledge is essential for the universal and definite acceptance of the clinical usefulness of polyphenols in cardiovascular disease.

**Acknowledgments:** This study was supported by a grant from Italian Ministry of Defence, (GREAM project). Rosanna Mattera is a recipient of the Sapienza PhD program in Molecular Medicine.

**Author Contributions:** All authors of this paper have directly participated in the planning or drafting of this manuscript and have read and approved the final version submitted.

**Conflicts of Interest:** The authors declare no conflict of interest.

## References

1. Townsend, N.; Wilson, L.; Bhatnagar, P.; Wickramasinghe, K.; Rayner, M.; Nichols, M. Cardiovascular disease in Europe: Epidemiological update 2016. *Eur. Heart J.* **2016**, *37*, 3232–3245. [CrossRef] [PubMed]
2. Zhou, S.; Sun, W.; Zhang, Z.; Zheng, Y. The role of Nrf2-mediated pathway in cardiac remodeling and heart failure. *Oxid. Med. Cell. Longev.* **2014**, *2014*, 260429. [CrossRef] [PubMed]
3. Ball, A.M.; Sole, M.J. Oxidative stress and the pathogenesis of heart failure. *Cardiol. Clin.* **1998**, *16*, 665–675. [CrossRef]
4. Dhalla, N.S.; Temsah, R.M.; Netticadan, T. Role of oxidative stress in cardiovascular diseases. *J. Hypertens.* **2000**, *18*, 655–673. [CrossRef] [PubMed]
5. Braunersreuther, V.; Jaquet, V. Reactive oxygen species in myocardial reperfusion injury: From physiopathology to therapeutic approaches. *Curr. Pharm. Biotechnol.* **2012**, *13*, 97–114. [CrossRef] [PubMed]
6. Takimoto, E.; Kass, D.A. Role of oxidative stress in cardiac hypertrophy and remodeling. *Hypertension* **2007**, *49*, 241–248. [CrossRef] [PubMed]
7. Granger, D.N.; Kvietys, P.R. Reperfusion injury and reactive oxygen species: The evolution of a concept. *Redox Biol.* **2015**, *6*, 524–551. [CrossRef] [PubMed]
8. Walters, J.W.; Amos, D.; Ray, K.; Santanam, N. Mitochondrial redox status as a target for cardiovascular disease. *Curr. Opin. Pharmacol.* **2016**, *27*, 50–55. [CrossRef] [PubMed]
9. Giordano, F.J. Oxygen, oxidative stress, hypoxia, and heart failure. *J. Clin. Investig.* **2005**, *115*, 500–508. [CrossRef] [PubMed]

10. Sabri, A.; Hughie, H.H.; Lucchesi, P.A. Regulation of hypertrophic and apoptotic signaling pathways by reactive oxygen species in cardiac myocytes. *Antioxid. Redox Signal.* **2003**, *5*, 731–740. [CrossRef] [PubMed]

11. Vauzour, D.; Rodriguez-Mateos, A.; Corona, G.; Oruna-Concha, M.J.; Spencer, J.P. Polyphenols and human health: Prevention of disease and mechanisms of action. *Nutrients* **2010**, *2*, 1106–1131. [CrossRef] [PubMed]

12. Scalbert, A.; Manach, C.; Morand, C.; Rémésy, C.; Jiménez, L. Dietary polyphenols and the prevention of diseases. *Crit. Rev. Food Sci. Nutr.* **2005**, *45*, 287–306. [CrossRef] [PubMed]

13. Manach, C.; Scalbert, A.; Morand, C.; Rémésy, C.; Jiménez, L. Polyphenols: Food sources and bioavailability. *Am. J. Clin. Nutr.* **2004**, *79*, 727–747. [PubMed]

14. Benvenuto, M.; Fantini, M.; Masuelli, L.; De Smaele, E.; Zazzeroni, F.; Tresoldi, I.; Calabrese, G.; Galvano, F.; Modesti, A.; Bei, R. Inhibition of ErbB receptors, Hedgehog and NF-kappaB signaling by polyphenols in cancer. *Front. Biosci.* **2013**, *18*, 1290–1310. [CrossRef]

15. Fantini, M.; Benvenuto, M.; Masuelli, L.; Frajese, G.V.; Tresoldi, I.; Modesti, A.; Bei, R. In vitro and in vivo antitumoral effects of combinations of polyphenols, or polyphenols and anticancer drugs: Perspectives on cancer treatment. *Int. J. Mol. Sci.* **2015**, *16*, 9236–9282. [CrossRef] [PubMed]

16. Benvenuto, M.; Mattera, R.; Taffera, G.; Giganti, M.G.; Lido, P.; Masuelli, L.; Modesti, A.; Bei, R. The potential protective effects of polyphenols in asbestos-mediated inflammation and carcinogenesis of mesothelium. *Nutrients* **2016**, *8*, E275. [CrossRef] [PubMed]

17. Marzocchella, L.; Fantini, M.; Benvenuto, M.; Masuelli, L.; Tresoldi, I.; Modesti, A.; Bei, R. Dietary flavonoids: molecular mechanisms of action as anti-inflammatory agents. *Recent Pat. Inflamm. Allergy Drug Discov.* **2011**, *5*, 200–220. [CrossRef] [PubMed]

18. Stedile, N.; Canuto, R.; Col, C.D.; Sene, J.S.; Stolfo, A.; Wisintainer, G.N.; Henriques, J.A.; Salvador, M. Dietary total antioxidant capacity is associated with plasmatic antioxidant capacity, nutrient intake and lipid and DNA damage in healthy women. *Int. J. Food Sci. Nutr.* **2016**, *67*, 479–488. [CrossRef] [PubMed]

19. Izzi, V.; Masuelli, L.; Tresoldi, I.; Sacchetti, P.; Modesti, A.; Galvano, F.; Bei, R. The effects of dietary flavonoids on the regulation of redox inflammatory networks. *Front. Biosci. (Landmark Ed.)* **2012**, *17*, 2396–2418. [CrossRef] [PubMed]

20. Grosso, G.; Micek, A.; Godos, J.; Pajak, A.; Sciacca, S.; Galvano, F.; Giovannucci, E.L. Dietary flavonoid and lignan intake and mortality in prospective cohort studies: Systematic review and dose-response meta-analysis. *Am. J. Epidemiol.* **2017**, 1–13. [CrossRef] [PubMed]

21. Grosso, G.; Godos, J.; Lamuela-Raventos, R.; Ray, S.; Micek, A.; Pajak, A.; Sciacca, S.; D'Orazio, N.; Del Rio, D.; Galvano, F. A comprehensive meta-analysis on dietary flavonoid and lignan intake and cancer risk: Level of evidence and limitations. *Mol. Nutr. Food Res.* **2017**, *61*. [CrossRef] [PubMed]

22. Yordi, E.G.; Pérez, E.M.; Matos, M.J.; Villares, E.U. Antioxidant and pro-oxidant effects of polyphenolic compounds and structure-activity relationship evidence. In *Nutrition, Well-Being and Health*; Bouayed, J., Bohn, T., Eds.; InTech: Rijeka, Croatia, 2012; Chapter 2; pp. 23–48.

23. Halliwell, B. Are polyphenols antioxidants or pro-oxidants? What do we learn from cell culture and in vivo studies? *Arch. Biochem. Biophys.* **2008**, *476*, 107–112. [CrossRef] [PubMed]

24. Stevenson, D.E.; Hurst, R.D. Polyphenolic phytochemicals-just antioxidants or much more? *Cell. Mol. Life Sci.* **2007**, *64*, 2900–2916. [CrossRef] [PubMed]

25. Chiva-Blanch, G.; Visioli, F. Polyphenols and health: Moving beyond antioxidants. *J. Berry Res.* **2012**, *2*, 63–71.

26. Forman, H.J.; Davies, K.J.; Ursini, F. How do nutritional antioxidants really work: Nucleophilic tone and para-hormesis versus free radical scavenging in vivo. *Free Radic. Biol. Med.* **2014**, *66*, 24–35. [CrossRef] [PubMed]

27. Mattson, M.P. Dietary factors, hormesis and health. *Ageing Res. Rev.* **2008**, *7*, 43–48. [CrossRef] [PubMed]

28. Visioli, F. Xenobiotics and human health: A new view of their pharma-nutritional role. *PharmaNutrition* **2015**, *3*, 60–64. [CrossRef]

29. Calabrese, V.; Cornelius, C.; Dinkova-Kostova, A.T.; Iavicoli, I.; Di Paola, R.; Koverech, A.; Cuzzocrea, S.; Rizzarelli, E.; Calabrese, E.J. Cellular stress responses, hormetic phytochemicals and vitagenes in aging and longevity. *Biochim. Biophys. Acta* **2012**, *1822*, 753–783. [CrossRef] [PubMed]

30. Crespo, M.C.; Tomé-Carneiro, J.; Burgos-Ramos, E.; Loria Kohen, V.; Espinosa, M.I.; Herranz, J.; Visioli, F. One-week administration of hydroxytyrosol to humans does not activate Phase II enzymes. *Pharmacol. Res.* **2015**, *95–96*, 132–137. [CrossRef] [PubMed]

31. Schiano, C.; Vietri, M.T.; Grimaldi, V.; Picascia, A.; De Pascale, M.R.; Napoli, C. Epigenetic-related therapeutic challenges in cardiovascular disease. *Trends Pharmacol. Sci.* **2015**, *36*, 226–235. [CrossRef] [PubMed]

32. Bladé, C.; Baselga-Escudero, L.; Salvadó, M.J.; Arola-Arnal, A. miRNAs, polyphenols, and chronic disease. *Mol. Nutr. Food Res.* **2013**, *57*, 58–70. [CrossRef] [PubMed]

33. Vaiserman, A.M. Hormesis and epigenetics: Is there a link? *Ageing Res. Rev.* **2011**, *10*, 413–421. [CrossRef] [PubMed]

34. Pan, M.H.; Lai, C.S.; Wu, J.C.; Ho, C.T. Epigenetic and disease targets by polyphenols. *Curr. Pharm. Des.* **2013**, *19*, 6156–6185. [CrossRef] [PubMed]

35. Russo, G.L.; Vastolo, V.; Ciccarelli, M.; Albano, L.; Macchia, P.E.; Ungaro, P. Dietary polyphenols and chromatin remodelling. *Crit. Rev. Food Sci. Nutr.* **2015**. [CrossRef]

36. Chistiakov, D.A.; Orekhov, A.N.; Bobryshev, Y.V. Treatment of cardiovascular pathology with epigenetically active agents: Focus on natural and synthetic inhibitors of DNA methylation and histone deacetylation. *Int. J. Cardiol.* **2017**, *227*, 66–82. [CrossRef] [PubMed]

37. Wojtala, M.; Pirola, L.; Balcerczyk, A. Modulation of the vascular endothelium functioning by dietary components, the role of epigenetics. *Biofactors* **2017**, *43*, 5–16. [CrossRef] [PubMed]

38. Wang, R.; Li, N.; Zhang, Y.; Ran, Y.; Pu, J. Circulating microRNAs are promising novel biomarkers of acute myocardial infarction. *Intern. Med.* **2011**, *50*, 1789–1795. [CrossRef] [PubMed]

39. D'Alessandra, Y.; Devanna, P.; Limana, F.; Straino, S.; di Carlo, A.; Brambilla, P.G.; Rubino, M.; Carena, M.C.; Spazzafumo, L.; de Simone, M.; et al. Circulating microRNAs are new and sensitive biomarkers of myocardial infarction. *Eur. Heart J.* **2010**, *31*, 2765–2773. [CrossRef] [PubMed]

40. Menghini, R.; Casagrande, V.; Cardellini, M.; Martelli, E.; Terrinoni, A.; Amati, F.; Vasa-Nicotera, M.; Ippoliti, A.; Novelli, G.; Melino, G.; et al. MicroRNA 217 modulates endothelial cell senescence via silent information regulator 1. *Circulation* **2009**, *120*, 1524–1532. [CrossRef] [PubMed]

41. Fichtlscherer, S.; De, R.S.; Fox, H.; Schwietz, T.; Fischer, A.; Liebetrau, C.; Weber, M.; Hamm, C.W.; Röxe, T.; Müller-Ardogan, M.; et al. Circulating microRNAs in patients with coronary artery disease. *Circ. Res.* **2010**, *107*, 677–684. [CrossRef] [PubMed]

42. Visioli, F.; Davalos, A. Polyphenols and cardiovascular disease: A critical summary of the evidence. *Mini Rev. Med. Chem.* **2011**, *11*, 1186–1190. [CrossRef] [PubMed]

43. Mukhopadhyay, P.; Mukherjee, S.; Ahsan, K.; Bagchi, A.; Pacher, P.; Das, D.K. Restoration of altered microRNA expression in the ischemic heart with resveratrol. *PLoS ONE* **2010**, *5*, e15705. [CrossRef] [PubMed]

44. Angeloni, C.; Leoncini, E.; Malaguti, M.; Angelini, S.; Hrelia, P.; Hrelia, S. Role of quercetin in modulating rat cardiomyocyte gene expression profile. *Am. J. Physiol. Heart Circ. Physiol.* **2008**, *294*, H1233–H1243. [CrossRef] [PubMed]

45. Daubney, J.; Bonner, P.L.; Hargreaves, A.J.; Dickenson, J.M. Cardioprotective and cardiotoxic effects of quercetin and two of its in vivo metabolites on differentiated H9c2 cardiomyocytes. *Basic Clin. Pharmacol. Toxicol.* **2015**, *116*, 96–109. [CrossRef] [PubMed]

46. Park, E.S.; Kang, J.C.; Jang, Y.C.; Park, J.S.; Jang, S.Y.; Kim, D.E.; Kim, B.; Shin, H.S. Cardioprotective effects of rhamnetin in H9c2 cardiomyoblast cells under $H_2O_2$-induced apoptosis. *J. Ethnopharmacol.* **2014**, *153*, 552–560. [CrossRef] [PubMed]

47. Thomas, C.J.; Lim, N.R.; Kedikaetswe, A.; Yeap, Y.Y.; Woodman, O.L.; Ng, D.C.; May, C.N. Evidence that the MEK/ERK but not the PI3K/Akt pathway is required for protection from myocardial ischemia-reperfusion injury by 3′,4′-dihydroxyflavonol. *Eur. J. Pharmacol.* **2015**, *758*, 53–59. [CrossRef] [PubMed]

48. Dong, Q.; Chen, L.; Lu, Q.; Sharma, S.; Li, L.; Morimoto, S.; Wang, G. Quercetin attenuates doxorubicin cardiotoxicity by modulating Bmi-1 expression. *Br. J. Pharmacol.* **2014**, *171*, 4440–4454. [CrossRef] [PubMed]

49. Sun, J.; Sun, G.; Meng, X.; Wang, H.; Luo, Y.; Qin, M.; Ma, B.; Wang, M.; Cai, D.; Guo, P.; et al. Isorhamnetin protects against doxorubicin-induced cardiotoxicity in vivo and in vitro. *PLoS ONE* **2013**, *8*, e64526. [CrossRef] [PubMed]

50. Xiao, J.; Sun, G.B.; Sun, B.; Wu, Y.; He, L.; Wang, X.; Chen, R.C.; Cao, L.; Ren, X.Y.; Sun, X.B. Kaempferol protects against doxorubicin-induced cardiotoxicity in vivo and in vitro. *Toxicology* **2012**, *292*, 53–62. [CrossRef] [PubMed]

51. Zhu, H.; Luo, P.; Fu, Y.; Wang, J.; Dai, J.; Shao, J.; Yang, X.; Chang, L.; Weng, Q.; Yang, B.; et al. Dihydromyricetin prevents cardiotoxicity and enhances anticancer activity induced by adriamycin. *Oncotarget* **2015**, *6*, 3254–3267. [CrossRef] [PubMed]

52. Jing, Z.; Wang, Z.; Li, X.; Li, X.; Cao, T.; Bi, Y.; Zhou, J.; Chen, X.; Yu, D.; Zhu, L.; et al. Protective effect of quercetin on posttraumatic cardiac injury. *Sci. Rep.* **2016**, *6*, 30812. [CrossRef] [PubMed]

53. Tang, L.; Peng, Y.; Xu, T.; Yi, X.; Liu, Y.; Luo, Y.; Yin, D.; He, M. The effects of quercetin protect cardiomyocytes from A/R injury is related to its capability to increasing expression and activity of PKCε protein. *Mol. Cell. Biochem.* **2013**, *382*, 145–152. [CrossRef] [PubMed]

54. Guo, Z.; Liao, Z.; Huang, L.; Liu, D.; Yin, D.; He, M. Kaempferol protects cardiomyocytes against anoxia/reoxygenation injury via mitochondrial pathway mediated by SIRT1. *Eur. J. Pharmacol.* **2015**, *761*, 245–253. [CrossRef] [PubMed]

55. Wang, S.; Dusting, G.J.; May, C.N.; Woodman, O.L. 3′,4′-Dihydroxyflavonol reduces infarct size and injury associated with myocardial ischaemia and reperfusion in sheep. *Br. J. Pharmacol.* **2004**, *142*, 443–452. [CrossRef] [PubMed]

56. Guo, H.; Zhang, X.; Cui, Y.; Zhou, H.; Xu, D.; Shan, T.; Zhang, F.; Guo, Y.; Chen, Y.; Wu, D. Taxifolin protects against cardiac hypertrophy and fibrosis during biomechanical stress of pressure overload. *Toxicol. Appl. Pharmacol.* **2015**, *287*, 168–177. [CrossRef] [PubMed]

57. Ozbek, N.; Bali, E.B.; Karasu, C. Quercetin and hydroxytyrosol attenuates xanthine/xanthine oxidase-induced toxicity in H9c2 cardiomyocytes by regulation of oxidative stress and stress-sensitive signaling pathways. *Gen. Physiol. Biophys.* **2015**, *34*, 407–414. [CrossRef] [PubMed]

58. Chen, C.; He, H.; Luo, Y.; Zhou, M.; Yin, D.; He, M. Involvement of Bcl-2 signal pathway in the protective effects of apigenin on anoxia/reoxygenation-induced myocardium injury. *J. Cardiovasc. Pharmacol.* **2016**, *67*, 152–163. [CrossRef] [PubMed]

59. Dong, L.Y.; Chen, Z.W.; Guo, Y.; Cheng, X.P.; Shao, X. Mechanisms of vitexin preconditioning effects on cultured neonatal rat cardiomyocytes with anoxia and reoxygenation. *Am. J. Chin. Med.* **2008**, *36*, 385–397. [CrossRef] [PubMed]

60. Dong, L.; Fan, Y.; Shao, X.; Chen, Z. Vitexin protects against myocardial ischemia/reperfusion injury in Langendorff-perfused rat hearts by attenuating inflammatory response and apoptosis. *Food Chem. Toxicol.* **2011**, *49*, 3211–3216. [CrossRef] [PubMed]

61. Shao, Z.H.; Vanden Hoek, T.L.; Qin, Y.; Becker, L.B.; Schumacker, P.T.; Li, C.Q.; Dey, L.; Barth, E.; Halpern, H.; Rosen, G.M.; et al. Baicalein attenuates oxidant stress in cardiomyocytes. *Am. J. Physiol. Heart Circ. Physiol.* **2002**, *282*, H999–H1006. [CrossRef] [PubMed]

62. Cui, G.; Luk, S.C.; Li, R.A.; Chan, K.K.; Lei, S.W.; Wang, L.; Shen, H.; Leung, G.P.; Lee, S.M. Cytoprotection of baicalein against oxidative stress-induced cardiomyocytes injury through the Nrf2/Keap1 pathway. *J. Cardiovasc. Pharmacol.* **2015**, *65*, 39–46. [CrossRef] [PubMed]

63. Chang, W.T.; Li, J.; Vanden Hoek, M.S.; Zhu, X.; Li, C.Q.; Huang, H.H.; Hsu, C.W.; Zhong, Q.; Li, J.; Chen, S.J.; et al. Baicalein preconditioning protects cardiomyocytes from ischemia-reperfusion injury via mitochondrial oxidant signaling. *Am. J. Chin. Med.* **2013**, *41*, 315–331. [CrossRef] [PubMed]

64. Tu, I.H.; Yen, H.T.; Cheng, H.W.; Chiu, J.H. Baicalein protects chicken embryonic cardiomyocyte against hypoxia-reoxygenation injury via mu- and delta- but not kappa-opioid receptor signaling. *Eur. J. Pharmacol.* **2008**, *588*, 251–258. [CrossRef] [PubMed]

65. Dreger, H.; Lorenz, M.; Kehrer, A.; Baumann, G.; Stangl, K.; Stangl, V. Characteristics of catechin- and theaflavin-mediated cardioprotection. *Exp. Biol. Med. (Maywood)* **2008**, *233*, 427–433. [CrossRef] [PubMed]

66. Hsieh, S.R.; Hsu, C.S.; Lu, C.H.; Chen, W.C.; Chiu, C.H.; Liou, Y.M. Epigallocatechin-3-gallate-mediated cardioprotection by Akt/GSK-3β/caveolin signalling in H9c2 rat cardiomyoblasts. *J. Biomed. Sci.* **2013**, *20*, 86. [CrossRef] [PubMed]

67. Sheng, R.; Gu, Z.L.; Xie, M.L.; Zhou, W.X.; Guo, C.Y. EGCG inhibits cardiomyocyte apoptosis in pressure overload-induced cardiac hypertrophy and protects cardiomyocytes from oxidative stress in rats. *Acta Pharmacol. Sin.* **2007**, *28*, 191–201. [CrossRef] [PubMed]

68. Sheng, R.; Gu, Z.L.; Xie, M.L.; Zhou, W.X.; Guo, C.Y. Epigallocatechin gallate protects H9c2 cardiomyoblasts against hydrogen dioxides- induced apoptosis and telomere attrition. *Eur. J. Pharmacol.* **2010**, *641*, 199–206. [CrossRef] [PubMed]

69. Li, W.; Nie, S.; Xie, M.; Chen, Y.; Li, C.; Zhang, H. A major green tea component, (−)-epigallocatechin-3-gallate, ameliorates doxorubicin-mediated cardiotoxicity in cardiomyocytes of neonatal rats. *J. Agric. Food Chem.* **2010**, *58*, 8977–8982. [CrossRef] [PubMed]

70. Zheng, J.; Lee, H.C.; Bin Sattar, M.M.; Huang, Y.; Bian, J.S. Cardioprotective effects of epigallocatechin-3-gallate against doxorubicin-induced cardiomyocyte injury. *Eur. J. Pharmacol.* **2011**, *652*, 82–88. [CrossRef] [PubMed]

71. Li, J.; Liu, H.; Ramachandran, S.; Waypa, G.B.; Yin, J.J.; Li, C.Q.; Han, M.; Huang, H.H.; Sillard, W.W.; Vanden Hoek, T.L.; et al. Grape seed proanthocyanidins ameliorate Doxorubicin-induced cardiotoxicity. *Am. J. Chin. Med.* **2010**, *38*, 569–584. [CrossRef] [PubMed]

72. Townsend, P.A.; Scarabelli, T.M.; Pasini, E.; Gitti, G.; Menegazzi, M.; Suzuki, H.; Knight, R.A.; Latchman, D.S.; Stephanou, A. Epigallocatechin-3-gallate inhibits STAT-1 activation and protects cardiac myocytes from ischemia/reperfusion-induced apoptosis. *FASEB J.* **2004**, *18*, 1621–1623. [CrossRef] [PubMed]

73. Shao, Z.H.; Wojcik, K.R.; Dossumbekova, A.; Hsu, C.; Mehendale, S.R.; Li, C.Q.; Qin, Y.; Sharp, W.W.; Chang, W.T.; Hamann, K.J.; et al. Grape seed proanthocyanidins protect cardiomyocytes from ischemia and reperfusion injury via Akt-NOS signaling. *J. Cell. Biochem.* **2009**, *107*, 697–705. [CrossRef] [PubMed]

74. Hirai, M.; Hotta, Y.; Ishikawa, N.; Wakida, Y.; Fukuzawa, Y.; Isobe, F.; Nakano, A.; Chiba, T.; Kawamura, N. Protective effects of EGCg or GCg, a green tea catechin epimer, against postischemic myocardial dysfunction in guinea-pig hearts. *Life Sci.* **2007**, *80*, 1020–1032. [CrossRef] [PubMed]

75. Wei, H.; Meng, Z. Epigallocatechin-3-gallate protects Na+ channels in rat ventricular myocytes against sulfite. *Cardiovasc. Toxicol.* **2010**, *10*, 166–173. [CrossRef] [PubMed]

76. Wei, H.; Meng, Z. Protective effects of epigallocatechin-3-gallate against lead-induced oxidative damage. *Hum. Exp. Toxicol.* **2011**, *30*, 1521–1528. [CrossRef] [PubMed]

77. Kim, J.A.; Jung, Y.S.; Kim, M.Y.; Yang, S.Y.; Lee, S.; Kim, Y.H. Protective effect of components isolated from Lindera erythrocarpa against oxidative stress-induced apoptosis of H9c2 cardiomyocytes. *Phytother. Res.* **2011**, *25*, 1612–1617. [CrossRef] [PubMed]

78. Quintieri, A.M.; Baldino, N.; Filice, E.; Seta, L.; Vitetti, A.; Tota, B.; de Cindio, B.; Cerra, M.C.; Angelone, T. Malvidin, a red wine polyphenol, modulates mammalian myocardial and coronary performance and protects the heart against ischemia/reperfusion injury. *J. Nutr. Biochem.* **2013**, *24*, 1221–1231. [CrossRef] [PubMed]

79. Škėmienė, K.; Jablonskienė, G.; Liobikas, J.; Borutaitė, V. Protecting the heart against ischemia/reperfusion-induced necrosis and apoptosis: The effect of anthocyanins. *Medicina (Kaunas)* **2013**, *49*, 84–88. [PubMed]

80. Louis, X.L.; Thandapilly, S.J.; Kalt, W.; Vinqvist-Tymchuk, M.; Aloud, B.M.; Raj, P.; Yu, L.; Le, H.; Netticadan, T. Blueberry polyphenols prevent cardiomyocyte death by preventing calpain activation and oxidative stress. *Food Funct.* **2014**, *5*, 1785–1794. [CrossRef] [PubMed]

81. Ramprasath, T.; Senthamizharasi, M.; Vasudevan, V.; Sasikumar, S.; Yuvaraj, S.; Selvam, G.S. Naringenin confers protection against oxidative stress through upregulation of Nrf2 target genes in cardiomyoblast cells. *J. Physiol. Biochem.* **2014**, *70*, 407–415. [CrossRef] [PubMed]

82. Huang, H.; Wu, K.; You, Q.; Huang, R.; Li, S.; Wu, K. Naringin inhibits high glucose-induced cardiomyocyte apoptosis by attenuating mitochondrial dysfunction and modulating the activation of the p38 signaling pathway. *Int. J. Mol. Med.* **2013**, *32*, 396–402. [CrossRef] [PubMed]

83. Chen, J.; Guo, R.; Yan, H.; Tian, L.; You, Q.; Li, S.; Huang, R.; Wu, K. Naringin inhibits ROS-activated MAPK pathway in high glucose-induced injuries in H9c2 cardiac cells. *Basic Clin. Pharmacol. Toxicol.* **2014**, *114*, 293–304. [CrossRef] [PubMed]

84. Chen, J.; Mo, H.; Guo, R.; You, Q.; Huang, R.; Wu, K. Inhibition of the leptin-induced activation of the p38 MAPK pathway contributes to the protective effects of naringin against high glucose-induced injury in H9c2 cardiac cells. *Int. J. Mol. Med.* **2014**, *33*, 605–612. [CrossRef] [PubMed]

85. Chen, R.C.; Sun, G.B.; Wang, J.; Zhang, H.J.; Sun, X.B. Naringin protects against anoxia/reoxygenation-induced apoptosis in H9c2 cells via the Nrf2 signaling pathway. *Food Funct.* **2015**, *6*, 1331–1344. [CrossRef] [PubMed]

86. Han, X.; Ren, D.; Fan, P.; Shen, T.; Lou, H. Protective effects of naringenin-7-O-glucoside on doxorubicin-induced apoptosis in H9c2 cells. *Eur. J. Pharmacol.* **2008**, *581*, 47–53. [CrossRef] [PubMed]

87. Han, X.; Pan, J.; Ren, D.; Cheng, Y.; Fan, P.; Lou, H. Naringenin-7-O-glucoside protects against doxorubicin-induced toxicity in H9c2 cardiomyocytes by induction of endogenous antioxidant enzymes. *Food Chem. Toxicol.* **2008**, *46*, 3140–3146. [CrossRef] [PubMed]

88. Han, X.Z.; Gao, S.; Cheng, Y.N.; Sun, Y.Z.; Liu, W.; Tang, L.L.; Ren, D.M. Protective effect of naringenin-7-O-glucoside against oxidative stress induced by doxorubicin in H9c2 cardiomyocytes. *Biosci. Trends* **2012**, *6*, 19–25. [CrossRef] [PubMed]

89. Yang, Z.; Liu, Y.; Deng, W.; Dai, J.; Li, F.; Yuan, Y.; Wu, Q.; Zhou, H.; Bian, Z.; Tang, Q. Hesperetin attenuates mitochondria-dependent apoptosis in lipopolysaccharide-induced H9c2 cardiomyocytes. *Mol. Med. Rep.* **2014**, *9*, 1941–1946. [CrossRef] [PubMed]

90. Gang, C.; Qiang, C.; Xiangli, C.; Shifen, P.; Chong, S.; Lihong, L. Puerarin suppresses angiotensin II-induced cardiac hypertrophy by inhibiting NADPH oxidase activation and oxidative stress-triggered AP-1 signaling pathways. *J. Pharm. Pharm. Sci.* **2015**, *18*, 235–248. [CrossRef] [PubMed]

91. Liu, B.; Zhang, J.; Liu, W.; Liu, N.; Fu, X.; Kwan, H.; Liu, S.; Liu, B.; Zhang, S.; Yu, Z.; et al. Calycosin inhibits oxidative stress-induced cardiomyocyte apoptosis via activating estrogen receptor-$\alpha/\beta$. *Bioorg. Med. Chem. Lett.* **2016**, *26*, 181–185. [CrossRef] [PubMed]

92. Yuan, X.; Niu, H.T.; Wang, P.L.; Lu, J.; Zhao, H.; Liu, S.H.; Zheng, Q.S.; Li, C.G. Cardioprotective effect of licochalcone D against myocardial ischemia/reperfusion injury in Langendorff-perfused rat hearts. *PLoS ONE* **2015**, *10*, e0128375. [CrossRef] [PubMed]

93. Han, J.; Wang, D.; Yu, B.; Wang, Y.; Ren, H.; Zhang, B.; Wang, Y.; Zheng, Q. Cardioprotection against ischemia/reperfusion by licochalcone B in isolated rat hearts. *Oxid. Med. Cell. Longev.* **2014**, *2014*, 134862. [CrossRef] [PubMed]

94. Zhang, X.; Zhu, P.; Zhang, X.; Ma, Y.; Li, W.; Chen, J.M.; Guo, H.M.; Bucala, R.; Zhuang, J.; Li, J. Natural antioxidant-isoliquiritigenin ameliorates contractile dysfunction of hypoxic cardiomyocytes via AMPK signaling pathway. *Mediat. Inflamm.* **2013**, *2013*, 390890. [CrossRef] [PubMed]

95. Duan, J.L.; Wang, J.W.; Guan, Y.; Yin, Y.; Wei, G.; Cui, J.; Zhou, D.; Zhu, Y.R.; Quan, W.; Xi, M.M.; et al. Safflor yellow A protects neonatal rat cardiomyocytes against anoxia/reoxygenation injury in vitro. *Acta Pharmacol. Sin.* **2013**, *34*, 487–495. [CrossRef] [PubMed]

96. Liu, S.X.; Zhang, Y.; Wang, Y.F.; Li, X.C.; Xiang, M.X.; Bian, C.; Chen, P. Upregulation of heme oxygenase-1 expression by hydroxysafflor yellow A conferring protection from anoxia/reoxygenation-induced apoptosis in H9c2 cardiomyocytes. *Int. J. Cardiol.* **2012**, *160*, 95–101. [CrossRef] [PubMed]

97. Zhong, P.; Wu, L.; Qian, Y.; Fang, Q.; Liang, D.; Wang, J.; Zeng, C.; Wang, Y.; Liang, G. Blockage of ROS and NF-κB-mediated inflammation by a new chalcone L6H9 protects cardiomyocytes from hyperglycemia-induced injuries. *Biochim. Biophys. Acta* **2015**, *1852*, 1230–1241. [CrossRef] [PubMed]

98. Dludla, P.V.; Muller, C.J.; Louw, J.; Joubert, E.; Salie, R.; Opoku, A.R.; Johnson, R. The cardioprotective effect of an aqueous extract of fermented rooibos (*Aspalathus linearis*) on cultured cardiomyocytes derived from diabetic rats. *Phytomedicine* **2014**, *21*, 595–601. [CrossRef] [PubMed]

99. Johnson, R.; Dludla, P.; Joubert, E.; February, F.; Mazibuko, S.; Ghoor, S.; Muller, C.; Louw, J. Aspalathin, a dihydrochalcone C-glucoside, protects H9c2 cardiomyocytes against high glucose induced shifts in substrate preference and apoptosis. *Mol. Nutr. Food Res.* **2016**, *60*, 922–934. [CrossRef] [PubMed]

100. Li, F.; Wu, J.H.; Wang, Q.H.; Shu, Y.L.; Wan, C.W.; Chan, C.O.; Kam-Wah Mok, D.; Chan, S.W. Gui-ling-gao, a traditional Chinese functional food, prevents oxidative stress-induced apoptosis in H9c2 cardiomyocytes. *Food Funct.* **2013**, *4*, 745–753. [CrossRef] [PubMed]

101. Chiarini, A.; Micucci, M.; Malaguti, M.; Budriesi, R.; Ioan, P.; Lenzi, M.; Fimognari, C.; Gallina Toschi, T.; Comandini, P.; Hrelia, S. Sweet chestnut (*Castanea sativa* Mill.) bark extract: Cardiovascular activity and myocyte protection against oxidative damage. *Oxid. Med. Cell Longev.* **2013**, *2013*, 471790. [CrossRef] [PubMed]

102. Kim, D.E.; Kim, B.; Shin, H.S.; Kwon, H.J.; Park, E.S. The protective effect of hispidin against hydrogen peroxide-induced apoptosis in H9c2 cardiomyoblast cells through Akt/GSK-3β and ERK1/2 signaling pathway. *Exp. Cell Res.* **2014**, *327*, 264–275. [CrossRef] [PubMed]

103. Khurana, S.; Hollingsworth, A.; Piche, M.; Venkataraman, K.; Kumar, A.; Ross, G.M.; Tai, T.C. Antiapoptotic actions of methyl gallate on neonatal rat cardiac myocytes exposed to $H_2O_2$. *Oxid. Med. Cell. Longev.* **2014**, *2014*, 657512. [CrossRef] [PubMed]

104. Ku, H.C.; Lee, S.Y.; Yang, K.C.; Kuo, Y.H.; Su, M.J. Modification of caffeic acid with pyrrolidine enhances antioxidant ability by activating AKT/HO-1 pathway in heart. *PLoS ONE* **2016**, *11*, e0148545. [CrossRef] [PubMed]

105. Song, Y.; Wen, L.; Sun, J.; Bai, W.; Jiao, R.; Hu, Y.; Peng, X.; He, Y.; Ou, S. Cytoprotective mechanism of ferulic acid against high glucose-induced oxidative stress in cardiomyocytes and hepatocytes. *Food Nutr. Res.* **2016**, *60*, 30323. [CrossRef] [PubMed]

106. Atale, N.; Gupta, K.; Rani, V. Protective effect of Syzygium cumini against pesticide-induced cardiotoxicity. *Environ. Sci. Pollut. Res. Int.* **2014**, *21*, 7956–7972. [CrossRef] [PubMed]

107. Chlopcíková, S.; Psotová, J.; Miketová, P.; Sousek, J.; Lichnovský, V.; Simánek, V. Chemoprotective effect of plant phenolics against anthracycline-induced toxicity on rat cardiomyocytes. Part II. caffeic, chlorogenic and rosmarinic acids. *Phytother. Res.* **2004**, *18*, 408–413. [CrossRef] [PubMed]

108. Yin, Y.; Guan, Y.; Duan, J.; Wei, G.; Zhu, Y.; Quan, W.; Guo, C.; Zhou, D.; Wang, Y.; Xi, M.; et al. Cardioprotective effect of Danshensu against myocardial ischemia/reperfusion injury and inhibits apoptosis of H9c2 cardiomyocytes via Akt and ERK1/2 phosphorylation. *Eur. J. Pharmacol.* **2013**, *699*, 219–226. [CrossRef] [PubMed]

109. Yu, J.; Wang, L.; Akinyi, M.; Li, Y.; Duan, Z.; Zhu, Y.; Fan, G. Danshensu protects isolated heart against ischemia reperfusion injury through activation of Akt/ERK1/2/Nrf2 signaling. *Int. J. Clin. Exp. Med.* **2015**, *8*, 14793–14804. [PubMed]

110. Chiu, P.Y.; Chen, N.; Leong, P.K.; Leung, H.Y.; Ko, K.M. Schisandrin B elicits a glutathione antioxidant response and protects against apoptosis via the redox-sensitive ERK/Nrf2 pathway in H9c2 cells. *Mol. Cell. Biochem.* **2011**, *350*, 237–250. [CrossRef] [PubMed]

111. Chen, P.; Pang, S.; Yang, N.; Meng, H.; Liu, J.; Zhou, N.; Zhang, M.; Xu, Z.; Gao, W.; Chen, B.; et al. Beneficial effects of schisandrin B on the cardiac function in mice model of myocardial infarction. *PLoS ONE* **2013**, *8*, e79418. [CrossRef] [PubMed]

112. Chang, R.; Li, Y.; Yang, X.; Yue, Y.; Dou, L.; Wang, Y.; Zhang, W.; Li, X. Protective role of deoxyschizandrin and schisantherin A against myocardial ischemia-reperfusion injury in rats. *PLoS ONE* **2013**, *8*, e61590. [CrossRef] [PubMed]

113. Cho, S.; Cho, M.; Kim, J.; Kaeberlein, M.; Lee, S.J.; Suh, Y. Syringaresinol protects against hypoxia/reoxygenation-induced cardiomyocytes injury and death by destabilization of HIF-1$\alpha$ in a FOXO3-dependent mechanism. *Oncotarget* **2015**, *6*, 43–55. [CrossRef] [PubMed]

114. Su, S.; Li, Q.; Liu, Y.; Xiong, C.; Li, J.; Zhang, R.; Niu, Y.; Zhao, L.; Wang, Y.; Guo, H. Sesamin ameliorates doxorubicin-induced cardiotoxicity: Involvement of Sirt1 and Mn-SOD pathway. *Toxicol. Lett.* **2014**, *224*, 257–263. [CrossRef] [PubMed]

115. Zheng, S.G.; Ren, Y.N.; Zhao, M.Q.; Tao, S.J.; Kong, X.; Yang, J.R. Effect of serum containing sesamin on angiotensin II-induced apoptosis in rat cardiomyocytes. *Zhong Yao Cai* **2015**, *38*, 1013–1017. [PubMed]

116. Chen, C.J.; Fu, Y.C.; Yu, W.; Wang, W. SIRT3 protects cardiomyocytes from oxidative stress-mediated cell death by activating NF-κB. *Biochem. Biophys. Res. Commun.* **2013**, *430*, 798–803. [CrossRef] [PubMed]

117. Li, Y.G.; Zhu, W.; Tao, J.P.; Xin, P.; Liu, M.Y.; Li, J.B.; Wei, M. Resveratrol protects cardiomyocytes from oxidative stress through SIRT1 and mitochondrial biogenesis signaling pathways. *Biochem. Biophys. Res. Commun.* **2013**, *438*, 270–276. [CrossRef] [PubMed]

118. Huang, C.Y.; Ting, W.J.; Huang, C.Y.; Yang, J.Y.; Lin, W.T. Resveratrol attenuated hydrogen peroxide-induced myocardial apoptosis by autophagic flux. *Food Nutr. Res.* **2016**, *60*, 30511. [CrossRef] [PubMed]

119. Movahed, A.; Yu, L.; Thandapilly, S.J.; Louis, X.L.; Netticadan, T. Resveratrol protects adult cardiomyocytes against oxidative stress mediated cell injury. *Arch. Biochem. Biophys.* **2012**, *527*, 74–80. [CrossRef] [PubMed]

120. Li, W.; Wang, Y.P.; Gao, L.; Zhang, P.P.; Zhou, Q.; Xu, Q.F.; Zhou, Z.W.; Guo, K.; Chen, R.H.; Yang, H.T.; et al. Resveratrol protects rabbit ventricular myocytes against oxidative stress-induced arrhythmogenic activity and Ca$^{2+}$ overload. *Acta Pharmacol. Sin.* **2013**, *34*, 1164–1173. [CrossRef] [PubMed]

121. Chen, C.J.; Yu, W.; Fu, Y.C.; Wang, X.; Li, J.L.; Wang, W. Resveratrol protects cardiomyocytes from hypoxia-induced apoptosis through the SIRT1-FoxO1 pathway. *Biochem. Biophys. Res. Commun.* **2009**, *378*, 389–393. [CrossRef] [PubMed]

122. Becatti, M.; Taddei, N.; Cecchi, C.; Nassi, N.; Nassi, P.A.; Fiorillo, C. SIRT1 modulates MAPK pathways in ischemic-reperfused cardiomyocytes. *Cell. Mol. Life Sci.* **2012**, *69*, 2245–2260. [CrossRef] [PubMed]

123. Danz, E.D.; Skramsted, J.; Henry, N.; Bennett, J.A.; Keller, R.S. Resveratrol prevents doxorubicin cardiotoxicity through mitochondrial stabilization and the Sirt1 pathway. *Free Radic. Biol. Med.* **2009**, *46*, 1589–1597. [CrossRef] [PubMed]

124. Gao, R.Y.; Mukhopadhyay, P.; Mohanraj, R.; Wang, H.; Horváth, B.; Yin, S.; Pacher, P. Resveratrol attenuates azidothymidine-induced cardiotoxicity by decreasing mitochondrial reactive oxygen species generation in human cardiomyocytes. *Mol. Med. Rep.* **2011**, *4*, 151–155. [CrossRef] [PubMed]

125. Zhao, X.Y.; Li, G.Y.; Liu, Y.; Chai, L.M.; Chen, J.X.; Zhang, Y.; Du, Z.M.; Lu, Y.J.; Yang, B.F. Resveratrol protects against arsenic trioxide-induced cardiotoxicity in vitro and in vivo. *Br. J. Pharmacol.* **2008**, *154*, 105–113. [CrossRef] [PubMed]

126. Guo, S.; Yao, Q.; Ke, Z.; Chen, H.; Wu, J.; Liu, C. Resveratrol attenuates high glucose-induced oxidative stress and cardiomyocyte apoptosis through AMPK. *Mol. Cell. Endocrinol.* **2015**, *412*, 85–94. [CrossRef] [PubMed]

127. Das, S.K.; Wang, W.; Zhabyeyev, P.; Basu, R.; McLean, B.; Fan, D.; Parajuli, N.; DesAulniers, J.; Patel, V.B.; Hajjar, R.J.; et al. Iron-overload injury and cardiomyopathy in acquired and genetic models is attenuated by resveratrol therapy. *Sci. Rep.* **2015**, *5*, 18132. [CrossRef] [PubMed]

128. Dong, M.; Ding, W.; Liao, Y.; Liu, Y.; Yan, D.; Zhang, Y.; Wang, R.; Zheng, N.; Liu, S.; Liu, J. Polydatin prevents hypertrophy in phenylephrine induced neonatal mouse cardiomyocytes and pressure-overload mouse models. *Eur. J. Pharmacol.* **2015**, *746*, 186–197. [CrossRef] [PubMed]

129. Feng, J.; Yang, Y.; Zhou, Y.; Wang, B.; Xiong, H.; Fan, C.; Jiang, S.; Liu, J.; Ma, Z.; Hu, W.; et al. Bakuchiol attenuates myocardial ischemia reperfusion injury by maintaining mitochondrial function: The role of silent information regulator 1. *Apoptosis* **2016**, *21*, 532–545. [CrossRef] [PubMed]

130. Kang, B.Y.; Khan, J.A.; Ryu, S.; Shekhar, R.; Seung, K.B.; Mehta, J.L. Curcumin reduces angiotensin II mediated cardiomyocyte growth via LOX1 inhibition. *J. Cardiovasc. Pharmacol.* **2010**, *55*, 417–424. [CrossRef] [PubMed]

131. Kim, Y.S.; Kwon, J.S.; Cho, Y.K.; Jeong, M.H.; Cho, J.G.; Park, J.C.; Kang, J.C.; Ahn, Y. Curcumin reduces the cardiac ischemia-reperfusion injury: Involvement of the toll-like receptor 2 in cardiomyocytes. *J. Nutr. Biochem.* **2012**, *23*, 1514–1523. [CrossRef] [PubMed]

132. Yang, Y.; Duan, W.; Lin, Y.; Yi, W.; Liang, Z.; Yan, J.; Wang, N.; Deng, C.; Zhang, S.; Li, Y.; et al. SIRT1 activation by curcumin pretreatment attenuates mitochondrial oxidative damage induced by myocardial ischemia reperfusion injury. *Free Radic. Biol. Med.* **2013**, *65*, 667–679. [CrossRef] [PubMed]

133. Xu, P.; Yao, Y.; Guo, P.; Wang, T.; Yang, B.; Zhang, Z. Curcumin protects rat heart mitochondria against anoxia-reoxygenation induced oxidative injury. *Can. J. Physiol. Pharmacol.* **2013**, *91*, 715–723. [CrossRef] [PubMed]

134. Yu, W.; Zha, W.; Ke, Z.; Min, Q.; Li, C.; Sun, H.; Liu, C. Curcumin protects neonatal rat cardiomyocytes against high glucose-induced apoptosis via PI3K/Akt signalling pathway. *J. Diabetes Res.* **2016**, *2016*, 4158591. [CrossRef] [PubMed]

135. Nehra, S.; Bhardwaj, V.; Kalra, N.; Ganju, L.; Bansal, A.; Saxena, S.; Saraswat, D. Nanocurcumin protects cardiomyoblasts H9c2 from hypoxia-induced hypertrophy and apoptosis by improving oxidative balance. *J. Physiol. Biochem.* **2015**, *71*, 239–251. [CrossRef] [PubMed]

136. Nehra, S.; Bhardwaj, V.; Ganju, L.; Saraswat, D. Nanocurcumin prevents hypoxia induced stress in primary human ventricular cardiomyocytes by maintaining mitochondrial homeostasis. *PLoS ONE* **2015**, *10*, e0139121. [CrossRef] [PubMed]

137. Hardy, N.; Viola, H.M.; Johnstone, V.P.; Clemons, T.D.; Cserne Szappanos, H.; Singh, R.; Smith, N.M.; Iyer, K.S.; Hool, L.C. Nanoparticle-mediated dual delivery of an antioxidant and a peptide against the L-Type $Ca^{2+}$ channel enables simultaneous reduction of cardiac ischemia-reperfusion injury. *ACS Nano* **2015**, *9*, 279–289. [CrossRef] [PubMed]

138. Li, W.; Wu, M.; Tang, L.; Pan, Y.; Liu, Z.; Zeng, C.; Wang, J.; Wei, T.; Liang, G. Novel curcumin analogue 14p protects against myocardial ischemia reperfusion injury through Nrf2-activating anti-oxidative activity. *Toxicol. Appl. Pharmacol.* **2015**, *282*, 175–183. [CrossRef] [PubMed]

139. Tuck, K.L.; Hayball, P.J. Major phenolic compounds in olive oil: Metabolism and health effects. *J. Nutr. Biochem.* **2002**, *13*, 636–644. [CrossRef]

140. Bali, E.B.; Ergin, V.; Rackova, L.; Bayraktar, O.; Küçükboyaci, N.; Karasu, C. Olive leaf extracts protect cardiomyocytes against 4-hydroxynonenal-induced toxicity in vitro: Comparison with oleuropein, hydroxytyrosol, and quercetin. *Planta Med.* **2014**, *80*, 984–992. [CrossRef] [PubMed]

141. Zhang, H.S.; Wang, S.Q. Salvianolic acid B from Salvia miltiorrhiza inhibits tumor necrosis factor-alpha (TNF-alpha)-induced MMP-2 upregulation in human aortic smooth muscle cells via suppression of NAD(P)H oxidase-derived reactive oxygen species. *J. Mol. Cell. Cardiol.* **2006**, *41*, 138–148. [CrossRef] [PubMed]

142. Yang, T.L.; Lin, F.Y.; Chen, Y.H.; Chiu, J.J.; Shiao, M.S.; Tsai, C.S.; Lin, S.J.; Chen, Y.L. Salvianolic acid B inhibits low-density lipoprotein oxidation and neointimal hyperplasia in endothelium-denuded hypercholesterolaemic rabbits. *J. Sci. Food Agric.* **2011**, *91*, 134–141. [CrossRef] [PubMed]

143. Dutta, M.; Ghosh, A.; Rangari, V.; Jain, G.; Khobragade, S.; Chattopadhyay, A.; Bhowmick, D.; Das, T.; Bandyopadhyay, D. Silymarin protects against copper-ascorbate induced injury to goat cardiac mitochondria in vitro: Involvement of antioxidant mechanism(s). *Int. J. Pharm. Pharm. Sci.* **2014**, *6*, 422–429.

144. Anestopoulos, I.; Kavo, A.; Tentes, I.; Kortsaris, A.; Panayiotidis, M.; Lazou, A.; Pappa, A. Silibinin protects H9c2 cardiac cells from oxidative stress and inhibits phenylephrine-induced hypertrophy: Potential mechanisms. *J. Nutr. Biochem.* **2013**, *24*, 586–594. [CrossRef] [PubMed]

145. Gabrielová, E.; Křen, V.; Jabůrek, M.; Modrianský, M. Silymarin component 2,3-dehydrosilybin attenuates cardiomyocyte damage following hypoxia/reoxygenation by limiting oxidative stress. *Physiol. Res.* **2015**, *64*, 79–91. [PubMed]

146. Esmaeili, M.A.; Sonboli, A. Antioxidant, free radical scavenging activities of Salvia brachyantha and its protective effect against oxidative cardiac cell injury. *Food Chem. Toxicol.* **2010**, *48*, 846–853. [CrossRef] [PubMed]

147. Chen, R.C.; Xu, X.D.; Zhi Liu, X.; Sun, G.B.; Zhu, Y.D.; Dong, X.; Wang, J.; Zhang, H.J.; Zhang, Q.; Sun, X.B. Total flavonoids from *Clinopodium chinense* (Benth.) O. Ktze protect against doxorubicin-induced cardiotoxicity in vitro and in vivo. *Evid. Based Complement. Altern. Med.* **2015**, *2015*, 472565. [CrossRef]

148. Chang, W.T.; Shao, Z.H.; Yin, J.J.; Mehendale, S.; Wang, C.Z.; Qin, Y.; Li, J.; Chen, W.J.; Chien, C.T.; Becker, L.B.; et al. Comparative effects of flavonoids on oxidant scavenging and ischemia-reperfusion injury in cardiomyocytes. *Eur. J. Pharmacol.* **2007**, *566*, 58–66. [CrossRef] [PubMed]

149. Akhlaghi, M.; Bandy, B. Preconditioning and acute effects of flavonoids in protecting cardiomyocytes from oxidative cell death. *Oxid. Med. Cell. Longev.* **2012**, *2012*, 782321. [CrossRef] [PubMed]

150. Visioli, F.; de La Lastra, C.A.; Andres-Lacueva, C.; Aviram, M.; Calhau, C.; Cassano, A.; D'Archivio, M.; Faria, A.; Favé, G.; Fogliano, V.; et al. Polyphenols and human health: A prospectus. *Crit. Rev. Food Sci. Nutr.* **2011**, *51*, 524–546. [CrossRef] [PubMed]

151. Goszcz, K.; Deakin, S.J.; Duthie, G.G.; Stewart, D.; Leslie, S.J.; Megson, I.L. Antioxidants in cardiovascular therapy: Panacea or false hope? *Front. Cardiovasc. Med.* **2015**, *2*, 29. [CrossRef] [PubMed]

152. Ginsburg, I.; Kohen, R.; Koren, E. Microbial and host cells acquire enhanced oxidant-scavenging abilities by binding polyphenols. *Arch. Biochem. Biophys.* **2011**, *506*, 12–23. [CrossRef] [PubMed]

153. Khurana, S.; Venkataraman, K.; Hollingsworth, A.; Piche, M.; Tai, T.C. Polyphenols: Benefits to the cardiovascular system in health and in aging. *Nutrients* **2013**, *5*, 3779–3827. [CrossRef] [PubMed]

154. Bohn, T. Dietary factors affecting polyphenol bioavailability. *Nutr. Rev.* **2014**, *72*, 429–452. [CrossRef] [PubMed]

155. Manach, C.; Williamson, G.; Morand, C.; Scalbert, A.; Rémésy, C. Bioavailability and bioefficacy of polyphenols in humans. I. Review of 97 bioavailability studies. *Am. J. Clin. Nutr.* **2005**, *81*, 230S–242S. [PubMed]

156. Barteková, M.; Šimončíková, P.; Fogarassyová, M.; Ivanová, M.; Okruhlicová, L'.; Tribulová, N.; Dovinová, I.; Barančík, M. Quercetin improves postischemic recovery of heart function in doxorubicin-treated rats and prevents doxorubicin-induced matrix metalloproteinase-2 activation and apoptosis induction. *Int. J. Mol. Sci.* **2015**, *16*, 8168–8185. [CrossRef] [PubMed]

157. Zhou, M.; Ren, H.; Han, J.; Wang, W.; Zheng, Q.; Wang, D. Protective effects of kaempferol against myocardial ischemia/reperfusion injury in isolated rat heart via antioxidant activity and inhibition of glycogen synthase kinase-3β. *Oxid. Med. Cell. Longev.* **2015**, *2015*, 481405. [CrossRef] [PubMed]

158. Qu, D.; Han, J.; Ren, H.; Yang, W.; Zhang, X.; Zheng, Q.; Wang, D. Cardioprotective effects of astragalin against myocardial ischemia/reperfusion injury in isolated rat heart. *Oxid. Med. Cell. Longev.* **2016**, *2016*, 8194690. [CrossRef] [PubMed]

159. Bhandary, B.; Piao, C.S.; Kim, D.S.; Lee, G.H.; Chae, S.W.; Kim, H.R.; Chae, H.J. The protective effect of rutin against ischemia/reperfusion-associated hemodynamic alteration through antioxidant activity. *Arch. Pharm. Res.* **2012**, *35*, 1091–1097. [CrossRef] [PubMed]

160. Umarani, V.; Muvvala, S.; Ramesh, A.; Lakshmi, B.V.; Sravanthi, N. Rutin potentially attenuates fluoride-induced oxidative stress-mediated cardiotoxicity, blood toxicity and dyslipidemia in rats. *Toxicol. Mech. Methods* **2015**, *25*, 143–149. [CrossRef] [PubMed]

161. Panda, S.; Kar, A. Combined effects of vincristine and quercetin in reducing isoproterenol-induced cardiac necrosis in rats. *Cardiovasc. Toxicol.* **2015**, *15*, 291–299. [CrossRef] [PubMed]

162. Song, L.; Yang, H.; Wang, H.X.; Tian, C.; Liu, Y.; Zeng, X.J.; Gao, E.; Kang, Y.M.; Du, J.; Li, H.H. Inhibition of 12/15 lipoxygenase by baicalein reduces myocardial ischemia/reperfusion injury via modulation of multiple signaling pathways. *Apoptosis* **2014**, *19*, 567–580. [CrossRef] [PubMed]

163. Yang, X.; Yang, J.; Hu, J.; Li, X.; Zhang, X.; Li, Z. Apigenin attenuates myocardial ischemia/reperfusion injury via the inactivation of p38 mitogen-activated protein kinase. *Mol. Med. Rep.* **2015**, *12*, 6873–6878. [CrossRef] [PubMed]

164. Dong, L.Y.; Li, S.; Zhen, Y.L.; Wang, Y.N.; Shao, X.; Luo, Z.G. Cardioprotection of vitexin on myocardial ischemia/reperfusion injury in rat via regulating inflammatory cytokines and MAPK pathway. *Am. J. Chin. Med.* **2013**, *41*, 1251–1266. [CrossRef] [PubMed]

165. Yang, J.T.; Qian, L.B.; Zhang, F.J.; Wang, J.; Ai, H.; Tang, L.H.; Wang, H.P. Cardioprotective effects of luteolin on ischemia/reperfusion injury in diabetic rats are modulated by eNOS and the mitochondrial permeability transition pathway. *J. Cardiovasc. Pharmacol.* **2015**, *65*, 349–356. [CrossRef] [PubMed]

166. Jia, J.H.; Chen, K.P.; Chen, S.X.; Liu, K.Z.; Fan, T.L.; Chen, Y.C. Breviscapine, a traditional Chinese medicine, alleviates myocardial ischaemia reperfusion injury in diabetic rats. *Acta Cardiol.* **2008**, *63*, 757–762. [CrossRef] [PubMed]

167. Akhlaghi, M.; Bandy, B. Dietary green tea extract increases phase 2 enzyme activities in protecting against myocardial ischemia-reperfusion. *Nutr. Res.* **2010**, *30*, 32–39. [CrossRef] [PubMed]

168. Liou, Y.M.; Hsieh, S.R.; Wu, T.J.; Chen, J.Y. Green tea extract given before regional myocardial ischemia-reperfusion in rats improves myocardial contractility by attenuating calcium overload. *Pflugers Arch.* **2010**, *460*, 1003–1014. [CrossRef] [PubMed]

169. Khan, G.; Haque, S.E.; Anwer, T.; Ahsan, M.N.; Safhi, M.M.; Alam, M.F. Cardioprotective effect of green tea extract on doxorubicin-induced cardiotoxicity in rats. *Acta Pol. Pharm.* **2014**, *71*, 861–868. [PubMed]

170. Li, W.; Xu, B.; Xu, J.; Wu, X.L. Procyanidins produce significant attenuation of doxorubicin-induced cardiotoxicity via suppression of oxidative stress. *Basic Clin. Pharmacol. Toxicol.* **2009**, *104*, 192–197. [CrossRef] [PubMed]

171. Sheng, R.; Gu, Z.L.; Xie, M.L. Epigallocatechin gallate, the major component of polyphenols in green tea, inhibits telomere attrition mediated cardiomyocyte apoptosis in cardiac hypertrophy. *Int. J. Cardiol.* **2013**, *162*, 199–209. [CrossRef] [PubMed]

172. Nazimabashir, V.; Manoharan, V.; Miltonprabu, S. Cadmium induced cardiac oxidative stress in rats and its attenuation by GSP through the activation of Nrf2 signaling pathway. *Chem. Biol. Interact.* **2015**, *242*, 179–193. [CrossRef] [PubMed]

173. Wang, X.H.; Huang, L.L.; Yu, T.T.; Zhu, J.H.; Shen, B.; Zhang, Y.; Wang, H.Z.; Gao, S. Effects of oligomeric grape seed proanthocyanidins on heart, aorta, kidney in DOCA-salt mice: Role of oxidative stress. *Phytother. Res.* **2013**, *27*, 869–876. [CrossRef] [PubMed]

174. Liu, Y.; Tan, D.; Shi, L.; Liu, X.; Zhang, Y.; Tong, C.; Song, D.; Hou, M. Blueberry anthocyanins-enriched extracts attenuate cyclophosphamide-induced cardiac injury. *PLoS ONE* **2015**, *10*, e0127813. [CrossRef] [PubMed]

175. Gandhi, C.; Upaganalawar, A.; Balaraman, R. Protection against in vivo focal myocardial ischemia/reperfusion injury-induced arrhythmias and apoptosis by hesperidin. *Free Radic Res.* **2009**, *43*, 817–827. [CrossRef] [PubMed]

176. Agrawal, Y.O.; Sharma, P.K.; Shrivastava, B.; Ojha, S.; Upadhya, H.M.; Arya, D.S.; Goyal, S.N. Hesperidin produces cardioprotective activity via PPAR-γ pathway in ischemic heart disease model in diabetic rats. *PLoS ONE* **2014**, *9*, e111212. [CrossRef] [PubMed]

177. Rani, N.; Bharti, S.; Manchanda, M.; Nag, T.C.; Ray, R.; Chauhan, S.S.; Kumari, S.; Arya, D.S. Regulation of heat shock proteins 27 and 70, p-Akt/p-eNOS and MAPKs by naringin dampens myocardial injury and dysfunction in vivo after ischemia/reperfusion. *PLoS ONE* **2013**, *8*, e82577. [CrossRef] [PubMed]

178. Trivedi, P.P.; Kushwaha, S.; Tripathi, D.N.; Jena, G.B. Cardioprotective effects of hesperetin against doxorubicin-induced oxidative stress and DNA damage in rat. *Cardiovasc. Toxicol.* **2011**, *11*, 215–225. [CrossRef] [PubMed]

179. Deng, W.; Jiang, D.; Fang, Y.; Zhou, H.; Cheng, Z.; Lin, Y.; Zhang, R.; Zhang, J.; Pu, P.; Liu, Y.; et al. Hesperetin protects against cardiac remodelling induced by pressure overload in mice. *J. Mol. Histol.* **2013**, *44*, 575–585. [CrossRef] [PubMed]

180. Selvaraj, P.; Pugalendi, K.V. Hesperidin, a flavanone glycoside, on lipid peroxidation and antioxidant status in experimental myocardial ischemic rats. *Redox Rep.* **2010**, *15*, 217–223. [CrossRef] [PubMed]

181. Elavarasan, J.; Velusamy, P.; Ganesan, T.; Ramakrishnan, S.K.; Rajasekaran, D.; Periandavan, K. Hesperidin-mediated expression of Nrf2 and upregulation of antioxidant status in senescent rat heart. *J. Pharm. Pharmacol.* **2012**, *64*, 1472–1482. [CrossRef] [PubMed]

182. Mahmoud, A.M.; Ashour, M.B.; Abdel-Moneim, A.; Ahmed, O.M. Hesperidin and naringin attenuate hyperglycemia-mediated oxidative stress and proinflammatory cytokine production in high fat fed/streptozotocin-induced type 2 diabetic rats. *J. Diabetes Complications* **2012**, *26*, 483–490. [CrossRef] [PubMed]

183. Ren, M.; Wang, X.; Du, G.; Tian, J.; Liu, Y. Calycosin-7-*O*-β-D-glucoside attenuates ischemia-reperfusion injury in vivo via activation of the PI3K/Akt pathway. *Mol. Med. Rep.* **2016**, *13*, 633–640. [CrossRef] [PubMed]

184. Liu, S.; Ren, H.B.; Chen, X.L.; Wang, F.; Wang, R.S.; Zhou, B.; Wang, C.; Sun, Y.X.; Wang, Y.J. Puerarin attenuates severe burn-induced acute myocardial injury in rats. *Burns* **2015**, *41*, 1748–1757. [CrossRef] [PubMed]

185. Zhou, M.; Liu, L.; Wang, W.; Han, J.; Ren, H.; Zheng, Q.; Wang, D. Role of licochalcone C in cardioprotection against ischemia/reperfusion injury of isolated rat heart via antioxidant, anti-inflammatory, and anti-apoptotic activities. *Life Sci.* **2015**, *132*, 27–33. [CrossRef] [PubMed]

186. Annapurna, A.; Mudagal, M.P.; Ansari, A.; Rao, A.S. Cardioprotective activity of chalcones in ischemia/reperfusion-induced myocardial infarction in albino rats. *Exp. Clin. Cardiol.* **2012**, *17*, 110–114. [PubMed]

187. Pantsi, W.G.; Marnewick, J.L.; Esterhuyse, A.J.; Rautenbach, F.; van Rooyen, J. Rooibos (*Aspalathus linearis*) offers cardiac protection against ischaemia/reperfusion in the isolated perfused rat heart. *Phytomedicine* **2011**, *18*, 1220–1228. [CrossRef] [PubMed]

188. Tang, Y.; Wang, M.; Chen, C.; Le, X.; Sun, S.; Yin, Y. Cardiovascular protection with danshensu in spontaneously hypertensive rats. *Biol. Pharm. Bull.* **2011**, *34*, 1596–1601. [CrossRef] [PubMed]

189. Wu, L.; Qiao, H.; Li, Y.; Li, L. Protective roles of puerarin and Danshensu on acute ischemic myocardial injury in rats. *Phytomedicine* **2007**, *14*, 652–658. [CrossRef] [PubMed]

190. Li, L.; Pan, Q.; Han, W.; Liu, Z.; Li, L.; Hu, X. Schisandrin B prevents doxorubicin-induced cardiotoxicity via enhancing glutathione redox cycling. *Clin. Cancer Res.* **2007**, *13*, 6753–6760. [CrossRef] [PubMed]

191. Thandavarayan, R.A.; Giridharan, V.V.; Arumugam, S.; Suzuki, K.; Ko, K.M.; Krishnamurthy, P.; Watanabe, K.; Konishi, T. Schisandrin B prevents doxorubicin induced cardiac dysfunction by modulation of DNA damage, oxidative stress and inflammation through inhibition of MAPK/p53 signaling. *PLoS ONE* **2015**, *10*, e0119214. [CrossRef] [PubMed]

192. Li, W.X.; Kong, X.; Zhang, J.X.; Yang, J.R. Long-term intake of sesamin improves left ventricular remodelling in spontaneously hypertensive rats. *Food Funct.* **2013**, *4*, 453–460. [CrossRef] [PubMed]

193. Jin, Y.C.; Kim, K.J.; Kim, Y.M.; Ha, Y.M.; Kim, H.J.; Yun, U.J.; Bae, K.H.; Kim, Y.S.; Kang, S.S.; Seo, H.G.; et al. Anti-apoptotic effect of magnolol in myocardial ischemia and reperfusion injury requires extracellular signal-regulated kinase1/2 pathways in rat in vivo. *Exp. Biol. Med. (Maywood)* **2008**, *233*, 1280–1288. [CrossRef] [PubMed]

194. Dolinsky, V.W.; Chan, A.Y.; Robillard Frayne, I.; Light, P.E.; Des Rosiers, C.; Dyck, J.R. Resveratrol prevents the prohypertrophic effects of oxidative stress on LKB1. *Circulation* **2009**, *119*, 1643–1652. [CrossRef] [PubMed]

195. Wang, B.; Yang, Q.; Sun, Y.Y.; Xing, Y.F.; Wang, Y.B.; Lu, X.T.; Bai, W.W.; Liu, X.Q.; Zhao, Y.X. Resveratrol-enhanced autophagic flux ameliorates myocardial oxidative stress injury in diabetic mice. *J. Cell. Mol. Med.* **2014**, *18*, 1599–1611. [CrossRef] [PubMed]

196. Zhang, C.; Feng, Y.; Qu, S.; Wei, X.; Zhu, H.; Luo, Q.; Liu, M.; Chen, G.; Xiao, X. Resveratrol attenuates doxorubicin-induced cardiomyocyte apoptosis in mice through SIRT1-mediated deacetylation of p53. *Cardiovasc. Res.* **2011**, *90*, 538–545. [CrossRef] [PubMed]

197. Al-Harthi, S.E.; Alarabi, O.M.; Ramadan, W.S.; Alaama, M.N.; Al-Kreathy, H.M.; Damanhouri, Z.A.; Khan, L.M.; Osman, A.M. Amelioration of doxorubicin-induced cardiotoxicity by resveratrol. *Mol. Med. Rep.* **2014**, *10*, 1455–1460. [CrossRef] [PubMed]

198. Wang, H.L.; Cui, X.H.; Yu, H.L.; Wu, R.; Xu, X.; Gao, J.P. Synergistic effects of polydatin and vitamin C in inhibiting cardiotoxicity induced by doxorubicin in rats. *Fundam. Clin. Pharmacol.* **2016**. [CrossRef] [PubMed]

199. Bai, T.; Hu, X.; Zheng, Y.; Wang, S.; Kong, J.; Cai, L. Resveratrol protects against lipopolysaccharide-induced cardiac dysfunction by enhancing SERCA2a activity through promoting the phospholamban oligomerization. *Am. J. Physiol. Heart Circ. Physiol.* **2016**, *311*, H1051–H1062. [CrossRef] [PubMed]

200. Wang, J.; He, D.; Zhang, Q.; Han, Y.; Jin, S.; Qi, F. Resveratrol protects against Cisplatin-induced cardiotoxicity by alleviating oxidative damage. *Cancer Biother. Radiopharm.* **2009**, *24*, 675–680. [CrossRef] [PubMed]

201. González-Salazar, A.; Molina-Jijón, E.; Correa, F.; Zarco-Márquez, G.; Calderón-Oliver, M.; Tapia, E.; Zazueta, C.; Pedraza-Chaverri, J. Curcumin protects from cardiac reperfusion damage by attenuation of oxidant stress and mitochondrial dysfunction. *Cardiovasc. Toxicol.* **2011**, *11*, 357–364. [CrossRef] [PubMed]

202. Izem-Meziane, M.; Djerdjouri, B.; Rimbaud, S.; Caffin, F.; Fortin, D.; Garnier, A.; Veksler, V.; Joubert, F.; Ventura-Clapier, R. Catecholamine-induced cardiac mitochondrial dysfunction and mPTP opening: Protective effect of curcumin. *Am. J. Physiol. Heart Circ. Physiol.* **2012**, *302*, H665–H674. [CrossRef] [PubMed]

203. Soetikno, V.; Sari, F.R.; Sukumaran, V.; Lakshmanan, A.P.; Mito, S.; Harima, M.; Thandavarayan, R.A.; Suzuki, K.; Nagata, M.; Takagi, R.; et al. Curcumin prevents diabetic cardiomyopathy in streptozotocin-induced diabetic rats: Possible involvement of PKC-MAPK signaling pathway. *Eur. J. Pharm. Sci.* **2012**, *47*, 604–614. [CrossRef] [PubMed]

204. Imbaby, S.; Ewais, M.; Essawy, S.; Farag, N. Cardioprotective effects of curcumin and nebivolol against doxorubicin-induced cardiac toxicity in rats. *Hum. Exp. Toxicol.* **2014**, *33*, 800–813. [CrossRef] [PubMed]

205. Andreadou, I.; Sigala, F.; Iliodromitis, E.K.; Papaefthimiou, M.; Sigalas, C.; Aligiannis, N.; Savvari, P.; Gorgoulis, V.; Papalabros, E.; Kremastinos, D.T. Acute doxorubicin cardiotoxicity is successfully treated with the phytochemical oleuropein through suppression of oxidative and nitrosative stress. *J. Mol. Cell. Cardiol.* **2007**, *42*, 549–558. [CrossRef] [PubMed]

206. Andreadou, I.; Mikros, E.; Ioannidis, K.; Sigala, F.; Naka, K.; Kostidis, S.; Farmakis, D.; Tenta, R.; Kavantzas, N.; Bibli, S.I.; et al. Oleuropein prevents doxorubicin-induced cardiomyopathy interfering with signaling molecules and cardiomyocyte metabolism. *J. Mol. Cell. Cardiol.* **2014**, *69*, 4–16. [CrossRef] [PubMed]

207. El-Shitany, N.A.; El-Haggar, S.M.; El-desoky, K. Silymarin prevents adriamycin-induced cardiotoxicity and nephrotoxicity in rats. *Food Chem. Toxicol.* **2008**, *46*, 2422–2428. [CrossRef] [PubMed]

208. Cecen, E.; Dost, T.; Culhaci, N.; Karul, A.; Ergur, B.; Birincioglu, M. Protective effects of silymarin against doxorubicin-induced toxicity. *Asian Pac. J. Cancer Prev.* **2011**, *12*, 2697–2704. [PubMed]

209. El-Awady, el-S.E.; Moustafa, Y.M.; Abo-Elmatty, D.M.; Radwan, A. Cisplatin-induced cardiotoxicity: Mechanisms and cardioprotective strategies. *Eur. J. Pharmacol.* **2011**, *650*, 335–341. [CrossRef] [PubMed]

210. Taghiabadi, E.; Imenshahidi, M.; Abnous, K.; Mosafa, F.; Sankian, M.; Memar, B.; Karimi, G. Protective effect of silymarin against acrolein-induced cardiotoxicity in mice. *Evid. Based Complement Altern. Med.* **2012**, *2012*, 352091. [CrossRef] [PubMed]

211. Muthumani, M.; Prabu, S.M. Silibinin potentially attenuates arsenic-induced oxidative stress mediated cardiotoxicity and dyslipidemia in rats. *Cardiovasc. Toxicol.* **2014**, *14*, 83–97. [CrossRef] [PubMed]

212. Tomé-Carneiro, J.; Visioli, F. Polyphenol-based nutraceuticals for the prevention and treatment of cardiovascular disease: Review of human evidence. *Phytomedicine* **2016**, *23*, 1145–1174. [CrossRef] [PubMed]

213. Islam, M.A.; Alam, F.; Solayman, M.; Khalil, M.I.; Kamal, M.A.; Gan, S.H. Dietary phytochemicals: Natural swords combating inflammation and oxidation-mediated degenerative diseases. *Oxid. Med. Cell Longev.* **2016**, *2016*, 5137431. [CrossRef] [PubMed]

214. Magyar, K.; Halmosi, R.; Palfi, A.; Feher, G.; Czopf, L.; Fulop, A.; Battyany, I.; Sumegi, B.; Toth, K.; Szabados, E. Cardioprotection by resveratrol: A human clinical trial in patients with stable coronary artery disease. *Clin. Hemorheol. Microcirc.* **2012**, *50*, 179–187. [CrossRef] [PubMed]

215. Agarwal, B.; Campen, M.J.; Channell, M.M.; Wherry, S.J.; Varamini, B.; Davis, J.G.; Baur, J.A.; Smoliga, J.M. Resveratrol for primary prevention of atherosclerosis: Clinical trial evidence for improved gene expression in vascular endothelium. *Int. J. Cardiol.* **2012**, *8*, 9–11. [CrossRef] [PubMed]

216. Zunino, S.J.; Peerson, J.M.; Freytag, T.L.; Breksa, A.P.; Bonnel, E.L.; Woodhouse, L.R.; Storms, D.H. Dietary grape powder increases IL-1β and IL-6 production by lipopolysaccharide-activated monocytes and reduces plasma concentrations of large LDL and large LDL-cholesterol particles in obese humans. *Br. J. Nutr.* **2014**, *112*, 369–380. [CrossRef] [PubMed]

217. Zern, T.L.; Wood, R.J.; Greene, C.; West, K.L.; Liu, Y.; Aggarwal, D.; Shachter, N.S.; Fernandez, M.L. Grape polyphenols exert a cardioprotective effect in pre- and postmenopausal women by lowering plasma lipids and reducing oxidative stress. *J. Nutr.* **2005**, *135*, 1911–1917. [PubMed]
218. Vaisman, N.; Niv, E. Daily consumption of red grape cell powder in a dietary dose improves cardiovascular parameters: A double blind, placebo-controlled, randomized study. *Int. J. Food Sci. Nutr.* **2015**, *66*, 342–349. [CrossRef] [PubMed]
219. Mellen, P.B.; Daniel, K.R.; Brosnihan, K.B.; Hansen, K.J.; Herrington, D.M. Effect of muscadine grape seed supplementation on vascular function in subjects with or at risk for cardiovascular disease: A randomized crossover trial. *J. Am. Coll. Nutr.* **2010**, *29*, 469–475. [CrossRef] [PubMed]

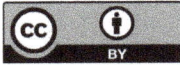

![nutrients logo] *nutrients*

MDPI

*Article*

# Seabuckthorn Leaves Extract and Flavonoid Glycosides Extract from Seabuckthorn Leaves Ameliorates Adiposity, Hepatic Steatosis, Insulin Resistance, and Inflammation in Diet-Induced Obesity

Eun-Young Kwon [1,2,†], Jeonghyeon Lee [1,†], Ye Jin Kim [1], Ara Do [1], Ji-Young Choi [1,2], Su-Jung Cho [1,2], Un Ju Jung [3], Mi-Kyung Lee [4], Yong Bok Park [5] and Myung-Sook Choi [1,2,*]

[1]  Department of Food Science and Nutrition, Kyungpook National University, 1370 San-Kyuk Dong Puk-Ku, Daegu 41566, Korea; savage20@naver.com (E.-Y.K.); wjdgus4411@naver.com (J.L.); freewilly59@hanmail.net (Y.J.K.); holy30000@hanmail.net (A.D.); jyjy31@hanmail.net (J.-Y.C.); chocrystalhihi@hanmail.net (S.-J.C.)
[2]  Center for Food and Nutritional Genomics Research, Kyungpook National University, 1370 San-Kyuk Dong Puk-Ku, Daegu 41566, Korea
[3]  Department of Food Science and Nutrition, Pukyong National University, Busan 608-737, Korea; jungunju@naver.com
[4]  Department of Food and Nutrition, Sunchon National University, Suncheon 540-950, Korea; leemk@sunchon.ac.kr
[5]  School of Life Sciences and Biotechnology, Kyungpook National University, 1370 San-Kyuk Dong Puk-Ku, Daegu 41566, Korea; parkyb@knu.ac.kr
*  Correspondence: mschoi@knu.ac.kr; Tel.: +82-53-950-6232; Fax: +82-53-958-1230
†  These authors contributed equally to this work.

Received: 26 April 2017; Accepted: 31 May 2017; Published: 2 June 2017

**Abstract:** The aim of the current study was to elucidate the effect of seabuckthorn leaves (SL) extract and flavonoid glycosides extract from seabuckthorn leaves (SLG) on diet-induced obesity and related metabolic disturbances, and additionally, to identify whether flavonoid glycosides and other components in SL can exert a possible interaction for the prevention of metabolic diseases by comparing the effect of SL and SLG. C57BL/6J mice were fed a normal diet (ND, AIN-93G purified diet), high-fat diet (HFD, 60 kcal% fat), HFD + 1.8% ($w/w$) SL (SL), and HFD + 0.04% ($w/w$) SLG (SLG) for 12 weeks. In high fat-fed mice, SL and SLG decreased the adiposity by suppressing lipogenesis in adipose tissue, while increasing the energy expenditure. SL and SLG also improved hepatic steatosis by suppressing hepatic lipogenesis and lipid absorption, whilst also enhancing hepatic fatty acid oxidation, which may be linked to the improvement in dyslipidemia. Moreover, SL and SLG improved insulin sensitivity by suppressing the levels of plasma GIP that were modulated by secreted resistin and pro-inflammatory cytokine, and hepatic glucogenic enzyme activities. SL, especially its flavonoid glycosides (SLG), can protect against the deleterious effects of diet-induced obesity (DIO) and its metabolic complications such as adiposity, dyslipidemia, inflammation, hepatic steatosis, and insulin resistance.

**Keywords:** flavonoid glycosides; hepatic steatosis; inflammation; insulin resistance; obesity; seabuckthorn

## 1. Introduction

The global prevalence of overweight and obesity has increased every decade in a number of countries and has been described as a global pandemic [1,2]. In 2014, according to world health organization (WHO), more than 1.9 billion adults were overweight and over 600 million of them were obese. Obesity is defined as excessive fat accumulation and is associated with various obesity-related metabolic syndromes such as adiposity, dyslipidemia, insulin resistance, and non-alcoholic fatty liver disease (NAFLD). Moreover, about 20–30% of severe obese patients have been diagnosed with NAFLD, so it has become an emerging issue for healthcare management [3]. NAFLD is a modern society health problem which ranges from the simple accumulation of triglycerides in the hepatocytes with no inflammation (hepatic steatosis), to steatosis along with liver inflammation (non-alcoholic steatohepatitis, NASH). Although the underlying mechanisms among adiposity, NAFLD, insulin resistance, and inflammation are not fully understood, the dysregulation of lipid metabolism in liver and adipose tissue is associated with adiposity and its complications [4].

Seabuckthorn (*Hippophae rhamnoides* L.) is a plant material and is in the family Elaeagnaceae. Seabuckthron is native to Europe and Asia, and the majority of the seabuckthorn plant's habitat is in northern Europe, China, Mongolia, Russia, and Canada. It is a unique and valuable plant currently cultivated in various parts of the world, and grows best in deep, well drained, sandy loam soil with ample organic matter. All parts of the seabuckthorn plant are considered to be a rich source of bioactive substances like isoflavones and flavonoids, which have various beneficial effects on health, such as anti-atherogenic, anti-oxidant, anti-cancer, and anti-bacterial effects [5]. In particular, its leaf extracts are reported to have marked anti-bacterial, anti-tumor, anti-inflammatory, and anti-oxidative activities [6–8]. This leaf extract contains a high content of flavonoid glycosides, including isorhamnetin 3-glucoside and quercetin 3-glucoside, which are known to prevent adiposity and dyslipidemia [9,10]. With the benefits of having various habitat and bioactive effects, seabuckthorn plays a significant part in the nutraceutical market. However, the potential anti-obesity effects of seabuckthorn leaves (SL) extract still remain unclear, and no studies have determined the effect of flavonoid glycosides extract from seabuckthorn leaves (SLG) on the lipid metabolism of adipose tissue and the liver in response to a high fat diet (HFD). Thus, the present study was undertaken to evaluate the effect of SL ethanol extract and flavonoid glycosides extract from SL (SLG) on adiposity, hepatic steatosis, insulin resistance, and inflammation in diet-induced obese (DIO) mice, and to identify whether flavonoid glycosides and other components in SL can exert a possible interaction for the prevention of metabolic diseases by comparing the effect of SL and SLG.

## 2. Materials and Methods

### 2.1. Preparation of Seabuckthorn Leaves (SL) Extract and Flavonoid Glycosides Extract from SL (SLG)

The dried seabuckthorn (*Hippophae rhamnoides* L.) leaves (1.15 kg) were extracted twice with 80% aqueous EtOH (10 L) under an ultrasonic cleaner (Power Sonic 420, Hwashintech, Incheon, Korea) for 2 h, filtered, and evaporated under reduced pressure. The concentrated EtOH extract (430.12 g) was obtained and isolated, and purified the flavonoids as follows. A portion (50 g) of the extract was solubilized in 20% aqueous EtOH and successively loaded into a Diaion HP-20 (Mitsubishi Chem. Co., Tokyo, Japan) column (5.5 × 50 cm). The column was eluted successively with 20%, 30%, and 50% aqueous EtOH, and each fraction was then evaporated to yield 20% EtOH fraction (Fr.) (32.3 g), 30% EtOH fr. (6.9 g), and 50% EtOH Fr. (3.0 g), respectively. All fractions were monitored by a UV-vis spectrophotometer and analytical HPLC to ascertain flavonoids. Among three fractions, the 30% EtOH Fr. was chromatographed on a silica gel (70–230 mesh, Merck, Damstadt, Germany) column (10.5 × 70 cm) with CHCl$_3$-MeOH-H$_2$O (65:35:7, *v*/*v*) as an eluent and obtained four fractions; Fr. 1 (0.35 g), Fr. 2 (0.92 g), Fr. 3 (0.85 g), and Fr. 4 (0.51 g). Fr. 2 and Fr. 3 were successively chromatographed on a ODS-A (YMC Inc., MA, USA) column (4.5 × 60 cm) with 25% aqueous EtOH, and a Sephadex LH-20 column (2.5 × 80 cm) with 80% aqueous EtOH, and yielded isorhamnetin 3-glucoside (4.7 mg) from Fr. 2 and quercetin 3-glucoside (5.3 mg) from Fr. 3, respectively. Finally, the two flavonoids were identified by NMR analysis (Table 1), and a comparison of the spectral data and the literature values was conducted [11].

**Table 1.** $^1$H- and $^{13}$C-NMR spectral data of two flavonoids isolated from seabuckthorn leaves (SL) (600 MHz).

| Position | Isorhamnetin 3-Glucoside | Quercetin 3-Glucoside |
|---|---|---|
| $^1$H-NMR | | |
| 6 | 6.43 (H, br s) | 6.45 (H, d, J = 2.4 Hz) |
| 8 | 6.72 (H, br s) | 6.73 (H, d, J = 2.4 Hz) |
| 2′ | 7.92 (H, d, J = 1.3 Hz) | 7.71 (H, d, J = 1.8 Hz) |
| 3′ | - | - |
| 5′ | 6.88 (H, d, J = 8.4 Hz) | 6.85 (H, d, J = 7.8 Hz) |
| 6′ | 7.60 (H, dd, J = 1.3 & 8.9 Hz) | 7.60 (H, dd, J = 1.8 & 7.8 Hz) |
| Glu 1″ | 5.44 (H, d, J = 6.6 Hz) | 5.20 (H, d, J = 7.2 Hz) |
| 2″~6″ | 3.18 ~3.70 | 3.21 ~3.72 |
| OCH$_3$ | 3.93 (3H, s) | |
| $^{13}$C-NMR | | |
| 2 | 157.57 | 158.00 |
| 3 | 135.32 | 135.72 |
| 4 | 177.79 | 179.68 |
| 5 | 161.71 | 162.85 |
| 6 | 100.06 | 100.58 |
| 7 | 165.12 | 163.63 |
| 8 | 94.95 | 95.47 |
| 9 | 158.63 | 159.60 |
| 10 | 105.66 | 105.03 |
| 1′ | 123.12 | 122.54 |
| 2′ | 114.38 | 116.13 |
| 3′ | 148.43 | 146.18 |
| 4′ | 150.88 | 150.68 |
| 5′ | 116.07 | 117.63 |
| 6′ | 123.81 | 122.54 |
| Glu 1 | 103.68 | 103.94 |
| 2 | 75.94 | 75.74 |
| 3 | 78.12 | 77.25 |
| 4 | 71.50 | 70.08 |
| 5 | 78.55 | 75.05 |
| 6 | 62.59 | 62.57 |
| OCH$_3$ | 56.77 | |

Chemical shift in δ ppm, coupling constant (J) expressed in Hz in parenthesis and measured in the solvent (MeOH-d$_4$). Taking TMS as an internal standard.

## 2.2. Experimental Animals and Diets

Male C57BL/6J mice (four-week-old) were obtained from The Jackson Laboratory (Bar Harbor, ME, USA). All mice were individually housed under a constant temperature (24 °C) and 12-h light/dark cycle, fed a normal chow diet for a one-week acclimation period, and subsequently randomly divided into four groups. The mice were fed a normal diet (ND, AIN-93G purified diet, $n$ = 10), HFD (60% of kilocalories from fat, $n$ = 10), HFD with 1.8% ($w/w$) of SL ($n$ = 10), and HFD with 0.04% ($w/w$) of SLG ($n$ = 10) for 12 weeks, respectively. A total of 1.8% ($w/w$) of SL contains 0.04% ($w/w$) of SLG. The experimental diets were prepared every week and stored at 4 °C. At the end of the experimental period, all mice were anesthetized with isoflurane (5 mg/kg body weight, Baxter, MN, USA) after 12 h of fasting. Blood was taken from the inferior vena cava to determine the plasma lipid, adipokine, and hormone concentrations. The liver and adipose tissue were removed, rinsed with physiological saline, weighed, immediately frozen in liquid nitrogen, and stored at −70 °C until analysis. The animal study protocols were approved by the Ethics Committee at Kyungpook National University (Approval No. KNU 2015-0020).

The energy expenditure, morphology of the liver and fat tissues, glucose metabolism markers, plasma lipid contents, hepatic and fecal lipid contents, glucose- and lipid-regulating enzyme activity, and analysis of gene expression were performed as stated in the Supplementary Materials on the materials and methods.

## 2.3. Energy Expenditure

Energy expenditure was measured using an indirect calorimeter (Oxylet; Panlab, Cornella, Spain). The mice were placed into individual metabolic chambers at 25 °C, with free access to food and water. $O_2$ and $CO_2$ analyzers were calibrated with highly purified gas standards. The oxygen consumption ($V_{O_2}$) and carbon dioxide production ($V_{CO_2}$) were recorded at 3-min intervals using a computer-assisted data acquisition program (Chart 5.2; AD Instrument, Sydney, Australia) over a 24-h period, and the data were averaged for each mouse. Energy expenditure (EE) was calculated according to the following formula: EE (kcal/day/kg of body weight$^{0.75}$) = $V_{O_2} \times 1.44 \times (3.815 + (1.232 \times V_{O_2}/V_{CO_2}))$.

## 2.4. Morphology of the Liver and Fat Tissues

The liver and epididymal while adipose tissue (eWAT) were removed from each mouse. Samples were subsequently fixed in 10% ($v/v$) paraformaldehyde/phosphate-buffered saline and embedded in paraffin for staining with hematoxylin and eosin. Stained areas were visualized using a microscope set at 200× magnification.

## 2.5. Plasma Biomarkers

Plasma lipid concentrations were determined with commercially available kits. Plasma free fatty acid (FFA) levels were measured using the Wako enzymatic kit (Wako Chemicals, Richmond, VA, USA), and triglyceride, total cholesterol, HDL-cholesterol, glutamic oxaloacetic transaminase (GOT), and glutamic pyruvic transaminase (GPT) levels were determined using Asan enzymatic kits (Asan, Seoul, Korea). Plasma apolipoprotein AI (apo AI; Eiken, Japan) and apolipoprotein B (apo B; Eiken, Japan) levels were also measured using enzymatic kits. The values of nonHDL-cholesterol, the ratio of HDL-cholesterol to total cholesterol (HTR), and the atherogenic index (AI) were calculated as follow: nonHDL-cholesterol = ((total-cholesterol) − (HDL-cholesterol) − (triglyceride/5)), HTR (%) = (HDL-cholesterol/total-cholesterol) × 100, AI = ((total-cholesterol) − (HDL-cholesterol))/(HDL-cholesterol). Plasma insulin, incretin hormone gastric inhibitory polypeptide (GIP), adipokines (resistin, leptin, and adiponectin), cytokines (tumor necrosis factor alpha (TNF-α), interleukin 1β (IL-1β), IL-6, and plasminogen activator inhibitor-1 (PAI-1)) were determined with a multiplex detection kit from Bio-Rad (Hercules, CA, USA). All samples were assayed in duplicate and analyzed with a Luminex 200 Labmap system (Luminex, Austin, TX, USA). Data analyses were done with the Bio-Plex Manager software version 4.1.1 (Bio-Rad, Richmond, CA, USA).

## 2.6. Fasting Blood Glucose, Intraperitoneal Glucose Tolerance Test, and Homeostatic Index of Insulin Resistance

The blood glucose concentration was measured by the glucose oxidase method using a glucose analyzer (Glucocard, Arkray, Japan) in whole blood obtained from the tail vein after food withholding for 12 h. The intraperitoneal glucose tolerance test (IPGTT) was performed at week 11. After 12 h of fasting, the mice were injected intraperitoneally with glucose (0.5 g/kg of body weight). The blood glucose level was determined from the tail vein at 0, 30, 60, and 120 min after the glucose injection. The homeostatic index of insulin resistance (HOMA-IR) was calculated according to the homeostasis assessment model as follows: HOMA-IR = (fasting glucose (mmol/L) × fasting insulin (IU/mL))/22.51.

## 2.7. Hepatic and Fecal Lipid Contents

Hepatic and fecal lipids were extracted as previously described [12], and then dried lipid residues were dissolved in 1 mL of ethanol for the triglyceride, cholesterol, and fatty acid (FA) assays. Triton X-100 and a sodium cholate solution in distilled water were added to 200 µL of a dissolved lipid solution for emulsification. Hepatic and fecal triglyceride, cholesterol, and FA contents were analyzed with the same enzymatic kits that were used for the plasma analysis.

## 2.8. Preparation of Hepatic Subcellular Fractions

Hepatic and adipocyte mitochondrial, cytosolic, and microsomal fractions were prepared as previously described [13]. The mitochondrial fraction was used to measure glucose-6-phosphatase (G6Pase) and β-oxidation, and the cytosolic fraction was used to measure glucose-6-phosphate dehydrogenase (G6PD), malic enzyme (ME), fatty acid synthase (FAS), glucokinase, and phosphoenolpyruvate carboxykinase (PEPCK) activities. The microsomal fraction was used to measure phosphatidate phosphohydrolase (PAP) and acyl-CoA:cholesterolacyltransferase (ACAT) activities. The protein concentrations were determined using the Bradford method.

## 2.9. Glucose- and Lipid-Regulating Enzyme Activity

Glucose-6-phosphate dehydrogenase (G6PD) [14], fatty acid synthase (FAS) [15], malic enzyme (ME) [16], and phosphatidate phosphohydrolase (PAP) [17] activities were measured as previously described. Glucose-6-phosphatase (G6Pase) activity was determined using the method of Alegre et al. [18]. Phosphoenolpyruvate carboxykinase (PEPCK) activity was monitored in the direction of oxaloacetate synthesis using a spectrophotometric assay developed by Bentle and Lardy [19]. Fatty acid β-oxidation was measured spectrophotometrically by monitoring the reduction of NAD to NADH in the presence of palmitoyl-CoA as described by Lazarow [15], with a slight modification.

## 2.10. Analysis of Gene Expression

The liver tissues were homogenized in the TRIzol reagent (Invitrogen, Grand Island, NY, USA), and the total RNA was isolated according to the manufacturer's instructions. The total RNA was converted to cDNA using the QuantiTect Reverse Transcription kit (Qiagen Gmbh, Hilden, Germany). mRNA expression was quantified by a quantitative real-time polymerase chain reaction (PCR) using the QuantiTect SYBR Green PCR kit (Qiagen) and SDS7000 sequence detection system (Applied Biosystems, CA, USA). Each cDNA sample was amplified using primers for the glyceraldehyde-3-phosphate dehydrogenase (GAPDH) gene labeled with SYBR green dye.

The amplification was performed as follows: 10 min at 90 °C, 15 s at 95 °C, and 60 s at 60 °C for a total of 40 cycles. The cycle threshold (Ct) was defined as the cycle at which a statistically significant increase in the SYBR green emission intensity occurred. The Ct data were normalized relative to those for the housekeeping gene, GAPDH, which is stably expressed in mice. The relative gene expression was calculated with the $2^{\Delta\Delta Ct}$ method [20].

## 2.11. Primer

The primer were designed using a Primer 5.0 software (Primer-E Ltd., Plymouth, UK), SREBP1c (Forward: 5′-GGA GCC ATG GAT TGC ACA TT-3′, Reverse: 5′-CCT GTC TCA CCC CCA GCA TA-3′), CPT1α (Forward: 5′-ATC TGG ATG GCT ATG GTC AAG GTC-3′, Reverse: 5′-GTG CTG TCA TGC GTT GGA AGT C-3′), ABCG5 (Forward: 5′-TCA ATG AGT TTT ACG GCC TGA A-3′, Reverse: 5′-GCA CAT CGG GTG ATT TAG CA-3′), ABCG8 (Forward: 5′-GCA ATG CCC TCT ACA ACT CCT T-3′, Reverse: 5′-GAG GAA CGA CAG CTT GGA GAT C-3′), IRS2 (Forward: 5′-CCC ATG TCC CGC CGT GAA G-3′, Reverse: 5′-CTC CAG TGC CAA GGT CTG AAG G-3′), and GAPDH (Forward: 5′-ACA ATG AAT ACG CT ACA GCA ACA G-3′, Reverse: 5′-GGT GGT CCA GGG TTT CTT ACT CC-3′).

## 2.12. Statistical Analysis

The parameter values were expressed as the mean (standard error of the mean (SEM)). Significant differences between the ND and HFD groups were determined by a student's *t*-test and significant differences among the HFD, SL, and SLG groups were determined by one-way ANOVA using the SPSS program (SPSS Inc., Chicago, IL, USA). The results were considered statistically significant at $p < 0.05$.

## 3. Results and Discussion

### 3.1. SL and SLG Supplement Lowered Body Weight Gain and Improved Plasma Lipid Profiles in DIO Mice

HFD generally induces adiposity, hepatic steatosis, and insulin resistance through multiple mechanisms. We also observed that HFD (60.3% energy from fat) feeding for 12 weeks promoted the development of obesity, as indicated by significant increases in body weight (BW), BW gain, and body fat mass, with increased energy intake (Figure 1A–E). The supplementation of SL and SLG significantly decreased BW after six weeks and eight weeks of high-fat feeding, respectively, without altering the energy intake (Figure 1A–D). Both SL and SLG also resulted in a significant decrease in weights for all white adipose tissue (WAT) depots (epididymal, perirenal, mesenteric, subcutaneous, and interscapular WAT), except for retroperitoneum WAT, which led to a decrease in the visceral WAT and total WAT weights compared to the HFD group (Figure 1E). Thus, it is plausible that both SL and SLG suppressed BW gain by regulating the expansion of fat mass. We also found that SL and SLG supplementation improved dyslipidemia by decreasing the levels of plasma total-cholesterol, nonHDL-cholesterol, triglyceride, FFA, ApoB, and AI, while increasing the Apo A-I/Apo B ratio compared to the HFD group (Figure 1F). This finding is supported by a previous study [21], which demonstrated the body fat and plasma lipid level lowering effects of powdered SL via the regulation of lipid and antioxidant metabolism in DIO mice.

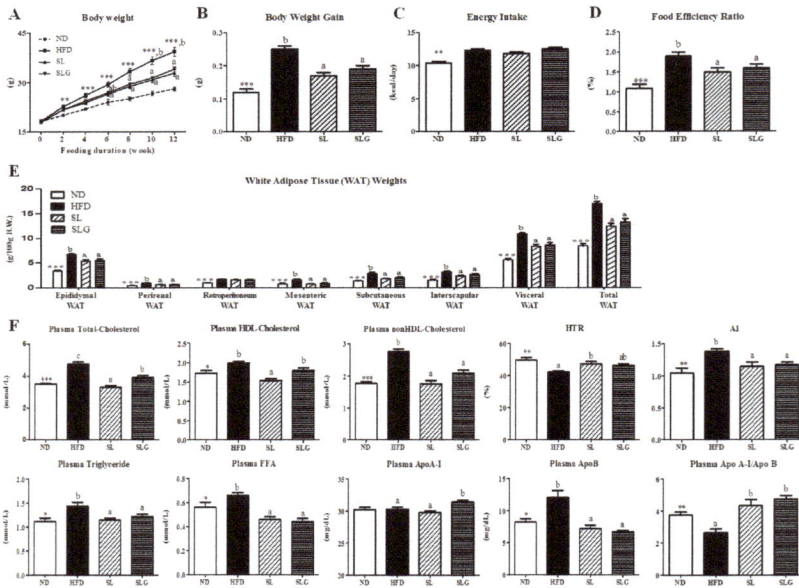

**Figure 1.** Effect of SL and SLG on body weight (**A**), body weight gain; (**B**), food intake; (**C**), food efficiency ratio; (**D**), white adipose tissue weights; (**E**) and plasma lipids levels; (**F**) in C57BL/6J mice fed HFD for 12 weeks. Data are shown as the mean ± SEM (*n* = 10). Significant differences between HFD versus ND are indicated; * *p* < 0.001, ** *p* < 0.01, *** *p* < 0.001. [abc] Means not sharing a common superscript are significantly different among the high-fat diet fed groups (HFD, SL, and SLG groups) at *p* < 0.05. ND, normal diet group; HFD, high-fat diet group; SL, HFD + 1.8% (*w*/*w*) ethanol extract of sea buckthorn leaves group; SLG, HFD + 0.04% (*w*/*w*) ethanol extract of flavonoid glycosides from sea buckthorn leaves group; Food Efficiency Ratio, body weight gain/Energy intakes per day; HTR, ratio of HDL-cholesterol to total cholesterol; AI, atherogenic index; FFA, free fatty acid; ApoA-I, apolipoprotein A-I; ApoB, apolipoprotein B.

### 3.2. SL and SLG Supplement Lowered Adiposity by Decreasing Lipogenesis in Adipose Tissue, While Increasing Energy Expenditure in DIO Mice

Lee et al. [21] and Pichiah et al. [22] demonstrated that the supplementation of powdered SL or SL ethanol extract effectively suppressed BW gain and the expansion of adipose tissue mass by modulating the plasma leptin level and hepatic lipid metabolism. However, these previous studies have not analyzed the markers associated with lipid metabolism in adipose tissue, despite the reduced body fat mass induced by the SL supplement. Thus, we measured the activities of enzymes for lipogenesis in epididymal fat and found that G6PD, ME, PAP, and ACAT enzyme activities were suppressed by SL and SLG supplements compared to the HFD group, which is likely associated with the reduced adiposity (Figure 2A,B). Notably, SL supplementation also markedly diminished the activities of FAS compared to the HFD group. Interestingly, SL and SLG supplements led to an increase in the reduced energy expenditure by HFD during both the light phase and dark phase (Figure 2C). These observations indicate that SL and SLG have the potential to regulate adipocyte lipid metabolism and energy expenditure, thereby ameliorating adiposity in DIO mice.

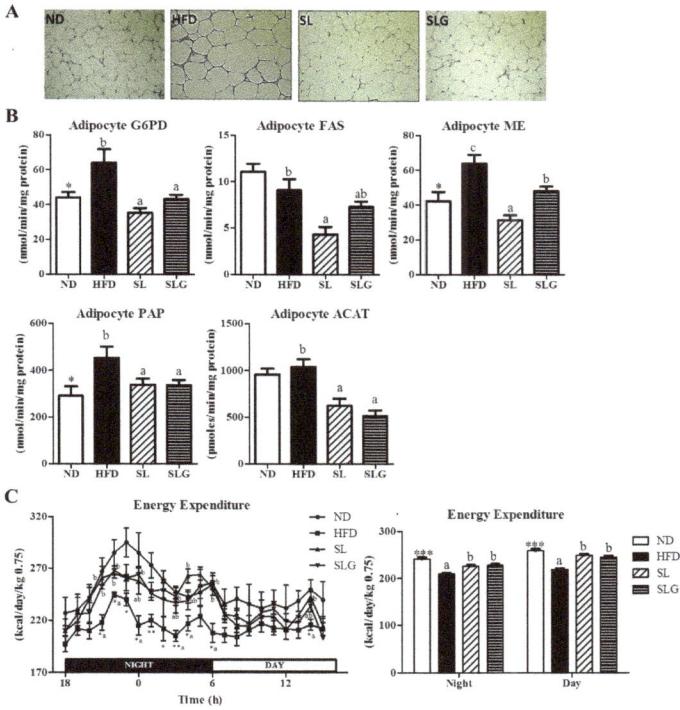

**Figure 2.** Effect of SL and SLG on adipocyte morphology (**A**) the activities of adipocyte lipogenic enzymes; (**B**) and energy expenditure in C57BL/6J mice fed HFD for 12 weeks. Data are shown as the mean $\pm$ SEM ($n = 10$). Significant differences between HFD versus ND are indicated; * $p < 0.001$, *** $p < 0.001$. [abc] Means not sharing a common superscript are significantly different among the high-fat diet fed groups (HFD, SL, and SLG groups) at $p < 0.05$. ND, normal diet group; HFD, high-fat diet group; SL, HFD + 1.8% ($w/w$) ethanol extract of sea buckthorn leaves group; SLG, HFD + 0.04% ($w/w$) ethanol extract of flavonoid glycosides from sea buckthorn leaves group; G6PD, glucose-6-phosphate dehydrogenase; FAS, fatty acid synthase; ME, malic enzyme; PAP, phosphatidate phosphohydrolase; ACAT, acyl-CoA:cholesterolacyltransferase.

*3.3. SL and SLG Supplement Lowered the Levels of Hepatic Lipids and Lipotoxicity Markers by Modulating Hepatic Lipid Regulating Enzume Activities and Gene Expressions, and Increasing Fecal Lipids in DIO Mice*

In general, a reduction of body fat mass and an improvement in dyslipidemia are highly correlated with improved hepatic steatosis [4,23]. SL and SLG supplementation improved hepatic steatosis, as well as adiposity, as evidenced by the reduced hepatic lipids accumulation and lipotoxicity markers (plasma GOT and GPT) compared with the HFD group (Figure 3A–C). SL and SLG supplementation markedly suppressed the hepatic lipogenic enzyme activities (FAS, ME, PAP, ACAT) and *SREBP1c* gene expression, and elevated the hepatic β-oxidation enzyme activity and *CPT1α* gene expression compared to the HFD group (Figure 3D,E), suggesting that SL and SLG may limit hepatic lipid availability by inhibiting lipogenesis and increasing fatty acid oxidation, thereby reducing hepatic lipotoxicity. Moreover, SLG supplementation significantly elevated fecal cholesterol, triglyceride, and FA levels with the mRNA expression of hepatic *ABCG5* and *ABCG8* (Figure 3F,G). Similarly, SL supplementation significantly increased fecal cholesterol and hepatic *ABCG5* and *ABCG8* mRNA expressions (Figure 3F,G). These could contribute to the inhibition of the hepatic lipid load by promoting biliary sterol excretion and decreasing the absorption of dietary fat.

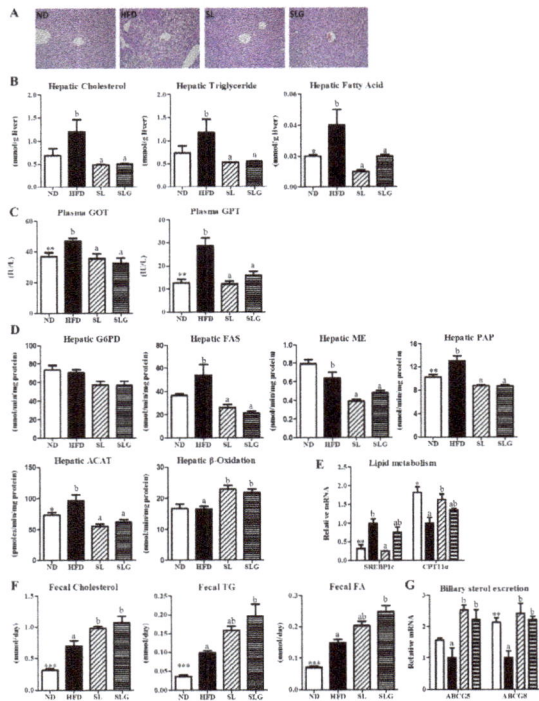

**Figure 3.** Effect of SL and SLG on hepatic morphology (**A**) hepatic lipids contents; (**B**) hepatic lipotoxicity markers; (**C**) hepatic lipid regulating enzyme activities; (**D**) and gene expressions; (**E**) fecal lipids contents; (**F**) and hepatic gene expression related with biliary sterol excretion in C57BL/6J mice fed HFD for 12 weeks. Data are shown as the mean ± SEM (*n* = 10). Significant differences between HFD versus ND are indicated; * *p* < 0.001, ** *p* < 0.01, *** *p* < 0.001. [ab] Means not sharing a common superscript are significantly different among the high-fat diet fed groups (HFD, SL, and SLG groups) at *p* < 0.05. ND, normal diet group; HFD, high-fat diet group; SL, HFD + 1.8% (*w/w*) ethanol extract of sea buckthorn leaves group; SLG, HFD + 0.04% (*w/w*) ethanol extract of flavonoid glycosides from sea buckthorn leaves group; GOT, glutamic oxaloacetic transaminase; GPT, glutamic pyruvic transaminase.

*3.4. SL and SLG Improved Insulin Resistance and Glucose Tolerance by Modulating Activities of Hepatic*

Glucose-Regulating Enzymes and Levels of Plasma Adipokines and Cytokines in DIO Mice

The striking improvement of hepatic steatosis coupled with the decreased adiposity in SL- and SLG- treated mice was associated with a normalization of the plasma glucose and insulin levels, which was a reflection of improved hepatic insulin sensitivity, as evidenced by the IPGTT and the reduced HOMA-IR (Figure 4A–D). In addition, SL and SLG supplementations suppressed the gluconeogenesis, as indicated by decreased hepatic G6Pase and PEPCK activities and the increased expression of hepatic *IRS2* mRNA (Figure 4E,F), which could be associated with the improved hepatic insulin sensitivity observed in SL- and SLG-supplemented DIO mice, similar to previous studies [17,18].

The incretin hormone GIP is a peptide hormone produced by the intestinal K cell and it acts directly on pancreatic islets to stimulate insulin secretion [24,25]. Fats strongly enhance GIP secretion [26], and its concentrations in obesity or obese type 2 diabetes mellitus (T2DM) patients are elevated [27]. GIP, in the presence of insulin, induces fatty acid uptake into adipose tissue and GIP receptor (GIPR)-deficient mice on HFD showed not only improved obesity by increasing the energy expenditure, but also insulin sensitivity, without differences in the energy intake compared to that of control mice [28]. Additionally, recent studies demonstrated that the binding of GIP to GIPR in the 3T3-L1 cells and adipose tissue of rats results in the increased secretion of resistin, and thus, GIP activates phosphoinositide 3-kinase (PI3K) and Akt/PKB (protein kinase B) through secreted resistin, thereby suppressing AMP-activated protein kinase (AMPK) in adipocytes, a key transcriptional factor in fatty acid oxidation [29,30]. Resistin is known as an adipose tissue-specific secretory factor, participating in the pathogenesis of insulin resistance, adipogenesis, and inflammation in mice [31,32]. Leptin is also a peptide hormone mainly expressed in adipose tissue, and can control the production and activation of pro-inflammatory cytokines such as TNF-α, IL-6, and IL-12 with the consequent amplification of inflammation and the development of liver fibrosis [33,34]. Previous human studies have shown that NAFLD patients have increased circulating resistin and leptin that it is correlated with insulin resistance, obesity, and the histological severity of the disease [34,35]. We also found that plasma GIP, resistin, and leptin levels, as well as the leptin/adiponectin ratio, were increased in HFD-fed mice, but SL and SLG reversed the HFD-induced increase in the plasma levels of GIP, resistin, and leptin, in addition to the leptin/adiponectin ratio (Figure 4G,H). The leptin/adiponectin ratio has been proposed as a potential surrogate biomarker for the diagnosis of metabolic diseases [36]. These observations suggest that the decrease in plasma GIP, resistin, and leptin levels is partially linked with glucose homeostasis, an increase in energy expenditure, and a decrease in the pro-inflammatory response, leading to the prevention of obesity, consequent insulin resistance, and hepatic steatosis induced by HFD.

An increase in obesity-associated inflammation can also contribute to the development of insulin resistance and hepatic steatosis [37]. It is well known that, in an obese state, the enlarged adipose tissue leads to the dysregulated secretion of adipokines and cytokines. The pro-cytokines reach metabolic tissues such as liver and muscle, and modify not only glucose and lipid metabolism, but also inflammatory responses, thereby contributing to metabolic syndrome. High levels of circulating TNF-α have been found in patients with obesity and NAFLD, and its levels are closely correlated with liver disease severity [38,39]. Moreover, circulating levels of IL-1β were demonstrated to predict T2DM when in conjunction with circulating IL-6 [40]. A previous study by Nov O [41] demonstrated that by promoting adipose inflammation and limiting fat tissue expandability, IL-1β supports ectopic fat accumulation in hepatocytes and adipose-tissue macrophages, contributing to impaired fat-liver crosstalk in nutritional obesity. In addition, IL-6 and PAI-1 are also pro-inflammatory cytokines synthesized by adipocyte, and its levels in plasma are increased in obesity and insulin resistance [42,43]. Interestingly, in the present study, SL and SLG significantly decreased plasma TNF-α, IL-1β, IL-6, and PAI-1 levels, resulting in a reduced inflammatory response, which was associated with the noticeable improvement in adiposity, insulin resistance, and hepatic steatosis by SL and SLG.

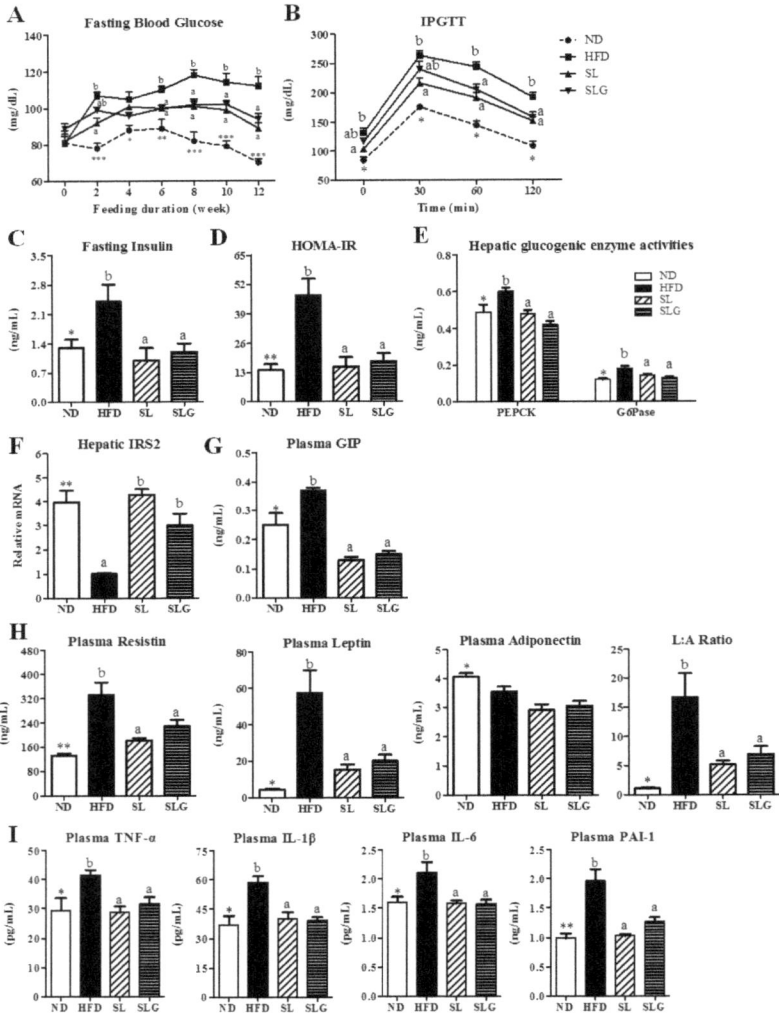

**Figure 4.** Effect of SL and SLG on fasting blood glucose (**A**) IPGTT; (**B**) fasting insulin; (**C**) HOMA-IR; (**D**) hepatic glucogenic enzymes; (**E**) hepatic IRS2 gene; (**F**) plasma GIP; (**G**) plasma adipokines; (**H**) and plasma pro-inflammatory cytokines in C57BL/6J mice fed HFD for 12 weeks. Data are shown as the mean ± SEM (*n* = 10). Significant differences between HFD versus ND are indicated; * *p* < 0.001, ** *p* < 0.01, *** *p* < 0.001. [a,b] Means not sharing a common superscript are significantly different among the high-fat diet fed groups (HFD, SL, and SLG groups) at *p* < 0.05. ND, normal diet group; HFD, high-fat diet group; SL, HFD + 1.8% (*w/w*) ethanol extract of sea buckthorn leaves group; SLG, HFD + 0.04% (*w/w*) ethanol extract of flavonoid glycosides from sea buckthorn leaves group; IPGTT, intraperitoneal glucose tolerance test; HOMA-IR, homeostasis model assessment-estimated insulin resistance; PEPCK, phosphoenolpyruvate carboxykinase; G6Pase, glucokinase, glucose-6-phosphatase; IRS2, insulin receptor substrate 2; GIP, incretin hormone gastric inhibitory polypeptide; L:A Ratio, leptin:adiponectin ratio; TNF-α, tumor necrosis factor α; IL, interleukin; PAI-1, plasminogen activator inhibitor-1.

## 4. Conclusions

The data obtained from our animal study indicate that SL and SLG can suppress DIO and modulate obesity-associated metabolic disorders such as insulin resistance and hepatic steatosis. SL and SLG prevent adiposity and dyslipidemia by suppressing the lipogenesis and the absorption of dietary fat, while increasing biliary sterol excretion and energy expenditure, which contributes to the improvement of both hepatic steatosis and lipotoxicity. SL and SLG also prevent insulin resistance by improving inflammation and decreasing gluconeogenesis. In this study, the anti-metabolic effect of SL and SLG are similarly presented, and these results thus suggest that the effect of seabuckthorn leaves may be caused by its flavonoid glycosides, including isorhamnetin-3-glucoside and quercetin-3-glucosdie. Moreover, there was no synergic effect between flavonoid glycosides and other components in seabuckthorn leaves. Figure 5 illustrates the possible mechanisms of the effects of SL and/or SLG for antiobesity. Taken together, the present findings suggest that seabuckthorn leaves, especially its flavonoid glycosides, ameliorates the deleterious effects of DIO and its metabolic complications such as adiposity, dyslipidemia, inflammation, hepatic steatosis, and insulin resistance.

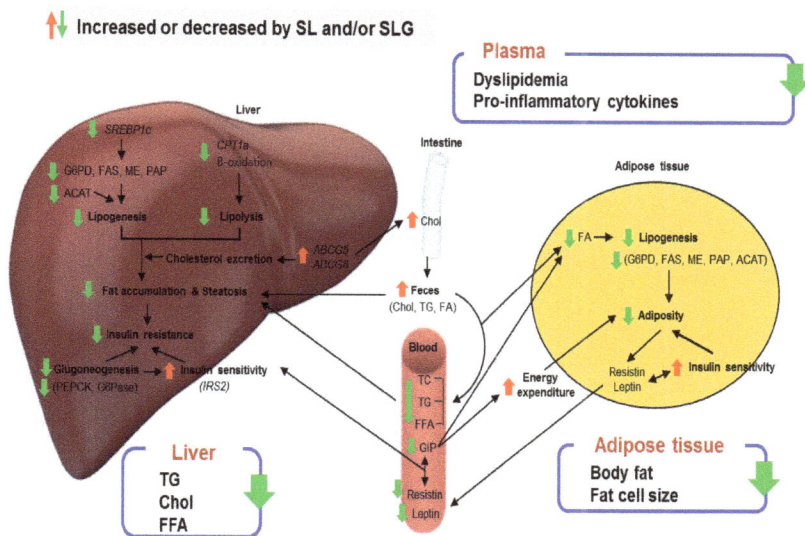

**Figure 5.** Proposed mechanism for SL and SLG regarding anti-obesity effects. SL and SLG altered the hepatic lipid and glucose metabolizing factors and decreased lipid absorption by increasing fecal lipid contents, thereby preventing hepatic steatosis via the reduction of the hepatic lipid load and eventually improving insulin resistance. In addition, SL and SLG reduced adiposity by suppressing adipocyte lipogenesis, while increasing the energy expenditure through decreasing the plasma GIP level, which is associated with a decrease in plasma pro-inflammatory cytokine levels.

**Supplementary Materials:** The following are available online at www.mdpi.com/2072-6643/9/6/569/s1.

**Acknowledgments:** This work was supported by the Kyungpook National University Bokhyeon Research Fund, 2015.

**Author Contributions:** J.L., E.-Y.L., and M.-S.C. carried out all animal studies and wrote the manuscript; Y.J.K., A.D., J.-Y.C., S.-J.C., and U.J.J. collected the data and reviewed the manuscript; and M.-K.L and Y.B.P. supervised the study.

**Conflicts of Interest:** The authors have declared no conflicts of interest.

## Abbreviations

| | |
|---|---|
| ABCG | ATP-binding cassette sub-family G member |
| ACAT | acyl-CoA:cholesterolacyltransferase |
| AI | atherogenic index |
| Apo | apolipoprotein |
| BW | body weight |
| CPT1$\alpha$ | carnitine palmitoyltransferase 1$\alpha$ |
| DIO | diet-induced obese |
| FAS | fatty acid synthase |
| FFA | free fatty acid |
| G6Pase | glucokinase, glucose-6-phosphatase |
| G6PD | glucose-6-phosphate dehydrogenase |
| GIP | incretin hormone gastric inhibitory polypeptide |
| GIPR | GIP receptor |
| HFD | high-fat diet |
| HOMA-IR | homeostasis model assessment-estimated insulin resistance |
| IL | interleukin |
| IPGTT | intraperitoneal glucose tolerance test |
| IRS2 | insulin receptor substrate 2 |
| ME | malic enzyme |
| ND | normal diet |
| PAI-1 | plasminogen activator inhibitor-1 |
| PAP | phosphatidate phosphohydrolase |
| PEPCK | phosphoenolpyruvate carboxykinase |
| SL | seabuckthorn leaf |
| SLG | flavonoid glycosides from seabuckthorn leaves |
| SREBP1c | sterol regulatory element-binding protein 1c |
| T2DM | type 2 diabetes mellitus |
| TNF-$\alpha$ | tumor necrosis factor $\alpha$ |
| WAT | white adipose tissue |

## References

1. Popkin, B.M.; Adair, L.S.; Ng, S.W. Global nutrition transition and the pandemic of obesity in developing countries. *Nutr. Rev.* **2012**, *70*, 3–21. [CrossRef] [PubMed]
2. Swinburn, B.A.; Sacks, G.; Hall, K.D.; McPherson, K.; Finegood, D.T.; Moodie, M.L.; Gortmaker, S.L. The global obesity pandemic: Shaped by global drivers and local environments. *Lancet* **2011**, *378*, 804–814. [CrossRef]
3. Vernon, G.; Baranova, A.; Younossi, Z.M. Systematic review: The epidemiology and natural history of non-alcoholic fatty liver disease and non-alcoholic steatohepatitis in adults. *Aliment. Pharmacol. Ther.* **2011**, *34*, 274–285. [CrossRef] [PubMed]
4. Kabir, M.; Catalano, K.J.; Ananthnarayan, S.; Kim, S.P.; Van Citters, G.W.; Dea, M.K.; Bergman, R.N. Molecular evidence supporting the portal theory: A causative link between visceral adiposity and hepatic insulin resistance. *Am. J. Physiol. Endocrinol. MeTable* **2005**, *288*, E454–E461. [CrossRef] [PubMed]
5. Suomela, J.P.; Ahotupa, M.; Yang, B.; Vasankari, T.; Kallio, H. Absorption of flavonols derived from sea buckthorn (*Hippophaë rhamnoides* L.) and their effect on emerging risk factors for cardiovascular disease in humans. *J. Agric. Food Chem.* **2006**, *54*, 7364–7369. [CrossRef] [PubMed]
6. Jain, M.; Ganju, L.; Katiyal, A.; Padwad, Y.; Mishra, K.P.; Chanda, S.; Karan, D.; Yogendra, K.M.; Sawhney, R.C. Effect of *Hippophae rhamnoides* leaf extract against Dengue virus infection in human blood-derived macrophages. *Phytomedicine* **2008**, *15*, 793–799. [CrossRef] [PubMed]
7. Geetha, S.; Sai Ram, M.; Singh, V.; Ilavazhagan, G.; Sawhney, R.C. Anti-oxidant and immunomodulatory properties of seabuckthorn (*Hippophae rhamnoides*)—An in vitro study. *J. Ethnopharmacol.* **2002**, *79*, 373–378. [CrossRef]

8.  Ganju, L.; Padwad, Y.; Singh, R.; Karan, D.; Chanda, S.; Chopra, M.K.; Bhatnagar, P.; Kashyap, R.; Sawhney, R.C. Anti-inflammatory activity of Seabuckthorn (*Hippophae rhamnoides*) leaves. *Int. Immunopharmacol.* **2005**, *5*, 1675–1684. [CrossRef] [PubMed]

9.  Lee, J.; Jung, E.; Lee, J.; Kim, S.; Huh, S.; Kim, Y.; Kim, Y.; Byun, S.Y.; Kim, Y.S.; Park, D. Isorhamnetin'represses adipogenesis in 3T3-L1 cells. *Obesity (Silver Spring)* **2009**, *17*, 226–232. [CrossRef] [PubMed]

10. Yan, S.X.; Li, X.; Sun, C.D.; Chen, K.S. Hypoglycemic and hypolipidemic effects of quercetin and its glycosides. *Zhongguo Zhong Yao Za Zhi* **2015**, *40*, 4560–4567. [PubMed]

11. Kim, J.S.; Kwon, Y.S.; Sa, Y.J.; Kim, M.J. Isolation and identification of sea buckthorn (*Hippophae rhamnoides*) phenolics with antioxidant activity and $\alpha$-glucosidase inhibitory effect. *J. Agric. Food Chem.* **2011**, *59*, 138–144. [CrossRef] [PubMed]

12. Folch, J.; Lees, M.; Sloan-Stanley, G.H. A simple method for isolation and purification of total lipids from animal tissues. *J. Biol. Chem.* **1957**, *226*, 497–509. [PubMed]

13. Davidson, A.L.; Arion, W.J. Factors underlying significant underestimations of glucokinase activity in crude liver extracts: Physiological implications of higher cellular activity. *Arch. Biochem. Biophys.* **1987**, *253*, 156–167. [CrossRef] [PubMed]

14. Rudack, D.; Chisholm, E.M.; Holten, D. Rat liver glucose 6-phosphate dehydrogenase. Regulation by carbohydrate diet and insulin. *J. Biol. Chem.* **1971**, *246*, 1249–1254. [PubMed]

15. Lazarow, P.B. Assay of peroxisomal beta-oxidation of fatty acids. *Methods Enzymol.* **1981**, *72*, 315–319. [PubMed]

16. Ochoa, S. Malic enzyme: Malic enzymes from pigeon and wheat germ. In *Methods in Enzymology*; Colowick, S.P., Kaplan, N.O., Eds.; Academic Press: New York, NY, USA, 1955; Volume 1, pp. 323–326.

17. Walton, P.A.; Possmayer, F. Mg2-dependent phosphatidate phosphohydrolase of rat lung: Development of an assay employing a defined chemical substrate which reflects the phosphohydrolase activity measured using membrane-bound substrate. *Anal. Biochem.* **1985**, *151*, 479–486. [CrossRef] [PubMed]

18. Alegre, M.; Ciudad, C.J.; Fillat, C.; Guinovart, J.J. Determination of glucose-6-phosphatase activity using the glucose dehydrogenase-coupled reaction. *Anal. Biochem.* **1988**, *173*, 185–189. [CrossRef] [PubMed]

19. Bentle, L.A.; Lardy, H.A. Interaction of anions and divalent metal ions with phosphoenolpyruvate carboxykinase. *J. Biol. Chem.* **1976**, *251*, 2916–2921. [PubMed]

20. Schmittgen, T.D.; Livak, K.J. Analyzing real-time PCR data by the comparative C(T) method. *Nat. Protoc.* **2008**, *3*, 1101–1108. [CrossRef] [PubMed]

21. Lee, H.I.; Kim, M.S.; Lee, K.M.; Park, S.K.; Seo, K.I.; Kim, H.J.; Kim, M.J.; Choi, M.S.; Lee, M.K. Anti-visceral obesity and antioxidant effects of powdered sea buckthorn (*Hippophae rhamnoides* L.) leaf tea in diet-induced obese mice. *Food Chem. Toxicol.* **2011**, *49*, 2370–2376. [CrossRef] [PubMed]

22. Pichiah, P.B.; Moon, H.J.; Park, J.E.; Moon, Y.J.; Cha, Y.S. Ethanolic extract of seabuckthorn (*Hippophae rhamnoides* L.) prevents high-fat diet-induced obesity in mice through down-regulation of adipogenic and lipogenic gene expression. *Nutr. Res.* **2012**, *32*, 856–864. [CrossRef] [PubMed]

23. Banerji, M.A.; Buckley, M.C.; Chaiken, R.L.; Gordon, D.; Lebovitz, H.E.; Kral, J.G. Liver fat, serum triglycerides and visceral adipose tissue in insulin-sensitive and insulin-resistant black men with NIDDM. *Int. J. Obes. Relat. Metab. Disord.* **1995**, *19*, 846–850. [PubMed]

24. Drucker, D.J. The biology of incretin hormones. *Cell. MeTable* **2006**, *3*, 153–165. [CrossRef] [PubMed]

25. Taminato, T.; Seino, Y.; Goto, Y.; Inoue, Y.; Kadowaki, S. Synthetic gastric inhibitory polypeptide. Stimulatory effect on insulin and glucagon secretion in the rat. *Diabetes* **1977**, *26*, 480–484. [CrossRef] [PubMed]

26. Carr, R.D.; Larsen, M.O.; Winzell, M.S.; Jelic, K.; Lindgren, O.; Deacon, C.F.; Ahrén, B. Incretin and islet hormonal responses to fat and protein ingestion in healthy men. *Am. J. Physiol. Endocrinol. MeTable* **2008**, *295*, E779–E784. [CrossRef] [PubMed]

27. Creutzfeldt, W.; Ebert, R.; Willms, B.; Frerichs, H.; Brown, J.C. Gastric inhibitory polypeptide (GIP) and insulin in obesity: Increased response to stimulation and defective feedback control of serum levels. *Diabetologia* **1978**, *14*, 15–24. [CrossRef] [PubMed]

28. Zhou, H.; Yamada, Y.; Tsukiyama, K.; Miyawaki, K.; Hosokawa, M.; Nagashima, K.; Toyoda, K.; Naitoh, R.; Mizunoya, W.; Fushiki, T.; et al. Gastric inhibitory polypeptide modulates adiposity and fat oxidation under diminished insulin action. *Biochem. Biophys. Res. Commun.* **2005**, *335*, 937–942. [CrossRef] [PubMed]

29. Kim, S.J.; Nian, C.; McIntosh, C.H. Resistin is a key mediator of glucose-dependent insulinotropic polypeptide (GIP) stimulation of lipoprotein lipase (LPL) activity in adipocytes. *J. Biol. Chem.* **2007**, *282*, 34139–34147. [CrossRef]

30. Kim, S.J.; Nian, C.; McIntosh, C.H. Activation of lipoprotein lipase by glucose-dependent insulinotropic polypeptide in adipocytes. A role for a protein kinase B, LKB1, and AMP-activated protein kinase cascade. *J. Biol. Chem.* **2007**, *282*, 8557–8567. [CrossRef] [PubMed]

31. Steppan, C.M.; Bailey, S.T.; Bhat, S.; Brown, E.J.; Banerjee, R.R.; Wright, C.M.; Patel, H.R.; Ahima, R.S.; Lazar, M.A. The hormone resistin links obesity to diabetes. *Nature* **2001**, *409*, 307–312. [CrossRef] [PubMed]

32. Steppan, C.M.; Lazar, M.A. The current biology of resistin. *J. Intern. Med.* **2004**, *255*, 439–447. [CrossRef] [PubMed]

33. Bekaert, M.; Verhelst, X.; Geerts, A.; Lapauw, B.; Calders, P. Association of recently described adipokines with liver histology in biopsy-proven non-alcoholic fatty liver disease: A systematic review. *Obes. Rev.* **2016**, *17*, 68–80. [CrossRef] [PubMed]

34. Polyzos, S.A.; Aronis, K.N.; Kountouras, J.; Raptis, D.D.; Vasiloglou, M.F.; Mantzoros, C.S. Circulating leptin in non-alcoholic fatty liver disease: A systematic review and meta-analysis. *Diabetologia* **2016**, *59*, 30–43. [CrossRef] [PubMed]

35. Shen, C.; Zhao, C.Y.; Wang, W.; Wang, Y.D.; Sun, H.; Cao, W.; Yu, W.Y.; Zhang, L.; Ji, R.; Li, M.; Gao, J. The relationship between hepatic resistin overexpression and inflammation in patients with nonalcoholic steatohepatitis. *BMC Gastroenterol.* **2014**, *14*, 39. [CrossRef] [PubMed]

36. López-Jaramillo, P.; Gómez-Arbeláez, D.; López-López, J.; López-López, C.; Martínez-Ortega, J.; Gómez-Rodríguez, A.; Triana-Cubillos, S. The role of leptin/adiponectin ratio in metabolic syndrome and diabetes. *Horm. Mol. Biol. Clin. Investig.* **2014**, *18*, 37–45. [CrossRef] [PubMed]

37. Chawla, A.; Nguyen, K.D.; Goh, Y.P. Macrophage-mediated inflammation in metabolic disease. *Nat. Rev. Immunol.* **2011**, *11*, 738–749. [CrossRef] [PubMed]

38. García-Ruiz, I.; Rodríguez-Juan, C.; Díaz-Sanjuan, T.; del Hoyo, P.; Colina, F.; Muñoz-Yagüe, T.; Solís-Herruzo, J.A. Uric acid and anti-TNF antibody improve mitochondrial dysfunction in ob/ob mice. *Hepatology* **2006**, *44*, 581–591. [CrossRef] [PubMed]

39. McCullough, A.J. Pathophysiology of nonalcoholic steatohepatitis. *J. Clin. Gastroenterol.* **2006**, *40*, S17–S29. [CrossRef] [PubMed]

40. Spranger, J.; Kroke, A.; Möhlig, M.; Hoffmann, K.; Bergmann, M.M.; Ristow, M.; Boeing, H.; Pfeiffer, A.F. Inflammatory cytokines and the risk to develop type 2 diabetes: Results of the prospective population-based European Prospective Investigation into Cancer and Nutrition (EPIC)-Potsdam Study. *Diabetes* **2003**, *52*, 812–817. [CrossRef] [PubMed]

41. Nov, O.; Shapiro, H.; Ovadia, H.; Tarnovscki, T.; Dvir, I.; Shemesh, E.; Kovsan, J.; Shelef, I.; Carmi, Y.; Voronov, E.; et al. Interleukin-1β regulates fat-liver crosstalk in obesity by auto-paracrine modulation of adipose tissue inflammation and expandability. *PLoS ONE* **2013**, *8*, e53626. [CrossRef] [PubMed]

42. Bastard, J.P.; Maachi, M.; Van Nhieu, J.T.; Jardel, C.; Bruckert, E.; Grimaldi, A.; Robert, J.J.; Capeau, J.; Hainque, B. Adipose tissue IL-6 content correlates with resistance to insulin activation of glucose uptake both in vivo and in vitro. *J. Clin. Endocrinol. MeTable* **2002**, *87*, 2084–2089. [CrossRef] [PubMed]

43. Juhan-Vague, I.; Alessi, M.C.; Mavri, A.; Morange, P.E. Plasminogen activator inhibitor-1, inflammation, obesity, insulin resistance and vascular risk. *J. Thromb. Haemost.* **2003**, *1*, 1575–1579. [CrossRef] [PubMed]

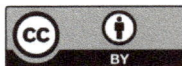

nutrients

MDPI

Article

# Antioxidant and Antihypertensive Effects of a Chemically Defined Fraction of Syrah Red Wine on Spontaneously Hypertensive Rats

Eugênia Abrantes de Figueiredo [1], Naiane Ferraz Bandeira Alves [1],
Matheus Morais de Oliveira Monteiro [1], Clenia de Oliveira Cavalcanti [1],
Tania Maria Sarmento da Silva [2], Telma Maria Guedes da Silva [2], Valdir de Andrade Braga [1] and
Eduardo de Jesus Oliveira [3],*

[1]  Centro de Biotecnologia, Programa de Pós Graduação em Produtos Naturais e Sintéticos Bioativos,
    Campus I, João Pessoa, PB 58051-970, Brazil; eugeniafigueiredo.farmacia@gmail.com (E.A.d.F.);
    naiferraz@gmail.com (N.F.B.A.); monteirommo@gmail.com (M.M.d.O.M.);
    cleniacavalcanti91@gmail.com (C.d.O.C.); valdir@cbiotec.ufpb.br (V.d.A.B.)
[2]  Departamento de Química, Laboratório de Bioprospecção Fitoquímica, Universidade Federal Rural de
    Pernambuco, Recife, PE 52171-900, Brazil; sarmento.silva@gmail.com (T.M.S.d.S.);
    guedes.meira@gmail.com (T.M.G.d.S.)
[3]  Departamento de Farmácia, Universidade Federal dos Vales do Jequitinhonha e Mucurí, Diamantina,
    MG 39100-000, Brazil
*   Correspondence: eduardo.oliveira@ufvjm.edu.br; Tel.: +55-38-3532-8863

Received: 27 January 2017; Accepted: 7 March 2017; Published: 3 June 2017

**Abstract:** A particularly phenolic-rich fraction extracted from red wine from the São Francisco valley (Northeastern Brazil) was chemically characterized and its hypotensive and antioxidant effects on spontaneously hypertensive rats were studied both in vitro and in vivo. The liquid-liquid pH dependent fractionation scheme afforded a fraction with high content of bioactive phenolics such as flavonols, flavonol glycosides, phenolic acids and anthocyanins, whose identities were confirmed by liquid chromatography coupled to mass spectrometry analysis. Pretreatment of spontaneously hypertensive rats with this wine fraction at doses of 50 and 100 mg/kg by gavage for 15 days was able to decrease mean arterial pressure and heart rate as well as decrease serum lipid peroxidation. The fraction at concentrations of 0.01–1000 µg/mL induced concentration-dependent relaxation of isolated rat superior mesenteric artery rings pre-contracted with phenylephrine and this effect was not attenuated by endothelium removal. Our results demonstrate it is possible for phenolic constituents of red wine that are orally bioavailable to exert in vivo hypotensive and antioxidant effects on intact endothelial function.

**Keywords:** red wine; phenolics; hypertension; flavonoids

---

## 1. Introduction

Red wine is the result of grape fermentation processes, and is characterized by high levels of polyphenols, including flavonoids, such as flavonols, flavones, proanthocyanidins, anthocyanins, and catechins; and non-flavonoid compounds which include derivatives of hydroxycinnamic acid, benzoic acid, hydrolysable acids and stilbenes, such as resveratrol [1,2].

Climactic factors such as temperature, humidity and solar radiation exert great influence on the development, production and quality of grapes and therefore wine, as well as their phenolic compound contents. Located in the Northeastern region of Brazil between the states of Pernambuco and Bahia, at latitude 8 to 9° S and longitude 40° W, the São Francisco Valley (SFV) is a recently developed wine-producing region in the country. This area has a tropical semi-arid climate with high temperatures, high brightness, abundant water for irrigation, sand-clay ground and annual rainfall of 300–800 mm [3]. These climactic characteristics allow producers to harvest twice a year and red wines from the region are marked by high levels of bioactive phenolic compounds [4]. Previous studies by our group with red wines from this region have demonstrated that these wines present considerably higher levels of phenolic compounds than those reported in the literature for red wines in general [4].

The mechanisms involved in the pathophysiology of arterial hypertension are complex but an increasing body of evidence mainly accumulated in the last decade by us and others suggests the participation of reactive oxygen species (ROS) in the development and maintenance of high blood pressure [5–7]. Oxidative stress is involved in the development of hypertension through different mechanisms [8–12]. These mechanisms include for example the inactivation of nitric oxide by superoxide, leading to endothelium dysfunction and vasoconstriction [13] and the effect of oxidative stress on the oxidation of low density lipoproteins [14].

Several studies have demonstrated an association between the consumption of food and/or beverages rich in phenolic compounds and a reduction on the risk of cardiovascular diseases [15–17]. A large number of existing epidemiological studies showed an inverse association between consumption of a number of phenolic compounds and risk of hypertension. This evidence comes not only from cross-sectional studies [18–20] but also from prospective ones [21,22]. The largest of these prospective studies [21] involved 156,957 subjects with a follow-up period of 14 years and revealed an 8% reduction in the risk of developing hypertension for those in the highest quintile of anthocyanin intake when compared with those in the lowest quintile. A similar reduction of 10% in the risk of developing hypertension for those in the highest quintile of flavonoid intake compared with those in the lowest quintile was seen in a prospective cohort of 40,574 French women with a follow-up period of 16 years [22]. Experimental evidence has implicated phenolic compounds in several different mechanisms relevant in the pathogenesis of hypertension, including the lowering of platelet aggregation [23], a decrease in the oxidation of low density lipoprotein [24], and an increase of endothelium nitric oxide [25].

Previous results with the high levels of phenolics in SFV wines prompted us to prepare a fraction from the Syrah red wine of SFV that concentrates biorelevant phenolic compounds (Fr 2 SySFV), to chemically characterize this fraction and study the antioxidant and antihypertensive activity in a variety of in vitro and in vivo assays using spontaneously hypertensive rats.

## 2. Materials and Methods

### 2.1. Standards and Reagents

Gallic acid, Folin–ciocalteu reagent, 1,1-diphenyl-2-picrylhydrazyl radical (DPPH), 2,20-azino-bis-3-ethylbenzothiazoline-6-sulphonic acid (ABTS), 6-hydroxy-2,5,7,8-tetramethylchroman-2-carboxylic acid (Trolox), potassium persulphate, quercetin, *trans*-resveratrol, ascorbic acid, phenylephrine (Phe), and acetylcholine chloride, were purchased from Sigma–Aldrich (St. Louis, MO, USA). Ethyl acetate and HPLC-grade acetonitrile was from Tedia (Tedia, Brazil). Water was purified through a Milliq1 water purification system (Millipore, Billerica, MA, USA) and the other solvents were all reagent-grade.

### 2.2. Wine Sample and Fractionation

The Fr 2 SySFV was obtained from a red wine produced in the São Francisco Valley region (Syrah variety, Rendeiras winery, harvest 2013). The Syrah variety was chosen because it displayed the highest phenolic content amongst different wines from SFV, Southern Brazil (Serra Gaucha) and Chile that were screened (results not shown). Liquid–liquid extraction methods according to Ghiselli et al. (1998) [26] were used to obtain several fractions containing different classes of polyphenolic compounds. Alcohol removal was performed by vacuum distillation (50 °C). In brief, the de-alcoholized wine (100 mL) had its pH adjusted to 2.0 and was first extracted with ethyl acetate (three times with 100 mL of EtOAc each). The aqueous phase was combined and concentrated under reduced pressure with ethanol addition (at 50 °C) until dryness, producing Fr 1 SySFV. The organic phase was concentrated to dryness, redissolved in water (100 mL), had its pH adjusted to 7.0 and was then further extracted with EtOAc (three times with 100 mL of EtOAc each). The combined organic phase from this second extraction was concentrated under reduced pressure (at 50 °C) until dryness to afford Fr 2 SySFV. The aqueous residue from this extraction was adjusted to pH 2.0 and extracted again with EtOAc (three times with 100 mL of EtOAc each). The resulting organic phase from this third extraction was combined and concentrated under reduced pressure (at 50 °C) to dryness, producing Fr 3 SySFV. The aqueous phase from the third extraction was discarded.

*2.3. Total Phenolic Content*

The total phenolic content of the fractions was determined by Folin-Ciocalteu reagent according to Waterhouse (2003) [27], with gallic acid as a standard, and expressed as milligrams of gallic acid equivalents/100 milligrams of fraction (mg GAE/100 mg). Briefly, a solution at 1 mg/mL of each wine fraction was transferred to a 5 mL volumetric flask together with 100 mL of the Folin-Ciocalteu reagent and 3 mL of Milliq® water; it was then agitated for 30 s. The volume was completed with Milliq® water and after 2 h the absorbance of the solution was measured at 760 nm in a ultraviolet/visible (UV/Vis) spectrophotometer. Solutions of gallic acid (ranging from 0.5 to 50 mg/mL) were analyzed in a similar manner to that described above and used to construct a calibration curve. Each sample (wine fraction) was analyzed in triplicate and the total phenolic content was expressed as milligrams of gallic acid equivalents/100 milligrams of fraction (mg GAE/100 mg).

*2.4. Antioxidant Assays*

The DPPH assay was used to measure the free radical-scavenging capacity of the wine fractions, according to a previously reported method [28]. After preliminary screening, solutions were prepared in methanol at final concentrations ranging from 3 to 30 µg/mL. Subsequently, 100 µL of the samples were transferred to 96-well plates and then 100 µL of the DPPH solution (118.2 µg/mL in MeOH) was added. The solutions were shaken and after 30 min of reaction at ambient temperature the absorbance of the samples was measured on a UV/Vis spectrophotometer at 517 nm. Each sample was tested in triplicate. The percentage radical-scavenging activity (%SA) was calculated using Equation (1) below:

$$\%SA = ((Abs_{control} - Abs_{sample}) \times 100)/Abs_{control},\tag{1}$$

where $Abs_{control}$ is the absorbance of a solution with DPPH and methanol alone, and $Abs_{sample}$ is the absorbance of the DPPH solution in the presence of the wine fractions or the standard used, i.e., ascorbic acid.

Trolox-equivalent antioxidant capacity (TEAC) and effective concentrations to sequester 50% of free radicals (EC$_{50}$ values) for the fractions against ABTS$^{•+}$ radical cation were determined following a previously published method [29], using 6-hydroxy 2,5,7,8-tetramethyl chroman 2-carboxylic acid (Trolox), a vitamin E water-soluble analog, as standard. Initially, the ABTS$^{•+}$ radical cation solution was prepared by mixing 2.5 mL of a solution of ABTS (7.0 mM) with 44 µL of a solution of potassium persulfate (140.0 mM), both in distilled water. The solution was kept protected from direct light at room temperature for a period of 12–16 h before use. Then, the solution of the ABTS$^{•+}$ radical was diluted with ethanol (approximately 1:80 *v/v*) obtaining an absorbance (A) of 0.7 ± 0.05 at the wavelength of 734 nm, using an UV/Vis spectrophotometer. The solutions of the samples were prepared in EtOH at concentrations of 0.5, 1.0 and 5.0 mg/mL. Through preliminary screening, appropriate quantities of the sample solutions and the ABTS$^{•+}$ solution were transferred to 2-mL Eppendorf tubes and the volume was completed to 500 µL with EtOH. Sample concentrations ranged from 5 to 200 µg/mL. Trolox was used as the standard substance at concentrations of 0.5, 1.0, 2.0, 3.0, 4.0, 5.0 and 6.0 µg/mL. The solutions were shaken and, after 6 min of reaction, the absorbance of the samples and the standard were measured on a UV/Vis spectrophotometer at a wavelength of 734 nm. Each concentration was tested in triplicate. The percentage of sequestering activity (% SA) was calculated as described for DPPH scavenging activity.

The results of the antioxidant assays were expressed as $EC_{50} \pm$ standard deviation (SD). $EC_{50}$ values for the fractions were obtained by linear regression (using the software Graphpad Prism, v. 5.0, Graphpad Software Inc., La Jolla, CA, USA) of the %SA values plotted against concentration and are expressed as µg of fraction/mL solution

### 2.5. Quantification of Trans-Resveratrol and Quercetin by HPLC-UV Analysis

The content of *trans* resveratrol and quercetin was determined in Fr 2 SySFV, the fraction with higher phenolic content and antioxidant activity. A reversed-phase chromatographic method to determine *trans*-resveratrol and quercetin has been previously described and validated [4]. The HPLC analyses were conducted on a Shimadzu liquid chromatograph system (Shimadzu Corp, Kyoto, Japan) equipped with a LC-10 ATvp pump, variable wavelength detector SPD 10AVvp, controller module SCL 10A vp, a LC-10AD vp pump, a vacuum degasser DGU-14A, and an autosampler. The analytes were separated on a Phenomenex C18 column (250 mm × 4.6 mm, 5 µm), using a gradient system of two eluents: acetonitrile and water containing 0.1% formic acid (35:65) at a flow rate of 1 mL/min. The detection wavelength was 307 nm for *trans*-resveratrol and 370 for quercetin. The injection volume was 20 µL. The concentration of each component of interest was calculated based on a calibration curve created from solutions of the *trans*-resveratrol standard at concentrations of 0.1, 0.3, 0.5, 1.0, 1.5 µg/mL and quercetin at concentrations of 0.5, 0.7, 1.0, 1.5, 2.0 µg/mL.

### 2.6. Chemical Characterization by Liquid Chromatography Coupled to Mass Spectrometry (LC–MS) Analysis

We investigated the chemical composition of the fraction with higher total phenolic content and highest antioxidant activity (Fr 2 SySFV). LC–MS analysis was performed on an ultra-performance liquid chromatograph ACQUITY UPLC H-Class (Waters Corporation, Milford, MA, USA) coupled to a quadrupole time-of-flight high-resolution mass spectrometer (Xevo G2-XS QTof, Waters, Manchester, UK) with electrospray ionization (UPLC-ESI-QTOF-HRMS). The mass spectrometer was connected to the ACQUITY UPLC system via an electrospray ionization (ESI) interface. Chromatographic separation of compounds was performed on the ACQUITY UPLC with a conditioned autosampler at 4 °C, using an Acquity BEH C18 column (50 mm × 2.1 mm i.d., 1.7-µm particle size) (Waters, Milford, MA, USA). The column temperature was maintained at 40 °C. The mobile phase consisting of water with 0.1% formic acid in water (solvent A) and acetonitrile (solvent B) was pumped at a flow rate of 0.4 mL min$^{-1}$. The gradient elution program was as follows: 0–5 min, 5%–10% B; 5–9 min, 10%–95% B. The injection volume was 10 µL. MS analysis was performed in the negative ion mode. The scan range was from 50 to 1200 *m/z* for data acquisition. In addition, $MS^E$ experiments were carried out allowing both precursor and product ion data to be acquired simultaneously in one injection. Source conditions were as follows: capillary voltage, 2.0 kV; sample cone, source temperature, 100 °C; desolvation temperature 250 °C; cone gas flow rate 20 L h$^{-1}$; desolvation gas (N$_2$) flow rate 600 L h$^{-1}$. All analyses were performed using the lockspray probe, which ensured accuracy and reproducibility. Leucine–enkephalin (5 ng mL$^{-1}$) was used as a standard or reference compound to calibrate the mass spectrometer during analysis and introduced using the lockspray probe at 10 µL min$^{-1}$ for accurate mass acquisition. All the acquisition and analysis of data were controlled using Waters MassLynx v 4.1 software (Waters, Milford, MA, USA). Simultaneous detection using a photodiode array detector (DAD) was performed monitoring absorbance at wavelengths ranging from 210 to 500 nm.

### 2.7. Animals and Treatment

Thirty-two adult male spontaneously hypertensive rats rats (270–320 g) were housed in a temperature-controlled room, set to a 12:12-h light–dark cycle with free access to standard rat chow (Labina®, Purina, Paulinea, SP, Brazil) and water. When the animals aged 12 weeks, they were treated with a daily dose of Fr 2 SySFV (50 and 100 mg/kg, p.o. by gavage) or saline (0.9% NaCl) for fifteen days. All procedures described in the present study are in agreement with the rules set forth by the Institutional Animal Care and Use Committee of the Federal University of Paraiba (CEUA/UFPB protocol n° 0601/13).

### 2.8. Blood Pressure and Heart Rate Recordings

One day before the experiments, rats were anesthetized with ketamine and xylazine (75 and 10 mg/kg, respectively, both by intraperitoneal injection (i.p.)) and fitted with femoral venous and arterial catheters for drug injection and arterial pressure recordings, respectively. Blood pressure measurements were performed 24 h after catheter implantation as previously described [30]. Changes in blood pressure and heart rate were recorded in conscious rats using a pressure transducer (MLT0380/D, ADInstruments, Sydney, Australia) connected to a computer (Mikro-tip Blood pressure system, ADInstruments, Australia) running the LabChart software (ADInstruments, Australia).

### 2.9. Tiobarbituric Acid Reactive Species (TBARS) Assay

TBARS levels in samples were measured by a spectrophotometric assay that quantifies a chromogen produced by the reaction of thiobarbituric acid with malondialdehyde (MDA), which is the end product of lipid peroxidation, and reacts with TBA as a TBARS to produce a red colored complex with peak absorbance at 532 nm as described previously [31]. Initially, 250 µL of serum was collected from each group and stored at 37 °C for 1 h, after which 400 µL of 35% perchloric acid was added, and the mixture was centrifuged at 14,000 rpm for 20 min at 4 °C. The supernatant was removed, mixed with 400 µL of 0.6% thiobarbituric acid and incubated at 60 °C for 1 h. After cooling, the absorbance at 532 nm was measured. A standard curve was generated using 1,1,3,3-tetramethoxypropane. The results were expressed as nmol of MDA/mL of serum.

### 2.10. Vascular Reactivity Studies in Isolated Rat Superior Mesenteric Artery Rings

Rats were euthanized and the superior mesenteric artery was removed and cleaned from connective tissue and fat. Rings (1–2 mm) were obtained and whenever appropriated, the endothelium was removed by gently rubbing the intimal surface of the vessels and placed in physiological Tyrode's solution. The Tyrode's solution composition was (in mmol/L): 158.3 NaCl; 4.0 KCl; 2.0 CaCl$_2$; 1.05 MgCl$_2$; 0.42 NaH$_2$PO$_4$; 10.0 NaHCO$_3$; 5.6 glucose, kept at 37 °C and gassed with a carbogenic mixture (95% O$_2$ and 5% CO$_2$) and maintained at pH 7.4. All preparations were stabilized under a resting tension of 0.75 g for 1 h. The solution was replaced every 15 min to prevent the accumulation of metabolites. Tension was recorded by a force transducer (PowerLab, ADInstruments, Australia). The presence of functional endothelium was assessed by the ability of acetylcholine (10 mM) to induce 85% relaxation of vessels pre-contracted with Phe (10 mM). Less than 10% of relaxation to acetylcholine was taken as evidence that the vessel segments were functionally denuded of endothelium.

The rings were again contracted with Phe (10 µM) and after about 30 min, increasing and cumulative concentrations of Fr 2 SySFV (0.01, 0.03, 0.1, 0.3, 1, 3, 10, 30, 100, 300, and 1000 µg/mL) were added to obtain a contraction-response curve. The maximal relaxation was calculated using as reference the maximum contracting response obtained to Phe (10 mM) when used at its highest concentration.

### 2.11. Statistical Analysis

Values were expressed as mean ± standard error of mean (SEM) unless otherwise stated. When appropriate, the data were analyzed by Student's *t*-test or two-way ANOVA followed by Tukey's post-test for multiple comparisons, using GraphPad Prism software (v. 5.0, GraphPad Software Inc., San Jose, CA, USA). Values of $p < 0.05$ were considered statistically significant.

## 3. Results

### 3.1. Phenolic Content and Antioxidant Activity

The fractionation of red wine using liquid-liquid extraction afforded three fractions (Fr 1 SySFV, Fr 2 SySFV and Fr 3 SySFV). The total phenolic content of these fractions as well as their antioxidant activity expresssed as $EC_{50}$ values are shown in Table 1. The total phenolic content of the fractions ranged from $5.57 \pm 0.01$ to $58.45 \pm 0.01$ mg GAE/100 mg. The fraction with the highest phenolic content was Fr 2 SySFV with $58.45 \pm 0.01$ mg GAE/100 mg. This fraction was obtained at neutral pH and concentrates flavonoids, phenolic acids and flavonoid glycosides [26], compounds with known antioxidant activity. It was thus expected that Fr 2 SySFV would display the highest radical scavenging activity on antioxidant assays. The antioxidant activity against DPPH radical expressed as $EC_{50}$ values varied from $3.4 \pm 0.03$ to $56,27 \pm 5.50$ µg/mL. Fr 2 SySFV was the most active of the three fractions tested ($EC_{50} = 3.4 \pm 0.03$ µg/mL), while Fr 1 SySFV was the least active. Ascorbic acid had an $EC_{50}$ value of $4.38 \pm 0.07$ µg/mL, thus showing that Fr 2 SySFV had radical-scavenging activities comparable to this standard. Similar results were found for the ABTS radical-scavenging assay (Table 1), with Fr 2 SySFV again displaying the highest antioxidant activity ($EC_{50} = 4.65 \pm 0.04$ µg/mL). A strong correlation ($r^2 = 0.9999$) was obtained between the $EC_{50}$ values of the fractions on the two radical-scavenging assays. Also, negative and strong correlations were obtained between total phenolic content of the fractions and their $EC_{50}$ values at DPPH or ABTS radical-scavenging assays ($r^2 = -0.8447$ and $r^2 = -0.8385$, respectively). The content of trans-resveratrol and quercetin in Fr 2 SySFV as determined by HPLC was $1.11 \pm 0.009$ and $8.56 \pm 0.078$ µg/mL, respectively.

**Table 1.** Total phenolic content of the wine fractions (expressed as gallic acid equivalents, GAE/100 mg fraction) and their antioxidant radical scavenging activity (as $EC_{50}$ values). DPPH: 1,1-diphenyl-2-picrylhydrazyl radical; ABTS: 2,20-azino-bis-3-ethylbenzothiazoline-6-sulphonic acid.

| Samples | Total Phenolic Content (mg GAE/100 mg) | $EC_{50}$ (µg/mL) | |
|---|---|---|---|
| | | DPPH | ABTS |
| Fr 1 SySFV | $5.57 \pm 0.01$ | $56.27 \pm 5.50$ | $90.48 \pm 1.34$ |
| Fr 2 SySFV | $58.45 \pm 0.01$ | $3.4 \pm 0.03$ | $4.65 \pm 0.04$ |
| Fr 3 SySFV | $26.29 \pm 0.03$ | $13.25 \pm 0.07$ | $11.47 \pm 0.55$ |
| Ascorbic acid | - | $4.38 \pm 0.07$ | - |
| Trolox | - | - | $3.77 \pm 0.02$ |

### 3.2. Chemical Characterization of Fr 2 SySFV by UPLC-ESI-QTOF-HRMS

The chemical characterization of Fr 2 Sy SFV confirmed that this fraction concentrated flavonols, phenolic acids and flavonol glycosides. Figure 1 shows the total ion chromatogram with the marked peaks of the main compounds identified. The identification was based on comparison of the predicted versus theoretical exact mass of the compounds and also on the presence of characteristic fragment ions (Table 2) on the mass spectrum. Twenty five compounds in total were thus identified and the chemical classes included as major constituents flavonoids and its glycosides (myricetin, myricetin hexoside, dihydroquercetin hexoside, quercetin hexoside, myricetin methyl ether hexoside, dihydrokaempferol hexoside, myricetin dimethyl ether hexoside, dihydrokaempferol rhamnoside, quercetin, myricetin methyl ether, quercetin methyl ether and luteolin), but also phenolic acids and derivatives (caffeic acid, p-coumaric acid, syringic acid, dimethoxy-cinnamic acid, and methyl-methoxycinnamate), catechins (catechin, epicatechin, epigallocatechin-coumaroyl, and epigallocatechin-cinnamoyl) and anthocyanins (procyanidin dimer and procyanidin dimer monoglycoside). The presence of these classes of compounds in Fr 2 SySFV confirms the efficacy of the wine's liquid-liquid fractionation scheme to concentrate the main bioactive phenolics in the neutral acetate fraction.

Table 2. Identification of compounds present in the fraction Fr 2 SySFV by UPLC–QTOF/MS [E].

| * Peak | Retention Time (min) | λmax | Compounds | Molecular Formula | [M−H]⁻ | Fragments (m/z) | Calc. Mass | Error (ppm) |
|---|---|---|---|---|---|---|---|---|
| 1 | 4.15 | 278 | Catechin | $C_{15}H_{14}O_6$ | 289.0706 | 245.0816 | 289.0712 | 2.10 |
| 2 | 4.48 | 278 | Procyanidin dimer [a] | $C_{30}H_{26}O_{12}$ | 577.1352 | 407.0798, 305.0674 | 577.1352 | 1.04 |
| 3 | 4.48 | 278 | Procyanidin dimer [a] | $C_{30}H_{26}O_{12}$ | 577.1331 | 407.0758, 289.0720 | 577.1352 | 2.60 |
| 4 | 4.50 | 322 | Caffeic acid | $C_9H_8O_4$ | 179.0346 | 160.8423, 135.0452 | 179.0344 | 1.11 |
| 5 | 4.71 | 278 | Epicatechin | $C_{15}H_{14}O_6$ | 289.0710 | 245.0824 | 289.0712 | 0.72 |
| 6 | 4.98 | 282 | Procyanidin dimer monoglycoside | $C_{36}H_{36}O_{17}$ | 739.1848 | 577.1340, 455.1034 | 739.1879 | >10 |
| 7 | 5.14 | 285 | Myricetin hexoside | $C_{21}H_{20}O_{13}$ | 479.0822 | 316.0234 | 479.0825 | 0.63 |
| 8 | 5.21 | 285 | Dihydroquercetin hexoside | $C_{21}H_{22}O_{12}$ | 465.1012 | 319.0827, 301.0351 | 465.1033 | 4.51 |
| 9 | 5.31 | 308 | p-Coumaric acid | $C_9H_8O_3$ | 163.0399 | 119.0505 | 163.0395 | 2.45 |
| 10 | 5.56 | 272 | Syringic acid | $C_9H_{10}O_5$ | 197.0453 | 160.8495 | 197.0450 | 1.52 |
| 11 | 5.56 | 374 | Myricetin | $C_{15}H_{10}O_8$ | 317.0301 | 259.0278 | 317.0303 | 1.26 |
| 12 | 5.70 | ND | Epigallocatechin-coumaroyl [a] | $C_{24}H_{20}O_9$ | 451.1026 | 341.0581, 255.8171 | 451.1035 | 0.66 |
| 13 | 5.71 | 357 | Quercetin hexoside | $C_{21}H_{20}O_{12}$ | 463.0852 | 300.0280, 271.0253 | 463.0876 | 5.20 |
| 14 | 5.73 | 357 | Myricetin methyl ether hexoside | $C_{22}H_{22}O_{13}$ | 493.0988 | 449.1082, 333.0980 | 493.0988 | 1.22 |
| 15 | 5.75 | 286 | Dihydrokaempferol hexoside | $C_{21}H_{22}O_{11}$ | 449.1085 | 285.0404, 229.1086 | 449.1085 | 0.22 |
| 16 | 6.29 | 283 | Epigallocatechin-coumaroyl [a] | $C_{24}H_{20}O_9$ | 451.1018 | 341.0667, 271.0651 | 451.1035 | 2.43 |
| 17 | 6.34 | 358 | Myricetin dimethyl ether hexoside | $C_{23}H_{24}O_{13}$ | 507.1122 | 477.1027, 341.1033 | 417.1114 | 3.35 |
| 18 | 6.44 | 282 | Dihydrokaempferol-rhamnoside | $C_{21}H_{22}O_{10}$ | 433.1139 | 353.1249, 267.1602 | 433.1140 | 0.92 |
| 19 | 6.90 | 305 | Epigallocatechin-cinnamoyl | $C_{24}H_{20}O_8$ | 435.1063 | 341.0666, 285.0812 | 435.1085 | 3.90 |
| 20 | 7.63 | 371 | Quercetin | $C_{15}H_{10}O_7$ | 301.0345 | 273.0420, 197.8082 | 301.0348 | 1.33 |
| 21 | 7.71 | 374 | Myricetin methyl ether | $C_{16}H_{12}O_8$ | 331.0448 | 301.0353, 197.8083 | 331.0459 | 3.02 |
| 22 | 8.21 | 324 | Dimethoxy-cinnamic acid | $C_{11}H_{12}O_4$ | 207.0671 | 161.0255, 130.0462 | 207.0663 | 8.24 |
| 23 | 8.61 | 360 | Luteolin | $C_{15}H_{10}O_6$ | 285.0404 | 239.9008, 197.8085 | 285.0399 | 1.40 |
| 24 | 8.86 | 360 | Quercetin methyl ether | $C_{16}H_{12}O_7$ | 315.0510 | 300.0280, 197.8084 | 315.0510 | 1.58 |
| 25 | 9.41 | 309 | Methyl methoxycinnamate | $C_{11}H_{12}O_3$ | 191.0715 | 174.9576, 145.0302 | 191.0714 | 3.66 |

* Peak number as marked in the chromatogram shown in Figure 1; ND—representative fragments were not detected; [a] positional isomers.

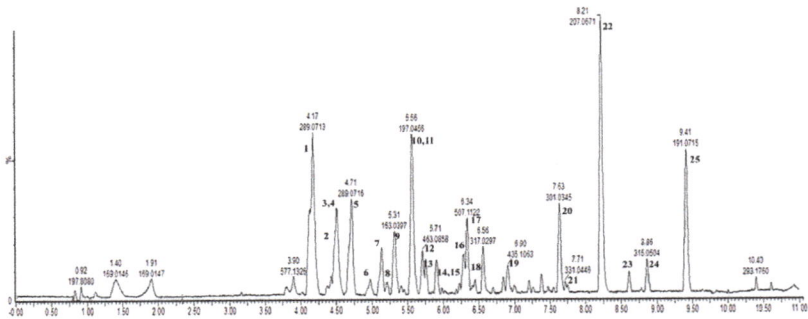

**Figure 1.** Base peak total ion chromatogram of the wine fraction (Fr 2 SySFV) obtained by an MS$^E$ data collection technique method using ultra performance liquid chromatography coupled with time of flight mass spectrometry (UPLC-QTOF/MS$^E$) in negative electrospray ionization mode (ESI$^-$).

### 3.3. Treatment with Fr 2 SySFV Reduces Blood Pressure in Spontaneoulsy Hypertensive Rats (SHR) In Vivo

Figure 2 shows representative tracings illustrating changes in pulse arterial pressure (PAP), mean arterial pressure (MAP) and heart rate (HR) in SHR groups pre-treated with Fr 2 SySFV and saline-treated controls. Treatment of animals with Fr 2 SySFV for fifteen days at 50 mg/kg by gavage (p.o) significantly reduced blood pressure when compared to the control group ($146.1 \pm 4.062$ $n = 7$ vs. $159.0 \pm 3.891$ mmHg, $n = 7$, respectively) as well as when administered at 100 mg/kg ($126.5 \pm 5.322$ $n = 8$ vs. $150.0 \pm 3.039$ mmHg, $n = 7$, respectively). Only the 100 mg/kg dose was able to significantly decrease the heart rate compared to the control group ($314.6 \pm 9.507$, $n = 8$, $358.6 \pm 15.00$ bpm, $n = 7$, respectively). These results are also shown in the group data in Figure 3.

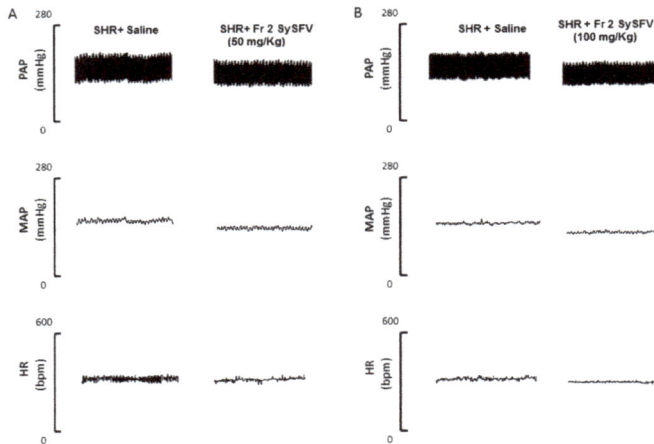

**Figure 2.** Representative tracings illustrating the changes in pulse arterial pressure (PAP, mmHg), mean arterial pressure (MAP, mmHg) and heart rate (HR, bpm) in spontaneously hypertensive rats (SHR) pretreated with Fr 2 SySFV at 50 mg/kg (**A**) and 100 mg/kg (**B**) p.o. and in saline-treated controls.

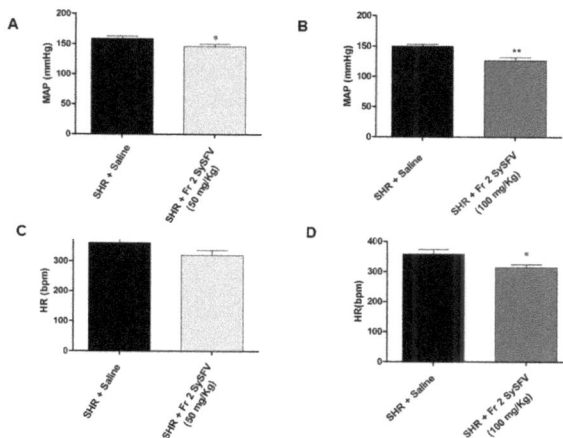

**Figure 3.** Effect of pre-treatment with Fr 2 SySFV on mean arterial pressure (MAP) of spontaneously hypertensive rats (SHR) at doses of 50 mg/kg p.o. (**A**) and 100 mg/kg p.o. (**B**) and on heart rate (HR) at 50 mg/kg p.o. (**C**) and 100 mg/kg p.o. (**D**) compared to saline-treated controls. * $p < 0.05$ and ** $p < 0.005$ when compared to SHR + saline group. Values are mean ± SEM., $n = 7$ for 50 mg/kg groups and $n = 8$ for 100 mg/kg groups

### 3.4. Treatment with Fr 2 SySFV Reduces Oxidative Stress in Spontaneoulsy Hypertensive Rats

We investigated whether pretreatment of SHR rats with Fr 2 SySFV by gavage for fifteen days at doses of 50 mg/kg and 100 mg/kg could affect the levels of serum lipid peroxidation as a measure of oxidative stress. Serum malondialdehyde levels were compared in animals pre-treated with Fr 2 SySFV for 15 days p.o. and saline-treated controls (Figure 4). Pre-treatment with Fr 2 SySFV was able to significantly decrease lipid peroxidation (0.9250 nmol/L ± 0.1750 $n = 4$ vs. 2.180 nmol/L ± 0.3891 $n = 5$) at the 100 mg/kg dose level but not at 50 mg/kg. This in vivo antioxidant effect confirms that the phenolic compounds present in the wine fraction are bioavailable when administered by gavage for 15 days and effectively contribute to plasma total antioxidant capacity.

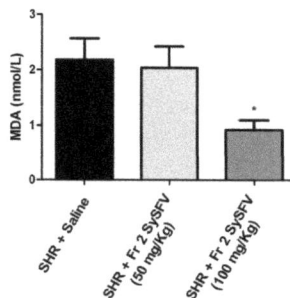

**Figure 4.** Levels of serum malondialdehyde (MDA) in spontaneously hypertensive rats pre-treated with Fr 2 SySFV for 15 days p.o. at doses of 50 mg/kg and 100 mg/kg and saline-treated controls. * $p < 0.05$, when compared to SHR + saline group. Values are mean ± SEM., $n = 5$ for each group.

### 3.5. Fr 2 Sy SFV Induces Endothelium-Independent Vasorelaxation in Isolated Rat Superior Mesenteric Rings

Red wine flavonoids are known to exert direct vasorelaxant activity. Thus, in order to investigate whether a direct decrease in peripheral resistance was contributing to the hypotensive effect of Fr 2

Sy SFV observed in spontaneously hypertensive rats, we tested in vitro the effect of the fraction on contractions induced by phenylephrine (PHE) on isolated rat superior mesenteric rings. In isolated rat mesenteric artery rings with intact endothelium, Fr 2 SySFV (at 0.01–1000 μg/mL) induced a concentration-dependent relaxation on the contractions induced by Phe (10 mM) (maximum relaxation to contractions by Phe 10 mM = 103.5 ± 9.9%, $n$ = 7) (Figure 5). After endothelium removal, the vasorelaxant effect elicited by Fr 2 SySFV was not significantly attenuated (Emax = 105.6 ± 5.9% $n$ = 6) (Figure 5). These results demonstrate that a decrease in peripheral resistance is probably involved in the hypotensive effects of Fr 2 SySFV observed in SHR and that the vasorelaxant effect of the fraction is not mediated by endothelium.

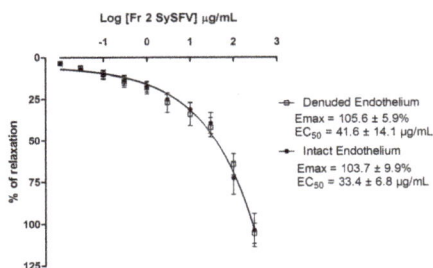

**Figure 5.** Concentration–response curves showing the relaxant effect induced by Fr 2 SySFV (0.01–1000 μg/mL) in rat mesenteric artery rings pre-contracted with phenylephrine (10 μM) in presence (–●–) and absence (–□–) of functional endothelium. Results are expressed as mean ± SEM; $n$ = 7 for rings with intact endothelium and $n$ = 8 for rings with denuded endothelium.

## 4. Discussion

Our results demonstrate that the fractionation of the red wine (Syrah variety) from the São Francisco Valley (SFV), yielded a fraction with high total phenolic content. In this work as in a previous study published by our group [4] the highest phenolic content as well as the highest antioxidant activity was found in the neutral (pH 7) acetate fraction (Fr 2 SySFV). According to Menkovic et al., (2014) [32] that used the same fractionation scheme as ours to study a red wine produced in Serbia from the Prokupac variety, the highest levels of phenolics were also observed in the EtOAc fraction obtained at pH 7.0. However, the value of total phenolics found in the study by Menkovic et al. for this fraction was almost half of what we found here for the Syrah red wine from the SFV, confirming the particularly high phenolic content of the red wines from the region. The climate conditions of the SFV and viticulture techniques including the use of controlled-stress irrigation, can contribute to the phenolic profile of these wines as demonstrated previously [33,34]. Our data also confirmed the correlation between the content of phenolic components and the radical scavenging activity of wine and its fractions which has been described in numerous studies [35–38], despite some authors reporting a lack of correlation between these variables and stressing the importance of the individual phenolic compounds in determining antioxidant activity [39].

The levels of *trans*-resveratrol and quercetin in Fr 2 Sy SFV were similar to those found in the literature for red wines [40–42], although higher levels of quercetin and trans-resveratrol have been reported in wines from warm climates such as in the SFV [43,44]. The concentration of *trans*-resveratrol is usually determined by the levels of biotic and abiotic stress in the grapes [45]. However, photoisomerization of *trans*-resveratrol into *cis*-resveratrol is known to occur with high sunlight exposure or during fermentation and storage [46–48]. Indeed, levels of cis-resveratrol up to five times those of trans-resveratrol were found in red wines from the SFV [4]. The fractionation of the wine sample proved to be efficient in concentrating bioactive phenolics, since the presence of expected chemical constituents in Fr 2 Sy SFV was confirmed by the experiments using UPLC/MS [26].

Ghiselli et al. (1998) [26] also reported the presence of some procyanidins, catechin, epicatechin, and quercetin-3-glucoside in the EtOAc extract at pH 7.0.

Evidence suggests that hypertensive animals have high levels of oxidative stress [6] and that free radical production can directly or indirectly play a major role in cellular processes implicated in cardiovascular diseases (CVD). Phenolic compounds have been largely considered dietary antioxidant compounds although much controversy still exists about their bioavailability [49]. In the present study the oral administration of Fr 2 Sy SFV in rats SHR for 15 days decreased arterial blood pressure at all doses tested and decreased heart rate at the highest dose (100 mg/kg). In addition, the treatment of animals with the fraction decreased oxidative stress as measured by serum malondialdehyde levels. These results are in line with previous studies, indicating that the antioxidant activity of phenolic compounds such as quercetin [31], vanillic acid [50], and rutin [51] are mainly responsible for the effects of these compounds on blood pressure in different models of hypertension. Recently, quercetin, one of the constituents of Fr 2 SySFV was shown to exert a reduction on blood pressure and on serum malondialdehyde levels in spontaneously hypertensive rats [52]. The antihypertensive effect of Fr 2 Sy SFV in reducing the mean arterial blood pressure is almost equipotent to that of the lyophilized Cabernet Sauvignon red wine from SFV as reported by Ribeiro et al., 2016 [53]. These authors demonstrated that the oral treatment of animals with 100 mg/kg lyophilized wine for 9 days reduced mean arterial blood pressure of chronically L-NAME-treated hypertensive Wistar rats by 29 mmHg compared to a reduction of 24 mmHg in our study. One of the hallmarks of the hypertensive pathophysiological process is endothelium dysfunction provoked by excessive reactive oxygen species production and vascular inflammation [54]. Although numerous studies indicate that red wine and polyphenols present in wine induce an endothelium-dependent vasorelaxant effects [55–57], our results have shown that Fr 2 SySFV at concentrations of 0.01–1000 µg/mL induced concentration-dependent relaxation of isolated rat superior mesenteric rings pre-contracted with phenylephrine, an effect which was not attenuated by removal of ring endothelium. In a previous study with a lyophilized red wine from SFV, Luciano et al. (2011) [25] demonstrated the vasorelaxant activity of the wine was significantly attenuated by endothelium removal. It seems plausible to hypothesize that in our work, the fractionation of red wine concentrated phenolic compounds with endothelium-independent vasorelaxant activity. Indeed, it was previously shown that resveratrol is able to induce endothelium-independent relaxation in human internal mammary artery [58]. Quercetin, a flavonoid abundant in most red wines has also been shown to produce endothelium-independent relaxation in arteries of resistance and conductance in rabbits [59].

Considering the 50 mg/kg dose in rats used in this study, Fr 2 SySFV corresponds to an intake of approximately one 750-mL bottle of wine in humans (for a person with an average weight of 70 kg). It is thus not very practical to consider this intake in terms of wine servings, although Fr 2 SySFV could easily be formulated into a dietary supplement or alcohol-free drink. Although we may contemplate vinification practices that could produce wines with chemical composition approaching that of Fr 2 SySFV, the wines would definitely have very different sensorial properties that could impact negatively on their acceptance and commercial viability. Thus, a dietary supplement would definitely be the most viable alternative to achieve an intake of phenolics in human diet that corresponds to the doses administered in this study.

## 5. Conclusions

Taken together our results demonstrate that it is possible to concentrate bioactive and bioavailable phenolics from red wine with important antioxidant and hypotensive activities that are not dependent on intact endothelium function. These results warrant further studies on the effects of individual phenolics on hypertension and on vascular reactivity. Of particular interest would be the identification of the individual phenolics responsible for the endothelium-independent vasorelaxation and hypotensive effects observed for the fraction.

**Acknowledgments:** Grant number PRONEM APQ-0741-1.06/14.

**Author Contributions:** E.J. Oliveira and V.A. Braga conceived the analyses and supervised and revised data analysis and manuscript preparation. E.A. de Figueiredo prepared the first draft of the manuscript and conducted experimental work. N.F.B. Alves, M.M. de Oliveira and C. de O. Cavalcanti conducted experimental work. T.M.S. Silva and T.M.G. da Silva helped with the LC/MS experiments.

**Conflicts of Interest:** The authors declare no conflict of interest.

## References

1. Cheynier, V. Polyphenols in foods are more complex than often thought. *Am. J. Clin. Nutr.* **2005**, *81*, 223S–229S. [PubMed]
2. Padilla, E.; Ruiz, E.; Redondo, S.; Gordillo-Moscoso, A.; Slowing, K.; Tejerina, T. Relationship between vasodilation capacity and phenolic content of Spanish wines. *Eur. J. Pharmacol.* **2005**, *517*, 84–91. [CrossRef] [PubMed]
3. Lima, M.d.S.; Silani, I.d.S.V.; Toaldo, I.M.; Corrêa, L.C.; Biasoto, A.C.T.; Pereira, G.E.; Bordignon-Luiz, M.T.; Ninow, J.L. Phenolic compounds, organic acids and antioxidant activity of grape juices produced from new Brazilian varieties planted in the northeast region of Brazil. *Food Chem.* **2014**, *161*, 94–103. [CrossRef] [PubMed]
4. Lucena, A.P.S.; Nascimento, R.J.B.; Maciel, J.A.C.; Tavares, J.X.; Barbosa-Filho, J.M.; Oliveira, E.J. Antioxidant activity and phenolics content of selected Brazilian wines. *J. Food Comp. Anal.* **2010**, *23*, 30–36. [CrossRef]
5. Botelho-Ono, M.S.; Pina, H.V.; Sousa, K.H.F.; Nunes, F.C.; Medeiros, I.A.; Braga, V.A. Acute superoxide scavenging restores depressed baroreflex sensitivity in renovascular hypertensive rats. *Auton. Neurosci.* **2011**, *159*, 38–44. [CrossRef] [PubMed]
6. Braga, V.A.; Medeiros, I.A.; Ribeiro, T.P.; França-Silva, M.S.; Botelho-Ono, M.S.; Guimarães, D.D. Angiotensin-ii-induced reactive oxygen species along the sfo-pvn-rvlm pathway: Implications in neurogenic hypertension. *Braz. J. Med. Biol. Res.* **2011**, *44*, 871–876. [CrossRef] [PubMed]
7. Porpino, S.K.P.; Zollbrecht, C.; Peleli, M.; Montenegro, M.F.; Brandão, M.C.R.; Athayde-Filho, P.F.; França-Silva, M.S.; Larsson, E.; Lundberg, J.O.; Weitzberg, E.; et al. Nitric oxide generation by the organic nitrate ndbp attenuates oxidative stress and angiotensin ii-mediated hypertension: Organic nitrate and hypertension. *Br. J. Pharmacol.* **2016**, *173*, 2290–2302. [CrossRef] [PubMed]
8. Lazartigues, E. Inflammation and neurogenic hypertension: A new role for the circumventricular organs? *Circ. Res.* **2010**, *107*, 166–167. [CrossRef] [PubMed]
9. Pedro-Botet, J.; Covas, M.I.; Martín, S.; Rubiés-Prat, J. Decreased endogenous antioxidant enzymatic status in essential hypertension. *J. Hum. Hypertens.* **2000**, *14*, 343–345. [CrossRef] [PubMed]
10. Romero, J.C.; Reckelhoff, J.F. Role of angiotensin and oxidative stress in essential hypertension. *Hypertension* **1999**, *34*, 943–949. [CrossRef] [PubMed]
11. Valko, M.; Leibfritz, D.; Moncol, J.; Cronin, M.T.D.; Mazur, M.; Telser, J. Free radicals and antioxidants in normal physiological functions and human disease. *Int. J. Biochem. Cell Biol.* **2007**, *39*, 44–84. [CrossRef] [PubMed]
12. Zimmerman, M.C.; Lazartigues, E.; Sharma, R.V.; Davisson, R.L. Hypertension caused by angiotensin II infusion involves increased superoxide production in the central nervous system. *Circ. Res.* **2004**, *95*, 210–216. [CrossRef] [PubMed]
13. Paravicini, T.M.; Touyz, R.M. Nadph oxidases, reactive oxygen species, and hypertension: Clinical implications and therapeutic possibilities. *Diabetes Care* **2008**, *31*, S170–S180. [CrossRef] [PubMed]
14. Dhawan, V.; Jain, S. Effect of garlic supplementation on oxidized low density lipoproteins and lipid peroxidation in patients of essential hypertension. *Mol. Cell. Biochem.* **2004**, *266*, 109–115. [CrossRef] [PubMed]
15. Arts, I.C.W.; Hollman, P.C.H. Polyphenols and disease risk in epidemiologic studies. *Am. J. Clin. Nutr.* **2005**, *81*, 317S–325S. [PubMed]
16. Habauzit, V.; Morand, C. Evidence for a protective effect of polyphenols-containing foods on cardiovascular health: An update for clinicians. *Ther. Adv. Chronic Dis.* **2012**, *3*, 87–106. [CrossRef] [PubMed]
17. Pandey, K.B.; Rizvi, S.I. Plant polyphenols as dietary antioxidants in human health and disease. *Oxid. Med. Cell. Longev.* **2009**, *2*, 270–278. [CrossRef] [PubMed]

18. Grosso, G.; Stepaniak, U.; Micek, A.; Stefler, D.; Bobak, M.; Pajak, A. Dietary polyphenols are inversely associated with metabolic syndrome in Polish adults of the hapiee study. *Eur. J. Nutr.* **2016**. [CrossRef] [PubMed]

19. Medina-Remon, A.; Zamora-Ros, R.; Rotches-Ribalta, M.; Andres-Lacueva, C.; Martinez-Gonzalez, M.A.; Covas, M.I.; Corella, D.; Salas-Salvado, J.; Gomez-Gracia, E.; Ruiz-Gutierrez, V.; et al. Total polyphenol excretion and blood pressure in subjects at high cardiovascular risk. *Nutr. Metab. Cardiovasc. Dis.* **2011**, *21*, 323–331. [CrossRef] [PubMed]

20. Miranda, A.M.; Steluti, J.; Fisberg, R.M.; Marchioni, D.M. Association between polyphenol intake and hypertension in adults and older adults: A population-based study in Brazil. *PLoS ONE* **2016**, *11*, e0165791. [CrossRef] [PubMed]

21. Cassidy, A.; O'Reilly, E.J.; Kay, C.; Sampson, L.; Franz, M.; Forman, J.P.; Curhan, G.; Rimm, E.B. Habitual intake of flavonoid subclasses and incident hypertension in adults. *Am. J. Clin. Nutr.* **2011**, *93*, 338–347. [CrossRef] [PubMed]

22. Lajous, M.; Rossignol, E.; Fagherazzi, G.; Perquier, F.; Scalbert, A.; Clavel-Chapelon, F.; Boutron-Ruault, M.C. Flavonoid intake and incident hypertension in women. *Am. J. Clin. Nutr.* **2016**, *103*, 1091–1098. [CrossRef] [PubMed]

23. Freedman, J.E.; Parker, C.; Li, L.; Perlman, J.A.; Frei, B.; Ivanov, V.; Deak, L.R.; Iafrati, M.D.; Folts, J.D. Select flavonoids and whole juice from purple grapes inhibit platelet function and enhance nitric oxide release. *Circulation* **2001**, *103*, 2792–2798. [CrossRef] [PubMed]

24. Apostolidou, C.; Adamopoulos, K.; Lymperaki, E.; Iliadis, S.; Papapreponis, P.; Kourtidou-Papadeli, C. Cardiovascular risk and benefits from antioxidant dietary intervention with red wine in asymptomatic hypercholesterolemics. *Clin. Nutr. ESPEN* **2015**, *10*, e224–e233. [CrossRef] [PubMed]

25. Luciano, M.N.; Ribeiro, T.P.; França-Silva, M.S.; do Nascimento, R.J.B.; de Jesus Oliveira, E.; França, K.C.; Antunes, A.A.; Nakao, L.S.; Aita, C.A.M.; Braga, V.A.; et al. Uncovering the vasorelaxant effect induced by vale do são francisco red wine: A role for nitric oxide. *J. Cardiovasc. Pharmacol.* **2011**, *57*, 696–701. [CrossRef] [PubMed]

26. Ghiselli, N.; Nardini, N.; Baldi, N.; Scaccini, N. Antioxidant activity of different phenolic fractions separated from an Italian red wine. *J. Agric. Food Chem.* **1998**, *46*, 361–367. [CrossRef] [PubMed]

27. Waterhouse, A.L. Determination of total phenolics. In *Current Protocols in Food Analytical Chemistry*; Wrolstad, R.E., Acree, T.E., Decker, E.A., Penner, M.H., Reid, D.S., Schwartz, S.J., Shoemaker, C.F., Smith, D., Sporns, P., Eds.; John Wiley & Sons, Inc.: Hoboken, NJ, USA, 2003.

28. Garcez, F.R.; Garcez, W.S.; Hamerski, L.; Miguita, C.H. Fenilpropanóides e outros constituintes bioativos de nectandra megapotamica. *Quím. Nova* **2009**, *32*, 407–411. [CrossRef]

29. Re, R.; Pellegrini, N.; Proteggente, A.; Pannala, A.; Yang, M.; Rice-Evans, C. Antioxidant activity applying an improved abts radical cation decolorization assay. *Free Radic. Biol. Med.* **1999**, *26*, 1231–1237. [CrossRef]

30. Braga, V.A. Dietary salt enhances angiotensin-ii-induced superoxide formation in the rostral ventrolateral medulla. *Auton. Neurosci.* **2010**, *155*, 14–18. [CrossRef] [PubMed]

31. Monteiro, M.; França-Silva, M.; Alves, N.; Porpino, S.; Braga, V. Quercetin improves baroreflex sensitivity in spontaneously hypertensive rats. *Molecules* **2012**, *17*, 12997–13008. [CrossRef] [PubMed]

32. Menkovic, N.; Zivkovic, J.; Savikin, K.; Godjevac, D.; Zdunic, G. Phenolic composition and free radical scavenging activity of wine produced from Serbian autochtonous grape variety prokupac: A model approach. *J. Serb. Chem. Soc.* **2014**, *79*, 11–24. [CrossRef]

33. Chavarria, G.; Bergamaschi, H.; Silva, L.C.d.; Santos, H.P.d.; Mandelli, F.; Guerra, C.C.; Flores, C.A.; Tonietto, J. Relações hídricas, rendimento e compostos fenólicos de uvas cabernet sauvignon em três tipos de solo. *Bragantia* **2011**, *70*, 481–487. [CrossRef]

34. Peterlunger, E.; Sivilotti, P.; Colussi, V. Water stress increased polyphenolic quality in 'merlot' grapes. *Acta Hortic.* **2005**, *689*, 293–300. [CrossRef]

35. Fernández-Pachón, M.S.; Villaño, D.; García-Parrilla, M.C.; Troncoso, A.M. Antioxidant activity of wines and relation with their polyphenolic composition. *Anal. Chim. Acta* **2004**, *513*, 113–118. [CrossRef]

36. Leja, M.; Kamińska, I.; Kramer, M.; Maksylewicz-Kaul, A.; Kammerer, D.; Carle, R.; Baranski, R. The content of phenolic compounds and radical scavenging activity varies with carrot origin and root color. *Plant Foods Hum. Nutr.* **2013**, *68*, 163–170. [CrossRef] [PubMed]

37. Lingua, M.S.; Fabani, M.P.; Wunderlin, D.A.; Baroni, M.V. In vivo antioxidant activity of grape, pomace and wine from three red varieties grown in Argentina: Its relationship to phenolic profile. *J. Funct. Foods* **2016**, *20*, 332–345. [CrossRef]

38. Velioglu, Y.S.; Mazza, G.; Gao, L.; Oomah, B.D. Antioxidant activity and total phenolics in selected fruits, vegetables, and grain products. *J. Agric. Food Chem.* **1998**, *46*, 4113–4117. [CrossRef]

39. Rice-Evans, C.A.; Miller, N.J. Antioxidant activities of flavonoids as bioactive components of food. *Biochem. Soc. Trans.* **1996**, *24*, 790–795. [CrossRef] [PubMed]

40. De Souza Dias, F.; Silva, M.F.; David, J.M. Determination of quercetin, gallic acid, resveratrol, catechin and malvidin in Brazilian wines elaborated in the vale do são francisco using liquid–liquid extraction assisted by ultrasound and GC-MS. *Food Anal. Method* **2013**, *6*, 963–968. [CrossRef]

41. Dias, F.d.S.; David, J.M.; David, J.P. Determination of phenolic acids and quercetin in brazilian red wines from vale do são francisco region using liquid-liquid ultrasound-assisted extraction and HPLC-DAD-MS. *J. Braz. Chem. Soc.* **2015**, *27*. [CrossRef]

42. Shalashvili, A.; Ugrekhelidze, D.; Mitaishvili, T.; Targamadze, I.; Zambakhidze, N. Phenolic compounds of wines from georgian autochthonous grapes, rkatsiteli and saperavi, prepared by georgian (kakhetian) technology. *ResearchGate* **2012**, *6*, 99–103.

43. Goldberg, D.M.; Tsang, E.; Karumanchiri, A.; Soleas, G.J. Quercetin and p-coumaric acid concentrations in commercial wines. *Am. J. Enol. Vitic.* **1998**, *49*, 142–151.

44. Price, S.F.; Breen, P.J.; Valladao, M.; Watson, B.T. Cluster sun exposure and quercetin in pinot noir grapes and wine. *Am. J. Enol. Vitic.* **1995**, *46*, 187–194.

45. Careri, M.; Corradini, C.; Elviri, L.; Nicoletti, I.; Zagnoni, I. Direct HPLC analysis of quercetin and *trans*-resveratrol in red wine, grape, and winemaking byproducts. *J. Agric. Food Chem.* **2003**, *51*, 5226–5231. [CrossRef] [PubMed]

46. Lamuela-Raventos, R.M.; Romero-Perez, A.I.; Waterhouse, A.L.; de la Torre-Boronat, M.C. Direct HPLC analysis of *cis*- and *trans*-resveratrol and piceid isomers in Spanish red vitis vinifera wines. *J. Agric. Food Chem.* **1995**, *43*, 281–283. [CrossRef]

47. Montsko, G.; Nikfardjam, M.S.P.; Szabo, Z.; Boddi, K.; Lorand, T.; Ohmacht, R.; Mark, L. Determination of products derived from *trans*-resveratrol UV photoisomerisation by means of HPLC–APCI-MS. *J. Photochem. Photobiol. A* **2008**, *196*, 44–50. [CrossRef]

48. Tříska, J.; Vrchotová, N.; Olejníčková, J.; Jílek, R.; Sotolář, R. Separation and identification of highly fluorescent compounds derived from *trans*-resveratrol in the leaves of vitis vinifera infected by plasmopara viticola. *Molecules* **2012**, *17*, 2773–2783. [CrossRef] [PubMed]

49. Hu, M. Commentary: Bioavailability of flavonoids and polyphenols: Call to arms. *Mol. Pharm.* **2007**, *4*, 803–806. [CrossRef] [PubMed]

50. Kumar, S.; Prahalathan, P.; Raja, B. Vanillic acid: A potential inhibitor of cardiac and aortic wall remodeling in l-name induced hypertension through upregulation of endothelial nitric oxide synthase. *Environ. Toxicol. Pharmacol.* **2014**, *38*, 643–652. [CrossRef] [PubMed]

51. Mendes-Junior, L.d.G.; Monteiro, M.M.d.O.; Carvalho, A.D.S.; de Queiroz, T.M.; Braga, V.d.A. Oral supplementation with the rutin improves cardiovagal baroreflex sensitivity and vascular reactivity in hypertensive rats. *Appl. Physiol. Nutr. Metab.* **2013**, *38*, 1099–1106. [CrossRef] [PubMed]

52. Romero, M.; Jiménez, R.; Hurtado, B.; Moreno, J.M.; Rodríguez-Gómez, I.; López-Sepúlveda, R.; Zarzuelo, A.; Pérez-Vizcaino, F.; Tamargo, J.; Vargas, F.; et al. Lack of beneficial metabolic effects of quercetin in adult spontaneously hypertensive rats. *Eur. J. Pharmacol.* **2010**, *627*, 242–250. [CrossRef] [PubMed]

53. Ribeiro, T.P.; Oliveira, A.C.; Mendes-Junior, L.G.; França, K.C.; Nakao, L.S.; Schini-Kerth, V.B.; Medeiros, I.A. Cardiovascular effects induced by northeastern Brazilian red wine: Role of nitric oxide and redox sensitive pathways. *J. Funct. Foods* **2016**, *22*, 82–92. [CrossRef]

54. Dharmashankar, K.; Widlansky, M.E. Vascular endothelial function and hypertension: Insights and directions. *Curr. Hypertens. Rep.* **2010**, *12*, 448–455. [CrossRef] [PubMed]

55. De Moura, R.S.; Miranda, D.Z.; Pinto, A.C.A.; Sicca, R.F.; Souza, M.A.V.; Rubenich, L.M.S.; Carvalho, L.C.R.M.; Rangel, B.M.; Tano, T.; Madeira, S.V.F.; et al. Mechanism of the endothelium-dependent vasodilation and the antihypertensive effect of Brazilian red wine. *J. Cardiovasc. Pharmacol.* **2004**, *44*, 302–309. [CrossRef] [PubMed]

*Nutrients* **2017**, *9*, 574

56. Diebolt, M.; Bucher, B.; Andriantsitohaina, R. Wine polyphenols decrease blood pressure, improve no vasodilatation, and induce gene expression. *Hypertension* **2001**, *38*, 159–165. [CrossRef] [PubMed]

57. Porteri, E.; Rizzoni, D.; De Ciuceis, C.; Boari, G.E.M.; Platto, C.; Pilu, A.; Miclini, M.; Agabiti Rosei, C.; Bulgari, G.; Agabiti Rosei, E. Vasodilator effects of red wines in subcutaneous small resistance artery of patients with essential hypertension. *Am. J. Hypertens.* **2010**, *23*, 373–378. [CrossRef] [PubMed]

58. Novakovic, A.; Gojkovic-Bukarica, L.; Peric, M.; Nezic, D.; Djukanovic, B.; Markovic-Lipkovski, J.; Heinle, H. The mechanism of endothelium-independent relaxation induced by the wine polyphenol resveratrol in human internal mammary artery. *J. Pharmacol. Sci.* **2006**, *101*, 85–90. [CrossRef] [PubMed]

59. Rendig, S.V.; Symons, J.D.; Longhurst, J.C.; Amsterdam, E.A. Effects of red wine, alcohol, and quercetin on coronary resistance and conductance arteries. *J. Cardiovasc. Pharmacol.* **2001**, *38*, 219–227. [CrossRef] [PubMed]

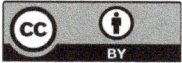

*nutrients*

MDPI

*Article*

# Influence of Hesperidin on the Systemic and Intestinal Rat Immune Response

Mariona Camps-Bossacoma [1,2], Àngels Franch [1,2], Francisco J. Pérez-Cano [1,2] and Margarida Castell [1,2,*]

[1] Section of Physiology, Department of Biochemistry and Physiology, Faculty of Pharmacy and Food Science, University of Barcelona (UB), 08028 Barcelona, Spain; marionacamps@ub.edu (M.C.-B.); angelsfranch@ub.edu (À.F.); franciscoperez@ub.edu (F.J.P.-C.)

[2] Nutrition and Food Safety Research Institute (INSA-UB), 08921 Santa Coloma de Gramenet, Spain

[*] Correspondence: margaridacastell@ub.edu; Tel.: +34-93-402-45-05; Fax: +34-93-403-59-01

Received: 21 April 2017; Accepted: 3 June 2017; Published: 6 June 2017

**Abstract:** Polyphenols, widely found in edible plants, influence the immune system. Nevertheless, the immunomodulatory properties of hesperidin, the predominant flavanone in oranges, have not been deeply studied. To establish the effect of hesperidin on in vivo immune response, two different conditions of immune system stimulations in Lewis rats were applied. In the first experimental design, rats were intraperitoneally immunized with ovalbumin (OVA) plus *Bordetella pertussis* toxin and alum as the adjuvants, and orally given 100 or 200 mg/kg hesperidin. In the second experimental design, rats were orally sensitized with OVA together with cholera toxin and fed a diet containing 0.5% hesperidin. In the first approach, hesperidin administration changed mesenteric lymph node lymphocyte (MLNL) composition, increasing the TCRαβ+ cell percentage and decreasing that of B lymphocytes. Furthermore, hesperidin enhanced the interferon (IFN)-γ production in stimulated MLNL. In the second approach, hesperidin intake modified the lymphocyte composition in the intestinal epithelium (TCRγδ+ cells) and the lamina propria (TCRγδ+, CD45RA+, natural killer, natural killer T, TCRαβ+CD4+, and TCRαβ+CD8+ cells). Nevertheless, hesperidin did not modify the level of serum anti-OVA antibodies in either study. In conclusion, hesperidin does possess immunoregulatory properties in the intestinal immune response, but this effect is not able to influence the synthesis of specific antibodies.

**Keywords:** antibody; flavanone; flavonoids; hesperidin; immune system; immunoregulatory; polyphenol

## 1. Introduction

Polyphenols are secondary metabolites of plants that are widely distributed in fruits (e.g., apple, grape, pear, cherry, berries), vegetables, nuts, flowers, cereals, legumes, chocolate, and beverages (tea, coffee, and wine) [1]. Polyphenols, named thus for the presence of various phenolic groups [2], are mainly classified according to their chemical structure into flavonoids (isoflavones, neoflavonoids, chalcones, flavones, flavonols, flavonones, flavononols, flavanols, proanthocyanidins, and anthocyanidins) or non-flavonoids (phenolic acids or phenolic amides) [3].

In the last 20 years, polyphenols have gained attention mainly due to their antioxidant properties [3,4], and a large number of beneficial effects have been reported such as on degenerative disease, cardiovascular disease, cancer, osteoporosis; and their influence on the immune system has also been shown [2,5,6]. Focusing on polyphenol immunomodulatory properties, a number of in vitro, in vivo, and clinical studies have confirmed the influence of various flavonoids on the innate and acquired immune response by attenuating immune function, thus showing their beneficial role in immune hypersensitivity [7]. Accordingly, flavonoid administration has been demonstrated to be useful in the prevention of allergic asthma and rhinitis [8].

Hesperidin (5,7,3-trihydroxy-4-methoxyflavanone-7-rhamnoglucoside) is a flavonoid belonging to the flavanone class [9], its aglycone form being hesperetin [10]. Hesperidin is mainly found in the fruits of the genus *Citrus* [1], particularly in the epicarp, mesocarp, endocarp, and juice of citrus fruits [11] and it is the predominant flavanone found in oranges [12,13]. The majority of the flavonoids found in citrus fruits are glycosides and just a little quantity of hesperitin is present [12].

To date, several pharmacological effects of hesperidin have been reported. It prevents hypercholesterolaemia and fatty liver [14], osteoporosis [15], hypertension, and cerebral thrombosis, among others [16]. In terms of its effects on the immune system, the role of hesperidin has been described in reducing Th2 cytokines in mouse models of asthma [9,17] and in stimulated macrophages [18]. Nevertheless, there are no in-depth studies concerning hesperidin's effect on immune tissues, including the intestinal lymphoid tissue, and on specific antibody synthesis. In this line, the study of such effects on animal models is of interest because it allows the arrival of hesperidin or its metabolites to the lymphoid tissues, and its analysis will contribute to a better understanding of a flavanone-enriched diet on human health. For this reason, the aim of the current study was to spotlight the effects of hesperidin on Th2 antibody production and on lymphoid tissues, focusing on the gut-associated lymphoid tissue (GALT), which is the first line of defence encountered by the hesperidin present in food. We have investigated this action under two different conditions triggering Th2 immune responses and using three different hesperidin dosages.

## 2. Materials and Methods

### 2.1. Chemicals

Hesperidin was provided by Ferrer HealthTech (Murcia, Spain), with a purity of 95.5% (High Performance Liquid Chromatography) containing 2% isonaringine, 1.5% didimine, and other impurities.

Carboxymethylcellulose (CMC), cholera toxin (CT), fetal bovine serum (FBS), L-glutamine, ovalbumin (OVA, grade V), penicillin-streptomycin, toxin from *Bordetella pertussis* (Bpt), and RPMI 1640 medium were provided by Sigma-Aldrich (Madrid, Spain). Imject™ alum adjuvant was obtained from Thermo Fisher Scientific (Barcelona, Spain). Biotin-conjugated anti-rat immunoglobulin (Ig)A, IgG1, IgG2a, IgG2b, and IgG2c monoclonal antibodies, anti-rat IgE monoclonal antibody, and anti-rat fluorochrome-conjugated monoclonal antibodies (detailed later) were purchased from BD Biosciences (Madrid, Spain), Biolegend (San Diego, CA, USA), or Novus Biologicals (Littleton, CO, USA). Peroxidase conjugated and unconjugated goat anti-rat IgA antibody and IgA standard were provided by Bethyl Laboratories (Montgomery, TX, USA). Peroxidase-conjugated anti-rat Ig was from DakoCytomation (Glostrup, Denmark). 2-β-mercaptoethanol was from Merck (Darmstadt, Germany). Ketamine was provided by Merial Laboratories S.A. (Barcelona, Spain) and xylazine by Bayer A.G. (Leverkusen, Germany).

### 2.2. Animals and Experimental Designs

Three-week-old Lewis rats (Janvier Labs, Saint Berthevin CEDEX, France) were maintained at the animal facility of the Faculty of Pharmacy and Food Science (University of Barcelona) housed in cages (three rats per cage) and kept under controlled conditions of temperature and humidity in a 12 h light-dark cycle. Animal procedures were approved by the Ethical Committee for Animal Experimentation at the University of Barcelona (CEEA/UB ref. 5988) and conducted in compliance with the Guide for the Care and Use of Laboratory Animals.

The effect of hesperidin on systemic and intestinal immune response was studied in two experimental designs (Figure 1). The first design studied the influence of hesperidin in a systemic immune response that was triggered by an intraperitoneal (i.p.) immunization, as previously described [19]. Briefly, rats received an i.p. injection with 0.5 mg of OVA plus 50 ng of *Bordetella pertussis* toxin (Bpt) in 0.5 mL of alum emulsion (1:3 alum:OVA+Bpt solution). Hesperidin was given by oral gavage three times per week at doses of 100 or 200 mg/kg of rat body weight (BW). Therefore, the first experimental design included three groups: the reference immunized group (OVAip group), the immunized group given 100 mg/kg hesperidin (H100 group), and the immunized group given 200 mg/kg hesperidin (H200 group). Hesperidin was prepared daily in 0.5% CMC as vehicle. The OVAip group received the vehicle. In the second design, the effect of hesperidin on the intestinal immune response was triggered in orally sensitized rats and was included in the rat food. For this, rats were orally sensitized with OVA and CT, as previously described [20], and animals were fed either a standard diet (AIN-93M, Harlan Teklad, Madison, WI, USA) (reference sensitized group: OVAoral group), or a diet containing 0.5% hesperidin (H0.5 group). In both designs, the animals had free access to water and food throughout the study. The consumption of water and food per cage was periodically registered and referred to as water or food consumed per 100 g of BW of the rats included in the cage.

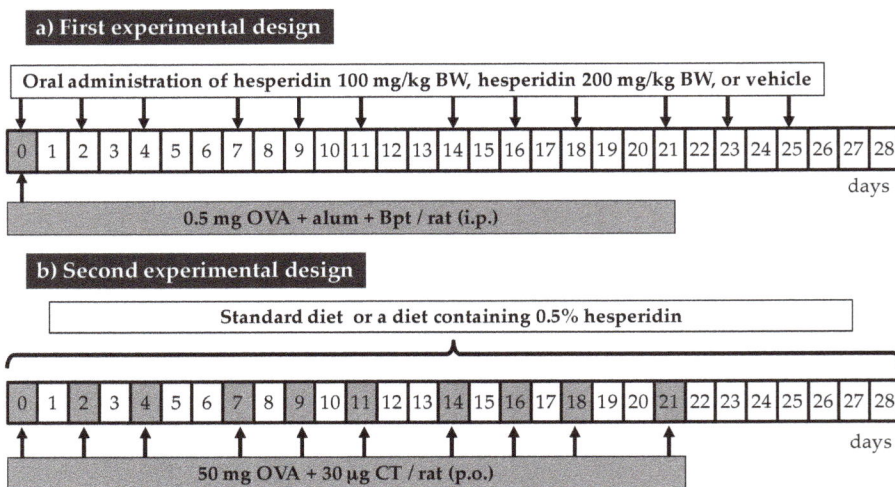

**Figure 1.** Experimental designs. (**a**) First experimental design: rats were immunized by intraperitoneal (i.p.) route the first day of the study (day 0), and hesperidin was given by oral gavage three times per week (indicated by arrows) for 4 weeks; (**b**) Second experimental design: rats were sensitized by oral route (*per os*, p.o.) three times per week (indicated by arrows), and hesperidin was included in the rat food throughout the 4 weeks. BW, body weight; OVA, ovalbumin; CT, cholera toxin.

### 2.3. Sample Collection and Processing

At the end of both studies, animals were anaesthetized by subcutaneous route with ketamine-xylazine. Apart from faecal and blood samples, the mesenteric lymph nodes (MLN) and the small intestine were collected. In the second design, the duodenal part of the intestine was discarded and the rest was opened lengthwise in order to separate the Peyer's patches (PP). From the ileum, intraepithelial lymphocytes (IEL) and lamina propria lymphocytes (LPL) were isolated, as reported previously [21]. From the resting tissue, gut lavage was obtained as previously described [21] and kept at $-20$ °C for IgA quantification and at $-80$ °C for cytokine determination.

The lymphocytes from MLN (MLNL) and from PP (PPL) were also isolated, as detailed in prior research [21,22]. Isolated lymphocyte counts and viability were determined by a Countess™ Automated Cell Counter (Invitrogen™, Thermo Fisher Scientific, Barcelona, Spain) in order to proceed with the staining for the flow cytometric analysis or the culture of MLNL.

Blood samples were centrifuged and serum was kept at $-20$ °C for antibody determination. From faeces, faecal homogenates supernatants were obtained and kept at $-20$ °C for intestinal IgA quantification. Briefly, faeces were dried, weighed, diluted with PBS pH 7.2 (20 mg/mL), homogenized with a Polytron (Kinematica, Lucerne, Switzerland), and, finally, the supernatants obtained after centrifugation were kept at −20 °C for intestinal IgA quantification.

## 2.4. Lymphocyte Phenotypic Analysis

MLNL, PPL, IEL, and LPL were stained with fluorescent-labelled antibodies, as previously described [22]. The following fluorochrome-conjugated antibodies were used: FITC-TCRαβ, FITC-CD8β, FITC-CD25, FITC-TLR4, FITC-CD103, PE-NKR-P1A, PE-TCRγδ, PE-TLR4, PerCP-CD8α, APC-CD4, and APC-Cy8-CD45RA. Data were acquired by Gallios Cytometer (Beckman Coulter, Miami, FL, USA) in the Scientific and Technological Centers of the University of Barcelona (CCiTUB) and the analysis was performed with FlowJo v.10 software (Tree Star, Inc., Ashland, OR, USA). Results are expressed as percentages of positive cells in the lymphocyte population selected according to their forward and side scatter characteristics.

## 2.5. Specific Anti-OVA Antibodies and Intestinal IgA Quantification

The levels of the specific anti-OVA antibodies (total, IgG1, IgG2a, IgG2b, and IgG2c isotypes) were determined by an indirect Enzyme-Linked ImmunoSorbent Assay (ELISA), as previously described [22]. Specific anti-OVA IgE was measured with a modified ELISA, as formerly reported [19]. In all cases, a pool of sera from immunized rats was used as positive control and all data were calculated in accordance with the arbitrary units (A.U.) assigned to this pool.

Total IgA concentration from serum, gut lavages, or faecal homogenates was determined with a sandwich ELISA using a Rat IgA ELISA Quantification Set (E110-102) from Bethyl Laboratories (Montgomery, TX, USA).

## 2.6. Cytokine Quantification

MLNL ($6 \times 10^6$/mL) were cultured in RPMI 1640 medium supplemented with 10% heat-inactivated FBS, 100 IU/mL penicillin-streptomycin, 2 mM L-glutamine, and 0.05 mM 2-β-mercaptoethanol and stimulated with 200 mg/mL of OVA in vitro. After 72 h, supernatants were collected to assess cytokine production.

The cytokines secreted by MLNL and from gut lavage were evaluated by ProcartaPlex® Multiplex Immunoassay (Affymetrix, eBioscience, San Diego, CA, USA) according to the manufacturer's protocol. The analysed cytokines were interleukin (IL)-10, IL-4, monocyte chemoattractant protein (MCP)-1, tumour necrosis factor (TNF)-α, and interferon (IFN)-γ, their detection limits being 11.08, 1.03, 17.99, 3.91, and 4.64 pg/mL, respectively.

## 2.7. Statistical Analysis

Statistical analysis of the data was performed with the software package SPSS version 22.0 (IBM Statistical Package for the Social Sciences, Chicago, IL, USA).

To assess the homogeneity of variance and the distribution of the results, Levene's and Shapiro-Wilk tests were performed, respectively. One-way ANOVA followed by Bonferroni's post hoc test were carried out in cases with homogenized and normally distributed variance from the data. Kruskal-Wallis and Mann-Whitney U tests were performed in cases with non-homogenized and/or non-normally distributed variance from the data. Significant differences were considered when $p \leq 0.05$.

## 3. Results

### 3.1. Effect of Hesperidin on Food and Water Intake and Body Weight

The administration of 100 or 200 mg/kg hesperidin by oral gavage altered neither food nor water consumption in comparison to the reference group (OVAip group) (Table 1). Likewise, the inclusion of hesperidin in the food did not produce any change among groups in food or water intake (Table 2). Moreover, the administration of hesperidin, both by oral gavage or in the food, did not affect BW increase (data not shown).

**Table 1.** Food and water intake in the first experimental design. These values were established per day and per cage and referred to 100 g of the total BW in the cage. Data are expressed as the range between the two values obtained from two cages. OVAip, the reference immunized group; H100, the immunized group given 100 mg/kg hesperidin; H200, the immunized group given 200 mg/kg hesperidin.

| | Food Intake (g/100 g BW/Day) | | | Water Intake (mL/100 g BW/Day) | | |
|---|---|---|---|---|---|---|
| | OVAip | H100 | H200 | OVAip | H100 | H200 |
| Day 4 | 13.06–13.97 | 12.80–13.07 | 13.59–13.92 | 11.73–11.74 | 11.52–15.78 | 11.95–12.11 |
| Day 11 | 13.51–13.57 | 7.75–8.64 | 10.20–10.47 | 11.31–12.66 | 11.26–12.39 | 12.15–12.74 |
| Day 18 | 11.60–12.03 | 11.94–12.02 | 11.82–12.24 | 10.39–11.03 | 11.07–13.83 | 11.42–12.11 |
| Day 25 | 9.32–9.34 | 9.35–9.35 | 9.07–9.08 | 11.01–11.20 | 12.68–14.55 | 13.19–14.85 |
| Day 28 | 9.58–10.16 | 9.38–10.03 | 9.73–9.85 | 11.77–12.87 | 13.95–15.61 | 14.05–15.05 |

**Table 2.** Food and water intake in the second experimental design. These values were established per day and per cage and referred to 100 g of the total BW in the cage. Data are expressed as the range between the two values obtained from two cages. OVAoral, animals were fed a standard diet; H0.5, a diet containing 0.5% hesperidin.

| | Food Intake (g/100 g BW/Day) | | Water Intake (mL/100 g BW/Day) | |
|---|---|---|---|---|
| | OVAoral | H0.5 | OVAoral | H0.5 |
| Day 7 | 10.93–11.37 | 10.74–10.97 | 16.84–24.85 | 14.93–20.67 |
| Day 14 | 11.65–11.70 | 11.28–11.52 | 11.39–14.45 | 11.05–16.23 |
| Day 21 | 10.25–10.60 | 10.76–10.77 | 9.01–10.57 | 9.95–14.33 |
| Day 28 | 8.33–8.55 | 7.90–8.57 | 9.57–10.52 | 8.24–12.44 |

### 3.2. Effect of 100–200 mg/kg Hesperidin on Mesenteric Lymph Node Lymphocyte Composition and Functionality

The influence of hesperidin administration on the lymphocyte composition of mesenteric lymph nodes was established (Figure 2). In comparison to the OVAip group, hesperidin, in both tested doses, increased the proportion of TCRαβ+ cells (107% in both doses) in MLNL and, consequently, decreased the proportion of B (CD45RA+) lymphocytes (81% and 77% for H100 and H200 doses, respectively) (Figure 2a), thus increasing the ratio of TCRαβ+/B cells (Figure 2b). The changes were not dose-dependent. No significant differences were seen in the two TCRαβ subsets, Th (TCRαβ+CD4+) and Tc (TCRαβ+CD8+) cells, meaning that both subsets were increased by hesperidin administration (Figure 2c–d). The expression of CD25 (a cell activation marker) was also determined in CD4+, CD8+, and B cells. A decrease in the proportion of CD8+CD25+ cells was observed only in the rats receiving the highest dose of hesperidin with respect to the OVAip group (Figure 2e).

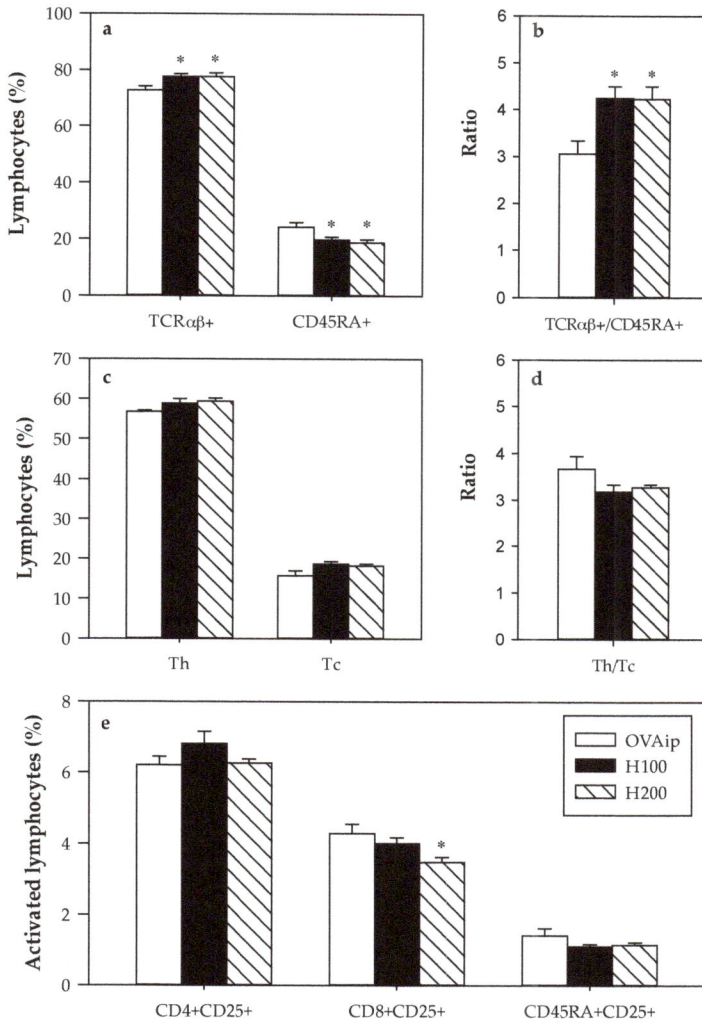

**Figure 2.** Proportion of mesenteric lymph node lymphocytes (MLNL) according to their phenotype in the first experimental design. (**a**) TCRαβ+ and CD45RA+ lymphocytes; (**b**) TCRαβ+/CD45RA+ ratio; (**c**) Th (TCRαβ+CD4+) and Tc (TCRαβ+CD8+) lymphocytes; (**d**) Th/Tc ratio; (**e**) CD25+ cells in CD4+, CD8+, and CD45RA+ lymphocytes. Data are expressed as mean ± standard error ($n = 6$). Statistical difference: * $p < 0.05$ (by Mann-Whitney U).

To establish the function of MLNL, the cytokine pattern secreted by these cells after in vitro stimulation with OVA was determined (Figure 3a). Hesperidin administration, in both doses, induced an increase in the release of IFN-γ (145% and 150% with respect to the OVAip group, for H100 and H200 doses, respectively), a Th1-related cytokine. No differences in the secretion of IL-4, IL-10, TNF-α, and MCP-1 were observed.

In addition, cytokines in gut lavage from the first experimental design were also determined, reflecting their spontaneous secretion (Figure 3f–j). In this compartment, hesperidin did not modify the production of the considered cytokines.

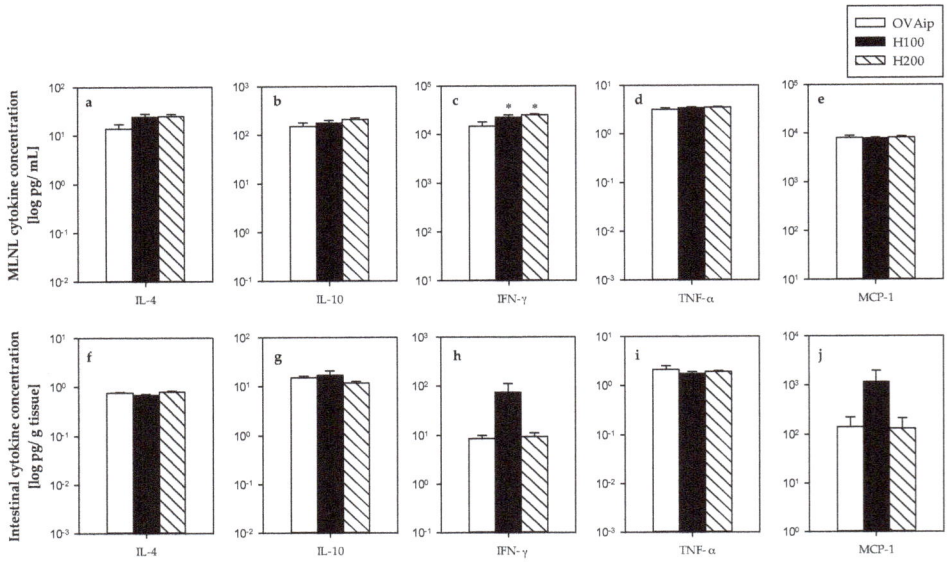

**Figure 3.** Cytokine concentrations in the second experimental design. Cytokines from stimulated MLNL (**a–e**) and gut lavage (**f–j**). Data are expressed as mean ± standard error (*n* = 6). Statistical difference: * *p* < 0.05 (by Mann-Whitney U).

### 3.3. Effect of 100–200 mg/kg Hesperidin on Antibody Synthesis and Intestinal IgA

The untreated i.p. immunized group (OVAip) developed systemic anti-OVA antibodies (Figure 4a) and no changes were seen after hesperidin administration. No serum IgE anti-OVA antibodies were detected in any of the studied groups.

Additionally, intestinal IgA was determined in gut lavage and in faeces (Figure 4b,c) but no modifications were produced as a result of the hesperidin administration.

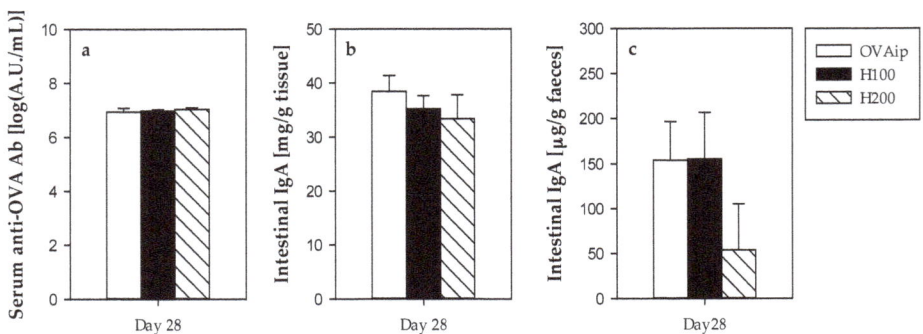

**Figure 4.** Anti-OVA antibodies (Ab) and total immunoglobulin (Ig)A levels from the first experimental design. (**a**) Serum anti-OVA Ab at the last day of the study; Total IgA from (**b**) gut lavage and (**c**) faecal homogenates from the last day of the study. Data are expressed as mean ± standard error (*n* = 6).

### 3.4. Effect of 0.5% Hesperidin on Intestinal Lymphocyte Composition

A second experimental design was then carried out focusing on the intestinal immune system, including both inductive (MLN, PP) and effector (IEL, LPL) compartments and using an oral sensitization process that challenged these specific sites. As the hesperidin intake in the first experimental design did not affect the synthesis of anti-OVA antibodies, the second approach applied hesperidin in a more continuous manner (included in the food) and using a higher dose. Therefore, the effect of 0.5% hesperidin intake on lymphocyte composition in a rat oral sensitization model was studied, analysing the phenotype of both inductive (MLNL and PPL) and effector sites (IEL and LPL) of the GALT.

No differences were seen as a result of the intake of the 0.5% hesperidin diet on MLNL or PPL (Table 3). In particular, in the mesenteric lymph nodes, the proportion of B (CD45RA+), T (TCRαβ+ and TCRγδ+), and natural killer (NK) cells, as well as that of TCRαβ+CD4+, TCRαβ+CD8+, TCRαβ+NK, CD4+CD25+, CD4+CD62L+, CD8+CD25+, and CD8+CD62L+ cells, was similar between the OVAoral and the H0.5 groups. Likewise, in the Peyer's patches, the proportion of B, T, and NK cells did not differ between groups, and that of TCRαβ+CD4+, TCRαβ+CD8+, TCRαβ+NK, TLR4+ (including CD45RA+TLR4+, CD4+TLR4+, CD8+TLR4+), CD45RA+CD25+, CD4+CD25+, and CD8+CD25+ cells also remained unchanged. Interestingly, the 0.5% hesperidin diet modified the proportion of the lymphocytes in the effector sites of the GALT (Table 3). In particular, hesperidin intake increased the percentage of TCRγδ+ cells in IEL (140%) in comparison to the reference group (OVAoral group), which was due to an increase in both TCRγδ+CD8αα+ and TCRγδ+CD8αβ+ subsets, although, in this compartment, hesperidin did not significantly modify other important lymphocytes such as TCRαβ+ (and any of their CD4+, CD8+, and natural killer T –NKT- cell subsets) and NK cells. With regard to LPL, the 0.5% hesperidin diet increased the proportion of B (CD45RA+) cells to 180% and decreased that of TCRγδ+ and NK cells (35% and 29%, respectively) with respect to orally sensitized animals (OVAoral group). In addition, although the total TCRαβ+ population was not significantly modified, the percentage of TCRαβ+CD4+ cells increased (132%), whereas that of TCRαβ+CD8+ cells and NKT cells decreased (52% and 42%, respectively) with respect to the OVAoral group. Likewise, the hesperidin-enriched diet intake decreased the percentage of both CD4+ and CD8+ LPL expressing the CD103+ (50% and 60%, respectively, from that found in the OVAoral group).

### 3.5. Effect of 0.5% Hesperidin on Antibody Synthesis and Total IgA

The oral sensitization procedure applied induced the development of serum anti-OVA antibodies. However, as in the first experimental design, this immune response was not modified by hesperidin (Table 4). In order to find out what happened in Th1/Th2-associated antibody isotypes, the concentration of specific IgG1, IgG2a, IgG2b, IgG2c, and IgE antibodies was determined. The oral sensitization caused the synthesis of antibodies belonging to IgG1, IgG2a, and IgG2b isotypes, as previously reported [20,22]. The 0.5% hesperidin-enriched diet did not significantly modify the levels of these anti-OVA antibodies (Table 4). Specifically, IgG2c and IgE were not detectable in any group.

In addition, intestinal and serum IgA was assessed after four weeks of the nutritional intervention. In this approach, hesperidin intake produced an increase in intestinal IgA, whereas no changes were found with respect to serum IgA (Table 4).

Table 3. Proportion of MLNL, Peyer's patches lymphocytes (PPL), intraepithelial lymphocytes (IEL), and lamina propria lymphocytes (LPL) according to their phenotype in the second experimental design. Data are expressed as mean ± standard error (n = 6). Statistical difference: * p < 0.05 (by Mann-Whitney U).

| Lymphocytes (%) | MLNL | | PPL | | IEL | | LPL | |
|---|---|---|---|---|---|---|---|---|
| | OVAoral | H0.5 | OVAoral | H0.5 | OVAoral | H0.5 | OVAoral | H0.5 |
| CD45RA+ | 12.30 ± 0.38 | 12.20 ± 0.29 | 58.90 ± 4.29 | 59.81 ± 3.81 | 10.54 ± 2.88 | 10.89 ± 0.88 | 25.86 ± 6.25 | 46.10 ± 6.11 * |
| TCRαβ+ | 77.21 ± 0.66 | 77.15 ± 0.72 | 16.16 ± 0.61 | 17.74 ± 1.12 | 41.59 ± 2.27 | 37.72 ± 3.13 | 29.65 ± 4.12 | 21.00 ± 2.78 |
| TCRγδ+ | 1.50 ± 0.04 | 1.45 ± 0.03 | 0.67 ± 0.09 | 0.92 ± 0.10 | 11.60 ± 1.21 | 16.22 ± 1.63 * | 3.81 ± 0.60 | 1.32 ± 0.40 * |
| TCRγδ+CD8αα+ | | | | | 73.12 ± 4.60 | 80.50 ± 3.39 | | |
| TCRγδ+CD8αβ+ | | | | | 26.88 ± 4.60 | 19.49 ± 3.39 | | |
| NK | 0.32 ± 0.03 | 0.26 ± 0.03 | 3.31 ± 0.45 | 2.92 ± 0.27 | 24.33 ± 2.52 | 22.24 ± 1.82 | 13.81 ± 2.14 | 3.97 ± 1.06 * |
| TCRαβ+CD4+ | 77.03 ± 0.66 | 77.22 ± 0.62 | 65.28 ± 1.38 | 68.69 ± 1.76 | 22.10 ± 6.99 | 13.07 ± 3.60 | 60.45 ± 6.92 | 80.08 ± 5.55 * |
| TCRαβ+CD8+ | 22.76 ± 0.69 | 22.58 ± 0.49 | 24.73 ± 1.17 | 23.37 ± 1.32 | 71.88 ± 6.43 | 81.00 ± 3.45 | 34.63 ± 5.99 | 18.09 ± 1.45 * |
| TCRαβ+NK | 0.61 ± 0.02 | 0.58 ± 0.04 | 6.95 ± 0.98 | 5.33 ± 0.59 | 4.95 ± 0.63 | 4.47 ± 0.54 | 3.47 ± 0.76 | 1.46 ± 0.23 * |
| TLR4+ | | | 37.76 ± 2.33 | 33.04 ± 2.74 | 5.43 ± 0.65 | 7.83 ± 1.12 | 6.88 ± 1.60 | 7.39 ± 2.41 |
| CD45RA+TLR4+ | | | 41.41 ± 5.34 | 32.46 ± 4.10 | | | | |
| CD45RA+CD25+ | | | 3.96 ± 0.32 | 3.65 ± 0.61 | | | | |
| CD4+CD25+ | 5.58 ± 0.15 | 5.38 ± 0.21 | 10.79 ± 0.96 | 9.22 ± 0.86 | 5.99 ± 3.46 | 1.75 ± 0.81 | 1.77 ± 1.09 | 0.81 ± 0.21 |
| CD4+CD62L+ | 66.99 ± 2.15 | 64.42 ± 4.29 | | | 91.09 ± 4.56 | 96.03 ± 0.98 | 19.02 ± 2.30 | 9.62 ± 1.59 * |
| CD4+CD103+ | | | 13.41 ± 2.12 | 11.15 ± 1.43 | | | | |
| CD4+TLR4+ | | | | | | | | |
| CD8+CD25+ | 3.95 ± 0.13 | 4.21 ± 0.32 | 53.01 ± 0.98 | 54.87 ± 3.98 | 38.92 ± 8.70 | 19.18 ± 7.76 | 1.34 ± 0.49 | 1.77 ± 0.61 |
| CD8+CD62L+ | 63.78 ± 2.99 | 60.35 ± 5.99 | | | 11.83 ± 2.74 | 15.36 ± 2.37 | 77.70 ± 5.86 | 46.69 ± 11.97 * |
| CD8+CD103+ | | | 36.48 ± 5.30 | 34.03 ± 3.89 | | | | |
| CD8+TLR4+ | | | | | | | | |

**Table 4.** Serum and intestinal anti-OVA and total antibodies from the second experimental design after 0.5% hesperidin diet. Data are expressed as mean ± standard error (*n* = 6). ND: not detectable. Statistical difference: * *p* < 0.05 (by ANOVA).

| | Group | |
|---|---|---|
| | **OVAoral** | **H0.5** |
| Serum total Ig anti-OVA [log(U.A./mL)] | 3.45 ± 0.32 | 3.16 ± 0.34 |
| Serum IgG1 anti-OVA [log(U.A./mL)] | 1.52 ± 0.26 | 1.86 ± 0.29 |
| Serum IgG2a anti-OVA [log(U.A./mL)] | 1.40 ± 0.34 | 1.21 ± 0.50 |
| Serum IgG2b anti-OVA [log(U.A./mL)] | 1.48 ± 0.05 | 1.65 ± 0.23 |
| Serum IgG2c anti-OVA | ND | ND |
| Serum IgE anti-OVA | ND | ND |
| Serum total IgA (µg/mL) | 5.72 ± 0.15 | 5.36 ± 0.24 |
| Intestinal total IgA (µg/g faeces) | 34.60 ± 6.79 | 58.07 ± 7.61 * |

## 4. Discussion

The current study shows the effect of hesperidin in two different approaches related to Th2 immune responses to ovalbumin: an i.p. immunization with the allergen Bpt and alum, and an oral sensitization with the allergen plus cholera toxin. It was found that the administration of hesperidin in i.p. immunized rats modified MLNL composition and functionality. Moreover, in orally sensitized rats, this flavanone changed the proportions of IEL and LPL and increased intestinal IgA content. However, hesperidin did not affect anti-OVA antibody production in any of the studied immune system stimulations.

First of all, we wanted to establish the effect of the hesperidin administration in an i.p. immunization model, triggering a systemic immune response. The hesperidin doses in this case were in accordance with the quantity given to rats to protect against gentamicin nephrotoxicity [23]. The i.p. immunization was performed using the adjuvants alum (enhancer of Th2 response [24]) and Bpt (considered a potent agent to elicit IgE response [25]), as was previously reported in Brown Norway rats [19]. However, this i.p. immunization in Lewis rats was not able to induce the production of anti-OVA IgE, contrary to when using the Brown Norway strain, a high IgE responder [26]. In addition, although a specific antibody response was induced, hesperidin did not modify the levels of such antibodies.

In order to establish the influence of hesperidin on the lymphocyte composition and function, MLNL were analysed. We observed that both doses of hesperidin used here were able to increase TCRαβ+ cell percentage and decrease that of B lymphocytes. This effect was opposite to results observed after cocoa flavonoids intake [22]. The imbalance between the proportions of TCRαβ+ cells and B cells could be due to an increase in the number of TCRαβ+ lymphocytes and/or a decrease in the number of B lymphocytes. In agreement with these results, some flavonoids have demonstrated their ability to reduce B cell viability [2,27]. In particular, catechin, a green tea flavanol, induces apoptosis of human malignant B cells [28]. Therefore, the effect of hesperidin on reducing B cell numbers may not be disregarded, although it is not reflected in antibody production. Consequently, further studies are necessary to confirm the potential of hesperidin in expanding TCRαβ+ cells or reducing B cell numbers.

Apart from the TCRαβ+ and B lymphocyte proportions, other TCRαβ+ subsets were determined. No changes in the Th (TCRαβ+CD4+) and Tc (TCRαβ+CD8+) cells were observed as a result of hesperidin administration, but a significant decrease in the proportion of CD8+CD25+ cells was found after the administration of 200 mg/kg hesperidin. The surface CD25 molecule is expressed in activated cells, and an increased number of blood T CD25+ cells in asthmatic patients has been reported [29]. Although we did not use a model of asthma, our results in terms of Tc CD25+ cell proportion would correspond with the anti-asthmatic effects of hesperidin [9].

On the other hand, stimulated MLNL induced the production of cytokines related to Th1 and Th2 responses. The administration of either 100 or 200 mg/kg hesperidin increased the amount of IFN-γ released from stimulated MLNL, although no changes were found in Th2 cytokines. IFN-γ is a product of Th1 cells that exerts inhibitory properties on Th2 differentiation [30], and its downregulation seems crucial for the development of allergic diseases [31]. Therefore, the increase of this type of Th1 cytokine suggests another hesperidin mechanism involved in the attenuation of allergic asthma. In addition, it has been reported that the administration of 5 mg/mL of hesperidin in a mouse model of allergic asthma inhibited the IL-4 production in splenocytes and the IL-5 concentration in the bronchoalveolar fluid [9]. Overall, these data suggest that hesperidin displays an anti-allergic action by increasing Th1 cytokines or decreasing Th2 cytokines.

Despite the results found after inducing a systemic immune response, we aimed to focus on the intestinal immune response, studying the effect of hesperidin on the GALT using a previously established model of oral sensitization [20]. As the applied doses of hesperidin did not influence antibody synthesis, we increased the dosage of flavanone, including it in the diet (0.5% hesperidin). This dosage was chosen because it has been used in previous reports, such as in the inhibition of bone loss in androgen-deficient male mice [15], in ovariectomized rats [32], and in senescent rats [33]. Considering the amount of food intake per rat, the diet with 0.5% hesperidin meant a consumption of about 360 mg/100 g BW of hesperidin per week, which was higher than that provided in the first experimental design (30 and 60 mg/100 g BW per week for 100 and 200 mg/kg hesperidin doses, respectively).

In the second approach, in contrast to the first, the hesperidin-enriched diet did not modify the composition of MLNL. Although in this second design we used a higher amount of flavanone than that used in the first approach (6- or 12-fold times higher), the inclusion of hesperidin in the food (meaning a slow intake) compared with the oral gavage (meaning a fast intake) and/or a different stimulation of MLNL (by i.p. route or by intestinal route) may affect the cellular composition of this lymphoid tissue differently. In addition, in this second approach, hesperidin did not affect the lymphocyte composition of another inductive site of the GALT, the PP. Interestingly, however, the hesperidin intake changed the proportion of cells found in the intraepithelial and the lamina propria compartments, the effector sites of the GALT. In particular, the hesperidin diet increased the proportion of TCRγδ+ lymphocytes in the intestinal epithelium, which is in line with previous results described after the intake of some polyphenol-enriched foods such as unripe apple [34] and cocoa [21]. TCRγδ+ IEL have an important role in maintaining the epithelial homeostasis, and several studies have related this cellular type with mucosa-associated tolerance [21,34–37]. However, it has been recently suggested that TCRγδ+ IEL triggered by CT exhibit antigen-presenting cell activity in recipient mice fed an oral antigen and contribute to breaking tolerance and inducing a Th2 response [38]. In particular, the oral administration of CT in mice caused the migration of TCRγδ+ IEL to LPL, where they produce IL-10 and IL-17 [38]. Our results regarding rats orally sensitized with OVA together with CT showed that hesperidin produced an opposite effect in the proportion of TCRγδ+ cells both in IEL and LPL, suggesting a protective action of hesperidin in the migration of these cells induced by CT. The hesperidin decrease in TCRγδ+ LPL is in line with the lower proportion of CD8+CD103+ cells in this compartment. The integrin CD103 (also known as αE) binds to E-cadherin and mediates T cell adhesion to the intestine [39], and is highly expressed at the mucosal sites [40], thus suggesting that CD8+CD103+ LPL would move to the intraepithelial compartment (although CD8+CD103+ IEL proportion did not significantly increase).

In addition, after the intake of 0.5% hesperidin diet, LPL showed a relative higher proportion of B cells, which could be related to the enhanced action of hesperidin in the antibody intestinal response, thereby increasing intestinal IgA content, which is in line with other dietary polyphenols [41,42]. In addition, a rise of the Th/Tc proportion in the hesperidin-fed group was found, in agreement with the results reported for LPL after a cocoa-enriched diet using the same rat oral sensitization model [21].

Despite all these lymphocyte composition changes, the specific antibody immune response was not modified in the animals fed the hesperidin diet. In addition, when Th1- and Th2-related antibodies

*Nutrients* **2017**, *9*, 580

were studied (IgG2b, and IgG1 and IgG2a, respectively) [19], no particular effects were observed, contrary to the impact of the intake of cocoa, a rich source of flavonoids, in the same oral sensitization model [21,22]. A wide range of polyphenols has been demonstrated to play a role in decreasing specific antibody production in allergy models [8] and it has also been reported that hesperidin attenuated the OVA-specific IgE production in asthma models [9,17,43]. Nevertheless, in the current study, no differences were detected in serum anti-OVA antibodies in either the first or the second experimental designs.

## 5. Conclusions

In summary, the present results show that hesperidin administration in i.p. immunized rats influences MLNL composition (increasing TCRαβ+ lymphocyte proportion and decreasing that of B and CD8+CD25+ cells) and functionality (increasing IFN-γ synthesis). Moreover, a diet containing 0.5% hesperidin in orally sensitized rats increases intestinal IgA content and also modifies IEL and LPL composition, suggesting the prevention of cell changes triggered by oral CT. However, this hesperidin immunomodulation is not associated with the attenuation of specific antibodies induced by both systemic and intestinal sensitization. Finally, it must be taken into account that this study shows the properties of hesperidin alone; further studies must focus on establishing the effect of hesperidin-enriched food and also the dosage of such foods to achieve these immune effects.

**Acknowledgments:** The authors would like to thank Ferrer HealthTech for providing the hesperidin. This study was financially supported by funding from the Spanish Ministry of Economy and Competitiveness (AGL2011-24279). The authors would like to thank students involved in this study for their help with the laboratory work (Patricia Ruiz, Ana Trenas, Eva Saenz, and Pilar Martínez). M.C.-B. is the recipient of a fellowship from the University of Barcelona (APIF2014).

**Author Contributions:** M.C., A.F. and F.J.P.-C. conceived and designed the experiments; M.C.-B. performed the experiments, analysed the data, and wrote the paper; M.C. reviewed the manuscript. All the authors approved the final version of the manuscript.

**Conflicts of Interest:** The authors declare no conflict of interest.

## References

1. Garg, A.; Garg, S.; Zaneveld, L.J.D.; Singla, A.K. Chemistry and pharmacology of the citrus bioflavonoid hesperidin. *Phyther. Res.* **2001**, *15*, 655–669. [CrossRef] [PubMed]
2. Cuevas, A.; Saavedra, N.; Salazar, L.A.; Abdalla, D.S.P. Modulation of immune function by polyphenols: possible contribution of epigenetic factors. *Nutrients* **2013**, *5*, 2314–2332. [CrossRef] [PubMed]
3. Tsao, R. Chemistry and biochemistry of dietary polyphenols. *Nutrients* **2010**, *2*, 1231–1246. [CrossRef] [PubMed]
4. Gabriele, M.; Frassinetti, S.; Caltavuturo, L.; Montero, L.; Dinelli, G.; Longo, V.; Di Gioia, D.; Pucci, L. Citrus bergamia powder: Antioxidant, antimicrobial and anti-inflammatory properties. *J. Funct. Foods* **2017**, *31*, 255–265. [CrossRef]
5. Scalbert, A.; Manach, C.; Morand, C.; Rémésy, C. Dietary polyphenols and the prevention of diseases. *Crit. Rev. Food Sci. Nutr.* **2005**, *45*, 287–306. [CrossRef] [PubMed]
6. Scalbert, A.; Johnson, I.T.; Saltmarsh, M. Polyphenols: Antioxidants and beyond. *Am. J. Clin. Nutr.* **2005**, *81*, 215S–217S. [PubMed]
7. Pérez-Cano, F.J.; Franch, À.; Pérez-Berezo, T.; Ramos-Romero, S.; Castellote, C.; Castell, M. The effects of flavonoids on the immune system. *Bioact. Food Diet. Interv. Arthr. Relat. Inflamm. Dis.* **2014**, *12*, 205–210.
8. Castell, M.; Perez-Cano, F.; Abril-Gil, M.; Franch, À. Flavonoids on allergy. *Curr. Pharm. Des.* **2014**, *20*, 973–987. [CrossRef] [PubMed]
9. Kim, S.-H.; Kim, B.-K.; Lee, Y.-C. Antiasthmatic effects of hesperidin, a potential Th2 cytokine antagonist, in a mouse model of allergic asthma. *Med. Inflamm.* **2011**, *2011*, 485402. [CrossRef] [PubMed]
10. Parhiz, H.; Roohbakhsh, A.; Soltani, F.; Rezaee, R.; Iranshahi, M. Antioxidant and Anti-inflammatory properties of the citrus flavonoids hesperidin and hesperetin: an updated review of their molecular mechanisms and experimental models. *Phyther. Res.* **2015**, *29*, 323–331. [CrossRef] [PubMed]

11. Kawaguchi, K.; Mizuno, T.; Aida, K.; Uchino, K. Hesperidin as an inhibitor of lipases from porcine pancreas and Pseudomonas. *Biosci. Biotechnol. Biochem.* **1997**, *61*, 102–104. [CrossRef] [PubMed]

12. Kobayashi, S.; Tanabe, S.; Sugiyama, M.; Konishi, Y. Transepithelial transport of hesperetin and hesperidin in intestinal Caco-2 cell monolayers. *Biochim. Biophys. Acta Biomembr.* **2008**, *1778*, 33–41. [CrossRef] [PubMed]

13. Hemanth Kumar, B.; Dinesh Kumar, B.; Diwan, P.V. Hesperidin, a citrus flavonoid, protects against L-methionine-induced hyperhomocysteinemia by abrogation of oxidative stress, endothelial dysfunction and neurotoxicity in Wistar rats. *Pharm. Biol.* **2017**, *55*, 146–155. [CrossRef] [PubMed]

14. Qian, W.; Hasegawa, J.; Cai, X.; Yang, J.; Ishihara, Y.; Ping, B.; Tsuno, S.; Endo, Y.; Matsuda, A.; Miura, N. Effects of hesperidin on the progression of hypercholesterolemia and fatty liver induced by high-cholesterol diet in rats. *Yonago Acta Med.* **2016**, *59*, 67–80. [PubMed]

15. Chiba, H.; Kim, H.; Matsumoto, A.; Akiyama, S.; Ishimi, Y.; Suzuki, K.; Uehara, M. Hesperidin prevents androgen deficiency-induced bone loss in male mice. *Phyther. Res.* **2014**, *28*, 289–295. [CrossRef] [PubMed]

16. Ikemura, M.; Sasaki, Y.; Giddings, J.C.; Yamamoto, J. Preventive effects of hesperidin, glucosyl hesperidin and naringin on hypertension and cerebral thrombosis in stroke-prone spontaneously hypertensive Rats. *Phyther. Res.* **2012**, *26*, 1272–1277. [CrossRef] [PubMed]

17. Wei, D.; Ci, X.; Chu, X.; Wei, M.; Hua, S.; Deng, X. Hesperidin suppresses ovalbumin-induced airway inflammation in a mouse allergic asthma model. *Inflammation* **2012**, *35*, 114–121. [CrossRef] [PubMed]

18. Dourado, G.K.Z.S.; Ribeiro, L.C.D.A.; Carlos, I.Z.; César, T.B. Orange juice and hesperidin promote differential innate immune response in macrophages ex vivo. *Int. J. Vitam. Nutr. Res.* **2014**, *83*, 162–167. [CrossRef] [PubMed]

19. Abril-Gil, M.; Massot-Cladera, M.; Pérez-Cano, F.J.; Castellote, C.; Franch, A.; Castell, M. A diet enriched with cocoa prevents IgE synthesis in a rat allergy model. *Pharmacol. Res.* **2012**, *65*, 603–608. [CrossRef] [PubMed]

20. Camps-Bossacoma, M.; Abril-Gil, M.; Franch, À.; Pérez-Cano, F.J.; Castell, M. Induction of an oral sensitization model in rats. *Clin. Immunol. Endocr. Metab. Drugs* **2014**, *1*, 1–10. [CrossRef]

21. Camps-Bossacoma, M.; Pérez-Cano, F.J.; Franch, À.; Untermayr, E.; Castell, M. Effect of a cocoa diet on the small intestine and gut-associated lymphoid tissue composition in a rat oral sensitization model. *J. Nutr. Biochem.* **2017**, *42*, 182–193. [CrossRef] [PubMed]

22. Camps-Bossacoma, M.; Abril-Gil, M.; Saldaña-Ruiz, S.; Franch, À.; Pérez-Cano, F.J.; Castell, M. Cocoa diet prevents antibody synthesis and modifies lymph node composition and functionality in a rat oral sensitization model. *Nutrients* **2016**, *8*, 242. [CrossRef] [PubMed]

23. Jain, D.; Somani, R. Antioxidant potential of hesperidin protects gentamicin induced nephrotoxicity in experimental rats. *Austin J. Pharmacol. Ther.* **2015**, *3*, 1071.

24. Eisenbarth, S.C. Use and limitations of alum-based models of allergy. *Clin. Exp. Allergy* **2008**, *38*, 1572–1575. [CrossRef] [PubMed]

25. Dong, W.; Selgrade, M.J.K.; Gilmour, M.I. Systemic administration of *Bordetella pertussis* enhances pulmonary sensitization to house dust mite in juvenile rats. *Toxicol. Sci.* **2003**, *72*, 113–121. [CrossRef] [PubMed]

26. Pilegaard, K.; Madsen, C. An oral Brown Norway rat model for food allergy: Comparison of age, sex, dosing volume, and allergen preparation. *Toxicology* **2004**, *196*, 247–257. [CrossRef] [PubMed]

27. Hassanain, E.; Silverberg, J.I.; Norowitz, K.B.; Chice, S.; Bluth, M.H.; Brody, N.; Joks, R.; Durkin, H.G.; Smith-Norowitz, T.A. Green tea (Camelia sinensis) suppresses B cell production of IgE without inducing apoptosis. *Ann. Clin. Lab. Sci.* **2010**, *40*, 135–143. [CrossRef] [PubMed]

28. Nakazato, T.; Ito, K.; Ikeda, Y.; Kizaki, M. Green tea component, catechin, induces apoptosis of human malignant B cells via production of reactive oxygen species. *Clin. Cancer Res.* **2005**, *11*, 6040–6049. [CrossRef] [PubMed]

29. Domínguez Ortega, J.; León, F.; Martínez Alonso, J.C.; Alonso Llamazares, A.; Roldán, E.; Robledo, T.; Mesa, M.; Bootello, A.; Martínez-Cócera, C. Fluorocytometric analysis of induced sputum cells in an asthmatic population. *J. Investig. Allergol. Clin. Immunol.* **2004**, *14*, 108–113. [PubMed]

30. Chung, F. Anti-inflammatory cytokines in asthma and allergy: Interleukin-10, interleukin-12, interferon-γ. *Med. Inflamm.* **2001**, *10*, 51–59. [CrossRef] [PubMed]

31. Teixeira, L.K.; Fonseca, B.P.; Barboza, B.A.; Viola, J.P. The role of interferon-gamma on immune and allergic responses. *Mem. Inst. Oswaldo Cruz* **2005**, *100*, 137–144. [CrossRef] [PubMed]

32. Horcajada, M.N.; Habauzit, V.; Trzeciakiewicz, A.; Morand, C.; Gil-Izquierdo, A.; Mardon, J.; Lebecque, P.; Davicco, M.J.; Chee, W.S.S.; Coxam, V.; et al. Hesperidin inhibits ovariectomized-induced osteopenia and shows differential effects on bone mass and strength in young and adult intact rats. *J. Appl. Physiol.* **2008**, *104*, 648–654. [CrossRef] [PubMed]

33. Habauzit, V.; Sacco, S.M.; Gil-Izquierdo, A.; Trzeciakiewicz, A.; Morand, C.; Barron, D.; Pinaud, S.; Offord, E.; Horcajada, M.N. Differential effects of two citrus flavanones on bone quality in senescent male rats in relation to their bioavailability and metabolism. *Bone* **2011**, *49*, 1108–1116. [CrossRef] [PubMed]

34. Akiyama, H.; Sato, Y.; Watanabe, T.; Nagaoka, M.H.; Yoshioka, Y.; Shoji, T.; Kanda, T.; Yamada, K.; Totsuka, M.; Teshima, R.; et al. Dietary unripe apple polyphenol inhibits the development of food allergies in murine models. *FEBS Lett.* **2005**, *579*, 4485–4491. [CrossRef] [PubMed]

35. Hänninen, A.; Harrison, L.C. Gamma delta T cells as mediators of mucosal tolerance: The autoimmune diabetes model. *Immunol. Rev.* **2000**, *173*, 109–119. [CrossRef] [PubMed]

36. Paul, S.; Singh, A.K.; Shilpi Lal, G. Phenotypic and functional plasticity of gamma-delta (γδ) T cells in inflammation and tolerance. *Int. Rev. Immunol.* **2014**, *33*, 537–558. [CrossRef] [PubMed]

37. Bol-Schoenmakers, M.; Marcondes Rezende, M.; Bleumink, R.; Boon, L.; Man, S.; Hassing, I.; Fiechter, D.; Pieters, R.H.H.; Smit, J.J. Regulation by intestinal γδ T cells during establishment of food allergic sensitization in mice. *Allergy Eur. J. Allergy Clin. Immunol.* **2011**, *66*, 331–340. [CrossRef] [PubMed]

38. Frossard, C.P.; Asigbetse, K.E.; Burger, D.; Eigenmann, P.A. Gut T cell receptor-γδ+ intraepithelial lymphocytes are activated selectively by cholera toxin to break oral tolerance in mice. *Clin. Exp. Immunol.* **2015**, *180*, 118–130. [CrossRef] [PubMed]

39. Agace, W.W.; Higgins, J.M.; Sadasivan, B.; Brenner, M.B.; Parker, C.M. T-lymphocyte-epithelial-cell interactions: Integrin αE(CD103)β7, LEEP-CAM and chemokines. *Curr. Opin. Cell Biol.* **2000**, *12*, 563–568. [CrossRef]

40. Annacker, O.; Coombes, J.L.; Malmstrom, V.; Uhlig, H.H.; Bourne, T.; Johansson-Lindbom, B.; Agace, W.W.; Parker, C.M.; Powrie, F. Essential role for CD103 in the T cell-mediated regulation of experimental colitis. *J. Exp. Med.* **2005**, *202*, 1051–1061. [CrossRef] [PubMed]

41. Okazaki, Y.; Han, Y.; Kayahara, M.; Watanabe, T.; Arishige, H.; Kato, N. Consumption of curcumin elevates fecal immunoglobulin A, an index of intestinal immune function, in rats fed a high-fat diet. *J. Nutr. Sci. Vitaminol.* **2010**, *56*, 68–71. [CrossRef] [PubMed]

42. Taira, T.; Yamaguchi, S.; Takahashi, A.; Okazaki, Y.; Yamaguchi, A.; Sakaguchi, H.; Chiji, H. Dietary polyphenols increase fecal mucin and immunoglobulin A and ameliorate the disturbance in gut microbiota caused by a high fat diet. *J. Clin. Biochem. Nutr.* **2015**, *57*, 212–216. [CrossRef] [PubMed]

43. Chang, J.H. Anti-inflammatory effects and its mechanisms of hesperidin in an asthmatic mouse model induced by ovalbumin. *J. Exp. Biomed. Sci.* **2010**, *16*, 83–90.

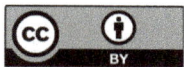

*nutrients*

MDPI

*Article*

# Kaempferol and Luteolin Decrease Claudin-2 Expression Mediated by Inhibition of STAT3 in Lung Adenocarcinoma A549 Cells

Hiroyuki Sonoki [1], Asami Tanimae [1], Satoshi Endo [1], Toshiyuki Matsunaga [1], Takumi Furuta [2], Kenji Ichihara [3] and Akira Ikari [1,*]

[1]   From the Laboratory of Biochemistry, Department of Biopharmaceutical Sciences, Gifu Pharmaceutical University, Gifu 501-1196, Japan; 116023@gifu-pu.ac.jp (H.S.); 125050@gifu-pu.ac.jp (A.T.); sendo@gifu-pu.ac.jp (S.E.); matsunagat@gifu-pu.ac.jp (T.M.)

[2]   Institute for Chemical Research, Kyoto University, Kyoto 611-0011, Japan; furuta@fos.kuicr.kyoto-u.ac.jp

[3]   Nagaragawa Research Center, API Co., Ltd., Gifu 502-0071, Japan; ichihara-kenji@api3838.co.jp

*    Correspondence: ikari@gifu-pu.ac.jp; Tel./Fax: +81-58-230-8124

Received: 8 April 2017; Accepted: 10 June 2017; Published: 13 June 2017

**Abstract:** Claudin-2 is highly expressed in human lung adenocarcinoma tissues and may be a novel target for cancer chemotherapy because knockdown of claudin-2 decreases cell proliferation. We found that flavonoids including kaempferol, chrysin, and luteolin concentration-dependently decrease claudin-2 expression in lung adenocarcinoma A549 cells.   Claudin-2 expression is up-regulated by mitogen-activated protein kinase kinase (MEK)/ extracellular signal-regulated kinase (ERK)/c-Fos and phosphoinositide 3-kinase (PI3K)/Akt/nuclear factor-κB (NF-κB) pathways, but these activities were not inhibited by kaempferol, chrysin, and luteolin. Promoter deletion assay using luciferase reporter vector showed that kaempferol and luteolin inhibit the function of transcriptional factor that binds to the region between −395 and −144 of claudin-2 promoter. The decrease in promoter activity was suppressed by mutation in signal transducers and activators of transcription (STAT)-binding site, which is located between −395 and −144. The phosphorylation level of STAT3 was not decreased, but the binding of STAT3 on the promoter region is suppressed by kaempferol and luteolin in chromatin immunoprecipitation assay. The inhibition of cell proliferation caused by kaempferol and luteolin was partially recovered by ectopic claudin-2 expression. Taken together, kaempferol and luteolin decreased claudin-2 expression and proliferation in A549 cells mediated by the inhibition of binding of STAT3 on the promoter region of claudin-2. The intake of foods and nutrients rich in these flavonoids may prevent lung adenocarcinoma development.

**Keywords:** lung adenocarcinoma; claudin-2; kaempferol; chrysin; STAT3

## 1. Introduction

Epithelial cells form tight junctions (TJs) at the most apical pole of the lateral membrane between neighboring cells. The TJs regulate the flux of ions and solutes through the paracellular pathway, cell proliferation, polarization, and differentiation [1–3]. Most solid cancers are derived from epithelial tissues and disruption of polarity accelerates cell proliferation and differentiation. Claudins are integral membrane proteins of TJs and comprise a large family of 27 subtypes in a mammal [4,5]. Dysregulation of claudins expression has been shown in various tumor tissues [6]. We have been reported that the expression of claudin-2 is up-regulated in human lung adenocarcinoma tissues [7]. Similarly, the elevation of claudin-2 expression is reported in liver [8], colon [9], and stomach cancer tissues [10]. The knockdown of claudin-2 decreases proliferation and migration in non-small-cell lung carcinoma cells [7,11]. Therefore, claudin-2 may be one of the targets for anticancer function of foods and drugs.

Anticancer activity is reported in polyphenols extracted from plants, fruits, vegetables, and bee propolis [12,13]. Polyphenols include many classes of compounds ranging from flavonoids, phenolic acids, and anthocyanins. Some flavonoids inhibit growth and invasion of cancer cells in various in vitro and in vivo models. A population-based case-control study in Montreal, Canada, reported that a low dietary intake of flavonoids increases the risk of lung cancer [14]. Antioxidant effect is one of the key factors to reduce cancer risk [15]. Flavonoids have a basic structure consisting of two aromatic rings linked by three carbon atoms that are confined in an oxygenated heterocycle ring, and clarified as flavonols, flavones, flavanones, flavanols, anthocyanidins, and isoflavones [16]. The antioxidant activity is affected by the number and position of hydroxyl substituents [17]. Quercetin, with $3',4'$ dihydroxy substituents in the B ring and conjugation between the A and B rings has strong antioxidant activity, and shows apoptotic and anti-proliferative effects in human cancer cells derived from lung [18], breast [19], gastrointestinal tract [20], and prostate [21]. We previously reported that quercetin decreases claudin-2 expression in human lung adenocarcinoma A549 cells [22]. However, other flavonoids that decrease claudin-2 expression have not been identified.

The expression of claudins is controlled by various transcriptional factors under physiological and pathophysiological conditions. Signal transducers and activators of transcription (STAT) forms a family with seven members in mammals (STAT1, STAT2, STAT3, STAT4, STAT5A, STAT5B, and STAT6) [23]. Among them, STAT3 and STAT5 are activated in a large number of human cancers and play major roles in proliferation, apoptosis, and angiogenesis [24]. The activation of tyrosine kinase signal promotes dimerization of STAT3 and its translocation into the nuclei. STAT3 binds to the promoter regions of tumor-related genes [25]. A few reports indicate that STATs are involved in the regulation of claudins expression. The activation of STAT1 and STAT3 decreases claudin-5 expression in human brain microvascular endothelial cells [26] and claudin-2 expression in Madin-Darby canine kidney (MDCK) II cells [27], respectively, but the binding site of STAT on the promoter region of claudins is unknown.

In the present study, we searched for new substances that can decrease claudin-2 expression in A549 cells and identified kaempferol, chrysin, and luteolin as the potential candidates. To clarify the mechanism, we examined the effects of these flavonoids on intracellular signaling factors, promoter activity of claudin-2, binding of transcriptional factor on promoter of claudin-2, and cell proliferation. Our results indicate that kaempferol and luteolin may decrease claudin-2 expression through inhibiting the interaction of STAT3 on promoter region of claudin-2 without affecting the phosphorylation of STAT3, resulting in suppression of cell proliferation.

## 2. Experimental Section

### 2.1. Materials

Rabbit anti-claudin-1 and mouse anti-claudin-2 antibodies were obtained from Thermo Fisher Scientific (Waltham, MA, USA). Goat anti-β-actin and rabbit anti-phosphorylated-c-Fos (p-c-Fos) antibodies were from Santa Cruz Biotechnology (Santa Cruz, CA, USA). Rabbit anti-p-Akt, rabbit anti-Akt, rabbit anti-ERK1/2, rabbit anti-c-Fos, rabbit anti-p-NF-κB p65 (Ser536), and rabbit anti-NF-κB p65 antibodies were from Cell Signaling Technology (Beverly, MA, USA). Mouse anti-p-STAT3, anti-STAT3, and anti-nucleoporin p62 antibodies were from BD Biosciences (San Jose, CA, USA). Apigenin, genistein, and quercetin were from Wako Pure Chemical Industries (Osaka, Japan). Chrysin, kaempferol, daidzein, and 7-hydroxyflavone were from Tokyo Kasei Kogyo (Tokyo, Japan). Hesperetin was from LKT Laboratories (St. Paul, MN, USA). Luteolin and 4'-hydroxyflavone were from INDOFINE Chemical Company (Hillsborough, NJ, USA). Flavonoids were dissolved in dimethyl sulfoxide (DMSO). All other reagents were of the highest grade of purity available.

## 2.2. Cell Culture and Transfection

The human lung adenocarcinoma A549 cell line was obtained from the RIKEN BRC through the National Bio-Resource Project of the MEXT, Japan. The cells were grown in Dulbecco's modified Eagle's medium (DMEM, Sigma-Aldrich, St. Louis, MO, USA) supplemented with 5% fetal calf serum (FCS, HyClone, Logan, UT, USA), 0.07 mg/mL penicillin-G potassium, and 0.14 mg/mL streptomycin sulfate in a 5% $CO_2$ atmosphere at 37 °C. The experiments were done in subconfluent culture condition (about 70–80% confluent), because the expression of claudin-2 decreased in 100% confluent condition [11]. The cells were treated with vehicle DMSO (control) and flavonoids (1–50 μM) for 24 h in FCS-free DMEM. The vector containing human claudin-2 cDNA was prepared as described previously [11]. The FLAG-tagged claudin-2 was sub-cloned into pTRE2-hyg vector and transfected into A549 cells with Lipofectamine 2000 as recommended by the manufacturer. Stable transfectants were selected with 500 ng/mL hygromycin B and maintained in the continuous presence of 50 ng/mL hygromycin B.

## 2.3. SDS-Polyacrylamide Gel Electrophoresis (SDS-PAGE) and Immunoblotting

Cells were scraped into cold phosphate-buffered saline and precipitated by centrifugation. They were lysed in a radioimmunoprecipitation assay lysis buffer containing 150 mM NaCl, 0.5 mM ethylenediaminetetraacetic acid, 1% Triton X-100, 0.1% sodium dodecyl sulfate, 50 mM Tris-HCl (pH 8.0), a protease inhibitor cocktail (Sigma-Aldrich), and sonicated for 20 s. The aliquots were used as whole cell extracts. After centrifugation at $6000 \times g$ for 5 min, the supernatants were collected and used as cell lysates which including plasma membrane and cytoplasmic proteins. Nuclear fractions were prepared using NE-PER nuclear and cytoplasmic fraction reagents as recommended by the manufacturer (Thermo Fisher Scientific). Samples were applied to SDS-PAGE and blotted onto a polyvinylidene difluoride membrane. The membrane was then incubated with each primary antibody (1:1000 dilution) at 4 °C for 16 h, followed by a peroxidase-conjugated secondary antibody (1:5000 dilution) at room temperature for 1 h. Finally, the blots were incubated in Pierce Western Blotting Substrate (Thermo Fisher Scientific) and exposed to film, or incubated in ECL Prime Western Blotting Detection System (GE healthcare, Chalfont St Giles, UK) and scanned with a C-DiGit Blot Scanner (LI-COR Biotechnology, Lincoln, NE, USA). Blots were further stripped and reprobed with anti-β-actin antibody. Band density was quantified with ImageJ software (National Institute of Health software, NIH, Bethesda, MD, USA). The signals were normalized for the loading control β-actin or nucleoporin p62. The expression levels were represented relative to the values in the absence of flavonoids.

## 2.4. Measurement of $O_2{}^-$ Scavenging Activity

Antioxidant activity of flavonoids and antioxidants was measured using the hypoxanthine-xanthine oxidase system as the source of superoxide anion [28]. Reaction solution contains 10 μM 2-methyl-6-p-methoxyphenyl ethynylimidazopyrazynone, 0.02 units/mL xanthine oxidase, 0.12 mM hypoxanthine, and 20 mM $KH_2PO_4$ (pH 7.5). Test compounds were mixed in the reaction buffer at the final concentration of 50 μM. A chemiluminescence intensity was measured with a luminometer (AB-2270 Luminescencer Octa, ATTO, Tokyo, Japan). $O_2{}^-$ scavenging activity was calculated by the following formula: Scavenging activity (%) = $(1 - CL_S/CL_C) \times 100$; where $CL_C$, chemiluminescence of control, $CL_A$, chemiluminescence of sample.

### 2.5. RNA Isolation and Polymerase Chain Reaction (PCR)

Total RNA was isolated from A549 cells using TRI reagent (Sigma-Aldrich). Reverse transcription was carried out with ReverTra Ace qPCR RT Kit (Toyobo Life Science, Osaka, Japan). Semi-quantitative PCR was carried out with DNA Engine Dyad Cycler (Bio-Rad, Richmond, CA, USA) using GoTaq DNA polymerase (Promega, Madison, WI, USA). The PCR product was visualized with ethidium bromide after electrophoretic separation on a 2% agarose gel. The size of PCR product was 86 bp (claudin-2) and 100 bp (β-actin). Quantitative real-time PCR was performed with a Thermal Cycler Dice Real-time System (TP700, Takara Bio, Shiga, Japan) or Eco Real-Time PCR system (AS One, Osaka, Japan) using KOD SYBR qPCR Mix (Toyobo Life Science). The primers used to PCR are listed in Table 1. The threshold cycle (Ct) for each PCR product was calculated with the instrument's software, and Ct values obtained for claudin-1 and -2 were normalized by subtracting the Ct values obtained for β-actin. The resulting ΔCt values were then used to calculate the relative change in mRNA expression as a ratio (R) according to the equation $R = 2^{-(\Delta Ct(treatment) - \Delta Ct(control))}$.

**Table 1.** Primers for polymerase chain reaction (PCR) amplification.

| Name | Direction | Sequence |
|------|-----------|----------|
| Claudin-1 | Forward | 5′-ATGAGGATGGCTGTCATTGG-3′ |
| Claudin-1 | Reverse | 5′-ATTGACTGGGGTCATAGGGT-3′ |
| Claudin-2 | Forward | 5′-ATTGTGACAGCAGTTGGCTT-3′ |
| Claudin-2 | Reverse | 5′-CTATAGATGTCACACTGGGTGATG-3′ |
| Occludin | Forward | 5′-TTTGTGGGACAAGGAACACA-3′ |
| Occludin | Reverse | 5′-TCATTCACTTTGCCATTGGA-3′ |
| E-cadherin | Forward | 5′-ACCCCCTGTTGGTGTCTTT-3′ |
| E-cadherin | Reverse | 5′-TTCGGGCTTGTTGTCATTCT-3′ |
| β-actin | Forward | 5′-CCTGAGGCACTCTTCCAGCCTT-3′ |
| β-actin | Reverse | 5′-TGCGGATGTCCACGTCACACTTC-3′ |

### 2.6. Luciferase Reporter Assay

Using the reporter plasmids containing fragments of −1031/+37, −393/+37, −143/+37, and −87/+37 of human claudin-2, luciferase reporter assay was carried out as described previously [29]. The mutant of putative STAT-binding site (−252/−230) was generated using the primer pairs (forward: 5′-GAATCTCGAGCAGCCACCTGTCTGGCTCCTGGC-3′ and reverse: 5′-AGGTGATGATGGCAGTGGTGGTTGTG-3′) and KOD-Plus-mutagenesis kit (Toyobo Life Science). The luminescence of luciferase was measured with a luminometer.

### 2.7. Chromatin Immunoprecipitation (ChIP) Assay

Cells were treated with 1% formaldehyde to crosslink the protein to the DNA. ChIP assay was carried out as described previously [29]. To co-immunoprecipitate the DNA, anti-STAT3 antibody or mouse IgG was used. The eluted DNA was amplified by quantitative PCR using the primer pairs for claudin-2 promoter (forward: 5′-ACTTGAGTTAACACAGCCACCA-3′ and reverse: 5′-ACTTTGAACGTGGAGCCAAAAT-3′). To confirm the same amounts of chromatins used in immunoprecipitation between groups, input chromatin was also used.

*2.8. Cell Proliferation*

Cells were seeded at $1 \times 10^5$ cells in 60-mm dishes. After 24, 48, and 72 h of culture, the cell images were captured with a light microscope (CKX53, Olympus, Tokyo, Japan). Cell proliferation was calculated by counting the number of cells using the CKX-CCSW software (Olympus).

*2.9. Statistics*

Results are presented as means ± S.E.M. Differences between groups were analyzed with a one-way analysis of variance, and corrections for multiple comparison were made using Tukey's multiple comparison test. Comparisons between two groups were made using Student's *t*-test. Statics were performed using KaleidaGraph version 4.5.1 software (Synergy Software, Reading, PA, USA). Significant differences were assumed at $p < 0.05$.

## 3. Results

*3.1. Effects of Flavonoids on Claudin-2 Expression in A549 Cells*

The protein level of claudin-2 in the cytoplasmic fraction was significantly decreased by quercetin, apigenin, kaempferol, chrysin, luteolin, and daizein at the concentration of 50 µM in A549 cells (Figure 1). The effects of kaempferol, chrysin, and luteolin were stronger than those of other flavonoids. Genistein and hesperetin showed no effect on claudin-2 expression. Hesperetin, kaempferol, and luteolin showed cytotoxicity at over 100 µM, but all flavonoids have little effect on cytotoxicity at the concentration of lower than 50 µM (Supplementary Figure S1). These results indicate that the decrease in claudin-2 expression is not due to cytotoxicity. The expression of other junctional proteins including claudin-1, occludin, and E-cadherin was not changed by these flavonoids. In the present study, we focused on the regulatory mechanism of which kaempferol, chrysin, and luteolin decrease claudin-2 expression because the effects of these flavonoids are the strongest.

*3.2. Effects of Antioxidant Capacity on Claudin-2 Expression*

The expression of claudin-2 was dose-dependently decreased by kaempferol, chrysin, and luteolin (Figure 2). The effects were significant over the concentration of 1 or 10 µM. Certain flavonoids have an antioxidant effect. Kaempferol, chrysin, and luteolin showed approximately 20% $O_2^-$ scavenging activity at 50 µM (Figure 3). 4′-Hydroxyflavonoe and 7-hydroxyflavone had little antioxidant activity, which is similar to previous report [30]. In contrast, *N*-acetyl cysteine (NAC, 1 mM) and reduced glutathione (GSH, 0.1 mM) had strong antioxidant activity. Although 4′-hydroxyflavonoe and 7-hydroxyflavone had little antioxidant activity, they decreased claudin-2 expression (Figure 4). In addition, claudin-2 expression was not decreased by NAC and GSH. These results indicate that antioxidant capacity may not be involved in the decrease in claudin-2 expression by flavonoids.

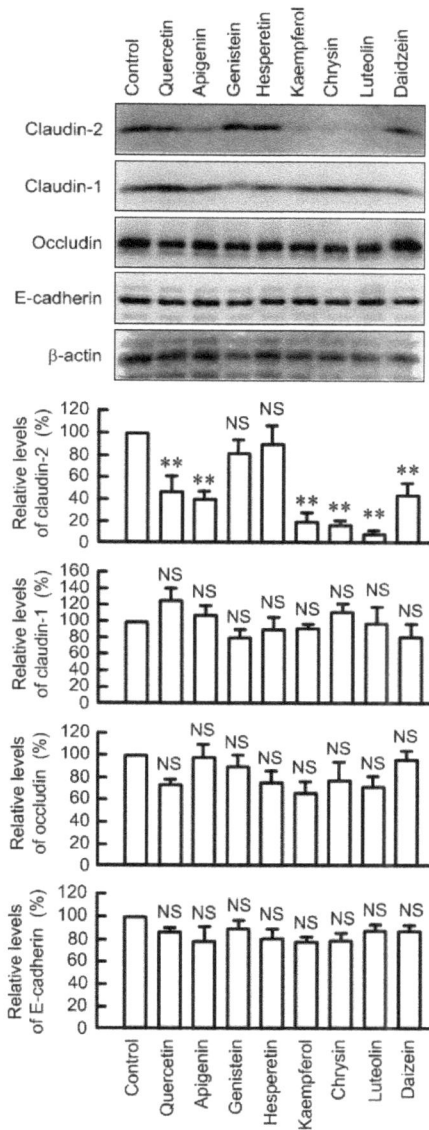

**Figure 1.** Effects of flavonoids on expression of junctional proteins in A549 cells. Cells were incubated in the absence and presence of 50 μM flavonoids including quercetin, apigenin, genistein, hesperetin, kaempferol, chrysin, luteolin, and daidzein for 24 h. Cell lysates were immunoblotted with anti-claudin-2, anti-claudin-1, anti-occludin, anti-E-cadherin, or anti-β-actin antibody. The expression levels were represented relative to the values in control. $n$ = 3–4. ** $p$ < 0.01 significantly different from control. NS, not significantly different.

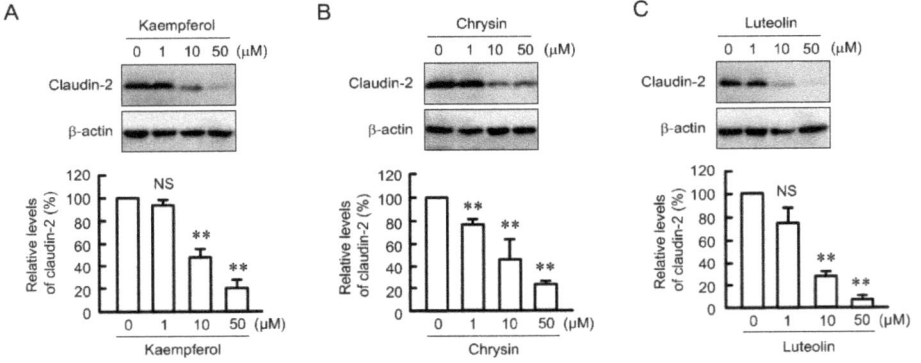

**Figure 2.** Dose-dependent effects of kaempferol, chrysin, and luteolin on claudin-2 expression. The cells were incubated in the absence and presence of kaempferol (**A**), chrysin (**B**), or luteolin (**C**) for 24 h at the concentration indicated. Cell lysates were immunoblotted with anti-claudin-2 or β-actin antibody. The expression levels of claudin-2 were represented relative to the values in 0 μM. $n = 3$–4. ** $p < 0.01$ significantly different from 0 μM. NS, not significantly different.

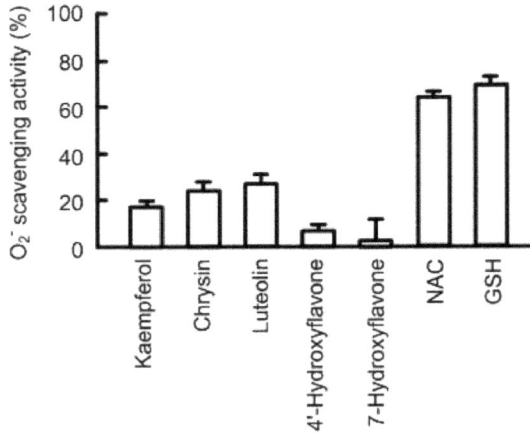

**Figure 3.** Antioxidant effects of flavonoids and antioxidants. $O_2^-$ scavenging activity was examined using the hypoxanthine-xanthine oxidase system. Flavonoids (50 μM), *N*-acetyl cysteine (NAC, 1 mM), and reduced glutathione (GSH, 0.1 mM) were mixed in the reaction buffer. $n = 4$.

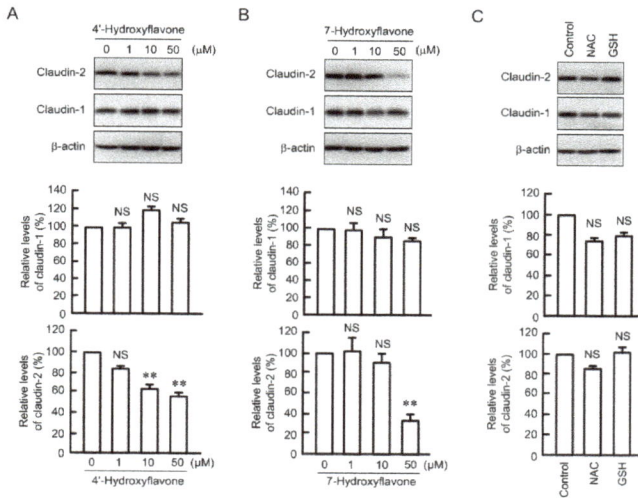

**Figure 4.** Effects of non-antioxidative flavones and antioxidants on claudin-2 expression. (**A,B**) The cells were incubated in the absence and presence of 4′-hydroxyflavone or 7-hydroxyflavone for 24 h at the concentration indicated. Cell lysates were immunoblotted with anti-claudin-1, claudin-2, or β-actin antibody. The expression levels of claudin-1 and -2 were represented relative to the values in 0 Mm; (**C**) Cells were incubated in the absence (control) and presence of NAC (1 mM) or GSH (0.1 mM) for 24 h. Cell lysates were immunoblotted with anti-claudin-1, claudin-2, or β-actin antibody. The expression levels of claudin-1 and -2 were represented relative to the values in control. $n = 3$. ** $p < 0.01$ significantly different from 0 μM or control. NS, not significantly different.

### 3.3. Effects of Flavonoids on mRNA Levels of Junctional Protein and Intracellular Signaling Pathway

Kaempferol, chrysin, and luteolin significantly decreased the mRNA level of claudin-2 without changing that of claudin-1 (Figure 5). These results coincide with those of Western blotting. In contrast, the mRNA level of occludin was increased by kaempferol and those of occludin and E-cadherin were decreased by luteolin. We previously reported that the transcriptional activity of claudin-2 is up-regulated by the MEK/ERK/c-Fos [29] and PI3K/Akt/NF-κB pathways [31]. Some flavonoids, including kaempferol, chrysin, and luteolin, increased the phosphorylation levels of ERK1/2 and/or c-Fos (Figure 6). On the contrary, these flavonoids had no effect on the phosphorylation of Akt and NF-κB p65. These results indicate that the MEK/ERK/c-Fos and PI3K/Akt/NF-κB pathways may not be involved in these flavonoids-induced decreases in claudin-2 expression.

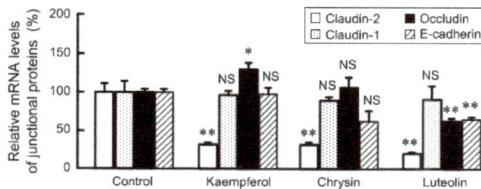

**Figure 5.** Effects of flavonoids on mRNA levels of junctional protein. The cells were incubated in the absence and presence of 50 μM flavonoids for 6 h. After isolation of total RNA, quantitative real-time PCR was performed using specific primers for claudin-1, claudin-2, occludin, and E-cadherin. $n = 4$. ** $p < 0.01$ and * $p < 0.05$ significantly different from control. NS, not significantly different.

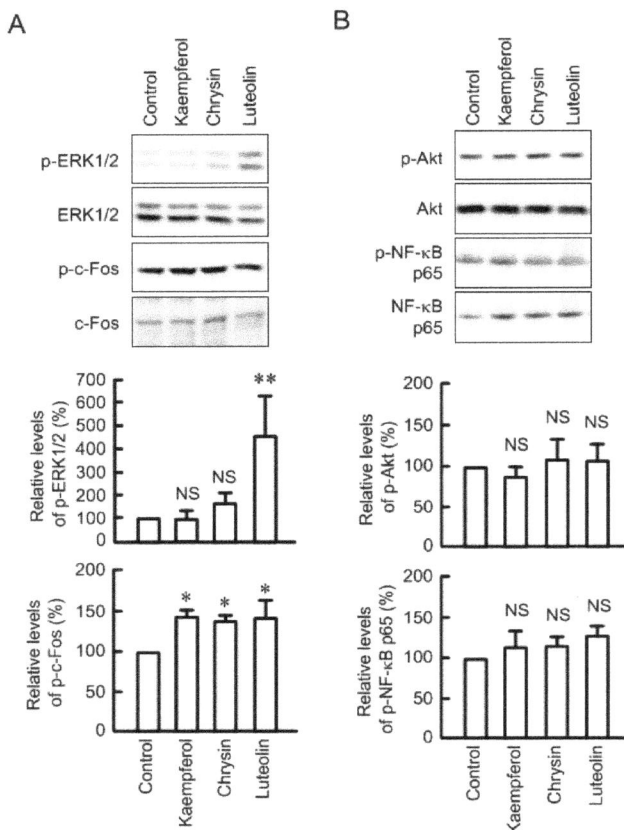

**Figure 6.** Effects of flavonoids on the phosphorylation of intracellular signaling pathways. The cells were incubated in the absence and presence of 50 μM flavonoids for 1 h. (**A**) Whole cell extracts were immunoblotted with anti-p-ERK1/2, ERK1/2, p-c-Fos, or c-Fos antibody; (**B**) Whole cell extracts were immunoblotted with anti-p-Akt, Akt, p-NF-κB p65, or NF-κB p65 antibody. The levels of p-ERK, p-c-Fos, p-Akt, and p-NF-κB p65 were represented relative to the values in control. $n = 3$. ** $p < 0.01$ and * $p < 0.05$ significantly different from control. NS, not significantly different.

### 3.4. Effects of Flavonoids on the Promoter Activity of Claudin-2

To clarify a major transcriptional factor involved in the flavonoids-induced decreases in claudin-2 expression, we performed the promoter deletion assay of human claudin-2. Apigenin, kaempferol, chrysin, and luteolin significantly decreased the promoter activity (Figure 7). These results coincide with those of Western blotting. In contrast, quercetin, genistein, hesperetin, and daidzein did not inhibit the promoter activity. Kaempferol, chrysin, and luteolin inhibited the activity of construct of −395/+37, but the inhibitory effects of kaempferol and luteolin disappeared in the constructs of −143/+37 and −87/+37. In contrast, the promoter activity of all deletion constructs was significantly inhibited by chrysin. These results indicate that the kaempferol- and luteolin-sensitive transcriptional factor may bind to the region between −395 and −144, and chrysin-sensitive one may bind to the region between −86 and −1. TFSEARCH showed that the region between −395 and −144 of claudin-2 promoter contains a putative STAT-binding site. The promoter activity of mutant of STAT-biding site was not significantly inhibited by kaempferol and luteolin. These results indicate that STAT may be involved in the decrease in claudin-2 expression by kaempferol and luteolin.

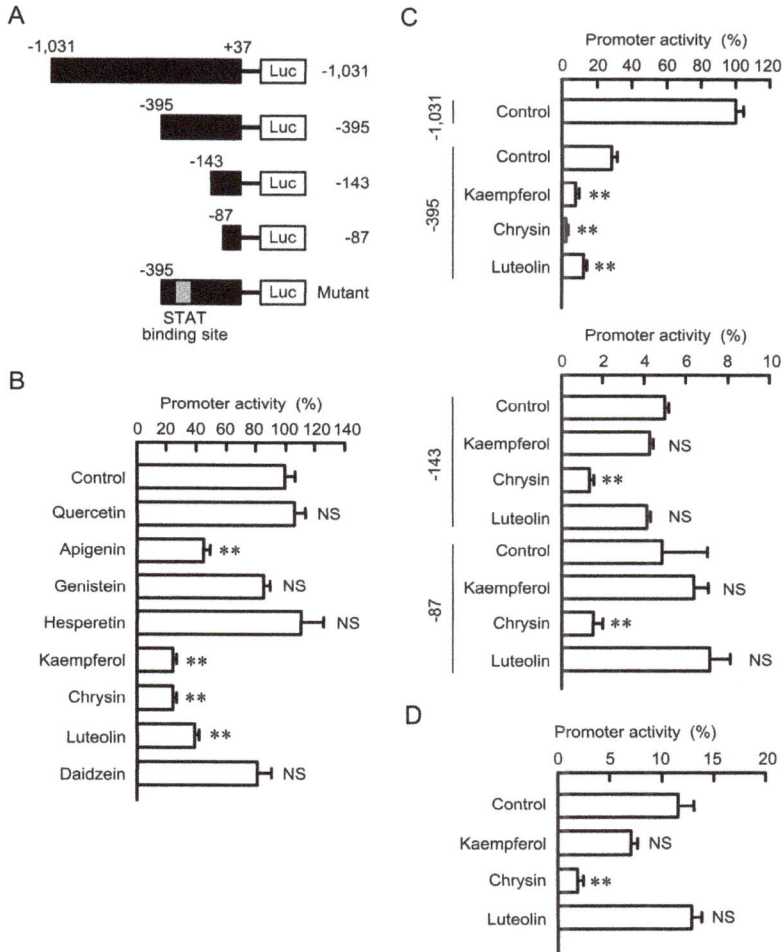

**Figure 7.** Effects of flavonoids on the promoter activity of human claudin-2. (**A**) Schematic drawing of human claudin-2 luciferase reporter vector; (**B**) The cells were co-transfected with luciferase −1031/pGL4.10 and pRL-TK vectors. After 24 h of transfection, the cells were incubated in the absence and presence of 50 μM flavonoids for 24 h. The promoter activity of claudin-2 was represented relative to the values in control; (**C**) The constructs of 5′-deletion series including −395, −143, and −87/pGL4 vector were co-transfected with the pRL-TK vector; (**D**) The construct of mutant of STAT-binding site was co-transfected with the pRL-TK vector. The relative promoter activity was represented relative to the values of control of −1031/pGL4 vector. $n$ = 3–4. ** $p < 0.01$ significantly different from vehicle. NS, not significantly different.

*3.5. Inhibition of Association between STAT3 and Claudin-2 Promoter by Flavonoids*

STAT3 is abundantly expressed in lung cancer cells and involved in the development of cancer [32]. The phosphorylation and nuclear localization of STAT3 were not inhibited by kaempferol, chrysin, and luteolin (Figure 8). In the ChIP assay, a primer pairs amplifying the STAT-binding site showed positive PCR signals in the control cells using anti-STAT3 antibody (Figure 8B). In the kaempferol, chrysin, and luteolin-treated cells, PCR signal was faint. The primer pairs amplifying STAT-binding site showed PCR bands using input samples. These results indicate that these flavonoids inhibit interaction between STAT3 and claudin-2 promoter. The interaction between transcriptional factor and promoter region is often regulated by epigenetic modification, such as histone acetylation [33]. However, three flavonoids did not change acetylation levels of histone H3 (Figure 8C), indicating that epigenetic mechanism may not be involved in the inhibition of association between STAT3 and claudin-2 promoter.

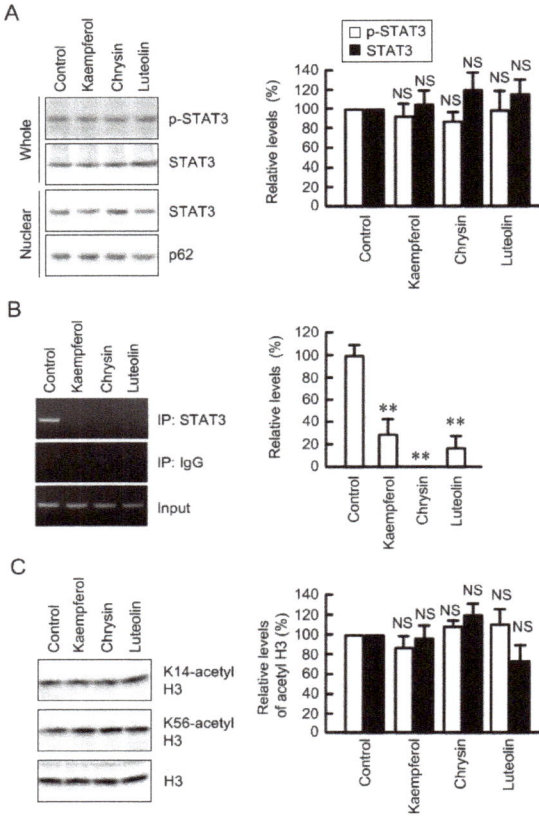

**Figure 8.** Effects of flavonoids on the binding of STAT3 to promoter region of claudin-2. The cells were incubated in the absence (control) and presence of 50 μM flavonoids for 1 h. (**A**) Whole cell extracts and nuclear fractions were immunoblotted with anti-p-STAT3, anti-STAT3, or anti-nucleoporin p62 antibody. The levels of p-STAT3 were represented relative to the values in control; (**B**) After immunoprecipitation of genomic DNA by anti-STAT3 antibody, semi-quantitative PCR (left images) and quantitative real-time PCR (right graphs) were performed using the primers amplifying the putative STAT-binding site of claudin-2 promoter. Mouse IgG was used for negative control. Input chromatin was used for normalization. The amount of PCR products is represented relative to the value of control cells; (**C**) Nuclear fractions were immunoblotted with anti-acetyl histone H3 (K14 or K56) or anti-histone H3 antibody. The levels of acetyl histone H3 were represented relative to the values in control. $n = 3$. ** $p < 0.01$ significantly different from control. NS, not significantly different.

### 3.6. Effects of Three Flavonoids and Ectopic Claudin-2 Expression on Cell Proliferation

Claudin-2 is partially involved in the regulation of proliferation in A549 cells [7,11]. Kaempferol, chrysin, and luteolin decreased claudin-2 expression, so we examined the effects of these flavonoids on cell proliferation. To avoid the effect of cytotoxicity, the cells were treated with these flavonoids at the concentration of 10 µM (Supplementary Figure S1). Cell number was not changed by overexpression of claudin-2 in the absence of flavonoids (Figure 9). Three flavonoids inhibited the increase in cell number and decreased the expression of claudin-2, which were rescued by ectopic claudin-2 expression. Therefore, these results indicate that kaempferol, chrysin, and luteolin may inhibit cell proliferation mediated by the decrease in claudin-2 expression.

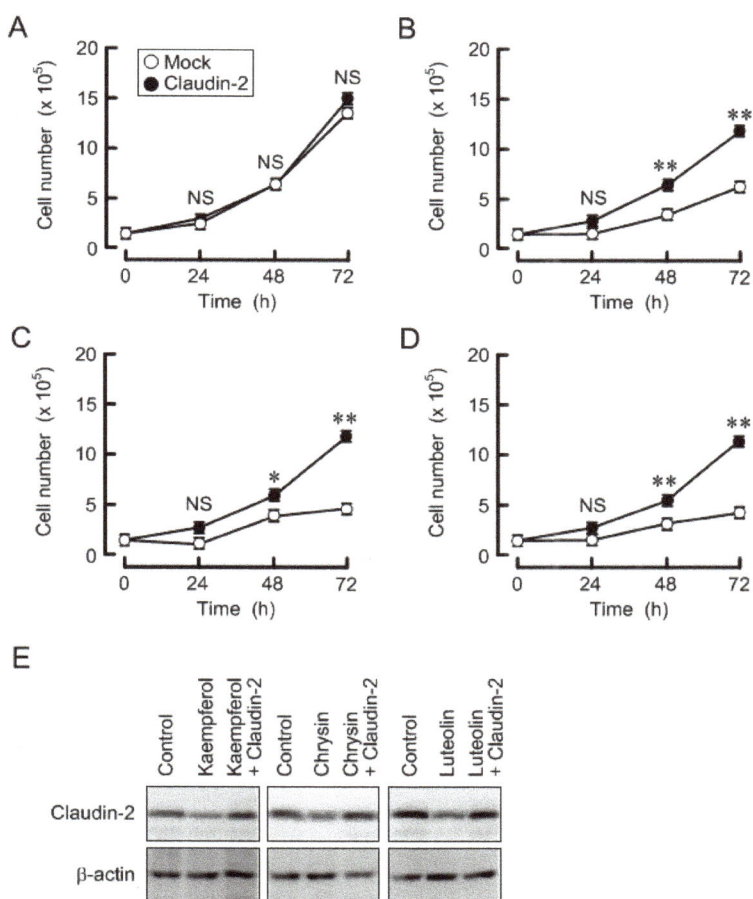

**Figure 9.** Rescue of cell proliferation by ectopic claudin-2 expression. Mock and claudin-2-overexpressing cells were cultured in the absence (**A**) and presence of 10 µM kaempferol (**B**); chrysin (**C**); or luteolin (**D**). Cell number was measured at 24, 48, and 72 h after inoculation; (**E**) Cell lysates were immunoblotted with anti-claudin-2 or β-actin antibody. $n = 3–4$. ** $p < 0.01$ and * $p < 0.05$ significantly different from mock. NS, not significantly different.

## 4. Discussion

The effects of flavonoids on the barrier function and expression of claudins have been examined in epithelial cells. Quercetin enhances intestinal barrier in Caco-2 cells through the elevation of claudin-4 [34] and through the assembly of zonula occludens-2, occludin, and claudin-1 [35]. Genistein and daidzein protect lipopolysaccharide-induced disruption of barrier function in glandular endometrial epithelial cells through the elevation of claudin-3, -4, and -8 [36]. In contrast, the effects of flavonoids on the pathophysiological function and expression of claudins in cancer cells have not been examined well. Here, we found that kaempferol, chrysin, and luteolin decrease the mRNA and protein levels of claudin-2 in lung adenocarcinoma A549 cells. The expression of claudin-2 is decreased by chemical inhibitors and dominant negative plasmids of MEK/ERK/c-Fos and PI3K/Akt/NF-κB pathways in A549 cells [7,31]. These factors of intracellular signaling pathway are activated in the lung cancer tissues [37,38]. However, kaempferol, chrysin, and luteolin did not inhibit the phosphorylation of ERK1/2 and Akt, but they surprisingly increased these phosphorylation. We suggest that kaempferol, chrysin, and luteolin decrease claudin-2 expression mediated by the different mechanisms from MEK/ERK/c-Fos and PI3K/Akt/NF-κB pathways.

The regulatory mechanism of claudin-2 expression is different in each tissue. Claudin-2 expression is down-regulated by the activation of MEK/ERK pathway in renal tubular Madin Darby canine kidney type II (MDCK II) cells [39]. The effect of MEK/ERK pathway in MDCK II cells is opposite to that in A549 cells [29]. At present, it is unknown why the MEK/ERK pathway has contrary effects on claudin-2 expression in both cells. In intestinal Caco-2 cells, claudin-2 is up-regulated by caudal-related homeobox 2 (cdx2) [40]. Cdx2 is an intestine-specific transcription factor highly expressed in the tissues of dysplasia and cancer, but is not expressed in the lung. Therefore, cdx2 should not be involved in the up-regulation of claudin-2 in lung cancer. To identify novel compounds that decrease claudin-2 expression, we had to search for them based on the novel mechanism of action.

It has been postulated that oxidative stress is closely associated with tumor formation, progression and metastasis. Numerous naturally occurring anti-oxidant compounds possess anti-cancer properties [12]. Oxidative stresses including hydrogen peroxide and nitric oxide decrease claudin-1 and -5 expression in colonic HT-29 cells [41], claudin-2 expression in MDCK II cells [42], and claudin-5 expression in ischemic brain [43], which are inhibited by antioxidants. Oxidative stress may be one of the key factors controlling claudins expression. Kaempferol, chrysin, and luteolin showed little antioxidative effect at the concentration used in the present study (Figure 3), whereas NAC and GSH had strong antioxidant activity. Nevertheless, both NAC and GSH did not decrease claudin-2 expression, whereas 4′-hydroxyflavonoe and 7-hydroxyflavone dose-dependently decreased. These results suggest that anti-oxidative capacity is not necessary to decrease claudin-2 expression in A549 cells, but the basic structure of flavones or flavonols is necessary.

Kaempferol, chrysin, and luteolin have been reported to inhibit properties of cancer mediated by inhibition of phosphorylation of STAT3: Kaempferol induces differentiation in partially differentiated colon cancer cells [44], chrysin suppresses hypoxia-induced metastasis of 4T1 mouse breast cancer cells [45], and luteolin inhibits hypoxia-induced vascular endothelial factor expression [46]. In contrast, our results indicated that these flavonoids do not inhibit the phosphorylation of STAT3, but they block the interaction between STAT3 and the promoter region of claudin-2. The direct inhibition of the binding of transcriptional factor and DNA are reported by some flavonoids. Apigenin, chrysin, and kaempferol bind to peroxisome proliferator-activated receptor γ and suppress inducible cyclooxygenase (COX) and nitric oxide synthase promoter activity in mouse macrophages [47]. Chrysin binds to nuclear factor for IL-6 and suppresses COX-2 expression in lipopolysaccharide-activated Raw 264.7 cells [48]. The binding site of flavonoids on STAT3 is unknown, but kaempferol, chrysin, and luteolin could interfere the interaction between STAT3 and promoter region of claudin-2.

The pharmacological inhibitor and dominant-negative isoform of STAT3 have been reported to induce cell cycle arrest in A549 cells [32]. So far, we reported that knockdown of claudin-2 inhibits cell cycle G1/S transition without affecting cytotoxicity [11]. In the present study, kaempferol, chrysin, and luteolin showed little cytotoxicity (Supplementary Figure S1) and decreased cell number. The flavonoids-induced decrease in cell number was significantly rescued by ectopic claudin-2 expression. Therefore, we suggest that these flavonoids inhibit cell proliferation mediated by the reduction of claudin-2 expression.

## 5. Conclusions

In the present study, we found that kaempferol, chrysin, and luteolin decrease claudin-2 expression in A549 cells. Kaempferol and luteolin inhibited the promoter activity of human claudin-2, which was rescued by deletion or mutation of STAT-binding site. The phosphorylation and nuclear localization of STAT3 were not inhibited by kaempferol and luteolin, but the interaction between STAT3 and the promoter region of claudin-2 was inhibited, indicating that kaempferol and luteolin may directly block the interaction of STAT3 on DNA. Chrysin also inhibited the promoter activity of claudin-2, which was not rescued by deletion of STAT-binding site. Other important transcriptional factors, which bind to the region between −86 and −1 of claudin-2 promoter, should be involved in the inhibitory effect of chrysin. Some foods that abundantly include these flavonoids may be useful to prevent development of lung adenocarcinoma.

**Supplementary Materials:** The following are available online at www.mdpi.com/2072-6643/9/6/597/s1, Figure S1: Effects of flavonoids on cell viability.

**Acknowledgments:** This work was supported in part by grants from the Takeda Science Foundation, the Futaba Electronics Memorial Foundation, and the Takahashi Sangyo-Keizai Research Foundation, and collaborative research grant from API Co., Ltd. (Gifu, Japan).

**Author Contributions:** H.S. and A.T. performed experiments and analyzed the data. S.E., T.M., T.F. and K.I. contributed the experiment plan and discussion of the manuscript. A.I. contributed to supervision of the project, interpretation of the data and writing the paper.

**Conflicts of Interest:** The authors declare no conflict of interest.

## Abbreviations

| | |
|---|---|
| cdx2 | caudal-related homeobox 2 |
| ChIP | chromatin immunoprecipitation |
| COX | cyclooxygenase |
| DMEM | Dulbecco's Modified Eagle's medium |
| DMSO | Dimethyl sulfoxide |
| ERK | extracellular signal-regulated kinase |
| FCS | fetal calf serum |
| NAC | *N*-acetyl cysteine |
| MDCK | Madin Darby canine kidney |
| MEK | mitogen-activated protein kinase kinase |
| NF-κB | nuclear factor-κB |
| PCR | polymerase chain reaction |
| PI3K | phosphoinositide 3-kinase |
| SDS-PAGE | SDS-polyacrylamide gel electrophoresis |
| STAT | signal transducers and activators of transcription |
| TJs | tight junctions |

## References

1. Tsukita, S.; Yamazaki, Y.; Katsuno, T.; Tamura, A. Tight junction-based epithelial microenvironment and cell proliferation. *Oncogene* **2008**, *27*, 6930–6938. [CrossRef] [PubMed]
2. Powell, D.W. Barrier function of epithelia. *Am. J. Physiol. Gastrointest. Liver Physiol.* **1981**, *241*, G275–G288.
3. Matter, K.; Balda, M.S. Signalling to and from tight junctions. *Nat. Rev. Mol. Cell Biol.* **2003**, *4*, 225–236. [CrossRef] [PubMed]

4.  Mineta, K.; Yamamoto, Y.; Yamazaki, Y.; Tanaka, H.; Tada, Y.; Saito, K.; Tamura, A.; Igarashi, M.; Endo, T.; Takeuchi, K.; et al. Predicted expansion of the claudin multigene family. *FEBS Lett.* **2011**, *585*, 606–612. [CrossRef] [PubMed]

5.  Turksen, K.; Troy, T.C. Barriers built on claudins. *J. Cell Sci.* **2004**, *117*, 2435–2447. [CrossRef] [PubMed]

6.  Ding, L.; Lu, Z.; Lu, Q.; Chen, Y.H. The claudin family of proteins in human malignancy: A clinical perspective. *Cancer Manag. Res.* **2013**, *5*, 367–375. [PubMed]

7.  Ikari, A.; Sato, T.; Takiguchi, A.; Atomi, K.; Yamazaki, Y.; Sugatani, J. Claudin-2 knockdown decreases matrix metalloproteinase-9 activity and cell migration via suppression of nuclear Sp1 in A549 cells. *Life Sci.* **2011**, *88*, 628–633. [CrossRef] [PubMed]

8.  Halasz, J.; Holczbauer, A.; Paska, C.; Kovacs, M.; Benyo, G.; Verebely, T.; Schaff, Z.; Kiss, A. Claudin-1 and claudin-2 differentiate fetal and embryonal components in human hepatoblastoma. *Hum. Pathol.* **2006**, *37*, 555–561. [CrossRef] [PubMed]

9.  Kinugasa, T.; Huo, Q.; Higashi, D.; Shibaguchi, H.; Kuroki, M.; Tanaka, T.; Futami, K.; Yamashita, Y.; Hachimine, K.; Maekawa, S.; et al. Selective up-regulation of claudin-1 and claudin-2 in colorectal cancer. *Anticancer Res.* **2007**, *27*, 3729–3734. [CrossRef]

10. Song, X.; Li, X.; Tang, Y.; Chen, H.; Wong, B.; Wang, J.; Chen, M. Expression of Cdx2 and claudin-2 in the multistage tissue of gastric carcinogenesis. *Oncology* **2007**, *73*, 357–365.

11. Ikari, A.; Watanabe, R.; Sato, T.; Taga, S.; Shimobaba, S.; Yamaguchi, M.; Yamazaki, Y.; Endo, S.; Matsunaga, T.; Sugatani, J. Nuclear distribution of claudin-2 increases cell proliferation in human lung adenocarcinoma cells. *Biochim. Biophys. Acta* **2014**, *1843*, 2079–2088. [CrossRef] [PubMed]

12. Zhou, Y.; Zheng, J.; Li, Y.; Xu, D.P.; Li, S.; Chen, Y.M.; Li, H.B. Natural Polyphenols for Prevention and Treatment of Cancer. *Nutrients* **2016**, *8*, 515. [CrossRef] [PubMed]

13. Sawicka, D.; Car, H.; Borawska, M.H.; Niklinski, J. The anticancer activity of propolis. *Folia Histochem Cytobiol.* **2012**, *50*, 25–37. [CrossRef] [PubMed]

14. Christensen, K.Y.; Naidu, A.; Parent, M.E.; Pintos, J.; Abrahamowicz, M.; Siemiatycki, J.; Koushik, A. The risk of lung cancer related to dietary intake of flavonoids. *Nutr. Cancer* **2012**, *64*, 964–974. [CrossRef] [PubMed]

15. Stefani, E.D.; Boffetta, P.; Deneo-Pellegrini, H.; Mendilaharsu, M.; Carzoglio, J.C.; Ronco, A.; Olivera, L. Dietary antioxidants and lung cancer risk: A case-control study in Uruguay. *Nutr. Cancer* **1999**, *34*, 100–110. [CrossRef] [PubMed]

16. Amararathna, M.; Johnston, M.R.; Rupasinghe, H.P. Plant Polyphenols as Chemopreventive Agents for Lung Cancer. *Int. J. Mol. Sci.* **2016**, *17*, 1352. [CrossRef] [PubMed]

17. Rice-Evans, C.A.; Miller, N.J.; Bolwell, P.G.; Bramley, P.M.; Pridham, J.B. The relative antioxidant activities of plant-derived polyphenolic flavonoids. *Free Radic. Res.* **1995**, *22*, 375–383. [CrossRef] [PubMed]

18. Nguyen, T.T.; Tran, E.; Nguyen, T.H.; Do, P.T.; Huynh, T.H.; Huynh, H. The role of activated MEK-ERK pathway in quercetin-induced growth inhibition and apoptosis in A549 lung cancer cells. *Carcinogenesis* **2004**, *25*, 647–659. [CrossRef] [PubMed]

19. Choi, J.A.; Kim, J.Y.; Lee, J.Y.; Kang, C.M.; Kwon, H.J.; Yoo, Y.D.; Kim, T.W.; Lee, Y.S.; Lee, S.J. Induction of cell cycle arrest and apoptosis in human breast cancer cells by quercetin. *Int. J. Oncol.* **2001**, *19*, 837–844. [CrossRef] [PubMed]

20. Yoshida, M.; Sakai, T.; Hosokawa, N.; Marui, N.; Matsumoto, K.; Fujioka, A.; Nishino, H.; Aoike, A. The effect of quercetin on cell cycle progression and growth of human gastric cancer cells. *FEBS Lett.* **1990**, *260*, 10–13. [CrossRef]

21. Vijayababu, M.R.; Kanagaraj, P.; Arunkumar, A.; Ilangovan, R.; Aruldhas, M.M.; Arunakaran, J. Quercetin-induced growth inhibition and cell death in prostatic carcinoma cells (PC-3) are associated with increase in p21 and hypophosphorylated retinoblastoma proteins expression. *J. Cancer Res. Clin. Oncol.* **2005**, *131*, 765–771. [CrossRef] [PubMed]

22. Sonoki, H.; Sato, T.; Endo, S.; Matsunaga, T.; Yamaguchi, M.; Yamazaki, Y.; Sugatani, J.; Ikari, A. Quercetin Decreases Claudin-2 Expression Mediated by Up-Regulation of microRNA miR-16 in Lung Adenocarcinoma A549 Cells. *Nutrients* **2015**, *7*, 4578–4592. [CrossRef] [PubMed]

23. Benekli, M.; Baumann, H.; Wetzler, M. Targeting signal transducer and activator of transcription signaling pathway in leukemias. *J. Clin. Oncol.* **2009**, *27*, 4422–4432. [CrossRef] [PubMed]

24. Yu, H.; Jove, R. The STATs of cancer—New molecular targets come of age. *Nat. Rev. Cancer* **2004**, *4*, 97–105. [CrossRef] [PubMed]

25. Darnell, J.E., Jr. STATs and gene regulation. *Science* **1997**, *277*, 1630–1635. [CrossRef] [PubMed]
26. Chaudhuri, A.; Yang, B.; Gendelman, H.E.; Persidsky, Y.; Kanmogne, G.D. STAT1 signaling modulates HIV-1-induced inflammatory responses and leukocyte transmigration across the blood-brain barrier. *Blood* **2008**, *111*, 2062–2072. [CrossRef] [PubMed]
27. Garcia-Hernandez, V.; Flores-Maldonado, C.; Rincon-Heredia, R.; Verdejo-Torres, O.; Bonilla-Delgado, J.; Meneses-Morales, I.; Gariglio, P.; Contreras, R.G. EGF regulates claudin-2 and -4 expression through Src and STAT3 in MDCK cells. *J. Cell. Physiol.* **2015**, *230*, 105–115. [CrossRef] [PubMed]
28. Shimomura, O.; Wu, C.; Murai, A.; Nakamura, H. Evaluation of five imidazopyrazinone-type chemiluminescent superoxide probes and their application to the measurement of superoxide anion generated by Listeria monocytogenes. *Anal. Biochem.* **1998**, *258*, 230–235. [CrossRef] [PubMed]
29. Ikari, A.; Sato, T.; Watanabe, R.; Yamazaki, Y.; Sugatani, J. Increase in claudin-2 expression by an EGFR/MEK/ERK/c-Fos pathway in lung adenocarcinoma A549 cells. *Biochim. Biophys. Acta* **2012**, *1823*, 1110–1118. [CrossRef] [PubMed]
30. Furusawa, M.; Tanaka, T.; Ito, T.; Nishikawa, A.; Yamazaki, N.; Nakaya, K.; Matsuura, N.; Tsuchiya, H.; Nagayama, M.; Iinuma, M. Antioxidant activity of hydroxyflavonoids. *J. Health Sci.* **2005**, *51*, 376–378. [CrossRef]
31. Hichino, A.; Okamoto, M.; Taga, S.; Akizuki, R.; Endo, S.; Matsunaga, T.; Ikari, A. Down-regulation of Claudin-2 Expression and Proliferation by Epigenetic Inhibitors in Human Lung Adenocarcinoma A549 Cells. *J. Biol. Chem.* **2017**, *292*, 2411–2421. [CrossRef] [PubMed]
32. Song, L.; Turkson, J.; Karras, J.G.; Jove, R.; Haura, E.B. Activation of Stat3 by receptor tyrosine kinases and cytokines regulates survival in human non-small cell carcinoma cells. *Oncogene* **2003**, *22*, 4150–4165. [CrossRef] [PubMed]
33. Ansari, J.; Shackelford, R.E.; El-Osta, H. Epigenetics in non-small cell lung cancer: From basics to therapeutics. *Transl. Lung Cancer Res.* **2016**, *5*, 155–171. [CrossRef] [PubMed]
34. Amasheh, M.; Andres, S.; Amasheh, S.; Fromm, M.; Schulzke, J.D. Barrier effects of nutritional factors. *Ann. N. Y. Acad. Sci.* **2009**, *1165*, 267–273. [CrossRef] [PubMed]
35. Suzuki, T.; Hara, H. Quercetin enhances intestinal barrier function through the assembly of zonnula occludens-2, occludin, and claudin-1 and the expression of claudin-4 in Caco-2 cells. *J. Nutr.* **2009**, *139*, 965–974. [CrossRef] [PubMed]
36. Kiatprasert, P.; Deachapunya, C.; Benjanirat, C.; Poonyachoti, S. Soy isoflavones improves endometrial barrier through tight junction gene expression. *Reproduction* **2015**, *149*, 269–280. [CrossRef] [PubMed]
37. Scrima, M.; De Marco, C.; Fabiani, F.; Franco, R.; Pirozzi, G.; Rocco, G.; Ravo, M.; Weisz, A.; Zoppoli, P.; Ceccarelli, M.; et al. Signaling networks associated with AKT activation in non-small cell lung cancer (NSCLC): New insights on the role of phosphatydil-inositol-3 kinase. *PLoS ONE* **2012**, *7*, e30427. [CrossRef] [PubMed]
38. Mossman, B.T.; Lounsbury, K.M.; Reddy, S.P. Oxidants and signaling by mitogen-activated protein kinases in lung epithelium. *Am. J. Respir. Cell Mol. Biol.* **2006**, *34*, 666–669. [CrossRef] [PubMed]
39. Lipschutz, J.H.; Li, S.; Arisco, A.; Balkovetz, D.F. Extracellular signal-regulated kinases 1/2 control claudin-2 expression in Madin-Darby canine kidney strain I and II cells. *J. Biol. Chem.* **2005**, *280*, 3780–3788. [CrossRef] [PubMed]
40. Suzuki, T.; Yoshinaga, N.; Tanabe, S. Interleukin-6 (IL-6) regulates claudin-2 expression and tight junction permeability in intestinal epithelium. *J. Biol. Chem.* **2011**, *286*, 31263–31271. [CrossRef] [PubMed]
41. Jeong, C.H.; Seok, J.S.; Petriello, M.C.; Han, S.G. Arsenic downregulates tight junction claudin proteins through p38 and NF-kappaB in intestinal epithelial cell line, HT-29. *Toxicology* **2017**, *379*, 31–39. [CrossRef] [PubMed]
42. Gonzalez, J.E.; DiGeronimo, R.J.; Arthur, D.E.; King, J.M. Remodeling of the tight junction during recovery from exposure to hydrogen peroxide in kidney epithelial cells. *Free Radic. Biol. Med.* **2009**, *47*, 1561–1569. [CrossRef] [PubMed]
43. Mohammadi, M.T. Overproduction of nitric oxide intensifies brain infarction and cerebrovascular damage through reduction of claudin-5 and ZO-1 expression in striatum of ischemic brain. *Pathol. Res. Pract.* **2016**, *212*, 959–964. [CrossRef] [PubMed]

Nutrients **2017**, *9*, 597

44. Nakamura, Y.; Chang, C.C.; Mori, T.; Sato, K.; Ohtsuki, K.; Upham, B.L.; Trosko, J.E. Augmentation of differentiation and gap junction function by kaempferol in partially differentiated colon cancer cells. *Carcinogenesis* **2005**, *26*, 665–671. [CrossRef] [PubMed]

45. Lirdprapamongkol, K.; Sakurai, H.; Abdelhamed, S.; Yokoyama, S.; Maruyama, T.; Athikomkulchai, S.; Viriyaroj, A.; Awale, S.; Yagita, H.; Ruchirawat, S.; et al. A flavonoid chrysin suppresses hypoxic survival and metastatic growth of mouse breast cancer cells. *Oncol. Rep.* **2013**, *30*, 2357–2364. [CrossRef] [PubMed]

46. Anso, E.; Zuazo, A.; Irigoyen, M.; Urdaci, M.C.; Rouzaut, A.; Martinez-Irujo, J.J. Flavonoids inhibit hypoxia-induced vascular endothelial growth factor expression by a HIF-1 independent mechanism. *Biochem. Pharmacol.* **2010**, *79*, 1600–1609. [CrossRef] [PubMed]

47. Liang, Y.C.; Tsai, S.H.; Tsai, D.C.; Lin-Shiau, S.Y.; Lin, J.K. Suppression of inducible cyclooxygenase and nitric oxide synthase through activation of peroxisome proliferator-activated receptor-gamma by flavonoids in mouse macrophages. *FEBS Lett.* **2001**, *496*, 12–18. [CrossRef]

48. Woo, K.J.; Jeong, Y.J.; Inoue, H.; Park, J.W.; Kwon, T.K. Chrysin suppresses lipopolysaccharide-induced cyclooxygenase-2 expression through the inhibition of nuclear factor for IL-6 (NF-IL6) DNA-binding activity. *FEBS Lett.* **2005**, *579*, 705–711. [CrossRef] [PubMed]

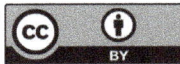

*nutrients*

MDPI

*Review*

# Fruits for Prevention and Treatment of Cardiovascular Diseases

Cai-Ning Zhao [1], Xiao Meng [1], Ya Li [1], Sha Li [2,*], Qing Liu [1], Guo-Yi Tang [1] and Hua-Bin Li [1,3,*]

[1] Guangdong Provincial Key Laboratory of Food, Nutrition and Health, Department of Nutrition, School of Public Health, Sun Yat-sen University, Guangzhou 510080, China; zhaocn@mail2.sysu.edu.cn (C.-N.Z.); mengx7@mail2.sysu.edu.cn (X.M.); liya28@mail2.sysu.edu.cn (Y.L.); liuq248@mail2.sysu.edu.cn (Q.L.); tanggy5@mail2.sysu.edu.cn (G.-Y.T.)

[2] School of Chinese Medicine, Li Ka Shing Faculty of Medicine, The University of Hong Kong, Hong Kong 999077, China

[3] South China Sea Bioresource Exploitation and Utilization Collaborative Innovation Center, Sun Yat-sen University, Guangzhou 510006, China

* Correspondence: u3003781@connect.hku.hk (S.L.); lihuabin@mail.sysu.edu.cn (H.-B.L.); Tel.: +852-3917-6498 (S.L.); +86-20-873-323-91 (H.-B.L.)

Received: 25 April 2017; Accepted: 9 June 2017; Published: 13 June 2017

**Abstract:** Cardiovascular diseases (CVDs) are leading global health problems. Accumulating epidemiological studies have indicated that consuming fruits was inversely related to the risk of CVDs. Moreover, substantial experimental studies have supported the protective role of fruits against CVDs, and several fruits (grape, blueberry, pomegranate, apple, hawthorn, and avocado) have been widely studied and have shown potent cardiovascular protective action. Fruits can prevent CVDs or facilitate the restoration of morphology and functions of heart and vessels after injury. The involved mechanisms included protecting vascular endothelial function, regulating lipids metabolism, modulating blood pressure, inhibiting platelets function, alleviating ischemia/reperfusion injury, suppressing thrombosis, reducing oxidative stress, and attenuating inflammation. The present review summarizes recent discoveries about the effects of fruits on CVDs and discusses potential mechanisms of actions based on evidence from epidemiological, experimental, and clinical studies.

**Keywords:** fruit; cardiovascular disease; coronary heart disease; stroke; hypertension; mechanisms of action

## 1. Introduction

Cardiovascular diseases (CVDs) are defined as disorders of the heart and vessels, and include coronary heart disease (CHD) and stroke. According to the WHO report, CVDs are responsible for 17.5 million deaths in 2012 (7.4 and 6.7 million due to CHD and stroke, respectively), accounting for 31% of all global deaths a year, constituting the leading causes of death worldwide [1]. Thus, studies on CVDs have drawn great attention around the world.

Diet represents the most important modifiable factor to prevent CVDs. There is evidence that plant-based dietary patterns are associated with lower risk of CVDs [2]. Among the most important key components, fruit has been suggested to play a major role in preventing CVDs [3]. Several epidemiological studies demonstrated that fruit intake was inversely associated with the risk of cardiovascular events [4–7]. It is estimated that a diet low in fruits is the third most important risk factor of CVDs following high blood pressure (BP) and cigarette smoking, accounting for more than 5 million deaths worldwide in 2010 [8]. In addition, much experimental evidence supports the protective role of fruit against CVDs. Furthermore, several fruits, such as grape, blueberry, pomegranate, apple, hawthorn, and avocado, have been widely studied and have shown strong cardiovascular protective effects. Additionally, the effectiveness of fruit intake in the primary prevention of CVDs has been revealed by growing clinical data in patients with high metabolic risk factors (hypertension, dyslipidemia, diabetes, and overweight/obesity). Currently, the common method of controlling CVDs is the use of long-term pharmacotherapy. Nevertheless, drugs are not effective on all patients and have side effects that may aggravate the patients' symptoms and signs. Some fruits (extract) possess similar or even more potent anti-hypertensive, lipid-lowering, and hypoglycemic activities, which has inspired many researchers to explore new therapies for CVDs [9–12]. The cardioprotective mechanisms of fruits are not entirely clear, but their outstanding antioxidant and free radical scavenging properties are considered principal [13]. In this context, people have paid more attention to natural products rich in polyphenols, a group of compounds characterized by the presence of an aromatic ring and phenolic hydroxyl groups [14–25]. Polyphenols are obtained through daily diets because they cannot be synthesized or stored in the human body, and fruit is one of the main dietary sources of polyphenols [26]. The richest sources of fruit polyphenols are dark berries, such as grapes and blueberries [27]. Further, pomegranate, apple, hawthorn, and avocado are also frequently consumed polyphenols-rich fruits. There is evidence that fruit rich in polyphenols helps to control CVDs.

This review aims to summarize the effects of fruit on CVDs based on evidence from epidemiological, experimental, and clinical studies, and special attention is paid to the mechanisms of action.

## 2. Epidemiological Studies

Epidemiological evidence supports that diets rich in fruit delay the onset, and attenuate the severity, of CVDs (Table 1).

Evidence from the China Kadoorie Biobank Study showed that consuming fresh fruits daily decreased systolic blood pressure (SBP) by 4.0 mmHg and blood glucose level by 0.5 mmol/L, which was inversely associated with the risks of cardiovascular death (hazard ratios (HRs): 0.60, 95% confidence intervals (CIs): 0.54–0.67) and major CVDs, i.e., CHD (HR: 0.66, 95% CI: 0.58–0.75), ischemic stroke (HR: 0.75, 95% CI: 0.72–0.79), and hemorrhagic stroke (HR: 0.64, 95% CI: 0.56–0.74), as compared with participants who never or rarely consumed fresh fruit [4]. In addition, two cohort studies of women aged 35–69 [5] and over 70 years [6], respectively, showed that consuming fruits reduced the risk of total CVD mortality. Additionally, a Japanese study suggested that frequent intake of citrus fruit protected against CVDs; the HR for near-daily intake versus infrequent intake of citrus fruit was 0.57 (95% CI: 0.33–1.01) in men and 0.51 (95% CI: 0.29–0.88) in women [7].

A cohort study of women in Shanghai showed a protective role of higher dietary total fruit and vegetable intake in CHD. Moreover, the study suggested that this association was primarily driven by fruit. The corresponding HRs for fruit and vegetable intake were 0.62 (95% CI: 0.37–1.03) and 0.94 (95% CI: 0.59–1.50), respectively [28]. In addition, a meta-analysis of 23 prospective cohort studies of 937,665 participants and 18,047 CHD patients showed that fruit consumption was inversely associated with a risk of CHD. Compared with those who consumed the lowest total fruits, the relative risk (RR) of CHD was 0.86 (95% CI: 0.82–0.91) for those consuming the highest, and the dose-response analysis indicated that the RR of CHD was 0.84 (95% CI: 0.75–0.93) per 300 g/day of total fruit intake [29]. For individual fruit, apple intake reduced the risk of acute coronary syndrome (ACS) by 3%, and the dose-response analysis indicated that the HR of ACS was 0.97 (95% CI: 0.93–1.01) per 25 g/day of apple intake [30].

In terms of stroke, cohorts of Swedish women and men suggested that consuming 3.1 servings/day of total fruits alleviated total stroke risk by 13% compared with 0.4 servings/day (95% CI: 0.78–0.97) [31]. Furthermore, the study also indicated that, among individual fruits, consumption of apple/pear particularly decreased the risk of total stroke (HR: 0.89, 95% CI: 0.80–0.98) [31], which was consistent with the result of a study in Netherlands of 20,069 adults [32]. The study in Netherlands also reported that consuming >120 g/day raw fruit decreased the risk of hemorrhagic stroke by 47% (95% CI: 0.28–1.01) compared with consuming ≤120 g/day raw fruits [33].

In addition, the Nurses' Health Study showed that high citrus fruit/juice intake was related to a reduced risk of ischemic stroke (RR: 0.90, 95% CI: 0.77–1.05) [34]. Additionally, a cohort study with 20,024 participants recruited also proved that citrus fruits/juice intake was inversely associated with risk of ischemic stroke (HR: 0.69, 95% CI: 0.53–0.91) [35].

Epidemiological studies have suggested that fruit consumption was related to a reduction in cardiovascular risk factors. Hypertension is an independent risk factor of CHD and total stroke [36]. Three cohort studies all reported that higher fruit intake was correlated with the decreased risk of hypertension [37–39]. A study of US women showed that total fruit and vegetables consumption attenuated the risk of hypertension. In addition, after adjusting for lifestyle factors and other food intake, total fruit ($p = 0.0004$) but not total vegetables ($p = 0.56$) remained significantly and inversely correlated with risk of hypertension [37]. In addition, a study on residents from Ohasama, Japan, revealed an association between fruit and vegetable intake and the risk of hypertension. In the sex- and BMI-adjusted analysis, the highest quartile of fruit intake was associated with a significantly lower risk of hypertension (HR: 0.40, 95% CI: 0.21–0.74), whereas no association was observed for vegetable intake [38]. Moreover, a study consisting of three large longitudinal cohorts, Nurses' Health Study, Nurses' Health Study II, and Health Professionals Follow-up Study, suggested that long-term and increased consumption of whole fruits reduced the risk of hypertension [39]. Additionally, a case–control study in Korea was also in line with this view [40]. Furthermore, cross-sectional studies of patients with type 2 diabetes demonstrated that higher fruit intake was correlated with a lower burden of CVDs by decreasing carotid intima-media thickness (IMT), the prevalence of carotid plaque [41] and high-sensitive C-reactive protein (hs-CRP) levels [42], which have been well-established predictors for cardiovascular incidents.

Epidemiological studies indicated that dietary intake of polyphenols was associated with a low incidence of CVDs. The Nurses' Health Study with 69,622 women involved showed that the RR for the fifth quintile of flavanone intake versus the lowest quintile was 0.81 (95% CI: 0.66–0.99) [34]. In addition, the relationship between flavonoids intake and CVDs in men was studied in the Health Professionals Follow-Up Study. The results revealed that higher anthocyanin intake was related with lower non-fatal myocardial infarction (MI) risk (HR: 0.87, 95% CI: 0.75–1.00), and higher flavanone intake was associated with decreased ischemic stroke risk (HR: 0.78, 95% CI: 0.62–0.97). The study also reported that over 90% dietary anthocyanins and flavanones came from fruits [43]. In addition, the association between flavonoid intake and ischemic stroke was evaluated in a cohort study of 20,024 participants. The study suggested that flavanone intake was inversely associated with a risk of ischemic stroke (HR: 0.72, 95% CI: 0.55–0.95) [35]. Furthermore, the cardiovascular benefits of flavonoid and stilbene were estimated in a cross-sectional study of 1393 Chinese adults. The study showed that fruits including apple, plum, pear, and peach were the richest sources of flavonoids and stilbenes. Higher anthocyanin intake was related with elevated serum HDL-C ($p = 0.001$), and total flavonoid and flavonol intake was inversely associated with serum TG ($p = 0.020$, $p = 0.035$) and TG/HDL-C ratios ($p = 0.040$, $p = 0.045$) in female subjects. However, significant relationships were not found in male subjects [44].

However, a cohort of Italian women indicated no significant association between fruit intake and the risk of CHD after adjusting for the consumption of vegetables [45]. In addition, a cohort of men aged 50–59 years in France and Northern Ireland reported that there was no significant association between fruit intake and ACS [46]. A large scale cohort of five ethnic groups, i.e., African American, Native Hawaiian, Japanese American, Latino, and Caucasian showed that the consumption of fruits did not protect against ischemic heart disease, and the results did not vary among ethnic groups [47,48]. Additionally, a cohort of Swedish women (aged 49–83 years) suggested that the highest quintile of fruit intake did not significantly decrease the risk of heart failure compared with the lowest [49]. Results are inconsistent maybe because data regarding fruit intake in these cohort studies were obtained on the basis of dietary recall. The actual consumption of fruits can only be rudely assessed, partly because the number of items and the information about portion size were limited.

**Table 1.** Fruit intake and CVD risk.

| Subject | Study Type | Dose | Disease | Risk Estimates (95%CI) | References |
|---|---|---|---|---|---|
| 512,891 Chinese adults (age: 30–79 years) | cohort study | daily vs. never/rarely fresh fruits | cardiovascular death | 0.60 (0.54–0.67) | [4] |
| | | | incident major coronary events | 0.66 (0.58–0.75) | |
| | | | ischemic stroke | 0.75 (0.72–0.79) | |
| | | | hemorrhagic stroke | 0.64 (0.56–0.74) | |
| 30,458 UK Women (age: 35–69 years) | cohort study | per 80 g/day total fruits | CVD | 0.94 (0.89–1.00) | [5] |
| | | | CHD | 0.93 (0.85–1.01) | |
| | | per 80 g/day fresh fruits | CVD | 0.92 (0.85–1.00) | |
| | | | CHD | 0.89 (0.79–1.00) | |
| 1456 women (age: >70 years) | cohort study | per 129 g/day total fruits | CVD | NA ($p < 0.05$) | [6] |
| 10,623 Japanese (4147 men, 6476 women) | cohort study | near-daily vs. infrequent citrus fruits | CVD | Men: 0.57 (0.33–1.01) Women: 0.51 (0.29–0.88) | [7] |
| 67,211 women in Shanghai, China (age: 40–70 years) | cohort study | 449 vs. 83 g/day fruits | CHD | 0.62 (0.37, 1.03) | [28] |
| 23 cohort studies of 937,665 participants and 18,047 patients with CHD | meta-analysis | the highest vs. the lowest of total fruits | CHD | 0.86 (0.82–0.91) | [29] |
| | | per 300 g/day fruits | | 0.84 (0.75–0.93) | |
| 25,065 men in Denmark (age: 50–64 years) | cohort study | per 25 g/day apples | ACS | 0.97 (0.94, 0.99) | [30] |
| 74,961 Swedish adults (34,670 women, 40,291 men; age: 45–83 years) | cohort study | 3.1 vs. 0.4 servings/day total fruits | total stroke | 0.87 (0.78–0.97) | [31] |
| | | 1.0 vs. 0.1 servings/day apples/pears | | 0.89 (0.80–0.98) | |
| 20,069 adults in the Netherlands (age: 20–65 years) | cohort study | >120 vs. ≤120 g/day raw fruits | hemorrhagic stroke | 0.53 (0.28–1.01) | [33] |
| | | per 25 g/day white fruits (usual apples and pears) | stroke | 0.91 (0.85–0.97) | [32] |
| 69,622 women from the Nurses' Health Study | cohort study | the fifth vs. the lowest quintile of citrus fruits/juices | ischemic stroke | 0.90 (0.77–1.05) | [34] |
| | | the fifth vs. the lowest quintile of flavanone | | 0.81 (0.66–0.99) | |

**Table 1.** *Cont.*

| Subject | Study Type | Dose | Disease | Risk Estimates (95%CI) | References |
|---|---|---|---|---|---|
| 20,024 participants without stroke history | cohort study | the highest vs. the lowest quintile of citrus fruits/juices | ischemic stroke | 0.69 (0.53–0.91) | [35] |
| | | the highest vs. the lowest quintile of flavonoid | | 0.72 (0.55–0.95) | |
| 28,082 US women (age: ≥39 years) | cohort study | ≥3 vs. <0.5 servings/day total fruits | hypertension | 0.89 (0.81–0.96) | [37] |
| 745 residents from Ohasama, Japan without hypertension at baseline (age: ≥35 years) | cohort study | the highest vs. the lowest quartile of fruits | hypertension | 0.40 (0.21–0.74) | [38] |
| 3 large longitudinal cohort studies of 187,453 subjects | cohort study | ≥4 vs. ≤4 servings/week of total whole fruits | hypertension | 0.92 (0.87–0.97) | [39] |
| 9791 subjects in Korea (3819 men, 5972 women) | case-control study | the fifth vs. the lowest quintile of fruits | hypertension | 0.73 (0.61–0.88) | [40] |
| 255 Chinese patients with type 2 diabetes (137 men, 118 women) | cross-sectional study | 92.6 ± 39.7 vs. 14.5 ± 8.6 g/day fruits | carotid IMT (0.97 ± 0.02 vs. 1.08 ± 0.03 mm) prevalence of carotid plaque (1.18 vs. 11.76%) | NA ($p$ = 0.046) NA ($p$ = 0.022) | [41] |
| 407 patients with type 2 diabetes (172 men, 235 women) | cross-sectional study | 101.3 ± 28.5 vs. 79.6 ± 24.2g/day fruits | carotid IMT hs-CRP | 0.92 (0.67–0.95) 0.69 (0.53–0.89) | [42] |
| 43,880 healthy men who had no prior diagnosed CVDs or cancer | cohort study | higher anthocyanin intake | MI | 0.87 (0.75–1.00) | [43] |
| | | higher flavanone intake | ischemic stroke | 0.78 (0.62–0.97) | |
| 1393 Chinese adults | cross-sectional study | higher anthocyanins intake | HDL-C | NA ($p$ = 0.001) (women) | [44] |
| | | higher total flavonoid intake | TG | NA ($p$ = 0.020) (women) | |
| | | | TG/HDL-C ratios | NA ($p$ = 0.040) (women) | |
| | | higher flavonol intake | TG | NA ($p$ = 0.035) (women) | |
| | | | TG/HDL-C ratios | NA ($p$ = 0.045) (women) | |
| 29,689 Italian women | cohort study | the highest vs. the lowest quartile of fruits | CHD | no significant association | [45] |
| 8060 men aged 50–59 years in France and Northern Ireland | cohort study | ≥1.29 vs. ≤0.57 times/day fruits | ACS | no significant association | [46] |
| 164,617 men and women from five ethnic groups | cohort study | >4.9 vs. <1.5 servings/day fruits | ischemic heart disease | no significant association | [47,48] |
| 34,319 Swedish women aged 49–83 years | cohort study | ≥2.6 vs. ≤0.8 servings/day total fruits | heart failure | no significant association | [49] |

NA, stands for not available.

### 3. Experimental Studies

There has been accumulating evidence in vivo and in vitro supporting the cardiovascular protective properties of fruits and investigating the underlying mechanisms (Table 2). Six fruits are discussed in detail below because they have been widely studied and have shown potent cardiovascular protective effects, while the fruits that were less investigated are discussed in the section entitled "Other Fruits."

*3.1. Grape*

Grapes are one of the most common and important fruits worldwide, and they are often consumed raw or after being converted to juice, wine, or jam.

3.1.1. Protecting Endothelial Function

In CVDs, endothelial dysfunction is a systemic pathology of the endothelium, is caused by an imbalance between vasodilator and vasoconstrictor substances produced by (or acting on) the endothelium, and presents as impaired vascular endothelium-dependent relaxation and compliance, which is the primary change in early hypertension [50]. Growing experimental and clinical data highlight the importance of oxidative stress on endothelial dysfunction. Grape plays an essential role in repairing endothelial impairment for its potent antioxidant and free radical scavenging capacities. In a study, vascular benefits of whole grape powder were studied using the spontaneously hypertensive rat (SHR). The results showed that grape treatment elicited a reduction in BP, improved arterial relaxation, and increased vascular compliance [51]. Moreover, the relationship between endothelial protective function of grape seed proanthocyanidin extracts (GSPEs) and oxidative stress was studied in SHR and deoxycorticosterone acetate (DOCA)-salt hypertensive mice. The study indicated that GSPEs reduced endothelin (ET)-1 production but increased nitric oxide (NO) production, which exhibited improved endothelial function. Moreover, GSPEs ameliorated oxidative stress by improving superoxide dismutase (SOD) and catalase (CAT) activities and reducing malondialdehyde (MDA) formation [52,53]. Similarly, enzymatic extract of grape pomace (GP-EE) also induced endothelium- and $NO^-$-dependent vasodilatation of both rat aorta and small mesenteric artery (SMA) segments, prevented contraction elicited by ET-1, and reduced superoxide anion radical ($O_2^-$) production [54]. Furthermore, another study showed that polyphenols in red grape skin and seeds increased endothelial progenitor cells viability, adhesion and migration, and prevented endothelial dysfunction by reducing reactive oxygen species (ROS) production [55]. In addition, red grape components increased the expression of endothelial nitric oxide synthase (eNOS) [56]. In vitro, human umbilical vein endothelial cells (HUVECs) were incubated with GSPEs to explore the signaling pathways of eNOS expression. The result suggested that the increased eNOS expression was attributed to the activation of 5′-AMP activated protein kinase (AMPK) and the increase in sirtuin-1 (SIRT-1) protein level, which was critical for transcription factor Krüpple like factor-2 (KLF-2) induction [57]. In addition, another study indicated that grape pomace extract (GPE) exerted antioxidant activity in endothelium (EA. hy926) through the increase of glutathione (GSH) levels due to increased gamma-glutamylcysteine synthetase (γ-GCS) levels and glutathione S-transferase (GST) activity [58]. Moreover, it was found that a low dose (1 µg/mL) of grape seed extract (GSE) potentiated the inhibitory action of HUVECs on platelet reactivity by about 10%, which accounted, at least partially, for the protective effects of grape products against CVDs. However, a high concentration (up to 10 µg gallic acid equivalent/mL) of GSE impaired endothelial cell proliferation in vitro [59].

3.1.2. Decreasing Blood Lipids

Hyperlipidemia can lead to lipoprotein deposition inside the vessel wall, and induce oxidative stress and the formation of oxidized low-density lipoprotein (Ox-LDL), which plays a key role in the pathogenesis of atherosclerosis. The GSE possesses potent lipid-lowering and antioxidant properties, which are beneficial to the prevention of atherosclerosis [60]. A study showed that plasma triglycerides (TG) were attenuated by red grape consumption [61]. The hypolipidemic effect of grape seed procyanidin extract at low doses was studied in hamsters, and results suggested that 25 mg/kg of the extract decreased body weight, protected against fat accumulation, lowered plasma free fatty acid (FFA), and reduced lipid and TG accumulation in the mesenteric white adipose tissue (MWAT). In addition, the extract exerted these effects in part through the activation of both β-oxidation and the glycerolipid (GL)/FFA cycle, mainly in the retroperitoneal white adipose tissue (RWAT) [62]. High-density lipoproteins (HDL) are responsible for transporting 20–30% of the total plasma cholesterol from tissues to the liver, as vehicles for reversing cholesterol transport, which help prevent or even regress atherosclerosis [63]. A study indicated that grape polyphenols modulated the activity of plasma HDL enzymes in old and obese rats. The result showed that grape polyphenols increased HDL paraoxonase (PON) and lecithin-cholesterol acyltransferase (LCAT) activity, reduced cholesteryl ester transfer protein (CETP) activity, and restored the function of HDL [64].

### 3.1.3. Decreasing Blood Pressure

The hypotensive effect of grape polyphenols has been detected in several studies [52,61]. Administration of GSPE markedly alleviated hypertension-induced arterial remodeling [51]. SHR were used to assess the anti-hypertensive effect of grape seed procyanidin extract. The results showed that the extract significantly decreased systolic and diastolic BP of SHR in a dose-dependent manner, and at the dose of 375 mg/kg, the decrease of both BP reached the maximum value. Moreover, the anti-hypertensive effect of the extract (375 mg/kg) in SHR was quite similar to that of Captopril (50 mg/kg), which has been considered as a very effective anti-hypertensive drug in clinical practice [9]. Another study suggested chronic administration of GSPE significantly blocked the BP increase in ouabain induced hypertensive rats model, and the improvement of the aortic NO production impaired by ouabain was the possible mechanisms involved [57]. Furthermore, a study investigated the anti-hypertensive effect and mechanism of red grape berry powder on rats with metabolic syndrome (MS). The study indicated that grape berry powder lowered BP via its ability of inhibiting ET-1 secretion and increasing eNOS levels of endothelium in a concentration-dependent manner [61].

### 3.1.4. Suppressing Platelets Function

Platelets play a pivotal role in physiological hemostasis. However, enhanced platelets activation, adhesion, and aggregation aggravate the formation of arteriosclerotic plaques. A study in vitro revealed the potential protective effects of GSE on hemostasis under the condition of hyperhomocysteinemia by reducing the toxicity action of homocysteine (Hcy) and its most reactive form homocysteine thiolactone (HTL) in blood. In human platelets incubated with Hcy (100 μM) or HTL (1 μM), GSE decreased platelet adhesion to collagen and fibrinogen, the platelet aggregation, and $O_2^-$ production in platelets [65]. Additionally, a study in vitro indicated that 1 μg/mL GSE reduced platelet reactivity by about 10% due to the direct effect of its polyphenol contents on HUVECs [59].

### 3.1.5. Alleviating Ischemia/Reperfusion Injury

A study investigated the cardio-protective effect of grape extracts rich in malvidin, an anthocyanin isolated from red grape skins, on isolated and Langendorff perfused rat heart. The result showed that malvidin elicited cardio-protective effect against ischemia/reperfusion (I/R) damages by activating the phosphatidylinositol 3-kinase (PI3K)/NO/cyclic guanosine monophosphate (cGMP)/protein kinase-G (PKG) pathway, increasing intracellular cGMP and the phosphorylation of eNOS, PI3K-AKT, extracellular regulated kinase1/2 (ERK1/2), and glycogen synthase kinase-3 β (GSK-3 β) [56]. In addition, grape extracts moderated cardiac and cerebral ischemia damages against I/R, which induced a drastic oxidative stress [56,66]. Moreover, a study investigated the relationship between grape seed and skin extract (GSSE) and ischemic stroke, and results showed that the extract not only reduced brain damage size and histology caused by I/R, but also inhibited oxidative stress, and improved transition metals associated enzyme activities [66]. Reperfusion arrhythmias (RA) are the most important causes of sudden death following reperfusion [67]. Another study analyzed the molecular mechanisms of protective effects of GSPE on RA. The study indicated that GSPE played an essential role in decreasing free radical generation for it increased the activity of $Na^+/K^+$-ATPase due to the upregulation of $Na^+/K^+$-ATPase $\alpha 1$ subunit [67].

### 3.1.6. Inhibiting Thrombosis

The dysfunction of vessel endothelial cells and platelets are major risk factors in the formation of atherosclerotic plaque. For the antithrombotic effect of proanthocyanidins, a study revealed that GSPE decreased the length and weight of thrombus, protected the integrity of endothelium, reduced thrombogenesis-promoting factors P-selectin, von Willebrand factor (vWF), and cellular adhesion molecules (CAMs), increased thrombogenesis-demoting factors CD34, vascular endothelial growth factor receptor-2 (VEGFR-2), and ADAMTS13 (a disintegrin and metalloproteinase with a thrombospondin type one motif, member 13), and downregulated inflammatory cytokines interleukine (IL)-6, IL-8, and tumor necrosis factor-alpha (TNF-α). Thus, GSPE facilitated endothelial protection and inhibited platelet aggregation, inflammatory responses, and thrombus formation [68].

Collectively, the consumption of grapes or products derived from grapes might reduce the incidence of CVDs through correcting endothelial dysfunction, reducing blood lipids, anti-hypertension, inhibiting oxidative stress, improving platelet function, alleviating I/R damages, protecting myocardial function, anti-thrombosis, and resisting inflammation. These effects might be due to several phytochemicals, such as resveratrol, anthocyanin, and proanthocyanidin.

### 3.2. Blueberry

Blueberry is a flavonoid-containing fruit and exerts cardiovascular benefits. The cardioprotective effects of blueberry (*Vaccinium ashei* Reade) extract were investigated in hypercholesterolemic rats for 14 days. The result showed that blueberry extract decreased aortic lesions, reduced serum lipid profiles (total cholesterol (TC), low-density lipoprotein cholesterol (LDL-C), and TG), and increased activities of antioxidant enzymes (CAT, SOD, and glutathione peroxidase (GSH-Px)) [69]. The effects of supplementation with blueberry for 10 weeks on endothelial function and BP were studied in rats fed a high-fat diet. The study showed that blueberry supplementation lowered SBP by 14% and improved endothelial dysfunction and aorta relaxation in response to acetylcholine [70]. Furthermore, a study evaluated the potential protective effects of seven phenolic acids, identified as metabolites of blueberry, on murine macrophage cell line RAW 264.7. The result indicated that phenolic acids decreased foam cell formation induced by Ox-LDL, Ox-LDL binding to macrophages, lipopolysaccharide (LPS)-induced mRNA expression, and protein levels of TNF-α and IL-6 via inhibiting the phosphorylation of mitogen-activated protein kinase (MAPK), Jun N-terminal kinase (JNK), p38, and ERK1/2, downregulated the mRNA expression and protein levels of scavenger receptor CD36, and upregulated the mRNA expression and protein levels of ATP-binding cassette transporter A1 (ABCA1), which facilitated cholesterol efflux and inhibited cholesterol accumulation in macrophages [71].

In conclusion, blueberry possesses commendably cardioprotective ability including anti-atherogenic properties, anti-inflammation, lowering BP, improving oxidative parameters, and vascular reactivity.

### 3.3. Pomegranate

The peel, seed, and juice of pomegranate are rich in antioxidants and have potent atheroprotective effect and antihypertensive properties. The major bioactive constituent of pomegranate is punicalagin, which is known to have cardiovascular protective ability for its antioxidant role as a scavenger and ferrous chelator of hydrogen peroxide [72]. A study found that pomegranate extract (PE) reducing aortic sinus and coronary artery atherosclerosis was associated with the reduced oxidative stress and inflammation in the vessel wall of SR-BI/apoE double KO mice [73]. The high level of oxidative stress in the paraventricular nucleus of the hypothalamus is essential in the pathogenesis of hypertension. A study investigated the antihypertensive properties of PE in a SHR model. The findings demonstrated that PE alleviated hypertension by reducing oxidative stress, increasing the antioxidant defense system, decreasing inflammation, and improving mitochondrial function in the paraventricular nucleus, thereby activating AMPK-nuclear factor-erythroid 2 p45-related factor 2 (Nrf2) pathway [74]. Similarly, the activation of the AMPK pathway by PE was studied in the heart of a rodent obesity model. The result showed that PE activated AMPK by quickly decreasing the cellular ATP/ADP ratio specifically in cardiomyocytes, and the activation of the AMPK pathway accounted for the prevention of mitochondrial loss by enhancing mitochondrial biogenesis and amelioration of oxidative stress via increasing the activity of phase II enzymes in high-fat diet-induced cardiac metabolic disorders [72]. In addition, pomegranate seed extract improved motor and cognitive deficits due to permanent cerebral hypoperfusion ischemia (CHI), which was most likely related at least in some part to its antioxidant and free radical scavenging actions [75].

### 3.4. Apple

Apple is the second most consumed fruit in the world following banana. In recent years, epidemiological studies have shown that eating apples is associated with the reduction of the occurrence of CVDs [30,31]. Apple is a major source of fiber and contains antioxidants such as vitamin C and good dietary polyphenols. Particularly, the reduced incidence of CVDs is related to apple consumption, probably as a result of the cholesterol-lowering effect of polyphenols, the main bioactive compounds of apple, which are concentrated in the fruit peel. The cholesterol-lowering effect of apple was detected in male Wistar rats fed with a cholesterol-enriched diet (2%). The study showed that Bravo de Esmolfe apple was able to decrease serum levels of TG, TC, LDL-C, and Ox-LDL by 27.2%, 21.0%, 20.4%, and 20.0%, respectively. It also indicated that the cholesterol-lowering ability of apple was mainly due to phytocompounds, such as catechin, epicatechin, procyanidin B1, and β-carotene [76]. The development of CVDs is related with the previous existence of MS. Another study suggested that apple peel reduced the biochemical parameters (glycaemia, TC, high-density lipoprotein cholesterol (HDL-C), LDL-C, TG, ureic nitrogen, insulin, and asymmetric dimethylarginine (ADMA)) in CF-1 mice with MS, diminished the cholesterol accumulation area, and reverted the progression of the atherogenesis in apoE$^{-/-}$ mice [77].

### 3.5. Hawthorn

Hawthorn (*Crataegus pinnatifida* Bge.) is a berry-like fruit from the species of *Crataegus*. It has been used as food or a traditional medicine to improve digestion for thousands of years. Moreover, during the last decades, hawthorn has received more attention because of its potential to treat CVDs, especially hyperlipidemia and atherosclerosis [78]. A study investigated the hypolipidemic effect of hawthorn fruit compounds (HFC, including hawthorn and kiwi fruit extract) in apoE$^{-/-}$ atherosclerotic mice with high blood lipid levels. The study indicated that HFC reduced TG and LDL-C/TC ratio. Moreover, the reduction of LDL-C was more evident in HFC than in Simvastatin (6 mg/kg/day), indicating HFC could be considered for the treatment of hyperlipidemia and the prevention of atherosclerosis [10]. Similarly, hawthorn pectin pentaoligosaccharide (HPPS) suppressed weight gain, decreased serum TG levels, increased lipid excretion in feces, upregulated the gene and protein expressions of peroxisome proliferator-activated receptor α (PPAR-a), and enhanced the hepatic fatty acid oxidation-related enzyme activities of acyl-CoA oxidase, carnitine palmitoyltransferase I, 3-ketoacyl-CoA thiolase, and 2,4-dienoyl-CoA reductase by 53.8%, 74.2%, 47.1%, and 24.2%, respectively, in the liver of hyperlipidemic mice [79]. The anti-atherosclerosis effect of hawthorn and the potential mechanisms were investigated in apoE$^{-/-}$ mice. The result showed that hawthorn decreased atherosclerotic lesions, serum TC and TG level, reduced the hepatic fatty acid synthase (FAS) and sterol regulatory element binding protein-1c (SREBP-1c) mRNA levels by 42% and 23%, and increased total antioxidant capacity (T-AOC), SOD and GSH-Px activities, and the mRNA expression levels of the antioxidant enzymes

SOD1, SOD2, glutathione peroxidase-3 (Gpx3) in the livers of mice fed with hawthorn fruit diet [80]. Another study indicated that aqueous extract of hawthorn (*Crataegus pinnatifida* var. Major) inhibited atherosclerosis progression in high-fat-diet-fed rats by improving lipid metabolism, decreasing inflammatory cytokine responses, and protecting endothelium. The result showed that aqueous extract of hawthorn inhibited artery lesion, decreased IMT, reduced TC, TG, LDL-C, and the levels of CRP, IL-1β, IL-8, and IL-18, increased HDL-C, ET, 6-keto-prostaglandin F1α (6-keto-PGF1α), and thromboxane B2 (TXB2). It also revealed that chlorogenic acid, procyanidin B2, (−)-epicatechin, rutin, and isoquercitrin were the main components of the extract [81].

### 3.6. Avocado

Avocado is an essential tropical fruit containing lipophilic compounds, i.e., monounsaturated fatty acids (MUFAs), polyphenols, carotenoids, vitamin E, phytosterols, and squalene, which have been recognized for cholesterol-lowering ability [82]. However, the antioxidant capacities of these lipophilic compounds have attracted far less attention compared with hydrophilic compounds in the fruit. In fact, the lipophilic extract of the fruit had higher antioxidant capacity than its hydrophilic extract [83]. A study indicated that avocado pulp, containing acetogenin compounds, inhibited platelet aggregation with a potential preventive effect on thrombus formation [84]. Moreover, avocado pulp contains variable oil contents and is widely used in many fields such as the pharmaceutical industry [82]. Another study evaluated the effects of avocado oil administration on inflammatory and lipid parameters in rats with metabolic changes induced by sucrose ingestion. The study demonstrated that avocado oil reduced hs-CRP and TG, very low-density lipoprotein (VLDL), and LDL levels [85]. In addition, the protective effects of dietary consuming avocado oil on biochemical markers of liver function in rats fed with sucrose were quite similar to olive oil [86]. Furthermore, a study has shown that avocado seeds improved hypercholesterolemia, and facilitated the prevention and treatment of hypertension, inflammatory conditions, and diabetes [87].

### 3.7. Other Fruits

Mango is rich in several bioactive components with antioxidant and anti-inflammatory properties, such as carotenoids, vitamin C, and phenolic compounds. A study demonstrated that two doses (1% and 10%) of freeze-dried mango pulp were effective in improving glucose tolerance and lipid profiles and reducing adiposity in mice fed with a high-fat diet. Additionally, the study also reported that the lower dose (1%) was more effective in modulating glucose than the higher dose (10%), and was more powerful in lowering blood glucose concentration than the hypoglycemic drug, rosiglitazone (50 mg/kg diet), in mice fed with a high-fat diet [11]. Moreover, the anti-hypertensive effects of the standardized methanolic extract of papaya (*Carica papaya*) were evaluated in SHR. The result showed that the angiotensin converting enzyme inhibitory effects of papaya (100 mg/kg) were similar to those of enalapril (10 mg/kg). The flavonoids, especially quercetin, rutin, nicotiflorin, clitorin, and manghaslin, were identified as bioactive components of the extract, which could be applied to the treatment of hypertension [12]. In addition, several studies revealed that cherry, Guangzao (*Choerospondias axillaris*), and acai (*Euterpe oleracea* Mart.) have significant cardioprotective effects and have been shown to play a beneficial role in improving myocardial infarction induced by I/R via anti-oxidative and anti-apoptotic activities [88–90]. In addition, bilberry, black raspberry, and sea buckthorn berries improved serum lipid profiles and promoted a hypocholesterolemic effect, which protected against hypercholesterolemia and prevented atherosclerosis [91–93]. Additionally, jujube (*Ziziphus jujuba*) and blackberry (*Rubus allegheniensis* Port.) inhibited foam cell formation in human monocyte-derived macrophages induced by acetylated LDL, which therefore were useful for the prevention of atherosclerosis [94,95]. In addition, yellow passion fruit and boysenberry decreased BP in SHR [96,97]. However, data on these individual fruits is still limited. Furthermore, the underlying mechanisms of protecting cardiovascular system remain to be investigated.

**Table 2.** The cardioprotective abilities of fruits.

| Fruit | Subject | Study Type | Dose | Main Effects | References |
|---|---|---|---|---|---|
| | | | **Grape** | | |
| freeze-dried grape powder | SHR and Wistar-Kyoto (WKY) rats | in vivo | 600 mg/day | BP↓, arterial relaxation↑, vascular compliance↑, cardiac hypertrophy↓ | [51] |
| GSPE | SHR | in vivo | 250 mg/kg/day | arterial remodeling↓, ET-1↓, NO↑, SOD↑, CAT↑, MDA↓ | [52] |
| oligomeric grape seed proanthocyanidins (GSPs) | mice treated with DOCA-salt to induce cardiovascular remodeling | in vivo | NA | heart weight/body weight ratio↓, kidney weight/body weight ratio↓, cross-sectional area of cardiomyocytes↓, collagen deposition in heart↓, histopathology injury↓, NO↑, SOD↑, MDA↓ | [53] |
| | isolated thoracic aorta ring | in vitro | | endothelial-dependent aorta ring relaxation↑ | |
| GP-EE | rat aorta and small mesenteric artery (SMA) segments | in vitro | 0.3 and 10 μM | endothelium- and NO-dependent vasodilatation↑, phenylephrine(Phe)-induced response in aortic rings↓, $O_2^-$↓, contraction elicited by ET-1↓ | [54] |
| red grape skin and seeds polyphenols | human endothelial progenitor cells (EPC) | in vitro | 5, 50 and 150 μg/mL | EPC viability and function↑, endothelial dysfunction↓, hyperglycemia effect↓, ROS production↓ | [55] |
| GSPE | ouabain induced hypertensive rats model | in vivo | 250 mg/kg/day | BP↓, aortic NO production↑ | [57] |
| GPE | endothelial (EA. hy926) cells | in vitro | 0.068 and 0.250 μg/mL | GCS levels↑, GST activity↑, antioxidant activity↑ | [58] |
| GSE | HUVECs | in vitro | 1 μg/mL | platelet reactivity↓ | [59] |
| red grape berry powder | rats with metabolic syndrome | in vivo | 200, 400 and 800 mg/kg/day | BP↓, plasma TG↓, insulin↓ | [61] |
| | HUVECs | in vitro | 20–1400 μg/mL | ET-1↓ | |
| | HUVECs | in vitro | 0.011, 0.058, 0.29, 1.46 and 3.66 mg/mL | eNOS level↑ | |
| grape seed procyanidin extract | hamster | in vivo | 25 mg/kg/day | body weight gain↓, adiposity index↓, weight of white adipose tissue depots↓, plasma phospholipids↓, plasma FFA↓, mesenteric lipid and triglyceride accumulation↓ | [62] |
| grape polyphenols from *Vitis vinifera* grapes | 24-month-old obese rats | in vivo | 90 mg/kg/day | plasma HDL PON activity↑, LCAT activity↑, CETP activity↑ | [64] |
| grape seed procyanidin extract | SHR | in vivo | 375 mg/kg | SBP↓, DBP↓, GSH activity↑ | [9] |
| GSE or black chokeberry (*Aronia melanocarpa*) extract | human platelets incubated with Hcy (100 μM) or HTL (1 μM) | in vitro | 2.5, 5, 10 μg/mL | platelet adhesion to collagen and fibrinogen↓, platelet aggregation↓, $O_2^{\bullet-}$ production in platelet↓ | [65] |
| malvidin-rich red grape skin extract | isolated and Langendorff perfused rat heart | in vitro | 1–1000 ng/mL | I/R damages↓, coronary dilation↑, active PI3K/NO/cGMP/PKG pathway, intracellular cGMP↑, eNOS, PI3K-AKT, ERK1/2, and GSK-3 β phosphorylation↑ | [56] |
| GSSE | a rat model of global ischemia | in vivo | 2.5 g/kg | brain damage size and histology↓, oxidative stress↓, transition metals associated enzyme activities↑ | [66] |
| GSPE | isolated rat hearts | in vitro | NA | RA↓, $Na^+/K^+$-ATPase activity↑, $Na^+/K^+$-ATPase α1 subunit↓, free radical↓ | [67] |
| GSPE | a rat model of deep vein thrombosis (DVT) | in vivo | 400 mg/kg/day | thrombus length and weight↓, protecte endothelium integrity, IL-6, IL-8 and TNF-α↓ | [68] |

**Table 2.** *Cont.*

| Fruit | Subject | Study Type | Dose | Main Effects | References |
|---|---|---|---|---|---|
| | | | **Blueberry** | | |
| blueberry extract (*Vaccinium ashei* Reade) | hypercholesterolemic rat | in vivo | 25, 50 mg/kg | aortic lesions↓, oxidative damage to lipids and proteins↓, TC↓, LDL-C↓, TG↓, activity of CAT, SOD and GSH-Px↑ | [69] |
| freeze-dried blueberry powder | rats fed a high-fat/cholesterol diet | in vivo | 2% (w/w) | SBP↓, aorta relaxation↑, endothelial dysfunction↓ | [70] |
| 7 phenolic acids of freeze-dried blueberry | murine macrophage cell line RAW 264.7 | in vitro | NA | TNF-α and IL-6 mRNA expression and protein levels↓, MAPK, JNK, p38, and Erk1/2 phosphorylation↓, mRNA expression and protein levels of scavenger receptor CD36↓, foam cell formation↓, expression and protein levels of ABCA1↑ | [71] |
| | | | **Pomegranate** | | |
| PE | SR-BI/apoE double KO mice | in vivo | 307.5 μL/L in water | aortic sinus and coronary artery atherosclerosis↓, oxidative stress and inflammation in the vessel wall↓ | [73] |
| PE containing 40% punicalagin | SHR | in vivo | 150 mg/kg/day | BP↓, cardiac hypertrophy↓, oxidative stress↓, antioxidant defense system↑, paraventricular nucleus inflammation↓, mitochondrial superoxide anion levels↓, mitochondrial function↑ | [74] |
| PE containing 40% punicalagin | heart of a high-fat diet-induced obesity rat model | in vivo | 150 mg/kg/day | mitochondrial biogenesis↑, oxidative stress↓, phase II enzymes↑, cardiac metabolic disorders↓ | [72] |
| pomegranate seed extract | CHI rat model | in vivo | 100, 200, 400, 800 mg/kg/day | motor and cognitive coordination↑ | [75] |
| | | | **Apple** | | |
| Bravo de Esmolfe apple | male Wistar rats fed a cholesterol-enriched diet (+2% cholesterol) | in vivo | 20% (w/w) = 5g/rat/day (~2–3 apples/person/day) for 30 days | serum TG↓, TC↓, LDL-C↓, oxLDL↓ | [76] |
| Fuji apple peel Granny Smith apple peel | CF-1 mice with MS apoE−/− mice | in vivo | 20% (w/w) for 43 days 20% (w/w) for 10 weeks | glycaemia↓, TC↓, HDL-C↓, LDL-C↓, ureic nitrogen↓, TG↓, insulin↓, ADMA↓, atherogenic progression↓, cholesterol accumulation area↓ | [77] |
| HPC | apoE−/− atherosclerotic mice with high blood lipid levels fed with a high cholesterol diet | in vivo | 0.5 mL/day | TG↓, LDL-C/TC ratio↓ | [10] |
| HPPS | the liver of high fat diet induced hyperlipidemic mice | in vivo | 150 mg/kg | weight gain↓, TG↓, lipid excretion in feces↑, mRNAs and activities of acyl-CoA oxidase, carnitine palmitoyltransferase I, 3-ketoacyl-CoA thiolase, and 2,4-dienoyl-CoA reductase↑, gene and protein expressions of PPAR-α↑ | [79] |
| | | | **Hawthorn** | | |
| freeze-dried hawthorn fruit (*Crataegus pinnatifida*) | apoE−/− mice | in vivo | 1% (w/w) | atherosclerotic lesions↓, TC↓, TG↓, T-AOC values↑, SOD and GSH-Px activities↑, hepatic FAS and SREBP-1c mRNA levels↓, hepatic SOD1, SOD2, Gpx3 mRNA levels↑ | [80] |
| sugar-free aqueous extract of hawthorn fruit (*Crataegus pinnatifida* var. Major) | high fat diet fed rats | in vivo | 72 and 288 mg/kg/day | TC, TG and LDL-C↓, HDL-C↑, CRP, IL-1β, IL-8 and IL-18↓, ET, 6-keto-PGF1α and TXB2↑, pathological changes in the arteries↓, IMT↓ | [81] |

**Table 2.** *Cont.*

| Fruit | Subject | Study Type | Dose | Main Effects | References |
|---|---|---|---|---|---|
| **Avocado** | | | | | |
| avocado pulp (*Persea americana*) extract | male adult CD 1 mice | in vivo | 25 mg/kg | thrombus formation↓ | [34] |
| | platelet | in vitro | 10 µL | platelet aggregation↓ | |
| avocado oil | rats ingested with sucrose | in vivo | 7.5% (*w/w*) | TG↓, VLDL↓, LDL↓, hs-CRP↓ | [35] |
| **Others** | | | | | |
| freeze-dried mango pulp | male C57BL/6J mice fed a high-fat diet | in vivo | 1% or 10% (*w/w*) | epididymal fat mass↓, percentage of body fat↓, improve glucose tolerance, insulin resistance↓ | [11] |
| methanolic extract of papaya (*Carica papaya*) | SHR | in vivo | 100 mg/kg (twice a day) | BP↓, angiotensin converting enzyme(ACE) activity↓, cardiac hypertrophy↓, improve baroreflex sensitivity | [12] |
| sour cherry seed kernel extract | hearts from Sprague-Dawley rats | in vitro | 30 mg/kg/day | post ischemic cardiac functions↑, infarct size↓, heme oxygenase-1 (HO-1)↑, Bcl-2↑ | [88] |
| total flavonoids of Guangzao (*Choerospondias axillaris*) | I/R male Sprague-Dawley rats | in vivo | 75, 150 and 300 mg/kg/day | cardiac function↑, heart pathologic lesion↓, CAT↑, GSH-Px↑, SOD↑, MDA↓, TUNEL-positive nuclear staining↓, Bcl-2-associated X protein (Bax)↓, caspase-3↓, Bcl-2↑, p38 MAPK activity↓, JNK activity↓ | [89] |
| hydroalcoholic extract of acai (*Euterpe oleracea* Mart.) seeds | male Wistar rats subjected to myocardial infarction | in vivo | 100 mg/kg/day | prevent the development of exercise intolerance, cardiac hypertrophy, fibrosis, and dysfunction | [90] |
| acai pulp | female Fischer rat of dietary-induced hypercholesterolemia | in vivo | 2% (*w/w*) | TC↓, LDL-C↓, atherogenic index↓, HDL-C↑, cholesterol excretion in feces↑, expression of the LDL-R, ABCG5, and ABCG8 genes↑ | [98] |
| bilberry (*Vaccinium myrtillus* L.) anthocyanin-rich extract | apoE$^{-/-}$ mice | in vivo | 0.02% (*w/w*) | improve hypercholesterolemia against atherosclerosis | [91] |
| unrefined black raspberry seed oils | male Syrian hamsters fed high-cholesterol (0.12%), high-fat (9%) diets | in vivo | NA | plasma and liver TG↓, hypertriglyceridemia↓ | [92] |
| polyphenols from sea buckthorn berry | rats with hyperlipidemia | in vivo | 7–28 mg/kg | serum lipids↓, TNF-α↓, IL-6↓, antioxidant enzymes activity↑, eNOS, ICAM-1, and LOX-1 mRNA expression and proteins in aortas↓ | [93] |
| Jujube (*Zizyphus jujuba*) fructus and semen extract | human macrophages | in vitro | NA | the foam cell formation induced by acetylated LDL↓, prevent atherosclerosis | [94] |
| methanol extract of blackberry (*Rubus allegheniensis* Port.) | human monocyte-derived macrophages induced by acetylated LDL | in vitro | 50 µM | foam cell formation↓ | [95] |
| yellow passion fruit pulp | SHR | in vivo | 5, 6 or 8 g/kg/day | SBP↓, GSH↑, thiobarbituric acid-reactive substances (TBARS)↓ | [96] |
| proanthocyanidins in boysenberry seed extract | SHR | in vivo | 100 and 200 mg/kg | SBP↓ | [97] |
| | rat aorta rings | in vitro | | vasorelaxant activity↑ | |
| methanolic extract of date palm (*Phoenix dactylifera* L.) | cerebral ischemia rats | in vivo | 100, 300 mg/kg | SOD↑, CAT↑, GSH↑, glutathione reductase↑, lipid peroxidation↓, oxidative stress↓, neuronal damage↓ | [99] |
| black chokeberry (*Aronia melanocarpa*) extract | bovine coronary artery endothelial cells | in vitro | 0.1 g/mL | NO↑, eNOS phosphorylation↑ | [100] |

**Table 2.** *Cont.*

| Fruit | Subject | Study Type | Dose | Main Effects | References |
|---|---|---|---|---|---|
| saskatoon berry powder | leptin receptor-deficient diabetic mice | in vivo | 5% (w/w) | monocyte adhesion to aorta↓, inflammatory, fibrinolytic or stress regulators in aorta or heart apex↓ | [101] |
| saskatoon berry powder | leptin receptor-deficient diabetic mice | in vivo | 5% (w/w) | endoplasmic reticulum stress (ERS)↓, unfolded protein response (UPR)↓ | [102] |
| | glycated LDL-treated HUVECs | in vitro | | | |
| 19 fruits widely consumed in central Chile | NA | in vitro | 1 mg/mL | anticoagulant activities: grape, raspberry fibrinolytic activity: raspberry | [103] |
| peach (*Prunus persica*) pulp ethylacetate extract | cultured vascular smooth muscle cells (VSMCs) | in vitro | 50, 100, or 200 µg/mL | Angiotensin II (Ang II) induced intracellular $Ca^{2+}$ elevation↓, generation of ROS↓ | [104] |
| methanolic extract of Lingonberry (*Vaccinium vitis-idaea* L.) | H9c2 rat myoblasts simulated IR | in vitro | 5 and 10 µM | apoptosis↓, markers of nuclei condensation, caspase-3 activation, and MAPK signaling↓ | [105] |
| blueberry anthocyanin fraction (BBA), blackberry anthocyanin fraction (BKA), and blackcurrant anthocyanin fraction (BCA) | RAW 264.7 macrophages treated by LPS bone marrow–derived macrophages from $Nrf2^{+/+}$ mice treated by LPS | in vitro | 0–20 µg/mL | IL-1 β mRNA levels↓, NF-κB p65 translocation to the nucleus↓, cellular ROS levels↓, IL-1β mRNA levels↓ | [106] |
| pomegranate juice, together with date fruit and date seeds extract | $apoE^{-/-}$ mice | in vivo | 0.5 µM gallic acid equivalents (GAE)/day | TC↓, TG↓, PON1 activity↑, mouse peritoneal macrophage (MPM) oxidative stress↓, MPM cholesterol content↓, and MPM LDL uptake↓, aortas lipid peroxide content↓, aortas PON lactonase activity↑ | [107] |

NA, stands for not available.

In conclusion, fruits such as grape, blueberry, pomegranate, apple, hawthorn, and avocado showed protective effects on cardiovascular function. Grape products markedly alleviated hypertension-induced cardiovascular remodeling and impaired endothelial function. Most fruits were effective in reducing oxidative stress, regulating lipids metabolism, and modulating BP. Additionally, some fruits attenuated platelet function, alleviated I/R injury, suppressed thrombosis, and inhibited inflammation (Figure 1).

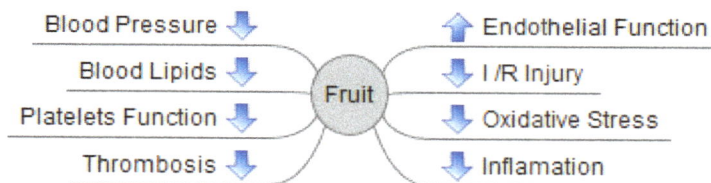

| Blood Pressure ⬇ | | Endothelial Function ⬆ |
| Blood Lipids ⬇ | Fruit | I /R Injury ⬇ |
| Platelets Function ⬇ | | Oxidative Stress ⬇ |
| Thrombosis ⬇ | | Inflamation ⬇ |

**Figure 1.** Effects and mechanisms of fruits on cardiovascular diseases (CVDs).

## 4. Clinical Trials

The anti-hypertensive effect of grape polyphenols in several randomized controlled trials (RCTs) was evaluated by a meta-analysis, and results showed that daily grape polyphenols intake significantly reduced SBP by 1.48 mmHg when compared with control subjects ($p = 0.03$). Contrarily, DBP was not significantly decreased [108]. Grapes have potent hypolipidemic and anti-oxidative effects. Several studies showed that grape reduced TC, LDL-C, and Ox-LDL and increased HDL-C in subjects with various risk factors of CVDs [60,109,110]. Additionally, a study conducted on 60 healthy volunteers indicated that supplying them with 700 mg polyphenol-rich grape extracts for 56 days modulated the lipid profiles in terms of cardiovascular risk indicators, lowered TC and LDL-C, and increased antioxidant capacity and vitamin E [111]. Moreover, a meta-analysis of 9 RCTs explored the endothelium protective effect of grape polyphenols supplementation in adults. The study suggested that consuming grape polyphenols improved endothelial function in healthy subjects, and the effect was more obvious in subjects with high cardiovascular risk factors [112]. Besides grapes, other berries such as strawberry, acai (*Euterpe oleracea* Mart.), Caucasian whortleberry (*Vaccinium arctostaphylos* L.), sea buckthorn, and bilberry also have a potent lipid-lowering effect [113–121]. The benefits of berries on the serum lipid metabolism might contribute to anthocyanin. The effects of berry-derived anthocyanin supplements on the serum lipid profiles were studied in 120 dyslipidemic patients. The results suggested that anthocyanin intake increased HDL-C and cellular cholesterol efflux to serum, and decreased LDL-C, possibly due to the inhibition of CETP [122].

A clinical trial evaluated the cardiovascular protective effects of consumption of 75 g (about two medium-sized apples) of dried apple for 1 year in 146 postmenopausal women. The study showed that dried apple significantly lowered serum levels of TC and LDL-Cl by 9% and 16%, respectively, at 3 months and further decreased by 13% and 24%, respectively, at 6 months, but stayed constant thereafter. Furthermore, consumption of dried apple also reduced lipid hydroperoxide and CRP [123]. In addition, a study compared the cholesterol-lowering effect of 5 different apple species, Red Delicious, Granny Smith, Fuji, Golden Delicious and Annurca apple, in mildly hypercholesterolaemic healthy subjects. The study detected that Annurca apples led to the most significant outcome, reduced TC and LDL-C levels by 8.3% and 14.5%, respectively, and an increased HDL-C level by 15.2% (all $p < 0.001$) [124]. Moreover, another study compared the effects of whole fresh apple and processed apple products (apple pomace, cloudy apple juice, or clear apple juice) on lipid profiles in healthy volunteers. The result showed that whole apple, pomace, and cloudy juice lowered serum TC and LDL-C; however, clear apple juice increased TC and LDL-C slightly, from which it could be concluded that the fiber component was necessary for the lipid-lowering effect of apple in healthy humans [125].

Additionally, the acute effects of apple on improving endothelial function were studied in some trials, showing that apple improved endothelial function by affecting NO metabolites [126,127].

Kiwifruit is a good source of antioxidants due to its wealth in vitamins C and E, folate, carotenoids, and phytochemicals and protects the body from endogenous oxidative damage [128]. A clinical trial conducted on 85 hypercholesterolemic men showed that consuming two green kiwifruits daily in conjunction with a healthy diet reduced inflammatory markers and lipid profiles in subjects with modestly elevated CRP [129], but there were no significant differences in BP [130]. In addition, a study of 43 subjects who had hyperlipidemia indicated that regular consumption of kiwifruit not only modulated lipids profiles but also exerted beneficial effects on the antioxidant status via decreasing LDL oxidation and oxidative stress [131]. Moreover, another study conducted on 118 subjects with moderately elevated BP or stage 1 hypertension (SBP: 130–159 mmHg, DBP: 85–99 mmHg) showed that mean 24 h ambulatory systolic/diastolic BP was lower in the group consuming three kiwifruits versus the group consuming one apple daily [132]. The hypotensive effect of kiwifruit, to some extent, was more notable in individuals with moderately elevated BP. Furthermore, the beneficial effects of consuming three kiwifruits per day on BP and platelet aggregation were studied in male smokers. The resulted showed that kiwifruits reduced the SBP and DBP by 10 mmHg ($p = 0.019$) and 9 mmHg ($p = 0.016$), respectively, decreased platelet aggregation by 15% ($p = 0.009$), and lowered ACE activity by 11% ($p = 0.034$) [133].

Avocados are a nutrient-dense source of MUFAs that can be used to replace saturated fatty acids (SFA) in a diet to lower LDL-C. A meta-analysis of 10 RCTs assessing the impacts of avocados on TC, LDL-C, HDL-C, and TG revealed that avocado decreased TC, LDL-C, and TG levels by 18.80 mg/dL, 16.50 mg/dL, and 27.20 mg/dL, respectively [134].

Finally, results from clinical trials are summarized in Table 3. Numerous clinical trials have demonstrated that grape, apple, kiwifruit, and avocado were potential candidates for cardiovascular protection due to their potent lipid-lowering efficiency. However, clinical studies on other fruits are relatively few, and more research is needed to investigate the potential in combating CVDs.

**Table 3.** Clinical trials of fruits against CVDs.

| Subject | Component | Treatment | Duration | Outcome | References |
|---|---|---|---|---|---|
| 152 patients with type 2 diabetes | low glycaemic index fruit | ~3.1 to 2.7 servings/day | 6 months | HbA1c↓, SBP↓, CHD risk↓ | [135] |
| 52 patients with mild hyperlipidemia | red grape seed extract (RGSE) | 200 mg/day | 8 weeks | TC↓, LDL-C↓, Ox-LDL↓ | [60] |
| 24 pre-hypertensive, overweight, and/or pre-diabetic subjects | whole grape extract (WGE) | 350 mg/day | 6 weeks | SOD↓, 8-isoprostane↓, Ox-LDL↓, TC/HDL-C ratios↓, HDL-C↑ | [109] |
| 69 patients with hyperlipidemia | Condori red grapes or Shahroodi white grapes | 500 g/day | 8 weeks | thiobarbituric acid reactive substances (TBARS)↓, total antioxidant capacity (TAC)↑, TC↓, LDL-C↓ | [110] |
| 60 healthy volunteers | polyphenol-rich grape extract supplementation | 700 mg/day | 56 days | TC↓, LDL-C↑, TAC↑, vitamin E↑ | [111] |
| 96 women aged 40–60 years who had at least one menopausal symptom | grape seed extract tablets | =100 or 200 mg proanthocyanidin/day | 4 weeks | SBP↓, DBP↓ | [136] |
| 70 untreated subjects with pre- and stage I hypertension (SBP: 120–159 mmHg) | grape seed extract (GSE) rich in low-molecular-weight polyphenolic compounds | 300 mg/day | 8 weeks | BP values were modestly, but not significantly, affected | [137] |
| 75 patients at high risk of CVD (with diabetes or hypercholesterolemia plus ≥1 other CV risk factor) and undergoing primary prevention of CVDs | resveratrol-rich grape supplementation | 350 mg/day = 8 mg resveratrol for the first 6 months and a double dose for the next 6 months | 12 months | hs-CRP↓, TNF-á↓, plasminogen activator inhibitor type 1 (PAI-1)↓, IL-6/IL-10 ratio↓, IL-10↑ | [138] |
| 75 stable patients with CHD treated according to currently accepted guidelines for secondary prevention of CVDs | resveratrol-rich grape supplementation | 350 mg/day = 8 mg resveratrol for the first 6 months and a double dose for the next 6 months | 12 months | serum adiponectin↑, PAI-1↓, inflammatory genes in peripheral blood mononuclear cells (PBMCs) | [139] |
| 48 participants with MS (4 men, 44 women; BMI: 37.8 ± 2.3 kg/m², age: 50.0 ± 3.0 years) | freeze-dried blueberry | 50 g (~350 g fresh)/day | 8 weeks | SBP↓, DBP↓, Ox-LDL↓, MDA↓, serum hydroxynonenal↓ | [140] |
| 58 postmenopausal women with pre-andstage 1-hypertension | freeze-dried blueberry powder | 22 g/day | 8 weeks | SBP↓, DBP↓, brachial-ankle pulse wave velocity↓, NO↑ | [141] |
| 25 sedentary men and postmenopausal women (age: 18–50 years) | whole blueberry powder | ~250 g berries/day | 6 weeks | natural killer(NK) cells↑, augmentation index (AIx)↓, aortic systolic pressures (ASPs)↓, diastolic pressures↓ | [142] |
| 18 male volunteers (age: 47.8 ± 9.7 years; BMI: 24.8 ± 2.6 kg/m²) | freeze-dried wild blueberries (*Vaccinium angustifolium*) powder | 25 g = 375 mg anthocyanins | 6 weeks | endogenously oxidized DNA bases↓, H₂O₂-induced DNA damage↓ | [143] |
| 23 healthy subjects (11 men, 12 women; age: 27 ± 3.2 years; weight: 63.5 ± 12.7 kg; BMI: 21.74 ± 2.5 kg/m²) | strawberries | 500 g/day | 1 month | TC↓, LDL-C↓, TG↓, MDA↓, urinary 8-OHdG↓, isoprostanes↓, TAC↑, spontaneous and oxidative hemolysis↓, activated platelets↓ | [113] |
| 60 volunteers (5 men, 55 women; age: 49 ± 10 years; BMI: 36 ± 5 kg/m²) | freeze-dried strawberries (FDS) | 25 or 50 g/day | 12 weeks | TC↓, LDL-C↓, MDA↓ | [114] |
| 27 subjects with MS (2 men, 25 women; age: 47.0 ± 3.0 years; BMI: 37.5 ± 2.15 kg/m²) | FDS | 50g (~3 cups fresh)/day | 8 weeks | TC↓, LDL-C↓, small LDL particles↓, vascular cell adhesion molecule-1(VCAM-1)↓ | [115] |

**Table 3.** *Cont.*

| Subject | Component | Treatment | Duration | Outcome | References |
|---|---|---|---|---|---|
| 36 subjects with type 2 diabetes (13 men, 23 women; age: 51.57 ± 10 years; BMI: 27.90 ± 3.7 kg/m²) | FDS | 50 g (~500 g fresh)/day | 6 weeks | CRP↓, MDA↓, HbA1c↓, TAC↑ | [144] |
| 24 overweight and obese subjects (10 men, 14 women; age: 50.9 ± 15 years; BMI: 29.2 ± 2.3 kg/m²) consumed high carbohydrate/fat meal | strawberry (Fragaria) beverage | =10 g FDS (~100 g fresh)/day | 6 weeks | TG↓, Ox-LDL↓, PAI-1↓, IL-1 β↓ | [116,117] |
| 10 overweight adults (BMI: 25–30 kg/m²) | acai pulp (*Euterpe oleracea* Mart.) | 100 g twice/day | 1 month | fasting glucose↓, postprandial plasma glucose↓, insulin↓, TC↓, LDL-C↓, TC/HDL-C ratio↓ | [118] |
| 23 healthy male volunteers (age: 30–65 years; BMI: 25–30 kg/m²) | acai-based smoothie | =694 mg total phenolics | 1 d | flow-mediated dilatation (FMD)↑ | [145] |
| 72 dyslipidemic patients | blackberry (*Morus nigra* L.) juice with pulp | 300 mL/day | 8 weeks | apo A-1↑, HDL↑, apo B↓, hs-CRP↓, SBP↓ | [146] |
| 40 hyperlipidemic patients (age: 20–60 years) | Caucasian whortleberry (*Vaccinium arctostaphylos* L.) fruit hydroalcoholic extract | 350 mg/8 h | 2 months | TC↓, TG↓, LDL-C↓, HDL-C↑ | [119] |
| 80 overweight and obese female volunteers (BMI: 29.6 ± 2.1 kg/m²) | sea buckthorn berries (SB), sea buckthorn oil (SBo), SB phenolic extract (SBe), bilberries (BB) | ~100 g/day fresh berries | 33–35 days | SB: TG and VLDL↓, waist circumference↓; SBo: total lipoprotein, intermediate-density lipoprotein (IDL), LDL and LDL-C↓, vascular cell adhesion molecule (VCAM)↓; SBe: VLDL fractions and serum TG↑, intercellular adhesion molecule (ICAM)↓; BB: improve serum lipids and lipoproteins, waist circumference↓, body weight↓, VCAM↓ | [120,121] |
| 120 dyslipidemic subjects (age: 40–65 years) | berry-derived anthocyanin | 160 mg twice/day | 12 weeks | LDL-C↓, HDL-C↑; cellular cholesterol efflux to serum↑, mass and activity of plasma CETP↓ | [122] |
| 160 postmenopausal women | dried apple | 75 g/day | 1 year | TC↓, LDL-C↓, lipid hydroperoxide↓, CRP↓ | [123] |
| 50 mildly hypercholesterolaemic healthy subjects (28 men, 22 women) | Annurca apple (*Malus pumila* Miller cv. Annurca) | 2/day | 4 months | TC↓, LDL-C↓, HDL-C↑ | [124] |
| 23 healthy volunteers | whole apples, apple pomace, clear apple juices, cloudy apple juices | 550 g/day, 22 g/day, 500 mL/day, 500 mL/day | 4 weeks | whole apple, pomace and cloudy juice lowered serum TC and LDL-C | [125] |

*Nutrients* **2017**, *9*, 598

**Table 3.** *Cont.*

| Subject | Component | Treatment | Duration | Outcome | References |
|---|---|---|---|---|---|
| 51 healthy adults (age: 40–60 years) | apple | 1/day | 4 weeks | Ox-LDL/$\beta_2$-glycoprotein I complex (Ox-LDL-$\beta_2$ GPI)↓ | [147] |
| 20 subjects (age: 21–29 years) | apple juice | two glasses (2 × 250 mL/day) | 4 weeks | plasma antioxidant activity (FRAP)↑, insulin↑, HOMA↑, total GSH↓ | [148] |
| 30 healthy subjects (6 men, 24 women; age: 47.3 ± 13.6 years) | flavonoid-rich apple | 120 g flesh + 80 g skin twice/day | 1 d | NO status↑, endothelial function↑, FMD↑, pulse pressure↓, SBP↓ | [126] |
| 14 subjects (age: 45–70 years) | drink containing epicatechin from an apple extract | ≈140 mg epicatechin/day | 1 d | NO metabolites | [127] |
| 30 hypercholesterolemic volunteers | polyphenol-rich apple | 40 g = 1.43 polyphenols/day | 4 weeks | did not improve vascular function | [149] |
| 85 hypercholesterolemic men consumed a healthy diet | green kiwifruit | 2/day | 8 weeks | plasma HDL-C↑, TC/HDL-C ratio↓, hs-CRP↓, IL-6↓ | [129] |
| | | | | did not improve BP and markers of cardiovascular function | [130] |
| 43 subjects who had hyperlipidemia in Taiwan (13 men, 30 women) | kiwifruit | 2/day | 8 weeks | HDL-C↑, LDL-C/HDL-C ratio↓, TC/HDL-C ratio↓, vitamin E↑, LDL oxidation↓, MDA↓, 4-hydroxy-2-nonenal↓ | [131] |
| 118 subjects with moderately elevated BP or stage 1 hypertension (SBP: 130–159 mmHg, DBP: 85–99 mmHg) | kiwifruit | 3/day | 8 weeks | 24-h ambulatory BP↓ | [132] |
| 102 male smokers (age: 44–74 years) | kiwifruit | 3/day | 8 weeks | SBP↓, DBP↓, platelet aggregation↓, ACE activity↓ | [133] |
| 45 overweight or obese participants with baseline LDL-C in the 25–90% | fresh Hass avocado | 1(≈36 g)/day | 5 weeks | LDL-C↓, LDL-particle number↓, small dense LDL-C↓, LDL-C/HDL-C ratio↓ | [150] |
| 74 overweight adults | fresh Rio-Red grapefruit | 0.5 with each meal (3x)/day | 6 weeks | waist circumference↓, SBP↓, TC↓, LDL↓ | [151] |
| 12 obese postmenopausal women (age: 57 ± 1 years; BMI: 38.1 ± 2.1 kg/m², SBP: 153 ± 4 mmHg) | L-citrulline-rich watermelon supplementation | ≈6 g L-citrulline/day | 6 weeks | arterial stiffness↓, aortic SBP↓, pressure wave reflection amplitude↓ | [152] |

## 5. Conclusions

The CVDs are greatly related to unbalanced diets. Several fruits can modulate metabolic risk factors such as hypertension, dyslipidemia, diabetes, and overweight/obesity, and inhibit atherosclerosis, which is the key pathological process of CHD and stroke. Many epidemiological studies investigating the relationship between fruit consumption and CVD risks yielded similar results regarding the protective effects of fruits on CVDs. Moreover, the majority of experimental studies also supported cardiovascular protecting properties of several fruits, such as grape, blueberry, pomegranate, apple, hawthorn, and avocado. The mechanisms of action mainly included the modulation of molecular events and signaling pathways associated with correcting endothelial dysfunction, reducing disorders in lipids metabolism, anti-hypertension, suppressing platelets function, alleviating I/R injury, inhibiting thrombosis, reducing oxidative stress, and inhibiting inflammation responses. In the future, the protective effects of a greater number of fruits on CVDs should be evaluated, and the bioactive components should be isolated and identified. Furthermore, the mechanisms of action should be further studied.

**Acknowledgments:** This work was supported by the National Natural Science Foundation of China (No. 81372976), Key Project of Guangdong Provincial Science and Technology Program (No. 2014B020205002), and the Hundred-Talents Scheme of Sun Yat-Sen University.

**Author Contributions:** Cai-Ning Zhao, Sha Li, and Hua-Bin Li conceived this paper; Cai-Ning Zhao, Xiao Meng, Ya Li, Qing Liu, and Guo-Yi Tang wrote this paper; Sha Li and Hua-Bin Li revised the paper.

**Conflicts of Interest:** The authors declare no conflict of interest.

## References

1. WHO. Cardiovascular Diseases (CVDs). Available online: http://www.who.int/cardiovascular_diseases/en/ (accessed on 13 March 2017).
2. Rodríguez-Monforte, M.; Flores-Mateo, G.; Sánchez, E. Dietary patterns and CVD: A systematic review and meta-analysis of observational studies. *Br. J. Nutr.* **2015**, *114*, 1341–1359. [CrossRef] [PubMed]
3. Grosso, G.; Marventano, S.; Yang, J.; Micek, A.; Pajak, A.; Scalfi, L.; Galvano, F.; Kales, S.N. A comprehensive meta-analysis on evidence of Mediterranean diet and cardiovascular disease: Are individual components equal? *Crit. Rev. Food Sci. Nutr.* **2017**, *57*, 3218–3232. [CrossRef] [PubMed]
4. Du, H.D.; Li, L.M.; Bennett, D.; Guo, Y.; Key, T.J.; Bian, Z.; Sherliker, P.; Gao, H.Y.; Chen, Y.P.; Yang, L.; et al. Fresh fruit consumption and major cardiovascular disease in China. *N. Engl. J. Med.* **2016**, *374*, 1332–1343. [CrossRef] [PubMed]
5. Lai, H.T.M.; Threapleton, D.E.; Day, A.J.; Williamson, G.; Cade, J.E.; Burley, V.J. Fruit intake and cardiovascular disease mortality in the UK Women's Cohort Study. *Eur. J. Epidemiol.* **2015**, *30*, 1035–1048. [CrossRef] [PubMed]
6. Hodgson, J.M.; Prince, R.L.; Woodman, R.J.; Bondonno, C.P.; Ivey, K.L.; Bondonno, N.; Rimm, E.B.; Ward, N.C.; Croft, K.D.; Lewis, J.R. Apple intake is inversely associated with all-cause and disease-specific mortality in elderly women. *Br. J. Nutr.* **2016**, *115*, 860–867. [CrossRef] [PubMed]
7. Yamada, T.; Hayasaka, S.; Shibata, Y.; Ojima, T.; Saegusa, T.; Gotoh, T.; Ishikawa, S.; Nakamura, Y.; Kayaba, K. Frequency of citrus fruit intake is associated with the incidence of cardiovascular disease: The jichi medical school cohort study. *J. Epidemiol.* **2011**, *21*, 169–175. [CrossRef] [PubMed]
8. Ezzati, M.; Riboli, E. Behavioral and dietary risk factors for noncommunicable diseases. *N. Engl. J. Med.* **2013**, *369*, 954–964. [CrossRef] [PubMed]
9. Quinones, M.; Guerrero, L.; Suarez, M.; Pons, Z.; Aleixandre, A.; Arola, L.; Muguerza, B. Low-molecular procyanidin rich grape seed extract exerts antihypertensive effect in males spontaneously hypertensive rats. *Food Res. Int.* **2013**, *51*, 587–595. [CrossRef]
10. Xu, H.; Xu, H.E.; Ryan, D. A study of the comparative effects of hawthorn fruit compound and simvastatin on lowering blood lipid levels. *Am. J. Chin. Med.* **2009**, *37*, 903–908. [CrossRef] [PubMed]

11. Lucas, E.A.; Li, W.J.; Peterson, S.K.; Brown, A.; Kuvibidila, S.; Perkins-Veazie, P.; Clarke, S.L.; Smith, B.J. Mango modulates body fat and plasma glucose and lipids in mice fed a high-fat diet. *Br. J. Nutr.* **2011**, *106*, 1495–1505. [CrossRef] [PubMed]

12. Brasil, G.A.; Ronchi, S.N.; Do Nascimento, A.M.; de Lima, E.M.; Romao, W.; Da Costa, H.B.; Scherer, R.; Ventura, J.A.; Lenz, D.; Bissoli, N.S.; et al. Antihypertensive effect of carica papaya via a reduction in ACE activity and improved baroreflex. *Planta Med.* **2014**, *80*, 1580–1587. [CrossRef] [PubMed]

13. Fu, L.; Xu, B.T.; Xu, X.R.; Gan, R.Y.; Zhang, Y.; Xia, E.Q.; Li, H.B. Antioxidant capacities and total phenolic contents of 62 fruits. *Food Chem.* **2011**, *129*, 345–350. [CrossRef]

14. Zhang, Y.J.; Gan, R.Y.; Li, S.; Zhou, Y.; Li, A.N.; Xu, D.P.; Li, H.B. Antioxidant phytochemicals for the prevention and treatment of chronic diseases. *Molecules* **2015**, *20*, 21138–21156. [CrossRef] [PubMed]

15. Song, F.L.; Gan, R.Y.; Zhang, Y.; Xiao, Q.; Kuang, L.; Li, H.B. Total phenolic contents and antioxidant capacities of selected chinese medicinal plants. *Int. J. Mol. Sci.* **2010**, *11*, 2362–2372. [CrossRef] [PubMed]

16. Gan, R.Y.; Xu, X.R.; Song, F.L.; Kuang, L.; Li, H.B. Antioxidant activity and total phenolic content of medicinal plants associated with prevention and treatment of cardiovascular and cerebrovascular diseases. *J. Med. Plants Res.* **2010**, *4*, 2438–2444.

17. Fu, L.; Xu, B.T.; Gan, R.Y.; Zhang, Y.; Xu, X.R.; Xia, E.Q.; Li, H.B. Total phenolic contents and antioxidant capacities of herbal and tea infusions. *Int. J. Mol. Sci.* **2011**, *12*, 2112–2124. [CrossRef] [PubMed]

18. Guo, Y.J.; Deng, G.F.; Xu, X.R.; Wu, S.; Li, S.; Xia, E.Q.; Li, F.; Chen, F.; Ling, W.H.; Li, H.B. Antioxidant capacities, phenolic compounds and polysaccharide contents of 49 edible macro-fungi. *Food Funct.* **2012**, *3*, 1195–1205. [CrossRef] [PubMed]

19. Deng, G.F.; Xu, X.R.; Zhang, Y.; Li, D.; Gan, R.Y.; Li, H.B. Phenolic compounds and bioactivities of pigmented rice. *Crit. Rev. Food Sci.* **2013**, *53*, 296–306. [CrossRef] [PubMed]

20. Deng, G.F.; Lin, X.; Xu, X.R.; Gao, L.L.; Xie, J.F.; Li, H.B. Antioxidant capacities and total phenolic contents of 56 vegetables. *J. Funct. Foods* **2013**, *5*, 260–266. [CrossRef]

21. Li, S.; Li, S.K.; Gan, R.Y.; Song, F.L.; Kuang, L.; Li, H.B. Antioxidant capacities and total phenolic contents of infusions from 223 medicinal plants. *Ind. Crops Prod.* **2013**, *51*, 289–298. [CrossRef]

22. Li, A.N.; Li, S.; Li, H.B.; Xu, D.P.; Xu, X.R.; Chen, F. Total phenolic contents and antioxidant capacities of 51 edible and wild flowers. *J. Funct. Foods* **2014**, *6*, 319–330. [CrossRef]

23. Xu, D.P.; Li, Y.; Meng, X.; Zhou, T.; Zhou, Y.; Zheng, J.; Zhang, J.J.; Li, H.B. Natural antioxidants in foods and medicinal plants: Extraction, assessment and resources. *Int. J. Mol. Sci.* **2017**, *18*, 96. [CrossRef] [PubMed]

24. Fu, L.; Xu, B.T.; Xu, X.R.; Qin, X.S.; Gan, R.Y.; Li, H.B. Antioxidant capacities and total phenolic contents of 56 wild fruits from South China. *Molecules* **2010**, *15*, 8602–8617. [CrossRef] [PubMed]

25. Manach, C.; Scalbert, A.; Morand, C.; Remesy, C.; Jimenez, L. Polyphenols: Food sources and bioavailability. *Am. J. Clin. Nutr.* **2004**, *79*, 727–747. [PubMed]

26. Ginter, E.; Simko, V. Plant polyphenols in prevention of heart disease. *Bratisl. Med. J.* **2012**, *113*, 476–480. [CrossRef]

27. Li, A.N.; Li, S.; Zhang, Y.J.; Xu, X.R.; Chen, Y.M.; Li, H.B. Resources and biological activities of natural polyphenols. *Nutrients* **2014**, *6*, 6020–6047. [CrossRef] [PubMed]

28. Yu, D.; Zhang, X.; Gao, Y.T.; Li, H.; Yang, G.; Huang, J.; Zheng, W.; Xiang, Y.B.; Shu, X.O. Fruit and vegetable intake and risk of CHD: Results from prospective cohort studies of Chinese adults in Shanghai. *Br. J. Nutr.* **2014**, *111*, 353–362. [CrossRef] [PubMed]

29. Gan, Y.; Tong, X.; Li, L.; Cao, S.; Yin, X.; Gao, C.; Herath, C.; Li, W.; Jin, Z.; Chen, Y.; et al. Consumption of fruit and vegetable and risk of coronary heart disease: A meta-analysis of prospective cohort studies. *Int. J. Cardiol.* **2015**, *183*, 129–137. [CrossRef] [PubMed]

30. Hansen, L.; Dragsted, L.O.; Olsen, A.; Christensen, J.; Tjonneland, A.; Schmidt, E.B.; Overvad, K. Fruit and vegetable intake and risk of acute coronary syndrome. *Br. J. Nutr.* **2010**, *104*, 248–255. [CrossRef] [PubMed]

31. Larsson, S.C.; Virtamo, J.; Wolk, A. Total and specific fruit and vegetable consumption and risk of stroke: A prospective study. *Atherosclerosis* **2013**, *227*, 147–152. [CrossRef] [PubMed]

32. Oude Griep, L.M.; Verschuren, W.M.M.; Kromhout, D.; Ocke, M.C.; Geleijnse, J.M. Colors of fruit and vegetables and 10-year incidence of stroke. *Stroke* **2011**, *42*, 3190–3195. [CrossRef] [PubMed]

33. Oude Griep, L.M.; Verschuren, W.M.M.; Kromhout, D.; Ocke, M.C.; Geleijnse, J.M. Raw and processed fruit and vegetable consumption and 10-year stroke incidence in a population-based cohort study in the Netherlands. *Eur. J. Clin. Nutr.* **2011**, *65*, 791–799. [CrossRef] [PubMed]

34. Cassidy, A.; Rimm, E.B.; O'Reilly, E.J.; Logroscino, G.; Kay, C.; Chiuve, S.E.; Rexrode, K.M. Dietary flavonoids and risk of stroke in women. *Stroke* **2012**, *43*, 946–975. [CrossRef] [PubMed]
35. Goetz, M.E.; Judd, S.E.; Hartman, T.J.; McClellan, W.; Anderson, A.; Vaccarino, V. Flavanone intake is inversely associated with risk of incident ischemic stroke in the REasons for geographic and racial differences in stroke (REGARDS) study. *J. Nutr.* **2016**, *146*, 2233–2243. [CrossRef] [PubMed]
36. Collins, R.; Peto, R.; MacMahon, S.; Hebert, P.; Fiebach, N.H.; Eberlein, K.A.; Godwin, J.; Qizilbash, N.; Taylor, J.O.; Hennekens, C.H. Blood pressure, stroke, and coronary heart disease. Part 2, Short-term reductions in blood pressure: Overview of randomised drug trials in their epidemiological context. *Lancet* **1990**, *335*, 827–838. [CrossRef]
37. Wang, L.; Manson, J.E.; Gaziano, J.M.; Buring, J.E.; Sesso, H.D. Fruit and vegetable intake and the risk of hypertension in middle-aged and older women. *Am. J. Hypertens.* **2012**, *25*, 180–189. [CrossRef] [PubMed]
38. Tsubota-Utsugi, M.; Ohkubo, T.; Kikuya, M.; Metoki, H.; Kurimoto, A.; Suzuki, K.; Fukushima, N.; Hara, A.; Asayama, K.; Satoh, H.; et al. High fruit intake is associated with a lower risk of future hypertension determined by home blood pressure measurement: The Ohasama study. *J. Hum. Hypertens.* **2011**, *25*, 164–171. [CrossRef] [PubMed]
39. Borgi, L.; Muraki, I.; Satija, A.; Willett, W.C.; Rimm, E.B.; Forman, J.P. Fruit and vegetable consumption and the incidence of hypertension in three prospective cohort studies. *Hypertension* **2016**, *67*, 288–293. [CrossRef] [PubMed]
40. Song, H.J.; Paek, Y.J.; Choi, M.K.; Lee, H.J. Gender differences in the relationship between risk of hypertension and fruit intake. *Prev. Med.* **2014**, *67*, 154–159. [CrossRef] [PubMed]
41. Chan, H.T.; Yiu, K.H.; Wong, C.Y.; Li, S.W.; Tam, S.; Tse, H.F. Increased dietary fruit intake was associated with lower burden of carotid atherosclerosis in Chinese patients with type 2 diabetes mellitus. *Diabetic Med.* **2013**, *30*, 100–108. [CrossRef] [PubMed]
42. Zhu, Y.; Zhang, Y.; Ling, W.; Feng, D.; Wei, X.; Yang, C.; Ma, J. Fruit consumption is associated with lower carotid intima-media thickness and C-reactive protein levels in patients with type 2 diabetes mellitus. *J. Am. Diet Assoc.* **2011**, *111*, 1536–1542. [CrossRef] [PubMed]
43. Cassidy, A.; Bertoia, M.; Chiuve, S.; Flint, A.; Forman, J.; Rimm, E.B. Habitual intake of anthocyanins and flavanones and risk of cardiovascular disease in men. *Am. J. Clin. Nutr.* **2016**, *104*, 587–594. [CrossRef] [PubMed]
44. Li, G.L.; Zhu, Y.N.; Zhang, Y.; Lang, J.; Chen, Y.M.; Ling, W.H. Estimated daily flavonoid and stilbene intake from fruits, vegetables, and nuts and associations with lipid profiles in chinese adults. *J. Acad. Nutr. Diet.* **2013**, *113*, 786–794. [CrossRef] [PubMed]
45. Bendinelli, B.; Masala, G.; Saieva, C.; Salvini, S.; Calonico, C.; Sacerdote, C.; Agnoli, C.; Grioni, S.; Frasca, G.; Mattiello, A.; et al. Fruit, vegetables, and olive oil and risk of coronary heart disease in Italian women: The EPICOR study. *Am. J. Clin. Nutr.* **2011**, *93*, 275–283. [CrossRef] [PubMed]
46. Dauchet, L.; Montaye, M.; Ruidavets, J.; Arveiler, D.; Kee, F.; Bingham, A.; Ferrieres, J.; Haas, B.; Evans, A.; Ducimetiere, P.; et al. Association between the frequency of fruit and vegetable consumption and cardiovascular disease in male smokers and non-smokers. *Eur. J. Clin. Nutr.* **2010**, *64*, 578–586. [CrossRef] [PubMed]
47. Sharma, S.; Vik, S.; Kolonel, L.N. Fruit and vegetable consumption, ethnicity and risk of fatal ischemic heart disease. *J. Nutr. Health Aging* **2014**, *18*, 573–578. [CrossRef] [PubMed]
48. Sangita, S.; Vik, S.A.; Pakseresht, M.; Kolonel, L.N. Adherence to recommendations for fruit and vegetable intake, ethnicity and ischemic heart disease mortality. *Nutr. Metab. Cardiovasc. Dis.* **2013**, *23*, 1247–1254. [CrossRef] [PubMed]
49. Rautiainen, S.; Levitan, E.B.; Mittleman, M.A.; Wolk, A. Fruit and vegetable intake and rate of heart failure: A population-based prospective cohort of women. *Eur. J. Heart Fail.* **2015**, *17*, 20–26. [CrossRef] [PubMed]
50. Deanfield, J.; Donald, A.; Ferri, C.; Giannattasio, C.; Halcox, J.; Halligan, S.; Lerman, A.; Mancia, G.; Oliver, J.J.; Pessina, A.C.; et al. Endothelial function and dysfunction. Part I: Methodological issues for assessment in the different vascular beds: A statement by the working group on endothelin and endothelial factors of the European Society of Hypertension. *J. Hypertens.* **2005**, *23*, 7–17. [CrossRef] [PubMed]
51. Thandapilly, S.J.; LeMaistre, J.L.; Louis, X.L.; Anderson, C.M.; Netticadan, T.; Anderson, H.D. Vascular and cardiac effects of grape powder in the spontaneously hypertensive rat. *Am. J. Hypertens.* **2012**, *25*, 1070–1076. [CrossRef] [PubMed]

52. Liang, Y.; Wang, J.; Gao, H.Q.; Wang, Q.Z.; Zhang, J.; Qiu, J. Beneficial effects of grape seed proanthocyanidin extract on arterial remodeling in spontaneously hypertensive rats via protecting against oxidative stress. *Mol. Med. Rep.* **2016**, *14*, 3711–3718. [CrossRef] [PubMed]

53. Wang, X.H.; Huang, L.L.; Yu, T.T.; Zhu, J.H.; Shen, B.; Zhang, Y.; Wang, H.Z.; Gao, S. Effects of oligomeric grape seed proanthocyanidins on heart, aorta, kidney in DOCA-salt mice: Role of oxidative stress. *Phytother. Res.* **2013**, *27*, 869–876. [CrossRef] [PubMed]

54. Rodriguez-Rodriguez, R.; Justo, M.L.; Claro, C.M.; Vila, E.; Parrado, J.; Herrera, M.D.; de Sotomayor, M.A. Endothelium-dependent vasodilator and antioxidant properties of a novel enzymatic extract of grape pomace from wine industrial waste. *Food Chem.* **2012**, *135*, 1044–1051. [CrossRef] [PubMed]

55. Felice, F.; Zambito, Y.; Di Colo, G.; D'Onofrio, C.; Fausto, C.; Balbarini, A.; Di Stefano, R. Red grape skin and seeds polyphenols: Evidence of their protective effects on endothelial progenitor cells and improvement of their intestinal absorption. *Eur. J. Pharm. Biopharm.* **2012**, *80*, 176–184. [CrossRef] [PubMed]

56. Quintieri, A.M.; Baldino, N.; Filice, E.; Seta, L.; Vitetti, A.; Tota, B.; De Cindio, B.; Cerra, M.C.; Angelone, T. Malvidin, a red wine polyphenol, modulates mammalian myocardial and coronary performance and protects the heart against ischemia/reperfusion injury. *J. Nutr. Biochem.* **2013**, *24*, 1221–1231. [CrossRef] [PubMed]

57. Cui, X.; Liu, X.; Feng, H.; Zhao, S.; Gao, H. Grape seed proanthocyanidin extracts enhance endothelial nitric oxide synthase expression through 5'-AMP activated protein kinase/surtuin 1-krupple like factor 2 pathway and modulate blood pressure in ouabain induced hypertensive rats. *Biol. Pharm. Bull.* **2012**, *35*, 2192–2197. [CrossRef] [PubMed]

58. Goutzourelas, N.; Stagos, D.; Housmekeridou, A.; Karapouliou, C.; Kerasioti, E.; Aligiannis, N.; Skaltsounis, A.L.; Spandidos, D.A.; Tsatsakis, A.M.; Kouretas, D. Grape pomace extract exerts antioxidant effects through an increase in GCS levels and GST activity in muscle and endothelial cells. *Int. J. Mol. Med.* **2015**, *36*, 433–441. [CrossRef] [PubMed]

59. Luzak, B.; Kosiorek, A.; Syska, K.; Rozalski, M.; Bijak, M.; Podsedek, A.; Balcerczak, E.; Watala, C.; Golanski, J. Does grape seed extract potentiate the inhibition of platelet reactivity in the presence of endothelial cells? *Adv. Med. Sci.* **2014**, *59*, 178–182. [CrossRef] [PubMed]

60. Razavi, S.M.; Gholamin, S.; Eskandari, A.; Mohsenian, N.; Ghorbanihaghjo, A.; Delazar, A.; Rashtchizadeh, N.; Keshtkar-Jahromi, M.; Argani, H. Red grape seed extract improves lipid profiles and decreases oxidized low-density lipoprotein in patients with mild hyperlipidemia. *J. Med. Food* **2013**, *16*, 255–258. [CrossRef] [PubMed]

61. Leibowitz, A.; Faltin, Z.; Perl, A.; Eshdat, Y.; Hagay, Y.; Peleg, E.; Grossman, E. Red grape berry-cultured cells reduce blood pressure in rats with metabolic-like syndrome. *Eur. J. Nutr.* **2014**, *53*, 973–980. [CrossRef] [PubMed]

62. Caimari, A.; Del Bas, J.M.; Crescenti, A.; Arola, L. Low doses of grape seed procyanidins reduce adiposity and improve the plasma lipid profile in hamsters. *Int. J. Obes.* **2013**, *37*, 576–583. [CrossRef] [PubMed]

63. Eren, E.; Yilmaz, N.; Aydin, O. High density lipoprotein and it's dysfunction. *Open Biochem. J.* **2012**, *6*, 78–93. [CrossRef] [PubMed]

64. Zagayko, A.L.; Kravchenko, G.B.; Krasilnikova, O.A.; Ogai, Y.O. Grape polyphenols increase the activity of HDL enzymes in old and obese rats. *Oxid. Med. Cell. Longev.* **2013**, *593761*. [CrossRef] [PubMed]

65. Malinowska, J.; Oleszek, W.; Stochmal, A.; Olas, B. The polyphenol-rich extracts from black chokeberry and grape seeds impair changes in the platelet adhesion and aggregation induced by a model of hyperhomocysteinemia. *Eur. J. Nutr.* **2013**, *52*, 1049–1057. [CrossRef] [PubMed]

66. Safwen, K.; Selima, S.; Mohamed, E.; Ferid, L.; Pascal, C.; Mohamed, A.; Ezzedine, A.; Meherzia, M. Protective effect of grape seed and skin extract on cerebral ischemia in rat: Implication of transition metals. *Int. J. Stroke* **2015**, *10*, 415–424. [CrossRef] [PubMed]

67. Zhao, G.; Gao, H.; Qiu, J.; Lu, W.; Wei, X. The molecular mechanism of protective effects of grape seed proanthocyanidin extract on reperfusion arrhythmias in rats in vivo. *Biol. Pharm. Bull.* **2010**, *33*, 759–767. [CrossRef] [PubMed]

68. Zhang, Y.; Shi, H.; Wang, W.; Ke, Z.; Xu, P.; Zhong, Z.; Li, X.; Wang, S. Antithrombotic effect of grape seed proanthocyanidins extract in a rat model of deep vein thrombosis. *J. Vasc. Surg.* **2011**, *53*, 743–753. [CrossRef] [PubMed]

69. Stroher, D.J.; Escobar, P.J.C.; Gullich, A.A.; Pilar, B.C.; Coelho, R.P.; Bruno, J.B.; Faoro, D.; Manfredini, V. 14 Days of supplementation with blueberry extract shows anti-atherogenic properties and improves oxidative parameters in hypercholesterolemic rats model. *Int. J. Food Sci. Nutr.* **2015**, *66*, 559–568. [CrossRef] [PubMed]

70. Rodriguez-Mateos, A.; Ishisaka, A.; Mawatari, K.; Vidal-Diez, A.; Spencer, J.P.; Terao, J. Blueberry intervention improves vascular reactivity and lowers blood pressure in high-fat-, high-cholesterol-fed rats. *Br. J. Nutr.* **2013**, *109*, 1746–1754. [CrossRef] [PubMed]

71. Xie, C.; Kang, J.; Chen, J.R.; Nagarajan, S.; Badger, T.M.; Wu, X. Phenolic acids are in vivo atheroprotective compounds appearing in the serum of rats after blueberry consumption. *J. Agric. Food Chem.* **2011**, *59*, 10381–10387. [CrossRef] [PubMed]

72. Cao, K.; Xu, J.; Pu, W.J.; Dong, Z.Z.; Sun, L.; Zang, W.J.; Gao, F.; Zhang, Y.; Feng, Z.H.; Liu, J.K. Punicalagin, an active component in pomegranate, ameliorates cardiac mitochondrial impairment in obese rats via AMPK activation. *Sci. Rep.* **2015**, *5*, 14014. [CrossRef] [PubMed]

73. Al-Jarallah, A.; Igdoura, F.; Zhang, Y.; Tenedero, C.B.; White, E.J.; MacDonald, M.E.; Igdoura, S.A.; Trigatti, B.L. The effect of pomegranate extract on coronary artery atherosclerosis in SR-BI/APOE double knockout mice. *Atherosclerosis* **2013**, *228*, 80–89. [CrossRef] [PubMed]

74. Sun, W.Y.; Yan, C.H.; Frost, B.; Wang, X.; Hou, C.; Zeng, M.Q.; Gao, H.L.; Kang, Y.M.; Liu, J.K. Pomegranate extract decreases oxidative stress and alleviates mitochondrial impairment by activating AMPK-Nrf2 in hypothalamic paraventricular nucleus of spontaneously hypertensive rats. *Sci. Rep.* **2016**, *6*, 34246. [CrossRef] [PubMed]

75. Hajipour, S.; Sarkaki, A.; Mohammad, S.; Mansouri, T.; Pilevarian, A.; RafieiRad, M. Motor and cognitive deficits due to permanent cerebral hypoperfusion/ischemia improve by pomegranate seed extract in rats. *Pak. J. Biol. Sci.* **2014**, *17*, 991–998. [PubMed]

76. Serra, A.T.; Rocha, J.; Sepodes, B.; Matias, A.A.; Feliciano, R.P.; de Carvalho, A.; Bronze, M.R.; Duarte, C.M.M.; Figueira, M.E. Evaluation of cardiovascular protective effect of different apple varieties—Correlation of response with composition. *Food Chem.* **2012**, *135*, 2378–2386. [CrossRef] [PubMed]

77. Gonzalez, J.; Donoso, W.; Sandoval, N.; Reyes, M.; Gonzalez, P.; Gajardo, M.; Morales, E.; Neira, A.; Razmilic, I.; Yuri, J.A.; et al. Apple peel supplemented diet reduces parameters of metabolic syndrome and atherogenic progression in ApoE$^{-/-}$ mice. *Evid. Based Complement. Altern.* **2015**, 918384. [CrossRef] [PubMed]

78. Hu, H.J.; Luo, X.G.; Dong, Q.Q.; Mu, A.; Shi, G.L.; Wang, Q.T.; Chen, X.Y.; Zhou, H.; Zhang, T.C.; Pan, L.W. Ethanol extract of Zhongtian hawthorn lowers serum cholesterol in mice by inhibiting transcription of 3-hydroxy-3-methylglutaryl-CoA reductase via nuclear factor-kappa B signal pathway. *Exp. Biol. Med.* **2016**, *241*, 667–674. [CrossRef] [PubMed]

79. Li, T.P.; Zhu, R.G.; Dong, Y.P.; Liu, Y.H.; Li, S.H.; Chen, G. Effects of pectin pentaoligosaccharide from hawthorn (*Crataegus pinnatifida* Bunge. Var. Major) on the activity and mRNA levels of enzymes involved in fatty acid oxidation in the liver of mice fed a high-fat diet. *J. Agric. Food Chem.* **2013**, *61*, 7599–7605. [CrossRef] [PubMed]

80. Zhang, Y.Y.; Zhang, L.; Geng, Y.; Geng, Y.H. Hawthorn fruit attenuates atherosclerosis by improving the hypolipidemic and antioxidant activities in apolipoprotein E-Deficient mice. *J. Atheroscler. Thromb.* **2014**, *21*, 119–128. [CrossRef] [PubMed]

81. Zhang, J.; Liang, R.; Wang, L.; Yan, R.; Hou, R.; Gao, S.; Yang, B. Effects of an aqueous extract of *Crataegus pinnatifida* Bge. Var. Major N.E.Br. fruit on experimental atherosclerosis in rats. *J. Ethnopharmacol.* **2013**, *148*, 563–569. [CrossRef] [PubMed]

82. Duarte, P.F.; Chaves, M.A.; Borges, C.D.; Mendonca, C. Avocado: Characteristics, health benefits and uses. *Cienc. Rural* **2016**, *46*, 747–754. [CrossRef]

83. Villa-Rodriguez, J.A.; Molina-Corral, F.J.; Ayala-Zavala, J.F.; Olivas, G.I.; Gonzalez-Aguilar, G.A. Effect of maturity stage on the content of fatty acids and antioxidant activity of 'Hass' avocado. *Food Res. Int.* **2011**, *44*, 1231–1237. [CrossRef]

84. Rodriguez-Sanchez, D.G.; Flores-Garcia, M.; Silva-Platas, C.; Rizzo, S.; Torre-Amione, G.; De la Pena-Diaz, A.; Hernandez-Brenes, C.; Garcia-Rivas, G. Isolation and chemical identification of lipid derivatives from avocado (*Persea americana*) pulp with antiplatelet and antithrombotic activities. *Food Funct.* **2015**, *6*, 193–203. [CrossRef] [PubMed]

85. Carvajal-Zarrabal, O.; Nolasco-Hipolito, C.; Aguilar-Uscanga, M.G.; Melo-Santiesteban, G.; Hayward-Jones, P.M.; Barradas-Dermitz, D.M. Avocado oil supplementation modifies cardiovascular risk profile markers in a rat model of sucrose-induced metabolic changes. *Dis. Markers* **2014**, *2014*, 386425. [CrossRef] [PubMed]

86. Carvajal-Zarrabal, O.; Nolasco-Hipolito, C.; Aguilar-Uscanga, M.G.; Santiesteban, G.M.; Hayward-Jones, P.M.; Barradas-Dermitz, D.M. Effect of dietary intake of avocado oil and olive oil on biochemical markers of liver function in sucrose-fed rats. *Biomed. Res. Int.* **2014**, 595479. [CrossRef] [PubMed]

87. Dabas, D.; Shegog, R.M.; Ziegler, G.R.; Lambert, J.D. Avocado (*Persea americana*) seed as a source of bioactive phytochemicals. *Curr. Pharm. Des.* **2013**, *19*, 6133–6140. [CrossRef] [PubMed]

88. Czompa, A.; Gyongyosi, A.; Czegledi, A.; Csepanyi, E.; Bak, I.; Haines, D.D.; Tosaki, A.; Lekli, I. Cardioprotection afforded by sour cherry seed kernel: The role of heme oxygenase-1. *J. Cardiovasc. Pharmacol.* **2014**, *64*, 412–419. [CrossRef] [PubMed]

89. Li, C.; He, J.; Gao, Y.; Xing, Y.; Hou, J.; Tian, J. Preventive effect of total flavones of *Choerospondias axillaries* on ischemia/reperfusion-induced myocardial infarction-related MAPK signaling pathway. *Cardiovasc. Toxicol.* **2014**, *14*, 145–152. [CrossRef] [PubMed]

90. Zapata-Sudo, G.; Da, S.J.; Pereira, S.L.; Souza, P.J.; de Moura, R.S.; Sudo, R.T. Oral treatment with *Euterpe oleracea* Mart. (acai) extract improves cardiac dysfunction and exercise intolerance in rats subjected to myocardial infarction. *BMC Complement. Altern. Med.* **2014**, *14*, 227. [CrossRef] [PubMed]

91. Mauray, A.; Felgines, C.; Morand, C.; Mazur, A.; Scalbert, A.; Milenkovic, D. Bilberry anthocyanin-rich extract alters expression of genes related to atherosclerosis development in aorta of apo E-deficient mice. *Nutr. Metab. Cardiovasc. Dis.* **2012**, *22*, 72–80. [CrossRef] [PubMed]

92. Ash, M.M.; Wolford, K.A.; Carden, T.J.; Hwang, K.T.; Carr, T.P. Unrefined and refined black raspberry seed oils significantly lower triglycerides and moderately affect cholesterol metabolism in male Syrian hamsters. *J. Med. Food* **2011**, *14*, 1032–1038. [CrossRef] [PubMed]

93. Yang, F.; Suo, Y.R.; Chen, D.L.; Tong, L. Protection against vascular endothelial dysfunction by polyphenols in sea buckthorn berries in rats with hyperlipidemia. *Biosci. Trends* **2016**, *10*, 188–196. [CrossRef] [PubMed]

94. Fujiwara, Y.; Hayashida, A.; Tsurushima, K.; Nagai, R.; Yoshitomi, M.; Daiguji, N.; Sakashita, N.; Takeya, M.; Tsukamoto, S.; Ikeda, T. Triterpenoids isolated from *Zizyphus jujuba* inhibit foam cell formation in macrophages. *J. Agric. Food Chem.* **2011**, *59*, 4544–4552. [CrossRef] [PubMed]

95. Ono, M.; Yasuda, S.; Komatsu, H.; Fujiwara, Y.; Takeya, M.; Nohara, T. Triterpenoids from the fruits and leaves of the blackberry (*Rubus allegheniensis*) and their inhibitory activities on foam cell formation in human monocyte-derived macrophage. *Nat. Prod. Res.* **2014**, *28*, 2347–2350. [CrossRef] [PubMed]

96. Konta, E.M.; Almeida, M.R.; Do, A.C.; Darin, J.D.; de Rosso, V.V.; Mercadante, A.Z.; Antunes, L.M.; Bianchi, M.L. Evaluation of the antihypertensive properties of yellow passion fruit pulp (*Passiflora edulis* Sims f. Flavicarpa Deg.) in spontaneously hypertensive rats. *Phytother. Res.* **2014**, *28*, 28–32. [CrossRef] [PubMed]

97. Furuuchi, R.; Sakai, H.; Hirokawa, N.; Watanabe, Y.; Yokoyama, T.; Hirayama, M. Antihypertensive effect of boysenberry seed polyphenols on spontaneously hypertensive rats and identification of orally absorbable proanthocyanidins with vasorelaxant activity. *Biosci. Biotechnol. Biochem.* **2012**, *76*, 1694–1701. [CrossRef] [PubMed]

98. De Souza, M.O.; Souza, E.S.L.; de Brito, M.C.; de Figueiredo, B.B.; Costa, D.C.; Silva, M.E.; Pedrosa, M.L. The hypocholesterolemic activity of acai (*Euterpe oleracea* Mart.) is mediated by the enhanced expression of the ATP-binding cassette, subfamily G transporters 5 and 8 and low-density lipoprotein receptor genes in the rat. *Nutr. Res.* **2012**, *32*, 976–984. [CrossRef] [PubMed]

99. Pujari, R.R.; Vyawahare, N.S.; Kagathara, V.G. Evaluation of antioxidant and neuroprotective effect of date palm (*Phoenix dactylifera* L.) against bilateral common carotid artery occlusion in rats. *Indian J. Exp. Biol.* **2011**, *49*, 627–633. [PubMed]

100. Varela, C.E.; Fromentin, E.; Roller, M.; Villarreal, F.; Ramirez-Sanchez, I. Effects of a natural extract of *Aronia melanocarpa* berry on endothelial cell nitric oxide production. *J. Food Biochem.* **2016**, *40*, 404–410. [CrossRef] [PubMed]

101. Zhao, R.Z.; Le, K.; Li, W.D.; Ren, S.; Moghadasian, M.H.; Beta, T.; Shen, G.X. Effects of Saskatoon berry powder on monocyte adhesion to vascular wall of leptin receptor-deficient diabetic mice. *J. Nutr. Biochem.* **2014**, *25*, 851–857. [CrossRef] [PubMed]

102. Zhao, R.Z.; Xie, X.P.; Le, K.; Li, W.D.; Moghadasian, M.H.; Beta, T.; Shen, G.X. Endoplasmic reticulum stress in diabetic mouse or glycated LDL-treated endothelial cells: Protective effect of Saskatoon berry powder and cyanidin glycans. *J. Nutr. Biochem.* **2015**, *26*, 1248–1253. [CrossRef] [PubMed]

103. Torres-Urrutia, C.; Guzman, L.; Schmeda-Hirschmann, G.; Moore-Carrasco, R.; Alarcon, M.; Astudillo, L.; Gutierrez, M.; Carrasco, G.; Yuri, J.A.; Aranda, E.; et al. Antiplatelet, anticoagulant, and fibrinolytic activity in vitro of extracts from selected fruits and vegetables. *Blood Coagul. Fibrinolysis* **2011**, *22*, 197–205. [CrossRef] [PubMed]

104. Kono, R.; Okuno, Y.; Nakamura, M.; Inada, K.; Tokuda, A.; Yamashita, M.; Hidaka, R.; Utsunomiya, H. Peach (*Prunus persica*) extract inhibits angiotensin II-induced signal transduction in vascular smooth muscle cells. *Food Chem.* **2013**, *139*, 371–376. [CrossRef] [PubMed]

105. Isaak, C.K.; Petkau, J.C.; O, K.; Debnath, S.C.; Siow, Y.L. Manitoba Lingonberry (*Vaccinium vitis-idaea*) bioactivities in ischemia-reperfusion injury. *J. Agric. Food Chem.* **2015**, *63*, 5660–5669. [CrossRef] [PubMed]

106. Lee, S.G.; Kim, B.; Yang, Y.; Pham, T.X.; Park, Y.K.; Manatou, J.E.; Koo, S.I.; Chun, O.K.; Lee, J.Y. Berry anthocyanins suppress the expression and secretion of proinflammatory mediators in macrophages by inhibiting nuclear translocation of NF-kappa B independent of NRF2-mediated mechanism. *J. Nutr. Biochem.* **2014**, *25*, 404–411. [CrossRef] [PubMed]

107. Rosenblat, M.; Volkova, N.; Borochov-Neori, H.; Judeinstein, S.; Aviram, M. Anti-atherogenic properties of date vs. Pomegranate polyphenols: The benefits of the combination. *Food Funct.* **2015**, *6*, 1496–1509. [CrossRef] [PubMed]

108. Li, S.H.; Zhao, P.; Tian, H.B.; Chen, L.H.; Cui, L.Q. Effect of grape polyphenols on blood pressure: A meta-analysis of randomized controlled trials. *PLoS ONE* **2015**, *10*, 0137665. [CrossRef] [PubMed]

109. Evans, M.; Wilson, D.; Guthrie, N. A randomized, double-blind, placebo-controlled, pilot study to evaluate the effect of whole grape extract on antioxidant status and lipid profile. *J. Funct. Foods* **2014**, *7*, 680–691. [CrossRef]

110. Rahbar, A.R.; Mahmoudabadi, M.; Islam, M.S. Comparative effects of red and white grapes on oxidative markers and lipidemic parameters in adult hypercholesterolemic humans. *Food Funct.* **2015**, *6*, 1992–1998. [CrossRef] [PubMed]

111. Yubero, N.; Sanz-Buenhombre, M.; Guadarrama, A.; Villanueva, S.; Carrion, J.M.; Larrarte, E.; Moro, C. LDL cholesterol-lowering effects of grape extract used as a dietary supplement on healthy volunteers. *Int. J. Food Sci. Nutr.* **2013**, *64*, 400–406. [CrossRef] [PubMed]

112. Li, S.H.; Tian, H.B.; Zhao, H.J.; Chen, L.H.; Cui, L.Q. The acute effects of grape polyphenols supplementation on endothelial function in adults: Meta-Analyses of controlled trials. *PLoS ONE* **2013**, *8*, 0069818. [CrossRef] [PubMed]

113. Alvarez-Suarez, J.M.; Giampieri, F.; Tulipani, S.; Casoli, T.; Di Stefano, G.; Gonzalez-Paramas, A.M.; Santos-Buelga, C.; Busco, F.; Quiles, J.L.; Cordero, M.D.; et al. One-month strawberry-rich anthocyanin supplementation ameliorates cardiovascular risk, oxidative stress markers and platelet activation in humans. *J. Nutr. Biochem.* **2014**, *25*, 289–294. [CrossRef] [PubMed]

114. Basu, A.; Betts, N.M.; Nguyen, A.; Newman, E.D.; Fu, D.; Lyons, T.J. Freeze-dried strawberries lower serum cholesterol and lipid peroxidation in adults with abdominal adiposity and elevated serum lipids. *J. Nutr.* **2014**, *144*, 830–837. [CrossRef] [PubMed]

115. Basu, A.; Fu, D.X.; Wilkinson, M.; Simmons, B.; Wu, M.; Betts, N.M.; Du, M.; Lyons, T.J. Strawberries decrease atherosclerotic markers in subjects with metabolic syndrome. *Nutr. Res.* **2010**, *30*, 462–469. [CrossRef] [PubMed]

116. Ellis, C.L.; Edirisinghe, I.; Kappagoda, T.; Burton-Freeman, B. Attenuation of meal-induced inflammatory and thrombotic responses in overweight men and women after 6-week daily strawberry (Fragaria) intake-a randomized placebo-controlled trial. *J. Atheroscler. Thromb.* **2011**, *18*, 318–327. [CrossRef] [PubMed]

117. Burton-Freeman, B.; Linares, A.; Hyson, D.; Kappagoda, T. Strawberry modulates LDL oxidation and postprandial lipemia in response to high-fat meal in overweight hyperlipidemic men and women. *J. Am. Coll. Nutr.* **2010**, *29*, 46–54. [CrossRef] [PubMed]

118. Udani, J.K.; Singh, B.B.; Singh, V.J.; Barrett, M.L. Effects of acai (*Euterpe oleracea* Mart.) berry preparation on metabolic parameters in a healthy overweight population: A pilot study. *Nutr. J.* **2011**, *10*, 45. [CrossRef] [PubMed]

119. Kianbakht, S.; Abasi, B.; Dabaghian, F.H. Improved lipid profile in hyperlipidemic patients taking vaccinium arctostaphylos fruit hydroalcoholic extract: A randomized double-blind placebo-controlled clinical trial. *Phytother. Res.* **2014**, *28*, 432–436. [CrossRef] [PubMed]

120. Larmo, P.S.; Kangas, A.J.; Soininen, P.; Lehtonen, H.M.; Suomela, J.P.; Yang, B.; Viikari, J.; Ala-Korpela, M.; Kallio, H.P. Effects of sea buckthorn and bilberry on serum metabolites differ according to baseline metabolic profiles in overweight women: A randomized crossover trial. *Am. J. Clin. Nutr.* **2013**, *98*, 941–951. [CrossRef] [PubMed]

121. Lehtonen, H.M.; Suomela, J.P.; Tahvonen, R.; Yang, B.; Venojarvi, M.; Viikari, J.; Kallio, H. Different berries and berry fractions have various but slightly positive effects on the associated variables of metabolic diseases on overweight and obese women. *Eur. J. Clin. Nutr.* **2011**, *65*, 394–401. [CrossRef] [PubMed]

122. Qin, Y.; Xia, M.; Ma, J.; Hao, Y.T.; Liu, J.; Mou, H.; Cao, L.; Ling, W.H. Anthocyanin supplementation improves serum LDL- and HDL-cholesterol concentrations associated with the inhibition of cholesteryl ester transfer protein in dyslipidemic subjects. *Am. J. Clin. Nutr.* **2009**, *90*, 485–492. [CrossRef] [PubMed]

123. Chai, S.C.; Hooshmand, S.; Saadat, R.L.; Payton, M.E.; Brummel-Smith, K.; Arjmandi, B.H. Daily apple versus dried plum: Impact on cardiovascular disease risk factors in postmenopausal women. *J. Acad. Nutr. Diet.* **2012**, *112*, 1158–1168. [CrossRef] [PubMed]

124. Tenore, G.C.; Caruso, D.; Buonomo, G.; D'Urso, E.; D'Avino, M.; Campiglia, P.; Marinelli, L.; Novellino, E. Annurca (*Malus pumila* Miller cv. Annurca) apple as a functional food for the contribution to a healthy balance of plasma cholesterol levels: Results of a randomized clinical trial. *J. Sci. Food Agric.* **2017**, *97*, 2107–2115. [CrossRef] [PubMed]

125. Ravn-Haren, G.; Dragsted, L.O.; Buch-Andersen, T.; Jensen, E.N.; Jensen, R.I.; Nemeth-Balogh, M.; Paulovicsova, B.; Bergstrom, A.; Wilcks, A.; Licht, T.R.; et al. Intake of whole apples or clear apple juice has contrasting effects on plasma lipids in healthy volunteers. *Eur. J. Nutr.* **2013**, *52*, 1875–1889. [CrossRef] [PubMed]

126. Bondonno, C.P.; Yang, X.; Croft, K.D.; Considine, M.J.; Ward, N.C.; Rich, L.; Puddey, I.B.; Swinny, E.; Mubarak, A.; Hodgson, J.M. Flavonoid-rich apples and nitrate-rich spinach augment nitric oxide status and improve endothelial function in healthy men and women: A randomized controlled trial. *Free Radic. Biol. Med.* **2012**, *52*, 95–102. [CrossRef] [PubMed]

127. Hollands, W.J.; Hart, D.J.; Dainty, J.R.; Hasselwander, O.; Tiihonen, K.; Wood, R.; Kroon, P.A. Bioavailability of epicatechin and effects on nitric oxide metabolites of an apple flavanol-rich extract supplemented beverage compared to a whole apple puree: A randomized, placebo-controlled, crossover trial. *Mol. Nutr. Food Res.* **2013**, *57*, 1209–1217. [CrossRef] [PubMed]

128. Stonehouse, W.; Gammon, C.S.; Beck, K.L.; Conlon, C.A.; von Hurst, P.R.; Kruger, R. Kiwifruit: Our daily prescription for health. *Can. J. Physiol. Pharm.* **2013**, *91*, 442–447. [CrossRef] [PubMed]

129. Gammon, C.S.; Kruger, R.; Conlon, C.A.; von Hurst, P.R.; Jones, B.; Stonehouse, W. Inflammatory status modulates plasma lipid and inflammatory marker responses to kiwifruit consumption in hypercholesterolaemic men. *Nutr. Metab. Cardiovas.* **2014**, *24*, 91–99. [CrossRef] [PubMed]

130. Gammon, C.S.; Kruger, R.; Brown, S.J.; Conlon, C.A.; von Hurst, P.R.; Stonehouse, W. Daily kiwifruit consumption did not improve blood pressure and markers of cardiovascular function in men with hypercholesterolemia. *Nutr. Res.* **2014**, *34*, 235–240. [CrossRef] [PubMed]

131. Chang, W.H.; Liu, J.F. Effects of kiwifruit consumption on serum lipid profiles and antioxidative status in hyperlipidemic subjects. *Int. J. Food Sci. Nutr.* **2009**, *60*, 709–716. [CrossRef] [PubMed]

132. Svendsen, M.; Tonstad, S.; Heggen, E.; Pedersen, T.R.; Seljeflot, I.; Bohn, S.K.; Bastani, N.E.; Blomhoff, R.; Holme, I.M.; Klemsdal, T.O. The effect of kiwifruit consumption on blood pressure in subjects with moderately elevated blood pressure: A randomized, controlled study. *Blood Press.* **2015**, *24*, 48–54. [CrossRef] [PubMed]

133. Karlsen, A.; Svendsen, M.; Seljeflot, I.; Laake, P.; Duttaroy, A.K.; Drevon, C.A.; Arnesen, H.; Tonstad, S.; Blomhoff, R. Kiwifruit decreases blood pressure and whole-blood platelet aggregation in male smokers. *J. Hum. Hypertens.* **2013**, *27*, 126–130. [CrossRef] [PubMed]

134. Peou, S.; Milliard-Hasting, B.; Shah, S.A. Impact of avocado-enriched diets on plasma lipoproteins: A meta-analysis. *J. Clin. Lipidol.* **2016**, *10*, 161–171. [CrossRef] [PubMed]

135. Jenkins, D.J.A.; Srichaikul, K.; Kendall, C.W.C.; Sievenpiper, J.L.; Abdulnour, S.; Mirrahimi, A.; Meneses, C.; Nishi, S.; He, X.; Lee, S.; et al. The relation of low glycaemic index fruit consumption to glycaemic control and risk factors for coronary heart disease in type 2 diabetes. *Diabetologia* **2011**, *54*, 271–279. [CrossRef] [PubMed]

136. Terauchi, M.; Horiguchi, N.; Kajiyama, A.; Akiyoshi, M.; Owa, Y.; Kato, K.; Kubota, T. Effects of grape seed proanthocyanidin extract on menopausal symptoms, body composition, and cardiovascular parameters in middle-aged women: A randomized, double-blind, placebo-controlled pilot study. *Menopause* **2014**, *21*, 990–996. [CrossRef] [PubMed]

137. Ras, R.T.; Zock, P.L.; Zebregs, Y.E.; Johnston, N.R.; Webb, D.J.; Draijer, R. Effect of polyphenol-rich grape seed extract on ambulatory blood pressure in subjects with pre- and stage I hypertension. *Br. J. Nutr.* **2013**, *110*, 2234–2241. [CrossRef] [PubMed]

138. Tome-Carneiro, J.; Gonzalvez, M.; Larrosa, M.; Yanez-Gascon, M.J.; Garcia-Almagro, F.J.; Ruiz-Ros, J.A.; Garcia-Conesa, M.T.; Tomas-Barberan, F.A.; Espin, J.C. One-year consumption of a grape nutraceutical containing resveratrol improves the inflammatory and fibrinolytic status of patients in primary prevention of cardiovascular disease. *Am. J. Cardiol.* **2012**, *110*, 356–363. [CrossRef] [PubMed]

139. Tome-Carneiro, J.; Gonzalvez, M.; Larrosa, M.; Yanez-Gascon, M.J.; Garcia-Almagro, F.J.; Ruiz-Ros, J.A.; Tomas-Barberan, F.A.; Garcia-Conesa, M.T.; Espin, J.C. Grape resveratrol increases serum adiponectin and downregulates inflammatory genes in peripheral blood mononuclear cells: A triple-blind, placebo-controlled, one-year clinical trial in patients with stable coronary artery disease. *Cardiovasc. Drug Ther.* **2013**, *27*, 37–48. [CrossRef] [PubMed]

140. Basu, A.; Du, M.; Leyva, M.J.; Sanchez, K.; Betts, N.M.; Wu, M.; Aston, C.E.; Lyons, T.J. Blueberries decrease cardiovascular risk factors in obese men and women with metabolic syndrome. *J. Nutr.* **2010**, *140*, 1582–1587. [CrossRef] [PubMed]

141. Johnson, S.A.; Figueroa, A.; Navaei, N.; Wong, A.; Kalfon, R.; Ormsbee, L.T.; Feresin, R.G.; Elam, M.L.; Hooshmand, S.; Payton, M.E.; et al. Daily blueberry consumption improves blood pressure and arterial stiffness in postmenopausal women with pre- and stage 1-hypertension: A randomized, double-blind, placebo-controlled clinical trial. *J. Acad. Nutr. Diet.* **2015**, *115*, 369–377. [CrossRef] [PubMed]

142. McAnulty, L.S.; Collier, S.R.; Landram, M.J.; Whittaker, D.S.; Isaacs, S.E.; Klemka, J.M.; Cheek, S.L.; Arms, J.C.; McAnulty, S.R. Six weeks daily ingestion of whole blueberry powder increases natural killer cell counts and reduces arterial stiffness in sedentary males and females. *Nutr. Res.* **2014**, *34*, 577–584. [CrossRef] [PubMed]

143. Riso, P.; Klimis-Zacas, D.; Del, B.C.; Martini, D.; Campolo, J.; Vendrame, S.; Moller, P.; Loft, S.; De Maria, R.; Porrini, M. Effect of a wild blueberry (*Vaccinium angustifolium*) drink intervention on markers of oxidative stress, inflammation and endothelial function in humans with cardiovascular risk factors. *Eur. J. Nutr.* **2013**, *52*, 949–961. [CrossRef] [PubMed]

144. Moazen, S.; Amani, R.; Homayouni, R.A.; Shahbazian, H.; Ahmadi, K.; Taha, J.M. Effects of freeze-dried strawberry supplementation on metabolic biomarkers of atherosclerosis in subjects with type 2 diabetes: A randomized double-blind controlled trial. *Ann. Nutr. Metab.* **2013**, *63*, 256–264. [CrossRef] [PubMed]

145. Alqurashi, R.M.; Galante, L.A.; Rowland, I.R.; Spencer, J.; Commane, D.M. Consumption of a flavonoid-rich acai meal is associated with acute improvements in vascular function and a reduction in total oxidative status in healthy overweight men. *Am. J. Clin. Nutr.* **2016**, *104*, 1227–1235. [CrossRef] [PubMed]

146. Aghababaee, S.K.; Vafa, M.; Shidfar, F.; Tahavorgar, A.; Gohari, M.; Katebi, D.; Mohammadi, V. Effects of blackberry (*Morus nigra* L.) consumption on serum concentration of lipoproteins, apo A-I, apo B, and high-sensitivity-C-reactive protein and blood pressure in dyslipidemic patients. *J. Res. Med. Sci.* **2015**, *20*, 684–691. [PubMed]

147. Zhao, S.; Bomser, J.; Joseph, E.L.; DiSilvestro, R.A. Intakes of apples or apple polyphenols decease plasma values for oxidized low-density lipoprotein/$\beta_2$-glycoprotein I complex. *J. Funct. Foods* **2013**, *5*, 493–497. [CrossRef]

148. Soriano-Maldonado, A.; Hidalgo, M.; Arteaga, P.; de Pascual-Teresa, S.; Nova, E. Effects of regular consumption of vitamin C-rich or polyphenol-rich apple juice on cardiometabolic markers in healthy adults: A randomized crossover trial. *Eur. J. Nutr.* **2014**, *53*, 1645–1657. [CrossRef] [PubMed]

149. Auclair, S.; Chironi, G.; Milenkovic, D.; Hollman, P.C.H.; Renard, C.M.G.C.; Megnien, J.; Gariepy, J.; Paul, J.; Simon, A.; Scalbert, A. The regular consumption of a polyphenol-rich apple does not influence endothelial function: A randomised double-blind trial in hypercholesterolemic adults. *Eur. J. Clin. Nutr.* **2010**, *64*, 1158–1165. [CrossRef] [PubMed]

150. Wang, L.; Bordi, P.L.; Fleming, J.A.; Hill, A.M.; Kris-Etherton, P.M. Effect of a moderate fat diet with and without avocados on lipoprotein particle number, size and subclasses in overweight and obese adults: A randomized, controlled trial. *J. Am. Heart Assoc.* **2015**, *4*, 001355. [CrossRef] [PubMed]

151. Dow, C.A.; Going, S.B.; Chow, H.; Patil, B.S.; Thomson, C.A. The effects of daily consumption of grapefruit on body weight, lipids, and blood pressure in healthy, overweight adults. *Metabolism* **2012**, *61*, 1026–1035. [CrossRef] [PubMed]

152. Figueroa, A.; Wong, A.; Hooshmand, S.; Sanchez-Gonzalez, M.A. Effects of watermelon supplementation on arterial stiffness and wave reflection amplitude in postmenopausal women. *Menopause* **2013**, *20*, 573–577. [CrossRef] [PubMed]

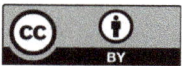

*nutrients*

MDPI

*Article*

# Effects of Epigallocatechin-3-Gallate on Autophagic Lipolysis in Adipocytes

Sang-Nam Kim [1,†], Hyun-Jung Kwon [1,†], Seun Akindehin [1], Hyun Woo Jeong [2] and Yun-Hee Lee [1,*]

[1]  College of Pharmacy, Yonsei Institute of Pharmaceutical Sciences, Yonsei University, Incheon 21983, Korea; sangnamik@nate.com (S.-N.K.); junek0603@gmail.com (H.-J.K.); akindehin@gmail.com (S.A.)
[2]  Vital Beautie Division, Amorepacific R&D Center, 314-1 Bora-dong, Giheung-gu, Yongin-si, Gyeonggi-do 17074, Korea; misterjay@amorepacific.com
*  Correspondence: yunhee.lee@yonsei.ac.kr; Tel.: +82-32-749-4522
†  These authors contributed equally to this work.

Received: 20 May 2017; Accepted: 22 June 2017; Published: 30 June 2017

**Abstract:** Previous studies demonstrated effects of green tea on weight loss; however, green tea-induced modulation of adipocyte function is not fully understood. Here, we investigated effects of the major green tea phytochemical, epigallocatechin-3-gallate (EGCG) on triglyceride contents, lipolysis, mitochondrial function, and autophagy, in adipocytes differentiated from $C_3H_{10}T1/2$ cells and immortalized pre-adipocytes in vitro. EGCG reduced the triglycerol content significantly in adipocytes by 25%, comparable to the nutrient starvation state. EGCG did not affect protein kinase A signaling or brown adipocyte marker expression in adipocytes; however, EGCG increased autophagy, as measured by autophagy flux analysis and immunoblot analysis of LC3B, ATG7, and Beclin1. EGCG treatment reduced mitochondrial membrane potential by 56.8% and intracellular ATP levels by 49.1% compared to controls. Although mammalian target of rapamycin signaling was not upregulated by EGCG treatment, EGCG treatment induced AMP-activated protein kinase phosphorylation, indicating an energy-depleted state. In addition, EGCG increased the association between RAB7 and lipid droplets, suggesting that lipophagy was activated. Finally, knockdown of *Rab7* attenuated the EGCG-dependent reduction in lipid contents. Collectively, these results indicated that EGCG upregulated autophagic lipolysis in adipocytes, supporting the therapeutic potential of EGCG as a caloric restriction mimetic to prevent obesity and obesity-related metabolic diseases.

**Keywords:** green tea; adipocytes; autophagy; epigallocatechin-3-gallate

## 1. Introduction

Green tea is consumed worldwide, and has been shown to have various health benefits [1], including effects on weight loss and metabolic health improvement [2,3] The major bioactive component in green tea is a polyphenolic catechin, epigallocatechin-3 gallate (EGCG) [1], to which the weight loss effects of green tea have been attributed [2]. Although obesity is clearly associated with metabolic syndrome [4], excessive fat mass per se does not appear to be the cause since lipodystrophic patients, who lack adequate fat mass, are also highly insulin resistant [4,5]. Rather, disease occurs when the functions of adipose tissues in metabolic homeostasis are impaired [4].

Adipocytes are a specialized cell type that can store energy in the form of neutral lipids, mainly triglycerides (TGs) [4]. In addition to this anabolic function, breakdown of TGs occur in adipocytes, contributing to mobilization of fatty acids from adipose tissues into circulation and other tissues [6]. Lipolysis can be defined as the hydrolysis of TGs into glycerol and fatty acids, and the three main lipolytic enzymes involved in TG hydrolysis have been identified, namely adipose triglyceride lipase (ATGL), hormone-sensitive lipase (HSL), and monoacylglycerol lipase (MGL) [7]. Lipolysis in adipocytes is controlled primarily by β-adrenergic stimulation [6], which mediates cAMP-dependent protein kinase A (PKA) downstream signaling [7]. In particular, phosphorylation of HSL by PKA increases the enzyme activity and translocation from the cytosol into lipid droplets [7]. Thus, understanding of impact of EGCG on adipocyte lipolysis is important to decipher the molecular mechanisms involved in the beneficial effects of green tea in metabolic health. However, the effects of green tea on adipocyte lipid metabolism have not yet been investigated.

In addition to lipolysis by cytosolic lipases, as mentioned above, autophagy of lipid droplets has been recognized as a complementary pathway for cellular lipid breakdown [8]. Autophagy is a process through which cells consume themselves and is induced by nutrient starvation, calorie restriction, and potential calorie restriction mimetics (CRMs) [9]. Recently, induction of autophagy by EGCG has been investigated in several cell types, including hepatocytes and vascular cells [8]; however, the effects of EGCG on autophagic lipolysis in adipocytes have not been examined.

To investigate the regulatory roles of EGCG in adipocyte lipid metabolism, we examined the effect of EGCG on the metabolic functions of adipocytes differentiated from $C_3H_{10}T1/2$ [10], 3T3-L1, and immortalized pre-adipocytes. We then investigated the role of EGCG in lipid catabolism pathways, including adrenergic activation of lipolysis, induction of brown adipocyte phenotypes, and autophagy-related degradation of lipid droplets in adipocytes. To further investigate the mechanisms by which EGCG reduces lipid contents in adipocytes, the mammalian target of rapamycin (mTOR) and AMP-activated protein kinase (AMPK) signaling pathways were analyzed. Finally, the involvement of autophagic lipolysis in the activation of lipid catabolism by EGCG was investigated by knockdown of *RAB7*, a lipophagy-related gene in adipocytes.

## 2. Materials and Methods

### 2.1. Cell Cultures

$C_3H_{10}T1/2$ cells and 3T3-L1 preadipocytes were obtained from ATCC (Manassas, VA, USA) and cultured, as previously described [11]. Briefly, cells were cultured to confluence in growth medium (Dulbecco's modified Eagle's medium (DMEM: Sigma, St. Louis, MO, USA) supplemented with 10% fetal bovine serum (FBS, Gibco, Thermo Fisher Scientific, Waltham, MA, USA) and 1% penicillin/streptomycin (Welgene, Gyeongsan-s, Gyongsangbuk-do, Korea) at 37 °C in a humidified atmosphere with 5% $CO_2$, and then exposed to adipogenic differentiation medium (DMEM containing BMP4 (20 ng/mL, R&D systems, Minneapolis, MN, USA), 0.125 mM indomethacin (Cayman, Ann Arbor, MI, USA), 2.5 mM isobutylmethylxanthine (IBMX, Cayman, Ann Arbor, MI, USA), 1 uM dexamethasone (Cayman, Ann Arbor, MI, USA), 10 ug/mL insulin (Sigma, St. Louis, MO, USA) and 1 nM triiodothyronine (T3, Cayman, Ann Arbor, MI, USA) for three days. For maintenance of adipogenic differentiation, cells were exposed to DMEM containing 10% FBS, 10 μg/mL insulin (Sigma, St. Louis, MO, USA) and 1 nM triiodothyronine (T3, Cayman, Ann Arbor, MI, USA) for three days.

To prepare immortalized preadipocytes with the potential to become brown adipocytes, interscapular brown adipose tissues were isolated from C57BL/6 mice [12]. Primary preadipocytes were collected in stromovascular factions by collagenase digestion and centrifugation, as previously described [12]. For retrovirus production, viral constructs for SV40 large and small T antigens (plasmid #13970, Addgene, Cambridge, MA, USA) were transfected into phoenix cells using Lipofectamin 2000. Immortalized preadipocytes are expanded in growth medium (DMEM with 10% FBS and 1% penicillin/streptomycin) and differentiated in adipogenic differentiation medium for three days. Cells were maintained in medium containing insulin for up to two weeks.

Fully differentiated adipocytes were exposed to DMEM supplemented with 10% FBS overnight and then treated with indicated concentration of EGCG (purity >95%; Sigma, St. Louis, MO, USA) or quercetin (purity >95%; Sigma, St. Louis, MO, USA). Earle's balanced Salt Solution (EBSS, Thermo Fisher, Waltham, MA, USA) was used for nutrient starvation. 8-bromoadenosine 3'5'-cyclic monophosphate (8-Br-cAMP) was used for PKA activation.

For inhibition of autophagy, chloroquine (an inhibitor of late phase (lysosomal degradation), 50 μM, Sigma, St. Louis, MO, USA) and 3-methyl adenine (3-MA, an inhibitor of early phase, 10 mM, Sigma, St. Louis, MO, USA) were used. Adipocytes were pretreated with inhibitors for 30 min before EGCG treatment.

For Rab7 knockdown, siRNA targeting Rab7 (cat. no. #EMU150241; Sigma, St. Louis, MO, USA) was transfected into adipocytes differentiated from $C_3H_{10}T1/2$ cells, using Lipofectamin2000 (Thermo Fisher, Waltham, MA, USA). Intracellular TG content was determined using a commercially available triglyceride colorimetric assay kit (Cayman Chemicals, Ann Arbor, MI, USA). ATP levels were measured with an ATP Assay Kit (Roche, Indianapolis, IN, USA). For the assays, $C_3H_{10}T1/2$ cells were plated on 12-well plates at a cell density of $10^5$ cells/mL and differentiated into adipocytes, as described above. Cell lysates were prepared in each sample buffer from the assay kit. 10 μL of cell lysate ($4 \times 10^4$ cells/assay) was used for analysis of TG contents, and 25 μL of cell lysate ($10^5$ cells/assay) was used for analysis of ATP levels. Data were normalized based on the protein concentration of the corresponding cell lysate.

## 2.2. Gene Expression Analysis

RNA was extracted using the TRIzol® reagent (Invitrogen, Carlsbad, CA, USA), and 1 μg of RNA was reverse transcribed using a cDNA synthesis kit (High-capacity cDNA Reverse Transcription kit; Applied Biosystems, Foster City, CA, USA). One hundred nanograms of cDNA was subjected to quantitative polymerase chain reaction (qPCR) in 20-μL reaction volumes (iQ SYBR Green Supermix; Bio-Rad, Hercules, CA, USA) with 100 nM primers. qRT-PCR was performed using SYBR Green dye and CFX Connect Real-time system (Bio-Rad, Hercules, CA, USA) for 45 cycles and fold change for all samples was calculated by using the $2^{-\Delta\Delta Ct}$ method. Peptidylprolyl Isomerase A (PPIA) was used as a housekeeping gene for mRNA expression analysis. Primers used for qRT-PCR were described previously [11].

## 2.3. Western Blotting

Protein were extracted in RIPA buffer (Thermo Fisher, Waltham, MA, USA) containing protease (Sigma, St. Louis, MO, USA) and phosphatase Roche, Indianapolis, IN, USA) inhibitors, as previously described [12]. Resolved proteins were transferred to polyvinylidene difluoride (PVDF) membranes, and membranes were blocked for 1 h at room temperature in 5% bovine serum albumin or 5% powdered skim milk in TBST. Then, the membranes were incubated with primary antibodies overnight at 4 °C. Blots were then washed, incubated with a secondary anti-rabbit horseradish peroxidase antibody (diluted 1:5000 in TBST; Cell Signaling Technology, Danvers, MA, USA) for 30 min at room temperature, and visualized with SuperSignal West Dura Substrate (Pierce-Invitrogen, Waltham, MA, USA). The following primary antibodies were used for Western blot analysis: anti-UCP1 (rabbit, Alpha Diagnostic International, San Antonio, TX, USA), anti-cytochrome c oxidase subunit IV (COX IV; rabbit, Cell Signaling, Danvers, MA, USA), phospho-HSL (Ser563, rabbit, Cell Signaling, Danvers, MA, USA), HSL (rabbit, Cell Signaling, Danvers, MA, USA), LC3B (rabbit, Cell Signaling, Danvers, MA, USA), anti-cAMP responsive element binding protein (CREB; rabbit, Cell Signaling, Danvers, MA, USA), phospho-CREB (Ser133, rabbit, Cell Signaling, Danvers, MA, USA), AMPK (rabbit, Cell signaling, Danvers, MA, USA), phospho-AMPK (Thr172, rabbit, Cell Signaling, Danvers, MA, USA), mTOR (rabbit, Cell Signaling, Danvers, MA, USA), phospho-mTOR (Ser2481, rabbit, Cell Signaling, Danvers, MA, USA), PLIN1 (rabbit, Santacruz, Dallas, TA, USA), RAB7 (rabbit, Cell Signaling, Danvers, MA, USA), anti-RAB7 (rabbit, Cell Signaling), anti-ATG7 (rabbit, Cell Signaling, Danvers, MA, USA), anti-BECLIN1 (rabbit, Cell Signaling, Danvers, MA, USA), and a/b tubulin (rabbit, Cell Signaling, Danvers, MA, USA).

*2.4. Analysis of Autophagic Flux*

For autophagic flux analysis, $C_3H_{10}T1/2$ cells were infected with pBABE-puro mCherry-EGFP-LC3B [13] (Plasmid #22418, Addgene, Cambridge, MA, USA, a gift from Jayanta Debnath) by using retrovirus infection as described previously. Autophagic flux was measured by quantifying the pH-sensitive decrease in green fluorescent protein (GFP) intensity over red fluorescent protein (RFP) intensity as an indication of autolysosome formation. For autophagic flux analysis by flow cytometry, analytic cytometry was performed using BD FACSAria III (BD Biosciences, San Jose, CA, USA). Raw data were processed using FlowJo software (Tree Star, Ashland, OR, USA). Alternatively, long-term live-cell imaging was performed every 1 h with IncuCyte ZOOM Live Cell Imaging equipment (Essen Bioscience, Ann Arbor, MI, USA), and the green and red fluorescence intensities of the images were analyzed using ImageJ (imagej.nih.gov, accessed on 1/22/2016).

*2.5. Analysis of Mitochondrial Function*

To measure mitochondrial membrane potential, adipocytes cultured in 24-well plates ($10^5$ cells/well) were incubated with 0.4 µM JC-1 (Sigma, St. Louis, MO, USA) for 30 min. The fluorescence signal was determined by using Tecan microplate reader at 485 nm excitation and 527 nm emission for green fluorescence, and 485 nm excitation and 590 nm emission for red fluorescence. To measure oxygen consumption, adipocytes differentiated from $C_3H_{10}T1/2$ cells ($5 \times 10^6$ cells/assay) were collected in a hypotonic medium containing 120 mM KCl, 5 mM $KH_2PO_4$, 3 mM HEPES, 1 mM EGTA and 1 mM $MgCl_2$ (pH 7.2) at 35 °C. Succinate (10 mM), digitonin (4 µg/mL), adenosine diphosphate (ADP, 1 mM), oligomycinA (0.2 uM), carbonyl cyanide-4-(trifluoromethoxy) phenylhydrazone (FCCP, 0.5 µM) and KCN (0.1 mM) were added sequentially. Oxygen concentrations and oxygen consumption rates were measured by the Oxygraph plus system (Hansatech, Norfolk, UK) with chart recording software. OCRs were normalized according to protein concentrations. Uncoupled respiration was calculated by subtraction of the KCN-induced OCR from the oligomycin A-induced OCR. ATP related respiration was calculated by subtraction of the oligomycin A-induced OCR from the basal OCR.

*2.6. Immunofluorescence Staining*

For immunofluorescence staining, cells were cultured in four-chamber cell culture slides (SPL), fixed with paraformaldehyde (4% in phosphate-buffered saline (PBS)) and subjected to immunocytochemical analysis as previously described [14]. Briefly, fixed cells were incubated with blocking buffer (5% normal goat serum in PBS) and permeabilization buffer (0.5% TritonX100 in PBS) for 30 min at room temperature. The slides were incubated with a primary antibody in blocking buffer overnight at 4 °C, washed, and then incubated with a secondary antibody in blocking buffer for 1 h at room temperature. Antibodies used for immunofluorescence detection were anti-RAB7 antibody (rabbit, 1:100, Cell Signaling, Danvers, MA, USA), PLIN2 (mouse, 1:100, Santacruz, Dallas, TA, USA), and LC3 (rabbit, 1:100, Cell signaling, Danvers, MA, USA). The secondary antibodies used were goat anti-rabbit-Alexa Fluor 488 and goat anti-mouse-Alexa Fluor 594 (1:500, Invitrogen, Carlsbad, CA, USA). For the negative control, primary antibodies were omitted. DAPI (Sigma) was used for nuclear counterstaining. Intracellular neutral lipid was stained with BODIPY® 493/503 (4,4-Difluoro-1,3,5,7,8-Pentamethyl-4-Bora-3a,4a-Diaza-s-Indacene, Thermo Fisher, Waltham, MA, USA) or HCS LipidTox Deep Red Neutral Lipid stain, for cellular imaging.

*2.7. Statistical Analysis*

Statistical analyses were performed using GraphPad Prism 5 software (GraphPad Software, La Jolla, CA, USA). Data are presented as mean ± standard errors of the means (SEMs). Statistical significance between two groups was determined by unpaired *t*-test, as appropriate. Comparisons among multiple groups was performed using a one-way or two-way analysis of variance (ANOVA), with Bonferroni post hoc tests to determine *p* values.

## 3. Results

### 3.1. EGCG Reduced Lipid Content in Adipocytes

To test the effect of EGCG on lipid contents, differentiated adipocytes from $C_3H_{10}T1/2$ cells were treated with EGCG under conditions that activate lipolysis (Figure 1). EGCG was used at concentration of 10 μM according to previous works [13]. Then 8Br-cAMP was used as a positive control that activates PKA and downstream events, including lipolysis. In addition, we included nutrient starvation medium. As expected, nutrient starvation and 8Br-cAMP treatment reduced neutral lipid contents significantly, as measured by BODIPY staining in live cells (Figure 1A) and reduced their intracellular TG contents (Figure 1B). EGCG reduced the neutral lipid TG content significantly, and this reduction was comparable with the levels in the nutrient starvation state (Figure 1A,B). The size of the lipid droplets (LDs) was also reduced in adipocytes treated with EGCG (Figure 1C: mean diameters of LDs: control (CTL) = 3.59 μm; EGCG = 2.72 μm; starvation = 2.62 μm; cAMP = 2.22 μm). PKA signaling is a well-known pathway that activates lipolysis in adipocytes [7,14]; therefore, we examined phosphorylation of the PKA downstream target proteins that are involved in upregulation of lipolysis: hormone sensitive lipase (HSL) and cAMP response element-binding protein (CREB). HSL is a primary lipolytic enzyme responsible for hydrolysis of diacylglycerol in adipocytes [7]. CREB is a transcription factor that can be activated by phosphorylation of the Ser133 residue by PKA activation and upregulates the expression of HSL as a downstream target [15]. We found that 8Br-cAMP increased the phosphorylation levels of HSL and CREB significantly (by three-fold and four-fold, respectively) compared with control conditions (Figure 1D,E). However, neither starvation nor EGCG treatment increased the phosphorylation levels. Interestingly, expression of HSL was significantly higher in the EGCG-treated groups than in the controls. The data suggested that EGCG reduced the lipid contents effectively in adipocytes; however, this phenomenon is independent of PKA signaling.

### 3.2. Effects of EGCG on Browning of Adipocytes

Non-shivering thermogenesis via uncoupling protein 1 (UCP1) expression in brown adipocytes is one of the mechanisms that activates catabolic metabolism to reduce the lipid content. Although it has been suggested that in vivo thermogenesis can be stimulated by green tea extract treatment (by upregulation of sympathetic tones) [16], the direct effects of EGCG on browning of white adipocytes has not been investigated. Therefore, we evaluated the effects of EGCG on browning of adipocytes differentiated from $C_3H_{10}T1/2$ cells (Figure 2A,B). In addition to EGCG, quercetin was tested because its browning effect has been reported previously [17].

EGCG treatment upregulated the UCP1 protein level by 2 fold (Figure 2A). However, the transcript levels of *UCP1* were not significantly induced by EGCG treatment (Figure 2B). In addition, Ucp1 mRNA levels were 300,000-fold lower than those in in vivo brown adipocytes (i.e., $C_3H_{10}T1/2$ *Ucp1* (% of *PPIA*) $0.01 \pm 0.005$ vs. BAT *Ucp1* (% of *PPIA*) = $3287 \pm 1100$, $n = 6$). Similarly, EGCG did not increase a brown adipocyte marker (*Dio2*) and genes involved in mitochondrial metabolism (i.e., *Ppargc1a, Acdam, Cox8b, Ucp2*) expression in adipocytes differentiated from $C_3H_{10}T1/2$ cells (Figure 2B). Analysis of oxygen consumption rate demonstrated that EGCG treatment did not affect either ATP-linked respiration or uncoupled respiration (Figure 2C,D). This suggested that upregulation of UCP1 expression or mitochondrial respiration does not seem to be a major contributor to the loss of lipids.

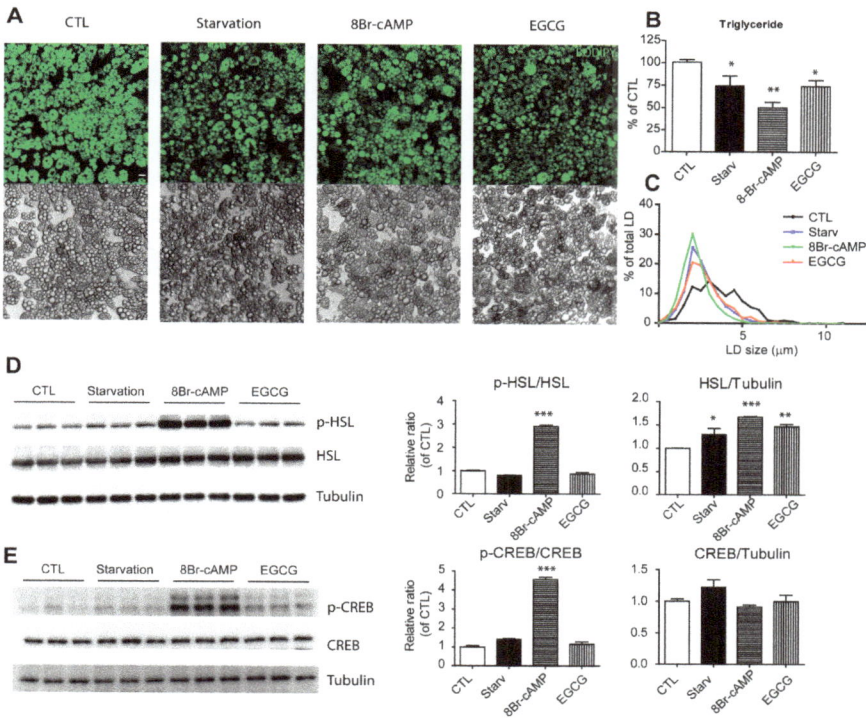

**Figure 1.** Effects of EGCG on lipid content and PKA signaling in adipocytes (**A–C**) BODIPY staining (**A**), intracellular triglyceride levels (**B**), dimeters of lipid droplets (**C**) in adipocyte differentiated from $C_3H_{10}T1/2$ cells treated with starvation medium, 8Br-cAMP (1 mM) and EGCG (10 μM) for 24 h (**D,E**) Immunoblot analysis of p-HSL, HSL, p-CREB, and CREB in adipocyte differentiated from $C_3H_{10}T1/2$ cells treated with starvation medium, 8Br-cAMP (1 mM) and EGCG (10 μM) for 24 h. *p* values were calculated using the two-tailed unpaired *t*-test (*n* = 3, means ± SE; * *p* < 0.05, ** *p* < 0.01, *** *p* < 0.001).

To test whether the minimal effect of UCP1 expression in adipocytes is related to cell type-specific gene expression machinery, we tested the effect of EGCG on brown adipocyte cell lines and 3T3L1 cells. We established brown adipocyte cell lines by immortalization of preadipocytes isolated from mouse interscapular BAT. As shown in Figure 3A, expression of UCP1 protein was confirmed in adipocytes differentiated from immortalized brown preadipocytes (Figure 3A). Ucp1 mRNA expression was approximately 1000 fold higher in the brown adipocytes, compared to the levels in 3T3L1 and $C_3H_{10}T1/2$ (Figure 3B). The gene expression patterns in adipocytes differentiated from 3T3L1 were similar to adipocytes from $C_3H_{10}T1/2$ cells resembling white adipocyte phenotypes (Figure 2B,C). In addition, EGCG did not increase Ucp1 expression and other genes involved in mitochondrial functions in brown adipocytes significantly (Figure 2D,E), which indicated that EGCG is not a thermogenic signal for the activation of brown adipocyte metabolism.

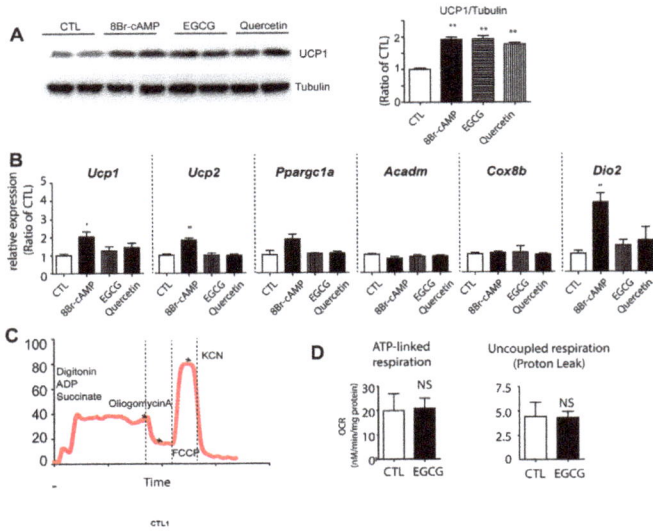

**Figure 2.** Effects of EGCG on brown adipocyte marker expression in adipocyte cultures. Immunoblot analysis of UCP1 expression (**A**) and quantitative PCR analysis (**B**) of genes involved in mitochondrial metabolism and brown adipocyte markers in adipocytes differentiated from $C_3H_{10}T1/2$ treated with 8Br-cAMP (1 mM), EGCG (10 μM) and quercetin (10 μM) for 24 h (**C,D**) Analysis of oxygen consumption of adipocytes differentiated from $C_3H_{10}T1/2$ cells treated with EGCG for 24 h; (**C**) An example of analysis of oxygen consumption rate (OCR) with a series of treatments of indicated drugs; (**D**) Comparisons of ATP-linked respiration and uncoupled respiration between cells treated with EGCG and vehicle controls. $p$ values were calculated using the two-tailed unpaired $t$-test ($n$ = 3, means ± SE; * $p < 0.05$, ** $p < 0.01$).

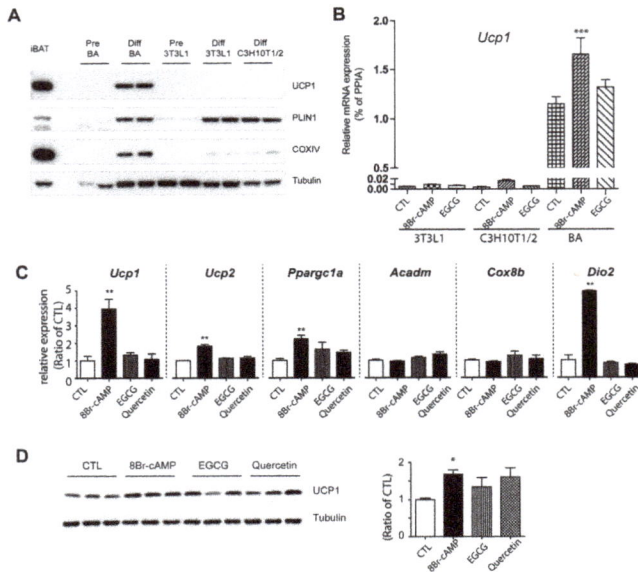

**Figure 3.** *Cont.*

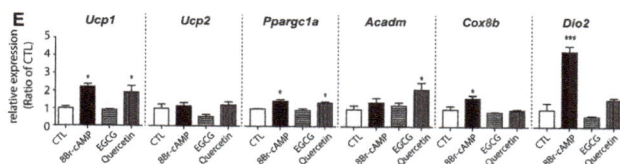

**Figure 3.** Establishment of BA cell lines and effects of EGCG on brown adipocyte marker expression in adipocyte cultures. Immunoblot analysis of UCP1, perilipin1 (PLIN1), and COXIV expression (**A**) and quantitative PCR analysis of UCP1 expression (**B**) in adipocytes differentiated from 3T3L1, $C_3H_{10}T1/2$, and immortalized preadipocytes isolated from iBAT. Two-way ANOVA revealed significant main effects of treatment ($p = 0.0165$) and cell types ($p < 0.0001$) in UCP1 expression and significant interaction of treatment and cell types ($p = 0.0060$). Significant differences between control and treated group were determined by post-hoc pairwise comparison with Bonferroni correction (mean ± SEM; $n = 4$ per condition, ***$p < 0.001$). (**C**) Quantitative PCR analysis of brown adipocyte gene expression in adipocytes differentiated from 3T3L1 treated with 8Br-cAMP (1 mM), EGCG (10 μM) and quercetin (10 μM) for 24 h. Immunoblot analysis of UCP1 expression (**D**) and quantitative PCR analysis (**E**) of brown adipocyte gene expression in adipocytes differentiated from BA cell lines treated with 8Br-cAMP (1 mM), EGCG (10 μM) and quercetin (10 μM) for 24 h. $p$ values were calculated using the two-tailed unpaired $t$-test ($n = 3$, means ± SE; * $p < 0.05$, ** $p < 0.01$, *** $p < 0.001$).

### 3.3. Effect of EGCG on Autophagy

EGCG reduced the lipid content in adipocytes without activation of HSL and PKA signaling; thus, we hypothesized that EGCG activates an alternative pathway to consume lipids. Autophagy has been reported as a novel regulator of lipolysis [8], acting as a lysosomal lipolytic pathway; therefore, we examined autophagic responses after EGCG treatment. Differentiated adipocytes from $C_3H_{10}T1/2$ cells were grown in nutrient starvation medium, and standard growth medium containing EGCG or 8-Br-cAMP. To measure autophagic flux, conversion of LC3B-I into LC3B-II was determined by Western blotting analysis. As shown in Figure 4A, an increased ratio of LC3B-II to LC3B-I was observed in all three conditions, including EGCG and 8Br-cAMP treatment. Interestingly, 8Br-cAMP treatment (i.e., PKA activation) increased LC3B-II generation to levels similar to that induced by starvation (Figure 4A). EGCG treatment increased other autophagy markers, Beclin1 and ATG7 expression (Figure S1). Treatment with chloroquine, an inhibitor of lysosomal degradation, increased accumulation of LC3bII in control and EGCG-treated groups, while 3-MA reduced LC3BII. In agreement with the immunoblotting analysis, immunofluorescence staining of adipocytes treated with EGCG showed punctuated patterns of LC3B staining (Figure 4B), which is a prominent feature of autophagy. In addition, EGCG increased the association between RAB7 and lipid droplets, indicating activation of lipophagy (Figure 4B). Next, autophagic flux was measured using LC3 tandemly tagged with fluorescent proteins that detect lysosomal degradation [18] in $C_3H_{10}T1/2$ cells. This system expresses a chimeric LC3 fused with eGFP and mCherry; thus, the pH-sensitive decrease in GFP intensity over RFP intensity indicates autolysosome formation. As shown in Figure 4C, long-term live cell imaging demonstrated that EGCG treatment induced a decrease in the green and red fluorescence intensity ratio during the course of the treatment (Figure 5C,D). Furthermore, flow cytometry analysis confirmed the decrease in green fluorescent intensity by EGCG treatment (Figure 3E). Collectively, analyses of the autophagic response supported the induction of autophagy by EGCG.

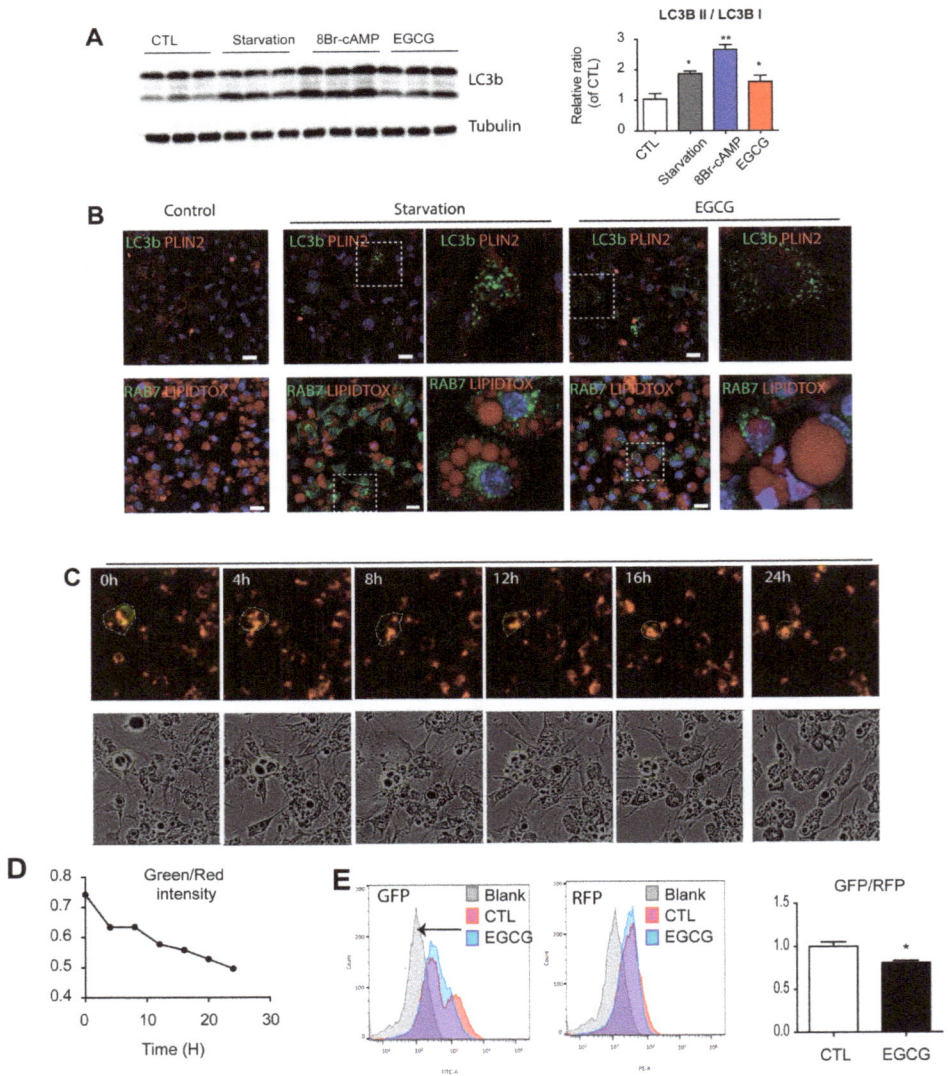

**Figure 4.** Effects of EGCG on autophagy responses in adipocytes. (**A**) Immunoblot analysis of LC3b expression in adipocytes differentiated from $C_3H_{10}T1/2$ treated with starvation medium, 8Br-cAMP (1 mM) and EGCG (10 μM) for 1 day. *p* values were calculated using the two-tailed unpaired *t*-test ($n$ = 3, means ± SE; * $p$ < 0.05, ** $p$ < 0.01); (**B**) Immunofluorescence staining of LC3b/PLIN2 or RAB7/LipidTox in adipocytes differentiated from $C_3H_{10}T1/2$ treated with 8Br-cAMP (1 mM) and EGCG (10 μM) for 24 h. Nuclei were counterstained with DAPI. Bars = 20 μm; (**C**) Representative images from long-term live imaging of adipocytes expressing LC3B-GFP-RFP reporters treated with EGCG; (**D**) Time course analysis of GFP/RFP ratio from (**C**); (**E**) Flow cytometric analysis of adipocytes expressing LC3B-GPF-RFP reporters treated with ECGC.

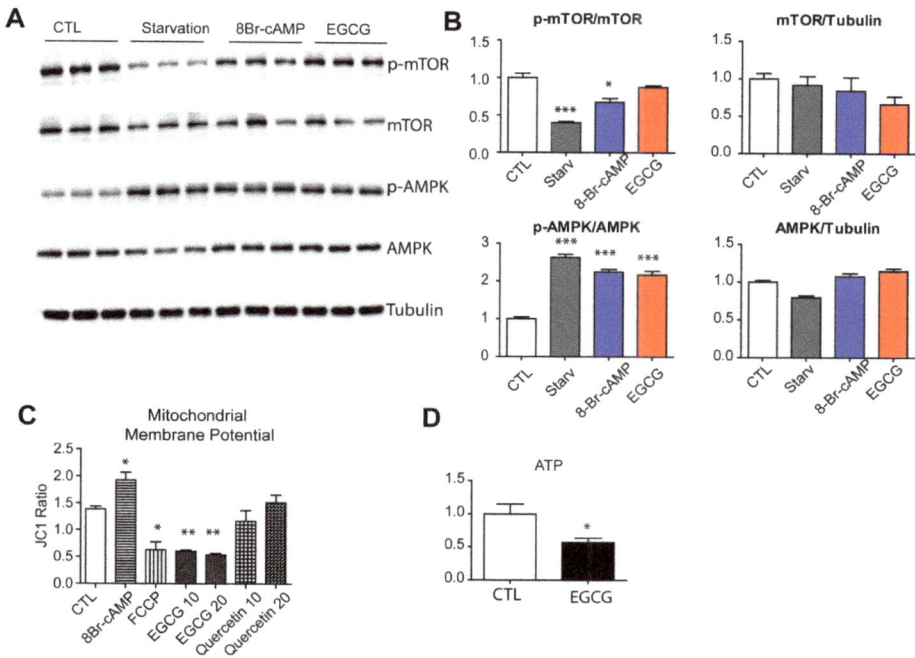

**Figure 5.** Effects of EGCG on activation of mTOR and AMPK in adipocytes. (**A,B**) Immunoblot analysis of phosphorylation of mTOR and AMPK in adipocytes differentiated from $C_3H_{10}T1/2$ treated with starvation medium, 8Br-cAMP (1 mM) and EGCG (10 μM) for 24 h. Mitochondrial membrane potential (**C**), and intracellular ATP (**D**) in adipocytes differentiated from $C_3H_{10}T1/2$ treated with 8Br-cAMP (1 mM), FCCP (0.5 μM), EGCG (10 or 20 μM) or quercetin (10 or 20 μM) for 2 h. *p* values were calculated using the two-tailed unpaired *t*-test ($n = 3$, means ± SE; * $p < 0.05$, ** $p < 0.01$, *** $p < 0.001$).

Autophagy can be activated by various extracellular and intracellular stimuli. Importantly, starvation can lead to inhibition of the mammalian target of rapamycin (mTOR) pathway, which is known as a nutrient sensing signaling pathway. To test whether EGCG mimics starvation by inhibiting of mTOR signaling, we examined the phosphorylation levels of mTOR using Western blotting. As shown in Figure 5A, starvation conditions and 8Br-cAMP treatment reduced mTOR phosphorylation significantly; however, EGCG treatment did not affect p-mTOR or total mTOR levels. AMP-activated protein kinase (AMPK) can directly phosphorylate UNC-51-Like kinase 1 (ULK1), a key regulator of autophagy induction during energy starvation; thus, we examined p-AMPK levels [15]. Starvation, 8Br-cAMP, and EGCG treatment increased the phosphorylation of AMPK, indicating depleted intracellular energy levels. Mitochondrial oxidative phosphorylation is the major pathway of ATP generation; thus, we examined the mitochondrial membrane potential. The data indicated that the membrane potential was reduced by EGCG treatment while it was increased by 8Br-cAMP treatment (Figure 5C). Consistent with this signaling status, EGCG treatment reduced intracellular ATP levels in adipocytes (Figure 5D).

Lipophagy has been described as a form of autophagy that is specialized for the degradation of lipid droplets, and RAB7 was reported as a key molecule that enables the specific recognition of LD proteins in the process of lipophagy [19]. Autophagy related genes, including *Rab7*, could affect the differentiation of adipocytes [20]; therefore, we silenced *Rab7* to transiently knockdown its expression using a siRNA after full differentiation. siRNA transfection knocked down *Rab7* expression by 45% compared with negative controls using a scrambled sequence (Figure 6A). As indicated in

Figure 6B, *Rab7* knockdown attenuated the reduction in the lipid content induced by EGCG treatment in adipocytes.

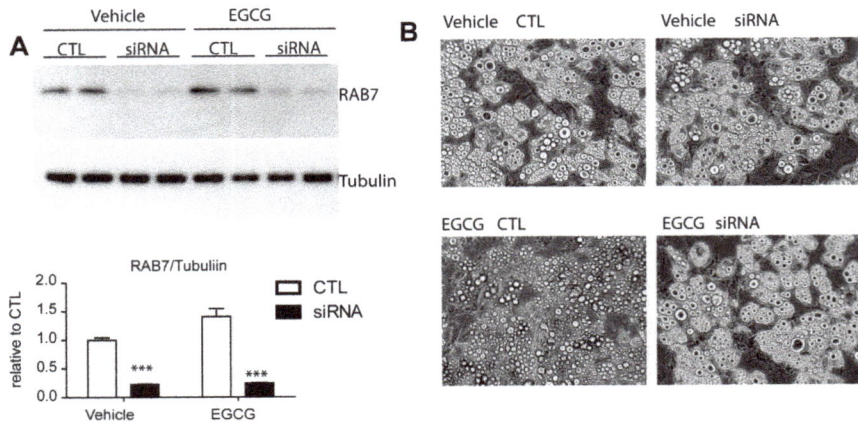

**Figure 6.** Effects of knockdown of RAB7 on EGCG induced reduction in lipid content in adipocytes. (**A**) Immunoblot analysis of RAB7 in adipocytes differentiated from $C_3H_{10}T1/2$ treated with siRNA or scrambled sequence controls. Two-way ANOVA revealed significant main effects of siRNA knockdown ($p < 0.0001$) and EGCG treatment ($p = 0.0122$) in RAB7 expression and significant interaction of siRNA knockdown and EGCG treatment ($p = 0.0206$). Significant differences between control and siRNA were determined by post-hoc pairwise comparison with Bonferroni correction (mean ± SEM; $n = 4$ per condition, *** $p < 0.001$) (**B**) Representative images of adipocytes differentiated from $C_3H_{10}T1/2$ treated with vehicle or EGCG (10 µM) for 24 h. ($n = 4$, means ± SE; *** $p < 0.001$).

## 4. Discussion

Metabolic disease is a multifactorial disease and the numerous health benefits of green tea, including its weight loss effects, have been proposed to have application in the prevention and/or treatment of obesity-related metabolic disease [21]. Among the various bioactive constituents in green tea, the polyphenolic catechin EGCG has been proposed to exert a weight loss effect [2,3,21]; however, the regulatory role of EGCG in adipocyte lipid metabolism remains unclear. In this study, we examined the direct effects of EGCG on adipocyte metabolism using in vitro adipocyte cultures, including its effects on lipolysis, thermogenic marker expression, mitochondrial metabolism, and autophagy. We demonstrated that EGCG reduced lipid contents by activating autophagy, partly via a reduction in intracellular ATP levels, mimicking the energy-depleted state.

The central finding in the current study was the demonstration of EGCG-induced autophagic lipolysis in adipocytes. Although this is not the first study to report the effects of EGCG on adipocyte function; previous works have focused on the inhibitory effects of EGCG on adipogenesis [22,23] but not on adipocyte lipid catabolism. The involvement of lipophagy in the clearance of lipid droplets has been investigated in several cell types, including hepatocytes and vascular cells [8]; however, the involvement of EGCG in the direct activation of lipophagy in adipocytes has not been investigated. The in vivo effects of EGCG on the autophagic lipolysis of adipose tissue were not addressed in this study, and further studies are required. In support of the effects of EGCG on weight loss, in vivo effects of green tea in mouse models have been shown to be related to the role of EGCG in the upregulation of sympathetic nervous system activity, leading to increased energy consumption, thermogenesis, and fat oxidation [21].

In this study, we found that lipophagy was an alternative pathway to reduce lipid contents without downstream activation of PKA and that EGCG could activate this process. Our findings also suggested that lipophagy activation in adipocytes could be involved in mediating the weight loss effects of EGCG. According to a previous pharmacokinetic analysis of green tea [24], the peak concentration of EGCG in the blood reaches 326 ng/mL after a single dose (4.5 g) of green tea consumption. Considering the high concentration of EGCG (10 μM) used in this study, further studies are required for the extrapolation of in vitro data to the in vivo situation, such as dose-response curves with lower doses and analysis of the tissue distribution of EGCG. Such studies will allow us to determine whether induction of autophagic lipolysis by EGCG can be achieved by green tea consumption or pharmacologic treatment with EGCG.

Under fasting conditions, stimulation of catecholamine release into systemic circulation is considered a major catabolic signal promoting the increase of lipid mobilization from adipocytes. In this study, we examined the effects of nutrient starvation on adipocyte lipid metabolism separately from catecholamine-stimulated β-adrenergic signaling. As expected, nutrient starvation increased autophagy and lipophagy to reduce the lipid content, without catecholamine-stimulated lipolysis. These data supported the view that the response of adipocytes to nutrient scarcity is integrated and coordinated at the organismal level via intrinsic cell properties and hormonal signals. Interestingly, the cAMP analog increased the levels of autophagy, and upregulation of mTOR signaling, and AMPK activation stimulated the autophagic response. Although not investigated in this study, determining the mechanism of PKA signaling in the induction of autophagy would be informative for subsequent studies of adipocyte metabolism.

The mechanisms of autophagy induction have been investigated intensively in various research areas related to chronic disease. In this study, we showed that reduction of ATP synthesis was the major initiating stimulus for autophagy induction by EGCG. Consistent with our observations, previous studies have reported that ATP synthase activity could be inhibited by resveratrol, several antioxidant flavonoids, and polyphenolic catechins, including EGCG [25].

The development of CRM is a promising approach to prevent aging and obesity-related metabolic diseases. In this regard, natural/pharmacological autophagy inducers have been investigated as CRMs that share molecular mechanisms of health improvement with calorie restriction [9]. In this regard, EGCG has been recognized as a CRM with acetyltransferase inhibitor activity [26]. Our findings demonstrated that EGCG induced autophagic lipolysis to reduce the lipid contents in adipocytes by inhibiting mitochondrial oxidative phosphorylation, and further supported the beneficial effects of EGCG as a CRM. Our results suggested that the adipocyte-specific effects of CRMs deserve further investigation as more favorable therapeutic targets for the reduction of adipocyte mass. Furthermore, investigation of the mechanisms involved in the specific lysosomal degradation of lipid droplets in adipocytes by other CRMs would lead to the identification of novel targets for drug discovery and CRMs.

**Supplementary Materials:** The following are available online at www.mdpi.com/2072-6643/9/7/680/s1, Figure S1: Effects of EGCG on autophagy responses in adipocytes.

**Acknowledgments:** This research was supported by the National Research Foundation of Korea (grant no. NRF-2014R1A6A3A04056472 to YHL). This work was performed within the program of the AMOREPACIFIC Open Research 'ORT19-01-16E705001' supported by a grant from AMOREPACIFIC.

**Author Contributions:** Y.H.L. conceived and designed the study. H.J.K., S.N.K., S.A., H.W.J. and Y.H.L. conducted the experiments, and H.J.K., S.N.K. and Y.H.L. analyzed the results. Y.H.L. wrote the manuscript. All authors reviewed the manuscript.

**Conflicts of Interest:** The authors declare that they have no conflict of interest.

## References

1. Reto, M.; Figueira, M.E.; Filipe, H.M.; Almeida, C.M. Chemical composition of green tea (Camellia sinensis) infusions commercialized in Portugal. *Plant Foods Hum. Nutr.* **2007**, *62*, 139–144. [CrossRef] [PubMed]
2. Thielecke, F.; Boschmann, M. The potential role of green tea catechins in the prevention of the metabolic syndrome—A review. *Phytochemistry* **2009**, *70*, 11–24. [CrossRef] [PubMed]

3. Hursel, R.; Viechtbauer, W.; Westerterp-Plantenga, M.S. The effects of green tea on weight loss and weight maintenance: A meta-analysis. *Int. J. Obes.* **2009**, *33*, 956–961. [CrossRef] [PubMed]

4. Gesta, S.; Tseng, Y.H.; Kahn, C.R. Developmental origin of fat: Tracking obesity to its source. *Cell* **2007**, *131*, 242–256. [CrossRef] [PubMed]

5. Fiorenza, C.G.; Chou, S.H.; Mantzoros, C.S. Lipodystrophy: Pathophysiology and advances in treatment. *Nat. Rev. Endocrinol.* **2011**, *7*, 137–150. [CrossRef] [PubMed]

6. Langin, D. Adipose tissue lipolysis as a metabolic pathway to define pharmacological strategies against obesity and the metabolic syndrome. *Pharmacol. Res.* **2006**, *53*, 482–491. [CrossRef] [PubMed]

7. Duncan, R.E.; Ahmadian, M.; Jaworski, K.; Sarkadi-Nagy, E.; Sul, H.S. Regulation of lipolysis in adipocytes. *Annu. Rev. Nutr.* **2007**, *27*, 79–101. [CrossRef] [PubMed]

8. Cingolani, F.; Czaja, M.J. Regulation and functions of autophagic lipolysis. *Trends Endocrinol. Metab.* **2016**, *27*, 696–705. [CrossRef] [PubMed]

9. Marino, G.; Pietrocola, F.; Madeo, F.; Kroemer, G. Caloric restriction mimetics: Natural/physiological pharmacological autophagy inducers. *Autophagy* **2014**, *10*, 1879–1882. [CrossRef] [PubMed]

10. Tseng, Y.-H.; Kokkotou, E.; Schulz, T.J.; Huang, T.L.; Winnay, J.N.; Taniguchi, C.M.; Tran, T.T.; Suzuki, R.; Espinoza, D.O.; Yamamoto, Y.; et al. New role of bone morphogenetic protein 7 in brown adipogenesis and energy expenditure. *Nature* **2008**, *454*, 1000–1004. [CrossRef] [PubMed]

11. Lee, Y.H.; Kim, S.N.; Kwon, H.J.; Maddipati, K.R.; Granneman, J.G. Adipogenic role of alternatively activated macrophages in beta-adrenergic remodeling of white adipose tissue. *Am. J. Physiol. Regul. Integr. Comp. Physiol.* **2016**, *310*, R55–R65. [CrossRef] [PubMed]

12. Lee, Y.H.; Petkova, A.P.; Konkar, A.A.; Granneman, J.G. Cellular origins of cold-induced brown adipocytes in adult mice. *FASEB J.* **2015**, *29*, 286–299. [CrossRef] [PubMed]

13. Kim, H.S.; Montana, V.; Jang, H.J.; Parpura, V.; Kim, J.A. Epigallocatechin gallate (EGCG) stimulates autophagy in vascular endothelial cells: A potential role for reducing lipid accumulation. *J. Biol. Chem.* **2013**, *288*, 22693–22705. [CrossRef] [PubMed]

14. Nielsen, T.S.; Jessen, N.; Jorgensen, J.O.; Moller, N.; Lund, S. Dissecting adipose tissue lipolysis: Molecular regulation and implications for metabolic disease. *J. Mol. Endocrinol.* **2014**, *52*, R199–R222. [CrossRef] [PubMed]

15. Choi, A.M.K.; Ryter, S.W.; Levine, B. Autophagy in human health and disease. *N. Engl. J. Med.* **2013**, *368*, 651–662. [CrossRef] [PubMed]

16. Gosselin, C.; Haman, F. Effects of green tea extracts on non-shivering thermogenesis during mild cold exposure in young men. *Br. J. Nutr.* **2013**, *110*, 282–288. [CrossRef] [PubMed]

17. Arias, N.; Pico, C.; Teresa Macarulla, M.; Oliver, P.; Miranda, J.; Palou, A.; Portillo, M.P. A combination of resveratrol and quercetin induces browning in white adipose tissue of rats fed an obesogenic diet. *Obesity* **2017**, *25*, 111–121. [CrossRef] [PubMed]

18. N'Diaye, E.N.; Kajihara, K.K.; Hsieh, I.; Morisaki, H.; Debnath, J.; Brown, E.J. Plic proteins or ubiquilins regulate autophagy-dependent cell survival during nutrient starvation. *EMBO Rep.* **2009**, *10*, 173–179. [CrossRef] [PubMed]

19. Schroeder, B.; Schulze, R.J.; Weller, S.G.; Sletten, A.C.; Casey, C.A.; McNiven, M.A. The small GTPase Rab7 as a central regulator of hepatocellular lipophy. *Hepatology* **2015**, *61*, 1896–1907. [CrossRef] [PubMed]

20. Singh, R.; Xiang, Y.; Wang, Y.; Baikati, K.; Cuervo, A.M.; Luu, Y.K.; Tang, Y.; Pessin, J.E.; Schwartz, G.J.; Czaja, M.J. Autophagy regulates adipose mass and differentiation in mice. *J. Clin. Investig.* **2009**, *119*, 3329–3339. [CrossRef] [PubMed]

21. Rains, T.M.; Agarwal, S.; Maki, K.C. Antiobesity effects of green tea catechins: A mechanistic review. *J. Nutr. Biochem.* **2011**, *22*, 1–7. [CrossRef] [PubMed]

22. Tang, W.; Song, H.; Cai, W.; Shen, X. Real time monitoring of inhibition of adipogenesis and angiogenesis by (−)-epigallocatechin-3-gallate in 3T3-L1 adipocytes and human umbilical vein endothelial cells. *Nutrients* **2015**, *7*, 8871–8886. [CrossRef] [PubMed]

23. Lin, J.; Della-Fera, M.A.; Baile, C.A. Green tea polyphenol epigalocatechin gallate inhibits adipogenesis and induces apoptosis in 3T3-L1 adipocytes. *Obes. Res.* **2005**, *13*, 982–990. [CrossRef] [PubMed]

24. Yang, C.S.; Chen, L.; Lee, M.J.; Balentine, D.; Kuo, M.C.; Schantz, S.P. Blood and urine levels of tea catechins after ingestion of different amounts of green tea by human volunteers. *Cancer Epidemiol. Biomark. Prev.* **1998**, *7*, 351–354.

25.  Zheng, J.; Ramirez, V.D. Inhibition of mitochondrial proton F0F1-ATPase/ATP synthase by polyphenolic phytochemicals. *Br. J. Pharmacol.* **2000**, *130*, 1115–1123. [CrossRef] [PubMed]

26.  Choi, K.C.; Jung, M.G.; Lee, Y.H.; Yoon, J.C.; Kwon, S.H.; Kang, H.B.; Kim, M.J.; Cha, J.H.; Kim, Y.J.; Jun, W.J.; et al. Epigallocatechin-3-gallate, a histone acetyltransferase inhibitor, inhibits EBV-induced B lymphocyte transformation via suppression of RelA acetylation. *Cancer Res.* **2009**, *69*, 583–592. [CrossRef] [PubMed]

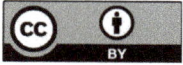

*nutrients*

MDPI

*Review*

# Dietary Natural Products for Prevention and Treatment of Breast Cancer

Ya Li [1], Sha Li [2,*], Xiao Meng [1], Ren-You Gan [3], Jiao-Jiao Zhang [1] and Hua-Bin Li [1,4,*]

[1] Guangdong Provincial Key Laboratory of Food, Nutrition and Health, Department of Nutrition, School of Public Health, Sun Yat-Sen University, Guangzhou 510080, China; liya28@mail2.sysu.edu.cn (Y.L.); mengx7@mail2.sysu.edu.cn (X.M.); zhangjj46@mail2.sysu.edu.cn (J.-J.Z.)

[2] School of Chinese Medicine, Li Ka Shing Faculty of Medicine, The University of Hong Kong, Hong Kong 999077, China

[3] School of Biological Sciences, The University of Hong Kong, Hong Kong 999077, China; ganry@connect.hku.hk

[4] South China Sea Bioresource Exploitation and Utilization Collaborative Innovation Center, Sun Yat-Sen University, Guangzhou 510006, China

* Correspondence: u3003781@connect.hku.hk (S.L.); lihuabin@mail.sysu.edu.cn (H.-B.L.); Tel.: +852-3917-6498 (S.L.); +86-20-8733-2391 (H.-B.L.)

Received: 29 April 2017; Accepted: 30 June 2017; Published: 8 July 2017

**Abstract:** Breast cancer is the most common cancer among females worldwide. Several epidemiological studies suggested the inverse correlation between the intake of vegetables and fruits and the incidence of breast cancer. Substantial experimental studies indicated that many dietary natural products could affect the development and progression of breast cancer, such as soy, pomegranate, mangosteen, citrus fruits, apple, grape, mango, cruciferous vegetables, ginger, garlic, black cumin, edible macro-fungi, and cereals. Their anti-breast cancer effects involve various mechanisms of action, such as downregulating ER-α expression and activity, inhibiting proliferation, migration, metastasis and angiogenesis of breast tumor cells, inducing apoptosis and cell cycle arrest, and sensitizing breast tumor cells to radiotherapy and chemotherapy. This review summarizes the potential role of dietary natural products and their major bioactive components in prevention and treatment of breast cancer, and special attention was paid to the mechanisms of action.

**Keywords:** breast cancer; soy; fruit; vegetable; anticancer; mechanism of action

## 1. Introduction

Globally, breast cancer is the most commonly diagnosed cancer and the major cause of cancer-related death among females [1]. In the United States alone, there are 255,180 new cases of breast cancer and 41,070 deaths projected to occur in 2017 [2]. Breast cancer is generally categorized into estrogen receptor (ER)-positive (such as MCF-7 and T47D cell lines) and ER-negative (such as MDA-MB-231, MDA-MB-468, SKBR3 and MDA-MB-453 cell lines) breast cancer. By using more biomarkers such as progesterone receptor (PR), and human epidermal growth factor receptor 2 (HER2), breast cancer is further divided into several molecular subtypes, such as luminal A, luminal B, basal-like and HER2-positive ones [3,4]. Basal-like breast cancer is also considered as triple-negative breast cancer (TNBC) in some cases, because TNBC is characterized as lacking the expression of these three biomarkers [5]. These distinct subtypes of breast tumor would response differently to treatment, which made breast cancer extremely intractable. Currently, surgical resection, adjuvant chemotherapy, radiotherapy and hormone therapy represent the main treatment options for early-stage breast cancer [6]. However, the development of drug resistance and major side effects has weakened the efficacy of these therapies [7,8]. Besides, triple-negative breast cancer does not respond to hormone therapy [9]. This situation urges the research of finding more effective prevention and treatment strategies with fewer side effects for breast cancer. Many exogenous and endogenous factors could affect the onset and development of breast cancer. Exogenous factors include reproductive, environmental and lifestyle factors, such as early menarche [10], nulliparity, oral contraceptive use [11], parity and lactation (never having or short duration of breast feeding) [12,13], use of hormone replacement therapy [14], alcohol consumption [15], diabetes [16,17], obesity [18], and night work (circadian disruption) [19]. Genetic risk factors, such as mutations on breast cancer susceptibility gene 1 (BRCA1) and BRCA2, only account for approximately 5–10% of all breast cancer incidences [20]. Therefore, the prevention of breast cancer is highly crucial.

Diet and nutrition have been considered as an effective preventive strategy for cancer. A bunch of dietary natural products have shown a potential role in prevention and treatment of cancers [21–26]. A recently published meta-analysis, which included 93 studies, pointed out that results on breast cancer were among the few reaching a convincing evidence of a protective effect of healthy dietary pattern and cancer risk, and the effect was especially prominent in postmenopausal, hormone receptor–negative women [27]. Furthermore, various epidemiological studies suggested that consumption of soy products, fruits, and vegetables (especially cruciferous vegetables) are associated with reduced risk of breast cancer [28,29], and high consumption of some dietary natural products might reduce the recurrence and increase the survival rate of breast cancer [30,31]. In addition, experimental studies indicated that many dietary natural products and their bioactive components showed inhibitory effects on breast cancer (Figure 1), through downregulating ER-α expression and activity, inhibiting proliferation, metastasis and angiogenesis of breast tumor cells, inducing apoptosis and cell cycle arrest, and sensitizing breast tumor cells to radiotherapy and chemotherapy [32–35]. Therefore, use of naturally occurring dietary substances could be a practical approach to prevention and treatment of breast cancer [36]. The objective of this review is to summarize the role of dietary natural products and their bioactive compounds in the prevention and treatment of breast cancer, and discuss the mechanisms of action.

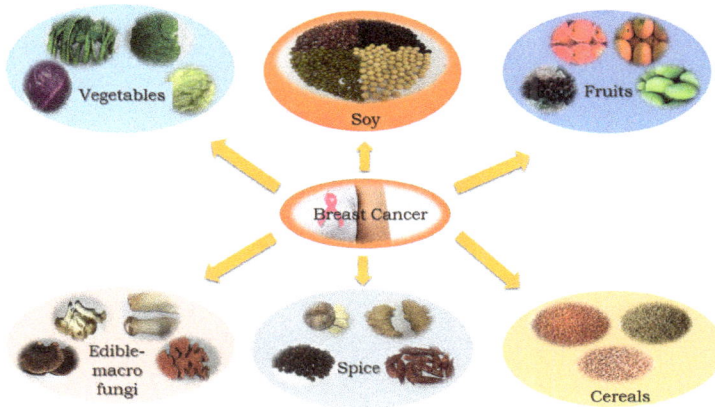

**Figure 1.** Dietary natural products that showed inhibitory effects on breast cancer.

## 2. Soy

Soy products have been widely consumed in Asian regions for centuries. Many potential health benefits have been linked with intake of soy products, such as lower incidences of coronary heart diseases [37], type 2 diabetes [38] and breast cancer [39]. Soy products are rich in isoflavones, and a meta-analysis of prospective studies indicated that intake of isoflavones was nearly significantly associated with decreased risk of breast cancer [40]. Besides, another meta-analysis, which included five cohort studies, found that post-diagnosis intake of soy food was associated with reduced mortality (HR for highest vs. lowest dose was 0.84, 95% CI = 0.71–0.99) and recurrence (HR = 0.74, 95% CI = 0.64–0.85) of breast cancer, indicating that soy food intake might be linked with better survival [41]. Indeed, numerous studies have supported the beneficial role of soy food intake for patients with breast cancer, although some reverse results were also observed. Given the vast number of studies, relevant peer-reviewed articles published in English within 5 years were included and discussed in this section.

## 2.1. Epidemiological Evidence

Most epidemiological studies have supported an inverse relationship between soy consumption and risk of breast cancer, though most studies were conducted in Asian population due to the different food preferences [39,42,43]. In recent years, epidemiological studies have widely investigated the effects of soy foods on breast cancer defined by different status. The amount of soy isoflavone consumption, estrogen receptor status of tumor, menopausal status of patients and timing of dietary exposure, could influence the soy-breast cancer association [44]. A recent study found an inverse association between adult soy intake and breast cancer risk (HR for fifth versus first quintile soy protein intake = 0.78; 95% CI = 0.63–0.97) of the population based in Shanghai Women's Health Study, with a predominance observed in premenopausal women (HR = 0.46; 95% CI: 0.29–0.74). Further stratified analyses found that soy intake during adulthood was significantly associated with decreased risk of ER−/PR− breast cancer in premenopausal women (HR = 0.46; 95% CI = 0.22–0.97) and decreased risk of ER+/PR+ breast cancer in postmenopausal women (HR = 0.72; 95% CI = 0.53–0.96). The HER2 status did not show a significant influence on the association [45]. Likewise, data extracted from the Takayama study in Japan pointed out that the relative risk of postmenopausal breast cancer was lower in women with larger consumption of soy (trend $p$ = 0.023) and isoflavone (trend $p$ = 0.046), although intake of soy and isoflavone did not affect the relative risks of premenopausal breast cancer [46]. In addition, it was found that high soy protein intake was associated with decreased breast cancer death (HR = 0.71, 95% CI = 0.52–0.98). Further stratified analysis pointed out that high intake of soy isoflavone was associated with a better prognosis of ER positive breast cancer (HR = 0.59, 95% CI = 0.40–0.93) [47]. Furthermore, data from the Korean Hereditary Breast Cancer Study reported that intake of soy products showed a lower risk of breast cancer in BRCA2 mutation carriers (HR: 0.39; 95% CI = 0.19–0.79 for the highest quartile) than noncarriers [48]. Besides, a study investigated the association between soy intake and tumor tissue miRNA and gene expression of TNBC patients, and found that long-term prediagnosis soy intake might be associated with elevated expression of tumor suppressors (such as miR-29a-3p and insulin-like growth factor 1 receptor (IGF1R)), and declined expression of oncogenes [49]. Ethnic diversity could also affect the soy-breast cancer association, thus some studies included participants from different ethnic groups or combined data from different cohort studies. A study combined 9514 breast cancer survivors from 2 US cohorts and 1 Chinese cohort. It was suggested that postdiagnosis soy food consumption ($\geq$10 mg isoflavones/day) was related to a significant decreased risk of recurrence (HR = 0.75; 95% CI = 0.61–0.92) and a nonsignificant lower risk of breast cancer specific mortality [30].

However, controversy still exists in this topic whether soy intake is associated with a reduced breast cancer risk. A multiethnic cohort study recruited women of African Americans, Latinos, Japanese Americans, Caucasians, and Native Hawaiians, and found that intake of prediagnosis soy was not associated with all-cause or breast cancer specific mortality [50]. Furthermore, no statistically significant relationship was observed between dietary isoflavone intake and overall risks of breast cancer across racial/ethnic groups in the same cohort [51]. Besides, a study showed that total soy food intake was not associated with an increased risk of cancer recurrence, but high intake of soy isoflavone increased the risk of cancer recurrence in HER2-positive breast cancer patients [52]. Moreover, according to a randomized phase II trial, a 6-month intervention of mixed soy isoflavones in high-risk or healthy adult Western women induced no reduction of breast epithelial proliferation, suggesting the poor efficacy of soy isoflavones for breast cancer prevention and an even possible adverse effect on premenopausal women [53]. The inconsistence of these results might be attributed to multiple reasons, such as the difference between food frequency questionnaires (FFQ) designed to capture the amount of soy intake [54].

*2.2. Experimental Evidence*

Despite the inconsistency in the abovementioned epidemiological studies, the fact that prevalence of breast cancers in Asia is much lower than that in North American and European countries has still raised an increasing interest in soy isoflavones as a potential therapeutic agent in breast cancer chemoprevention [55]. In fact, numerous experimental studies have demonstrated the inhibitory effects of soy products and soy isoflavones on breast cancer through various mechanisms of action.

In general, soy isoflavones (such as genistein and daidzein) exert their anti-breast cancer effects through the ER-dependent signaling pathways, due to the structural resemblance with 17-β-estradiol (Figure 2). For instance, genistein, one of the predominant soy isoflavones, could bind with both ERα and ERβ [56,57]. The ERα/ERβ ratio is a prognostic marker for breast tumors, and plays a vital role in the effect of soy isoflavones on breast cancer cells [58–60]. Genistein regulated the proliferation and mitochondrial functionality of breast cancer cells in an ERα/ERβ ratio-dependent way, since genistein treatment induced cell cycle arrest and improved mitochondrial functionality in T47D cells (low ERα/ERβ ratio), without affecting MCF-7 (high ERα/ERβ ratio) and MDA-MB-231 (ER-negative) cells [58]. Likewise, genistein regulated oxidative stress, uncoupling proteins, antioxidant enzymes and sirtuin, which was also dependent on ERα/ERβ ratio of breast cancer cells [59]. Furthermore, the synergetic effect of genistein with other anticancer drugs (cisplatin, paclitaxel or tamoxifen) was also dependent on ERα/ERβ ratio, judging by that the anticancer effect of combination treatment was more predominant in T47D cells than that in MCF-7 and MDA-MB-231 cells [60]. Additionally, in mouse mammary tumor virus erbB2 female transgenic mice administrated with different doses of 17β-oestradiol, it was found that the breast cancer incidence of mice was reduced by soybean diet in a high-oestrogen environment, but increased in a low-oestrogen environment [61].

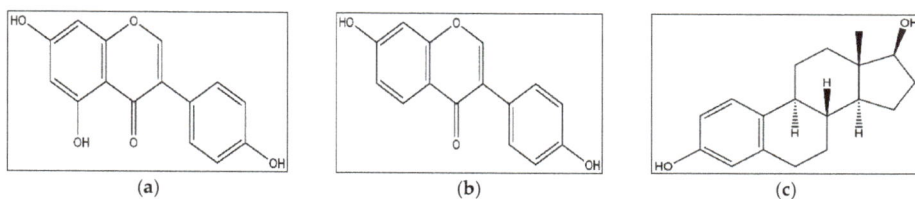

**Figure 2.** Structures of genistein (**a**); daidzein (**b**); 17-β-estradiol (**c**).

Soy isoflavones also showed inhibitory effects on the ER-negative MDA-MB-231 breast cancer cells [62,63], indicating that apart from interacting with ER, soy isoflavones also exert anti-breast cancer effect through various ER-independent mechanisms. For instance, soy products and soy isoflavones could induce apoptosis in both ER+ and ER− breast cancer cells. A water-soluble extract of long-term fermented doenjang (a fermented soybean product in Korea) induced cell cycle arrest, proliferation inhibition, and consequential apoptosis in breast cancer cells [64]. In addition, growth inhibition and apoptosis were induced by genistein in MCF-7-C3 and T47D cells, through downregulation of the cancerous inhibitor of protein phosphatase 2A, an oncogene found overexpressed in breast cancer [65]. Genistein also induced apoptosis in MCF-7 cells via the inactivation of the IGF-1R/p-Akt signaling pathway and decreasing the Bcl-2/Bax mRNA and protein expression [66]. Besides, 6,7,4′-trihydroxyisoflavone, a metabolite of daidzein, induced apoptosis in MCF10CA1a cells, through upregulation of DR4 expression and downregulation of XIAP, leading to the PARP cleavage. This metabolite also induced cell cycle arrest at S- and $G_2$/M phases by regulating cyclins and cyclin-dependent kinases (CDKs) [67]. Besides, extract of a soybean biotransformed by fungus induced cell death on MCF-7 cells, which was associated with the activation of caspase-3 and upregulation of proapoptotic molecule expression [68].

Soy isoflavones could also cause epigenetic alterations in breast cancer cells. Genistein inhibited DNA methylation and increased expression of some tumor suppressor genes in breast cancer cells, which might partly contribute to the anticancer effect of genistein [69]. In addition, quantitative phosphoproteomics revealed that genistein inhibited the growth of TNBC cell through modulating the DNA damage response and cell cycle in a more complex manner [70]. Furthermore, several prosurvival signalings in breast cancer cells were blocked by soy isoflavones. Genistein dose-dependently inhibited the growth of MDA-MB-231 cells by inhibiting activity of NF-κB via the Nocth-1 signaling pathway [71]. Genistein also decreased the breast cancer stem-like cell population both in vitro and in vivo, through downregulation of the Hedgehog-Gli1 signaling pathway [72]. Equol is a bacterial metabolite of daidzein. A study found that daidzein, R-(+)equol and S-(−)equol showed inhibition on the invasion of MDA-MB-231 cells through the downregulation of MMP-2 expression [63].

The controversy also exists in the results of experimental studies. Several recent studies challenged the inhibitory effect of soy isoflavones on breast cancer. For instance, a study found that isoflavone extracts of 51 commercial soybean cultivars were estrogenic and stimulated the growth of ER+ MCF-7 cells by 1.14 to 4.59 folds [73]. In addition, a study found that genistein at physiological concentration (5 μM) increased cellular levels of ROS and stimulated proliferation of breast cancer cell through the induction of CYP1B1 gene expression [74]. Moreover, long-term genistein treatment at low doses (≤500 ppm) promoted MCF-7 tumor growth and led to a more aggressive and advanced tumor growth phenotype after stimulus withdrawal [75]. Besides, in an experimental model of breast cancer with bone micro-tumors, soy isoflavones supplement (750 mg/kg) induced an increase of metastasis to lungs [76]. Furthermore, daidzein promoted growth of breast cancer cells in vitro (1 μg/mL) and stimulated estrogen-induced cell proliferation in rat uterus (0.066 mg/kg body weight (bw)), which suggested a caution for the use of daidzein in hormone replacement therapy [77]. Likewise, daidzein exposure promoted the expression of proto-oncogene BRF2 in ER+ breast cancer cells, through enhancing the demethylation and/or mRNA stabilization [78]. In addition, overexpression of ABC drug transporters is a contributor to multidrug resistance. Genistein treatment increased the expression of ABCC1 and ABCG2 at the protein level in MCF-7 cells, leading to an enhancement in doxorubicin and mitoxantrone efflux and resistance [79].

Collectively, most studies have supported a protective role of soy isoflavones against breast cancer, though some adverse effects have also been reported. Nevertheless, it should be noted that since the intrinsic cellular pathways often interfere or overlap, there was not a clear boundary between ER-dependent and ER-independent mechanisms under the anti-breast cancer action of soy isoflavones. Meanwhile, whether soy isoflavones promote or inhibit the growth of breast cancer seemed to be dependent on their doses [80], thus the dosage and long-term safety of soy isoflavones need to be further investigated before they are recommended as supplement for breast cancer patients.

## 3. Fruits

Fruits normally contain high content of polyphenols, which gives fruits great antioxidant activity and may help reduce risk of cancer [81–85]. In a meta-analysis which included fifteen prospective studies, high intake of fruits was associated with a weak reduction in risk of breast cancer (summary RR for the highest versus the lowest intake was 0.92, 95% CI = 0.86–0.98, $I^2$ = 9%) [86]. Besides, another meta-analysis suggested a borderline inverse association between pre-diagnostic fruit intake and the overall survival of breast cancer (summary HR for the highest versus the lowest intake was 0.83, 95% CI = 0.67–1.02, $I^2$ = 0%) [87]. Some fruits, such as pomegranate, mangosteen and citrus fruits, have shown inhibition on breast cancer cells.

## 3.1. Pomegranate

Pomegranate (*Punica granatum* L.) has been utilized for medicinal purposes for centuries and is described as "nature's power fruit" [88]. Pomegranate fruit contained a high content of polyphenols, among which ellagitannins predominate, and showed great antioxidant activity and anti-inflammatory properties [89,90]. Pomegranate extract (PE) inhibited MCF-7 breast cancer cell growth by inducing cell cycle arrest in $G_2/M$ phase and inducing apoptosis, and the effects might be associated with downregulation of homologous recombination, which could sensitize cancer cells to double strand breaks [91]. Another study revealed that PE exerted proapoptotic and antiproliferative effects on DMBA-inflicted rat mammary tumorigenesis, possibly through concurrent disruption of ER and Wnt/-catenin signaling pathways [92]. Furthermore, hydrophilic fraction of pomegranate seed oil significantly decreased cell viability of MCF-7 and MDA-MB-231 breast cancer cell lines and induced cell cycle arrest in $G_0/G_1$ phase [93]. Besides, pomegranate juice or combined with its components (luteolin + ellagic acid + punicic acid) could block the metastatic processes of breast cancer cells, as shown by inhibited cell growth, increased cell adhesion and decreased cell migration [94]. Another study indicated that PE showed anticancer activities on breast cancer cells, which was partly due to targeting microRNAs155 and 27a [95]. Additionally, pomegranate peel extract reduced cell proliferation and induced apoptosis on MCF-7 cancer cells, by increasing expression of Bax and decreasing the expression Bcl-2 [96]. Another study found that a pomegranate extract consisting of fermented juice and seed oil could inhibit invasion and motility of human breast cancer by inhibiting RhoC and RhoA protein expression. The bioactive components were identified as ellagitannins and phenolic acids in the aqueous extract, and conjugated octadecatrienoic acids in the lipid extract of seed [97]. Besides, pomegranate ellagitannin-derived compounds inhibited aromatase activity and proliferation of breast cancer cell line, indicating a potential for the prevention of estrogen-responsive breast cancers [98]. Furthermore, the whole pomegranate seed oil and fermented pomegranate juice polyphenols both inhibited the cancerous lesion formation induced by DMBA in a murine mammary gland organ culture, suggesting a chemopreventive property and adjuvant therapeutic potential of pomegranate [99,100].

## 3.2. Mangosteen

Mangosteen (*Garcinia mangostana* L.) known as "queen of fruits" is a common tropical fruit. Crude methanolic extract of mangosteen pericarp could inhibit proliferation and induce apoptosis on SKBR3 human breast cancer cell line [101]. In addition, phenolics from mangosteen fruit pericarp produced great cytotoxicities against MCF-7 human breast cancer cells [102].

Mangosteen pericarp is a rich source of xanthones, such as α- and γ-mangostin, which have a variety of bioactivities, such as antioxidant, anti-inflammatory, and anticancer activities [103]. In a study, twelve xanthone constituents were isolated from the pericarp of mangosteen, among which α-mangostin, γ-mangostin, garcinone D, and garcinone E, showed dose-dependent anti-aromatase activity in SK-BR-3 breast cancer cells, with γ-mangostin being the most potent [104]. Furthermore, a study showed that α-mangostin could induce apoptosis in T47D breast cancer cells through modulating HER2/PI3K/Akt and MAPK signaling pathways [105]. In addition, α-mangostin treatment on MDA-MB231 cell line carrying a p53 mutation induced mitochondria-mediated apoptosis and cell cycle alterations ($G_1$-phase arrest, upregulation of p21(cip1) expression and downregulation of cyclins, cdc(s), CDKs and PCNA) [106]. Besides, α-mangostin isolated from mangosteen exerted cytotoxicity on SKBR3 breast cancer cells and showed apoptotic bodies [107]. In addition, α-mangostin effectively inhibited fatty acid synthase (FAS) expression and intracellular FAS activity, and induced apoptosis in human breast cancer cells [108].

Furthermore, a study revealed that the presence of ERα is necessary for growth inhibition and apoptosis induced by α-mangostin in human breast cancer cells, as evidenced by that MDA-MB-231 cells (ER-α negative) is less sensitive to α-mangostin than MCF-7 cells (ERα positive), and that knockdown of ERα reduced the cell growth inhibition and caspase-7 activation induced by α-mangostin [109]. Besides, lymph node metastasis partly contributes to the lethality of breast cancer. In a study, α-mangostin treatment (20 mg/kg/day) significantly increased survival rate of mice carrying mammary tumors, and greatly suppressed tumor volume and the multiplicity of lymph node metastases. In vitro studies showed that α-mangostin induced mitochondria-mediated apoptosis and $G_1$- and S-phase cell cycle arrest, and decreased levels of phospho-Akt-threonine 308 (Thr308) [110]. Besides, treatment of panaxanthone (approximately 80% α-mangostin and 20% γ-mangostin) isolated from pericarp of mangosteen significantly suppressed mammary tumor volumes in mice, and decreased the multiplicity of lung metastasis and lymph node metastasis. These effects were associated with increases of apoptotic cell death, antiproliferation and antiangiogenesis. The in vitro analysis also confirmed that α-mangostin induced apoptosis on BJMC3879 cells [111].

### 3.3. Citrus Fruits

Citrus fruits include a large class of fruits, such as orange, lemon, grapefruit, pomelo and lime. Recently the anti-breast cancer activity of citrus fruits has attracted increasing attention. A meta-analysis of observational studies pointed out an inverse association between citrus fruits intake and the risk of breast cancer (OR, 0.90; 95% CI = 0.85–0.96; $p < 0.001$) [112].

Polysaccharides from Korean Citrus hallabong peels inhibited angiogenesis as shown by reducing tube formation of human umbilical vein vascular endothelial cells, and suppressed cell migration of MDA-MB-231 cells via downregulation of MMP-9 [113]. Besides, extracts from a citrus fruit named Phalsak induced apoptosis in anoikis-resistant breast cancer stem cell line MCF-7-SC [114]. In addition, lemon citrus extract induced apoptosis in MCF-7 breast cancer cells via upregulating the expression of bax and caspase-3 genes, and downregulating the expression of bcl-2 gene [115]. Furthermore, naringin, a flavonoid presenting abundantly in citrus fruits, inhibited cell proliferation, and promote cell apoptosis and $G_1$ cycle arrest in TNBC cell lines-based in vitro and in vivo models through modulating β-catenin pathway [116]. Besides, hesperidin, a flavonoid derived from citrus fruits, showed inhibitory effect on the proliferation of MCF-7-GFP-Tubulin cells [117].

### 3.4. Apple

Apple is widely consumed and an important part of the human diet. Flavonoids extracted from the peel and flesh of Pink Lady apples could both inhibit MCF-7 breast cancer cell growth, with $IC_{50}$ of 58.42 ± 1.39 mg/mL and 296.06 ± 3.71 mg/mL, respectively [118]. Besides, another study investigated an apple cultivar called Pelingo, and found that the Pelingo apple juice contained high content of polyphenol and exerted antiproliferative effect on MCF-7 and MDA-MB-231 cells. Pelingo juice also inhibited 12-o-tetra-decanoyl-phorbol-13-acetate (TPA)-induced tumorigenesis of pre-neoplastic cells, by inhibiting colony formation and TPA-induced ERK1/2 phosphorylation [119]. Additionally, apple extract showed a significant antiproliferative effect on MCF-7 and MDA-MB-231 cells at concentrations of 10–80 mg/mL ($p < 0.05$). Apple extract also significantly induced cell cycle arrest at $G_1$ phase in MCF-7 cells by decreasing cyclin D1 and Cdk4 proteins [120]. Another study showed that apple extract and 2α-hydroxyursolic acid isolated from apple peel could both inhibit NF-κB activation induced by TNF-α in MCF-7 cells through suppressing the proteasomal activities [121,122]. In addition, 2α-hydroxyursolic also showed antiproliferative and pro-apoptotic effects on MDA-MB-231 cells by regulating the p38/MAPK signal transduction pathway [123]. Furthermore, pectic acid isolated from apple could induce apoptosis and inhibit cell growth of 4T1 breast cancer cells in vitro, and prevent tumor metastasis in BALB/c mice via overexpression of p53 [124]. Results of another study indicated a synergistic inhibitory effect of the quercetin 3β-D-glucoside and apple extract combination on the proliferation of MCF-7 cells [125].

### 3.5. Grape

Grape and its products such as wine are well recognized healthy food consumed in the world. Dietary grape skin extract (0.5 and 1.0 mg/mL in drinking water) significantly inhibited the lung metastasis of breast tumor in Balb/c mice implanted with 4T1 cells. In vitro study revealed that grape skin polyphenols inhibited migration of 4T1 cells, which might be associated with blocking the PI3k/Akt and MAPK pathways [126]. Another study showed that grape seed extract suppressed migration and invasion of the highly metastatic MDA-MB231 cells, possibly through inhibiting β-catenin expression and localization, decreasing fascin and NF-κB expression and the activities of urokinase-type plasminogen activator (uPA), MMP-2 and MMP-9 [127]. In addition, a red grape wine polyphenol fraction showed selective cytotoxicity on MCF-7 cells, as evidenced by membrane damage, disrupted mitochondrial function and $G_2$/M cell cycle arrest [128]. Another study screened *Vitis amurensis* grape for active compounds to inhibit vascular endothelial growth factor (VEGF) production in tamoxifen-resistant MCF-7 cells, and amurensin G presented to be the most potent one. The effect was through blocking Pin1-mediated VEGF gene transcription [129]. Furthermore, muscadine grape skin extract could decrease cell invasion, migration and bone turnover in MCF-7 cells, via inhibiting expression of Snail and phosphorylated signal transducers and activators of transcription 3 (STAT3) and abrogating Snail-mediated CatL activity [130].

### 3.6. Mango

Mango (*Mangifera indica* L.) is a commonly cultivated tropical fruit and rich in polyphenolic compounds such as gallic acid and gallotannins. A study found that mango polyphenolics exhibited cytotoxic effects on BT474 cells in vitro, and decreased tumor volume by 73% in mice bearing BT474 xenograft compared with control group. These effects were partially regulated through the PI3K/AKT pathway and miR-126 [131]. Another study investigated three genetically diverse mango varieties, and found that the peel extract of Nam Doc Mai mango contained the highest amounts of polyphenols, inhibited cell viability of MCF-7 cells with an $IC_{50}$ of 56 μg/mL, and significantly ($p < 0.01$) stimulated cell death in MDA-MB-231 cells [132]. Furthermore, ethanolic extract of mango seed induced apoptosis in MCF-7 and MDA-MB-231 cells, through increasing pro-apoptotic proteins (cytochrome c, Bax, caspase-7, -8 and -9) and decreasing anti-apoptotic proteins (p53, Bcl-2, and glutathione). The effects were also associated with the activation of oxidative stress in breast cancer cells [133,134]. Besides, gallotannins in mango are generally not absorbable, therefore they are rarely studied for bioactivities. A study found that pyrogallol, the major microbial metabolite of gallotannins, and a mango polyphenols fraction could both inhibit breast cancer ductal carcinoma in situ proliferation in vitro, which was possibly through mediating the AKT/mTOR signaling pathway [135].

### 3.7. Other Fruits

Jujube (*Ziziphus jujube*) fruit has shown numerous medicinal and pharmacological effects, such as antioxidant and anti-inflammatory activities [136]. A study found that *Ziziphus jujube* extracts induced cell death by apoptosis in MCF-7 and SKBR3 breast cancer cells, without decreasing cell viability of nonmalignant breast epithelial MCF-10A cells or normal human fibroblasts BJ1-hTERT [137]. In addition, betulinic acid was isolated from sour jujube fruit, and microencapsulated betulinic acid could induce apoptosis in MCF-7 cells, through the mitochondria transduction pathway [138]. Furthermore, jujube aqueous extract treatment on MCF-7 cells exhibited antiproliferative and pro-apoptotic effects, through upregulating expression of Bax and downregulating Bcl2 gene [139].

Some berry fruits except for grape mentioned above also showed inhibitory effects on breast cancer cells. Methanolic extract of strawberry exerted cytotoxicity in T47D breast cancer cells in vitro, and inhibited the proliferation of tumor cells in mice bearing breast adenocarcinoma by activating apoptosis [140]. Besides, bilberry extract inhibited proliferation of MCF-7 cells in a concentration-dependent manner ($IC_{50}$ = 0.3–0.4 mg/mL), accompanied by induction of apoptotic cell death [141]. Furthermore, Jamun is the ripe purple and edible berries of the plant *Eugenia jambolana* Lam, and widely consumed in the United States. In a study, Jamun fruit extract showed great antiproliferative and pro-apoptotic effect on MCF-7aro and MDA-MB-231 cells, but only mild antiproliferative activity and no pro-apoptotic effect on the normal MCF-10A cells [142]. Additionally, cranberry extract could inhibit the proliferation of MCF-7 cells, which was partly attributed to the induction of apoptosis and $G_1$ phase arrest [143].

Polyphenolics from peach (*Prunus persica*) suppressed breast tumor growth and lung metastasis in a dose range of 0.8–1.6 mg/day in mice (about 370.6 mg/day for a human adult of 60 kg), which was regulated by inhibition of MMPs gene expression [144]. Another study investigated the anticancer effect of plums (*Prunus salicina*), and found that immature plums exhibited higher cytotoxic effects against MDA-MB-231 cells than mid-mature and mature plums, and contained higher levels of total phenolics and condensed tannins. The immature plums also induced apoptosis in MDA-MB-231 cells, associated with increased Bax levels, decreased Bcl-2 levels and the cleavage of caspases and PARP [145]. Besides, flavanols from Japanese quince (*Chaenomeles Japonica*) fruit exerted antiproliferative activity and inhibited invasiveness in MDA-MB-231 cells [146]. Additionally, a graviola fruit extract selectively inhibited the growth MDA-MB-468 breast cancer cells ($IC_{50}$ = 4.8 μg/mL), without affecting nontumorigenic MCF-10A breast epithelial cells in vitro. Furthermore, 5-week dietary treatment of this extract (200 mg/kg) inhibited tumor growth by 32% ($p$ < 0.01) in mouse xenograft model, through the EGFR/ERK signaling pathway [147]. In addition, litchi fruit pericarp extract inhibited cell growth ($IC_{50}$ = 80 μg/mL) of human breast cancer cells dose- and time-dependently in vitro, and 0.3 mg/mL oral administration of the extract for 10 weeks reduced tumor mass volume by 40.70% in mice, through multiple mechanisms [148]. Besides, bromelain isolated from the stems and immature fruits of pineapple induced cell death of GI-101A breast cancer cells in vitro by promoting apoptosis [149].

Collectively, the intake of fruits is generally beneficial for the prevention and treatment of breast cancer, and pomegranate, mangosteen, apple, citrus fruits, grape and mango have shown the most promising effects. The anti-breast cancer action of these fruits might be attributed to the presence of some bioactive component, such as ellagitannins in pomegranate and mangostin in mangosteen.

## 4. Vegetables

A meta-analysis of prospective studies indicated that high intake of fruits and vegetables combined was associated with a weak reduction in risk of breast cancer, with the summary relative risk (RR) for the highest versus the lowest intake of 0.89 (95% CI: 0.80–0.99, $I^2$ = 0%). However, no significant association was found between vegetable intake alone and risk of breast cancer [86]. In experimental studies, several vegetables, especially cruciferous vegetables, have shown inhibitory effect on breast cancer cells.

### 4.1. Cruciferous Vegetables

Cruciferous vegetables, such as broccoli, cauliflower, watercress and Brussel sprouts, are grown and consumed worldwide. According to a meta-analysis with 13 epidemiologic studies included, intake of cruciferous vegetables was inversely associated with risk of breast cancer (RR = 0.85, 95% CI = 0.77–0.94) [150]. Cruciferous vegetables have shown anti-breast cancer effect on experimental models, which might be attributed to its high contents of glucosinolates. When the vegetables are cut or chewed, the enzyme myrosinase is released, and glucosinolates would be degraded to form isothiocyanates. Isothiocyanates include a variety of compounds such as benzyl isothiocyanate, phenethyl isothiocyanate and sulforaphane, and have been long known to have chemopreventive activities for various neoplasms including breast cancer [151,152]. Besides, the indole-3-carbinol in cruciferous vegetables and its metabolite 3,3'-diindolylmethane also showed anti-breast cancer action [153,154].

#### 4.1.1. Isothiocyanates

Benzyl isothiocyanate (BITC)-induced inhibition on breast cancer cells is associated with apoptotic cell death, and inhibition of mitochondrial fusion was found to be an early and critical event involved in BITC-induced apoptosis [155]. Meanwhile, it was found that BITC-induced apoptosis in MCF-7 and

MDA-MB-231 cells was not p53-dependent, but mediated by suppression of XIAP expression [156]. In addition, in breast cancer cells treated with BITC, the proapoptotic proteins Bax and Bak were upregulated and the antiapoptotic proteins Bcl-2 and Bcl-xL were downregulated, indicating that apoptosis was induced by BITC. Generation of ROS and cleavage of caspase-9, caspase-8, and caspase-3 were also involved in this process [157]. BITC could also inhibit the migration and metastasis of human breast cancer cells. On the one hand, BITC markedly suppressed the invasion and migration of MDA-MB-231 cells, which was involved with reduced uPA activity, and suppression of Akt signaling [158]. On the other hand, epithelial-mesenchymal transition (EMT) process was triggered during progression of cancer to invasive state [159]. BITC treatment inhibited TGF β-/TNF α-induced migration via suppression on EMT process, as shown by the upregulated epithelial markers (E-cadherin and occludin), and downregulated mesenchymal markers (vimentin, fibronectin, snail, and c-Met), both in vitro and in vivo [160]. Besides, BITC exposure caused FoxO1-mediated autophagic death in breast cancer cells and MDA-MB-231 xenografts [161]. BITC could also act against the oncogenic effects of leptin on MDA-MB-231 and MCF-7 cells through suppressing activation of signal transducer and activator of transcription 3 [162]. BITC inhibited the growth of MDA-MB-231 xenografts by suppression on cell proliferation and neovascularization [163]. Additionally, BITC treatment inhibited breast cancer stem cells in vitro and in vivo, possibly by targeting Ron receptor tyrosine kinase [164].

Phenethyl isothiocyanate (PEITC), another natural isothiocyanate, also showed growth inhibition on breast cancer cells. Pharmacological concentrations of PEITC induced a PUMA-independent apoptosis on BRI-JM04 breast cancer cells, which was mediated by Bim [165]. Besides, PEITC suppressed adhesion, aggregation, migration and invasion of MCF-7 and MDA-MB-231 cells via modulation of HIF-1α [166]. Moreover, PEITC administration significantly prolonged the tumor-free survival and reduced the tumor incidence induced by N-methyl nitrosourea (NMU) in rats, since the tumor incidences were 56.6%, 25.0% and 17.2% for control, 50 μmol/kg, and 150 μmol/kg group, respectively. This chemopreventive activity might be attributed to its anti-angiogenic effects [167]. Besides, PEITC treatment (3 μM) to MCF-7 cells caused alterations in some genes in breast cancer, such as p57 Kip2, p53, BRCA2, IL-2, and ATF-2, which were involved in tumor suppression and cellular proliferation/apoptosis [168].

Sulforaphane (SFN), is also a potent inhibitor of mammary carcinogenesis through various mechanisms of action. SFN could downregulate ERα expression in MCF-7 cells, partially by blocking ERα mRNA transcription and increasing proteasome-mediated degradation [169]. SFN also induced cell type-specific apoptosis in breast cancer cells, since SFN-activated apoptosis in different breast cancer cell lines was initiated through different signaling pathways. To be specific, SFN activated apoptosis in MDA-MB-231 cells through induction of Fas ligand which led to activation of caspase-8, caspase-3 and poly (ADPribose) polymerase, while SFN induced apoptosis in the other breast cancer cell lines by reduction of Bcl-2 expression, release of cytochrome c into the cytosol, activation of caspase-3 and caspase-9, but not caspase-8, and poly (ADP-ribose) polymerase cleavage [170]. In addition, SFN suppressed the growth of KPL-1 human breast cancer cells both in vitro and in athymic mice [171], and the anti-metastatic action of SFN might be through inhibiting MMP-9 expression via the NF-κB signaling pathway [172]. Moreover, it was found that SFN showed antiproliferative effect on various TNBC cells through activating tumor suppressor Egr1 [173]. Besides, SFN also downregulated telomerase in breast cancer cells by inducing epigenetic repression of hTERT expression [174]. In addition, a study found that SFN showed anticancer efficacy in ER+ and COX-2 expressed breast cancer, which might be mediated by p38 MAP kinase and caspase-7 activations [175].

### 4.1.2. Indole-3-Carbinol

Indole-3-carbinol (I3C) is found at high concentrations in Brassica vegetables, and is a natural anti-carcinogenic compound. Studies have indicated that I3C showed anti-breast cancer action, since it could interact directly with the ERα and inhibit its activity, or through estrogen-independent actions, such as blocking cell cycle progression and metastasis, and inducing apoptosis. I3C (50 or 100 μM) could suppress the cell adhesion, migration, and invasion in vitro as well as the in vivo lung metastasis formation in MCF-7 and MDA-MB-468 cell lines, which was associated with upregulation of BRCA1 and E-cadherin/catenin complexes [176]. In addition, I3C pretreatment inhibited the migration through suppressing the EMT process and downregulating FAK expression [177]. I3C-induced inhibition on MMP-2 by blocking the ERK/Sp1-mediated gene transcription also contributed to its anti-invasive action on breast cancer cells [178]. Furthermore, I3C could induce inhibition on breast cancer bone metastasis by inhibiting CXCR4 and MMP-9 expression through downregulation of the NF-κB signaling pathway [179]. I3C could also regulate the cell cycle progression of breast cancer cells. For instance, I3C could inhibit CDK2 function in MCF-7 cells, by regulating cyclin E composition, the size distribution, and subcellular localization of the CDK2 protein complex [180]. Moreover, I3C suppressed CDK6 expression in MCF-7 cells, via targeting Sp1 at a composite DNA site in the CDK6 promoter [181]. Moreover, I3C downregulated expression of telomerase gene through disruption of the combined ERα- and Sp1-driven transcription of hTERT gene expression, leading to a cell cycle arrest in breast cancer cell [182]. Besides, I3C could induce apoptotic cell death in MDA-MB-435 and MCF10CA1a breast cancer cells, mainly through inducing overexpression and translocation of Bax to mitochondria, resulting in mitochondrial depolarization and activation of caspases [183,184]. In addition, I3C exerted antiproliferative action on estrogen-sensitive MCF-7 breast cancer cells, via suppressing the expression of IGF1R and IRS1, which was dependent on downregulation of ERα [185]. Furthermore, I3C induced stress fibers and focal adhesion formation through upregulation of Rho kinase activity, leading to an inhibited motility of MDA-MB-231 cell [186]. Interferon gamma (IFNγ) played a key role in prevention of the development of primary and transplanted tumors [187]. The anti-breast cancer effect of I3C might also be through stimulating expression of interferon gamma receptor 1 (IFNγR1) and augmenting the IFNγ response [188].

### 4.1.3. 3,3′-Diindolylmethane

3,3′-Diindolylmethane (DIM) is an in vivo acid-catalyzed condensation product of I3C and much more stable than I3C. DIM is also a promising anticancer agent. Multiple targets and underlying mechanisms of DIM-induced inhibition on breast cancer cells have been found. For instance, DIM induced apoptosis in MCF-7 and MDA-MB-231 breast cancer cells (Figure 3), by decreasing total transcript and protein levels of Bcl-2 and increasing Bax protein levels [189]. Apoptosis induced by DIM in MCF10CA1a breast cancer cells was also modulated by inactivation of Akt and NF-κB [190]. Another study revealed the upstream mechanism of DIM-induced inhibition on Akt in MDA-MB-231 breast cancer cells, which was through blockade of hepatocyte growth factor/c-Met signaling [191]. Meanwhile, DIM inhibited breast cancer cell proliferation and induced cell cycle arrest in $G_2/M$ phase in MCF-7 breast cancer cells, via enhancing miR-21-mediated Cdc25A degradation [192]. Meanwhile, DIM treatment markedly increased the portion of cells in $G_1$ phase through Sp1/Sp3-induced activation of p21 expression [193]. The upstream events leading to DIM-induced p21 overexpression were further studied, and results showed that DIM could act as a strong mitochondrial $H^+$-ATP synthase inhibitor. Hyperpolarization of mitochondrial inner membrane was induced by DIM treatment, which decreased cellular ATP level and markedly promoted mitochondrial ROS production, and in turn induced p21$^{Cip1/Waf1}$ expression [194]. Besides, DIM lowered the invasive and metastatic potential of breast cancer cells through downregulation of CXCR4 and CXCL12 [195]. In addition, survivin was found to be another target of cell growth inhibition and apoptosis induced by DIM in MDA-MB-231 breast cancer cells [196]. Like I3C, DIM could also stimulate the expression and secretion of IFNγ in MCF-7 cells through the activation of JNK and p38 pathways [197].

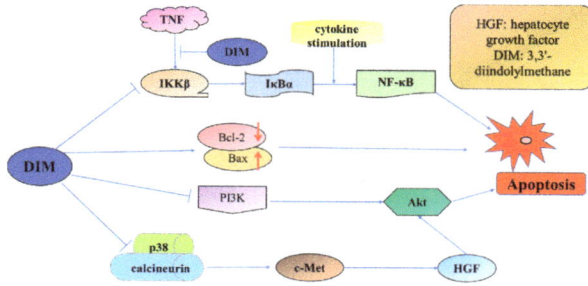

**Figure 3.** Signaling pathways involved in DIM-induced apoptosis in breast cancer cells.

## 4.2. Other Vegetables

It is reported that the extract of red beetroot (*Beta vulgaris* L.) exhibited a dose-dependent cytotoxic effect on MCF-7 cells in vitro [198]. Besides, a randomized study pointed out that daily intake of 8 ounces of fresh Balero or BetaSweet orange carrot juice increased plasma level of total carotenoid by 1.65 and 1.38 µM respectively in overweight breast cancer survivors. This increase in total plasma carotenoids was inversely associated with the level of 8-iso-PGFα, which was used as an oxidative stress marker (OR: 0.13; 95% CI = 0.20–0.75). These results indicated that daily intake of fresh carrot juice might benefit patients with breast cancer [199].

Collectively, cruciferous vegetables have shown a potential role in the prevention and treatment of breast cancer, and the main bioactive components are isothiocyanates (including BITC, PEITC, SFN), indole-3-carbinol and its metabolite 3,3'-diindolylmethane. The underlying mechanisms mainly include down-regulating ERα and repressing ER signaling, inducing apoptosis and cell cycle arrest, and inhibiting the metastasis of breast cancer cells.

## 5. Spices

Spices have been widely used in folk medicines and as food flavorings for a long time. In recent years, several spices and their bioactive constituents, such as gingerols and shogaols in ginger, organosulfur components in garlic, and thymoquinone in black cumin, have been suggested to possess anti-breast cancer activity.

### 5.1. Ginger

Ginger (*Zingiber officinale*) is a commonly used spice around the world for dietary and medicinal purpose since ancient period. Ginger has shown anti-breast cancer effect in recent researches. For instance, methanolic extract of ginger exhibited inhibitory effect on the proliferation and colony formation in MDA-MB-231 cells dose- and time-dependently [200]. Ginger extract also induced apoptosis in MCF-7 and MDA-MB-231 cells, via up-regulation of Bax, and downregulation of Bcl-2 proteins, NF-κB, Bcl-X, Mcl-1, survivin, cyclin D1 and CDK-4. Besides, the expression of c-Myc and hTERT, the two prominent molecular targets of cancer, was inhibited by ginger extract [201]. The anti-breast cancer property of ginger might be attributed to the bioactive constituents in ginger, such as gingerols and shogaols.

Gingerols showed inhibition on the proliferation and metastasis of breast cancer cells [202, 203]. 10-Gingerol inhibited proliferation of MDA-MB-231 through inhibition on cyclin-dependent kinases and cyclins, leading to a $G_1$ phase arrest. Invasion of cancer cell was also inhibited by 10-gingerol through suppression of Akt and p38 (MAPK) activity [202]. Besides, 6-gingerol exerted a concentration-dependent inhibition on migration and motility of MDA-MB-231 cells, accompanied with a decreased of expression and activities of MMP-2 and -9 [203].

Shogaols also inhibited metastasis of breast cancer cells through different mechanisms [204,205]. 6-Shogaol reduced expression of MMP-9 via blockade of NF-κB activation, leading to an inhibited invasion of MDA-MB-231 cells [204]. Besides, 6-shogaol inhibited invadopodium formation by decreasing levels of c-Src kinase, cortactin, and MT1-MMP, which are key modulators of invadopodium maturation, thereby inhibiting invasion of MDA-MB-231 cells [205]. Besides, 6-shogaol could inhibit the growth and sustainability of spheroid generated from adherent breast cancer cells. This effect was through γ-secretase-mediated downregulation of Notch signaling and induction of autophagic cell death [206]. 6-Dehydrogingerdione is also an active constituent of dietary ginger, and induced apoptosis and cell cycle arrest in $G_2$/M phase in MCF-7 and MDA-MB-231 cells through mediation of ROS/JNK pathways [207].

Furthermore, several clinical studies suggested a beneficial effect of ginger on patients with breast cancer. In patients receiving oral supplement of ginger, nausea severity and the number of vomiting episodes were significantly reduced than those of control group [208]. Besides, a single-blind, controlled, randomized cross-over study revealed that breast cancer patients who received ginger essential oil inhalation showed significantly lower nausea scores during acute phase, but no significant difference in overall treatment effect. Besides, ginger aromatherapy improved the baseline for global health status and appetite loss, while the vomiting was not improved [209].

## 5.2. Garlic

Garlic (*Allium sativum*) as a spice has been used worldwide. Meanwhile, it has been used in folk medicine to treat a variety of ailments [210]. A recent case-control study suggested that high consumption of certain *Allium* vegetables, especially garlic, is associated with a decreases risk of breast cancer, with adjusted ORs of 0.41 (95% CI = 0.20–0.83) [211]. Experimental studies indicated that the anti-breast cancer property of garlic might be attributed to organosulfur components, including diallyl disulfide [212], diallyl trisulfide [213], *S*-allyl mercaptocysteine [214], and allicin [215].

Diallyl disulfide (DADS) is one of the major organosulfur compounds isolated from garlic oil, and could induce apoptosis in MCF-7 breast cancer cells [216,217]. The pro-apoptotic effect might be through inhibition of histone deacetylation [216] and inhibition of ERK and the activation of the SAPK/JNK and p38 pathways [217]. Besides, DADS inhibited proliferation and metastasis of human breast cancer [218,219]. The DADS treatment upregulated expression of miR-34a, which led to inhibition on SRC expression and consequently triggered the blockade of the SRC/Ras/ERK pathway, ultimately led to an inhibitory effect on the proliferation and metastasis of MDA-MB-231 cells [218]. The DADS treatment also inhibited growth and metastatic potential of TNBC cells through inactivation of the β-catenin signaling pathway [219].

Diallyl trisulfide (DATS) also exhibited inhibitory effect on breast cancer by inducing apoptotic cell death [220,221]. It induced apoptosis in both MCF-7 cells and tumor xenografts by overproduction of ROS and subsequent activation of JNK and AP-1 [220]. The DATS also induced apoptosis in MCF-7 cells through upregulating the expression level of FAS, cyclin B1, cyclin D1, Bax and p53, and downregulating expression of Akt and Bcl-2 [221]. Furthermore, DATS inhibited migration and invasion of TNBC cells, through inhibiting MMP2/9 by suppressing NF-κB and ERK/MAPK signaling pathways [222]. Besides, a study indicated ERα might be a target of DATS in breast cancer cells, since DATS inhibited the expression and activity of ERα in MCF-7 and T47D cells. Peptidyl-prolyl *cis-trans* isomerase (Pin1) partially accounted for ERα protein suppression induced DATS treatment in MCF-7 cells [213]. Forkhead Box Q1 (FoxQ1) might be another novel target of DATS in breast cancer stem cell [223]. Pharmacological concentrations of DATS (2.5 and 5 μM) induced a dose-dependent inhibition on MCF-7 and SUM159 cells, which was associated with a decreased protein level of FoxQ1 [223].

S-allyl mercaptocysteine (SAMC), a water-soluble constituent derived from garlic, effectively inhibited cell growth of MCF-7 and MDA-MB-231 cells, by inducing apoptosis and cell cycle arrest in $G_0$/$G_1$ phase [214]. The mitochondrial apoptotic pathway was triggered by SAMC treatment, as shown by upregulation of Bax, downregulation of Bcl-2 and Bcl-X-L, and activation of caspase-9 and caspase-3 [214]. Another major component of garlic, allicin, inhibited the invasion and metastasis of MCF-7 cells induced by TNF-α, but not in MDA-MB-231 cells. The underlying mechanism was through suppressing the VCAM-1 through inhibiting ERK1/2 and NF-κB signaling pathways and increasing interaction between ERα and p65 [215].

### 5.3. Black Cumin

Black cumin (*Nigella sativa*) is a popular spice and has been used in folk medicine for over 1400 years. Recently, the anticancer effect of black cumin has attracted increasing attention. In a study, a supercritical $CO_2$ extract of black cumin exhibited pro-apoptotic and anti-metastatic effect on MCF-7 cells in vitro [224]. Another study pointed out that the antiproliferative ($IC_{50}$ = 62.8 μL/mL) and pro-apoptotic effects of black cumin extract were through mediating both the p53 and caspase pathways [225].

Thymoquinone (TQ) is the major bioactive component isolated from the seeds of *Nigella sativa*, and has shown potent chemopreventive and chemotherapeutic activities [226]. Firstly, studies indicated that TQ might be an Akt suppressor. Akt could be activated (phosphorylated) by PI3K, and promote cell survival by inhibiting apoptosis through inactivating downstream targets, such as Bcl-2 family member BAD and GSK-3β [227]. TQ induced cell cycle arrest and apoptosis in doxorubicin-resistant MCF-7 cells [228], and in T-47D and MDA-MB-468 cells [229], all by inhibiting Akt phosphorylation. TQ also inhibited tumor growth and induced apoptosis in mice bearing breast cancer xenograft, which might be through inducing p38 phosphorylation via ROS generation [230]. Besides, studies indicated that the antiproliferative effect of TQ on breast cancer might be through modulation of the PPAR-γ activation pathway [231], and by mediating expression of COX-2 and production of prostaglandin E2 through PI3K/p38 kinase pathway [232].

### 5.4. Other Spices

Red chili peppers of the genus *Capsicum* are popular spice worldwide, and contained certain amount of capsaicin (8-methyl-N-vanillyl-6-nonenamide), which has shown antiproliferative effect on breast cancer cells [233–235]. Capsaicin treatment for 24 h induced apoptosis in MCF-7 cells dose-dependently in vitro through a caspase-independent pathway [233]. Besides, capsaicin induced apoptosis in MCF-7 breast cancer cell, which was associated with inducing mitochondrial dysfunction [234]. In another study, capsaicin inhibited growth and blocked migration of MCF-7, MDA-MB231, T47D, SKBR-3 and BT-474 cell lines in vitro. In vivo, capsaicin decreased the volume of breast tumors in mice by 50% without noticeable drug side effects, and suppressed the progression of preneoplastic breast lesions by 80%. Mechanistically, these effects were through mediating the EGFR/HER-2 pathway [235]. However, it should be noted that the role of capsaicin in cancer is controversial. Some studies have indicated that capsaicin itself was mutagenic and promote tumor formation, and might increase the cancer risk in humans [236–238].

Piperine is an alkaloid isolated from black pepper (*Piper nigrum*), and has been reported to have anti-breast cancer activities. In a study, piperine exhibited growth, motility and metastasis inhibitory effects on TNBC cells in vitro, and suppressed the growth of TNBC xenografts in immune-deficient mice [239]. Another study found piperine induced cytotoxicity and apoptosis, and inhibited migration of HER2-overexpressing breast cancer cells in vitro. Piperine significantly inhibited HER2 and FAS expression, and downregulated EGF-induced MMP-9 expression via inactivation of AP-1 and NF-κB through modulating ERK1/2, p38 MAPK and Akt signaling pathways [240]. Moreover, piperine inhibited the growth of 4T1 cells (at doses of 35–280 pmol/L) time- and dose-dependently, and induced apoptosis (at doses of 70–280 pmol/L) in a dose-dependent manner, accompanying activation of caspase 3. Besides, injection of 5 mg/kg piperine dose-dependently inhibited the 4T1 tumor growth and significantly suppressed the lung metastasis in vivo [241].

Saffron (*Crocus sativus*), a well-known spice, is widely used in the Mediterranean, Indian and Chinese diet [242]. Saffron has showed anticancer effect in several studies, which was attributed to its bioactive compounds, such as crocin and crocetin [243,244]. According to an in vitro study, incubating the highly invasive MDA-MB-231 cells with crocetin (1 and 10 μM) significantly inhibited proliferation and invasion of cancer cells, and the effect was through downregulation of MMP expression [243]. Besides, a study found that crocin and crocetin both inhibited the incidence of *N*-methyl-*N*-nitrosourea (NMU)-induced breast tumors in rats. Moreover, crocetin was found to be a more effective chemopreventive agent than crocin at both the initiation and promotion stages [244]. Clove (*Syzygium aromaticum*) is commonly used as a spice and traditional Chinese medicine [245]. Eugenol is the major contributor to the bioactivities of clove. A study indicated that eugenol treatment inhibited the growth and proliferation of MCF-7 cells and induced apoptosis in vitro. Besides, the level of intracellular glutathione was decreased and the level of lipid peroxidation was elevated by eugenol treatment [246]. In another study, eugenol (2 μM) showed antiproliferative and proapoptotic activity both in vitro and in xenografted human breast tumors, which was mediated through targeting the E2F1/survivin pathway [247]. Besides, a supercritical fluid extract of rosemary (*Rosmarinus officinalis*) exhibited inhibitory effect on breast cancer cells through mediation of ERα and HER2 signaling pathways [248]. Wasabi (*Wasabia japonica*) is a popular spice in Japan. In a study, 6-(methylsulfinyl)hexyl isothiocyanate derived from wasabi exhibited proapoptotic effect on mice inoculated with MDA-MB-231 cells by inhibiting NF-κB and thus regulating the PI3K/AKT pathway [249]. Besides, coriander, a common culinary spice, has been reported for its health promoting effects. The coriander root extract exerted cytotoxicity on MCF-7 cells by affecting antioxidant enzymes, inducing $G_2$/M phase arrest and apoptotic cell death, which was associated with death receptor and mitochondrial apoptotic pathways [250]. It should be noted that the turmeric and its main bioactive component curcumin are not discussed in this section because their effects on breast cancer have been extensively reviewed [251–254].

Collectively, ginger, garlic and black cumin have shown the most promising anti-breast cancer effects among various spices. More attention has been paid to the effects of bioactive components in spices, such as gingerols and shogaols in ginger, diallyl disulfide and diallyl trisulfide in garlic. However, some adverse results have also been reported, such as the cancer-promoting effect of capsaicin isolated from red chili peppers.

## 6. Edible Macro-Fungi

Several kinds of edible macro-fungi have shown inhibitory effect on breast cancer, such as *Antrodia camphorate*, oyster mushroom (*Pleutorus eous*), and lingzhi mushroom (*Ganoderma lucidum*). In a case-control study conducted among Korean women, a significant inverse association between mushroom consumption and breast cancer incidence was found in postmenopausal women (OR = 0.17, 95% CI = 0.05–0.54, trend *p* = 0.0037 for average frequency; OR = 0.16, 95% CI = 0.04–0.54, trend *p* = 0.0058 for daily intake). No significant association was found in premenopausal women [255]. Besides, according to a meta-analysis with 7 observational studies included, mushroom intake might be inversely associated with risk of breast cancer (RR = 0.94, 95% CI = 0.91–0.97 for postmenopausal women; RR = 0.96, 95% CI = 0.91–1.00 for premenopausal women) [256].

*Antrodia camphorate* is a medicinal mushroom widely used in Taiwan [257]. Methyl antcinate A (MAA) is an ergostane-type triterpenoid isolated from the fruiting bodies of *A. camphorate*. MAA suppressed the population of cancer stem-like cells in MCF-7 cell line through inhibiting Hsp27 expression and increasing expression of p53 and IκBα [257]. Besides, a polysaccharide (SP1) with a molecular weight of 56 kDa was isolated from the fruiting body of mushroom Huaier (*Trametes robiniophila* Murr.). SP1 induced apoptosis in MCF-7 cells through downregulation of metadherin, which was overexpressed in most cancers [258]. Furthermore, an acidic polysaccharide, isolated from *Pleurotus abalonus* fruiting body, showed antiproliferative and proapoptotic effect on MCF-7 cells via ROS-mediated mitochondrial apoptotic pathway [259]. Treatment of this polysaccharide caused reduction in mitochondrial membrane potential, activation of caspase-9/3, increase of Bax/Bcl-2 ratio, overproduction of intracellular ROS, and degradation of PARP [259]. In addition, spores and unpurified fruiting body of *Ganoderma lucidum* inhibited invasion of MDA-MB-231 cells via inhibiting the expression of uPA and uPA receptor as well as the secretion of uPA [260]. The crude extract of *Ganoderma lucidum* fruiting body also caused both apoptosis and necrosis in estrogen-independent cell line, MDA-MB-435 [261]. Additionally, the aqueous extract of white button mushroom (*Agaricus bisporus*) dose-dependently suppressed the aromatase activity in MCF-7aro cells, which is an aromatase-transfected breast cancer cell line [262]. Besides, polysaccharides (50–250 µg/mL) isolated from oyster mushroom (*Pleurotus eous*) suppressed angiogenesis by downregulating VEGF, and induced apoptosis in MCF-7 cells through ROS-dependent JNK activation and mitochondrial mediated mechanisms [263].

Collectively, the anti-breast cancer effects of edible macro-fungi are mainly attributed to the polysaccharides with different molecular weights. Several mechanisms have been found to explain the anti-breast cancer effects of edible macro-fungi, such as inhibiting proliferation, inducing apoptosis and suppressing angiogenesis.

## 7. Cereals

Cereals are consumed worldwide, and rich in dietary fiber. A systematic review and meta-analysis of the evidence from prospective studies indicated an inverse association between cereal fiber intake and breast cancer risk (summary RR for the highest versus the lowest intake was 0.96, 95% CI = 0.90–1.02, $I^2$ = 5%) [264].

Sorghum (*Sorghum bicolor*) is a primary cereal food in some parts of the world [265]. A study showed that sorghum suppressed tumor growth, induced cell cycle arrest, and inhibited metastasis via the Jak2/STAT pathway in nude mice bearing breast cancer xenografts [266]. Furthermore, 3-deoxyanthocyanin extracted from red sorghum bran exhibited cytotoxicity on MCF-7 cells with a $CTC_{50}$ value of 300 µg/mL, and induced apoptosis mediated by upregulating the p53 gene and downregulating the Bcl-2 gene [267].

Barley (*Hordeum vulgare* L.) is widely consumed worldwide. A study showed that young barley (the grass of the barley plant) exhibited significant antiproliferative and proapoptotic activities in rat breast tumor model and in human breast cancer cells in vitro [268]. Wheat (*Triticum aestivum*) is a common kind of cereal, and contains rich nutritional constituents, such as starches and proteins (mainly in the endosperm), vitamins, minerals, phytochemicals and fibre (mainly in the wheat grain). A study showed that germinated wheat flour inhibited the growth of MCF-7 and MDA-MB-231 cells and induced apoptosis in vitro [269].

Collectively, sorghum, barley and wheat have shown the potential to inhibit the growth of breast cacer cells, mainly through inducing apoptosis and cell cycle arrest, and inhibiting metastasis.

## 8. Synergistic Effects of Dietary Natural Products with Anticancer Therapies

At present, chemotherapy and radiotherapy are frequently used in cancer treatment, but they are often accompanied with certain toxic adverse effects and drug resistance, which are common causes of chemotherapy failure and disease recurrence. Some dietary products and their bioactive components have shown synergistic effects with chemotherapy or radiotherapy, through enhancing their therapeutic effect or reducing side effects. For instance, combination of genistein and doxorubicin exerted a synergistic effect on MCF-7/Adr cells through stimulating the intracellular accumulation of doxorubicin and suppressing HER2/neu expression [270]. Besides, combination of genistein and centchroman (a selective estrogen receptor modulator) showed significantly higher cytotoxicity in human breast cancer cell lines compared to each drug used alone, and the nontumorigenic human mammary epithelial cell remained unaffected [271]. Moreover, equol enhanced the anticancer efficacy of tamoxifen in MCF-7 cells through inducing caspase-mediated apoptosis [272]. Equol could also be a potent radiosensitizer in both ER+ and ER− human breast cancer cells. It might be because equol enhanced cell death following irradiation and increased the DNA damage induced by remaining radiation, thereby reducing the surviving fraction of irradiated cells [273]. Furthermore, pomegranate extract enhanced tamoxifen-induced inhibition on cell viability of both sensitive and TAM-resistant MCF-7 cells by inducing cell death [274]. Meanwhile, DIM acted synergistically with Paclitaxel to inhibit growth of HER2/Neu human breast cancer cells via mediating the Her2/neu receptor and the downstream target ERK1/2. The cotreatment of DIM and Paclitaxel also enhanced apoptosis through the mitochondrial pathway (Bcl-2/PARP) [275]. Furthermore, DIM sensitized multidrug-resistant human breast cancer cells to $\gamma$-irradiation, judging from that $G_2/M$ phase cell cycle arrest was induced, intracellular ROS generation was increased and radiation-induced apoptosis was enhanced by DIM treatment (20 and 30 µM, 2 h before irradiation) [276]. Besides, the inactivation Akt/NF-$\kappa$B signaling induced by DIM also contributed to sensitization of breast cancer cells to Taxotere-induced apoptosis [277]. TQ could also enhance the efficacy of other antitumor agents. Combination treatment of TQ and tamoxifen synergistically reduced cells viability and induced apoptosis in both ER+ MCF-7 and ER- MDA-MB-231 cell lines in vitro [278]. Besides, a TQ-Paclitaxel combination treatment inhibited breast cancer growth in cell culture and in mice, through the interplay with apoptosis network [279]. Furthermore, piperine could enhance the efficacy of TRAIL-based therapies for TNBC cells, possibly through the inhibition of survivin and activation of p65 phosphorylation [280]. Moreover, piperine sensitized TNBC cells to the cytotoxicity induced by gamma radiation [239]. In addition, a supercritical fluid extract of rosemary enhanced the therapeutic effect of 3 anti-breast cancer agents, tamoxifen, trastuzumab, and Paclitaxel [248]. Rice bran is one of the byproducts of rice milling. A team found that a modified arabinoxylan from rice bran increased the sensitivity of MCF-7 and HCC70 breast cancer cells to daunorubicin through enhancing the accumulation of daunorubicin in cancer cells [281]. Later, they found that the modified arabinoxylan was also an effective chemosensitizer to Paclitaxel, as evidenced by increased susceptibility of MCF-7 and 4T1 cells to Paclitaxel by over 100 folds. Mechanistically, the synergistical effects were through enhancing apoptosis and DNA damage, and inhibiting cell proliferation [282]. Furthermore, a study showed that wheat grass juice (squeezed from the mature sprouts of wheat seeds) taken by breast cancer patients during FAC chemotherapy (5-fluorouracil, doxorubicin, and cyclophosphamide combination) could reduce myelotoxicity and the dose, without decreasing efficacy of the chemotherapy [283].

Finally, the epidemiological and experimental studies on dietary natural products for the prevention and treatment of breast cancer are summarized in Tables 1 and 2, respectively. In addition, some effects of dietary natural products against breast cancer and possible mechanisms are shown in Figure 4.

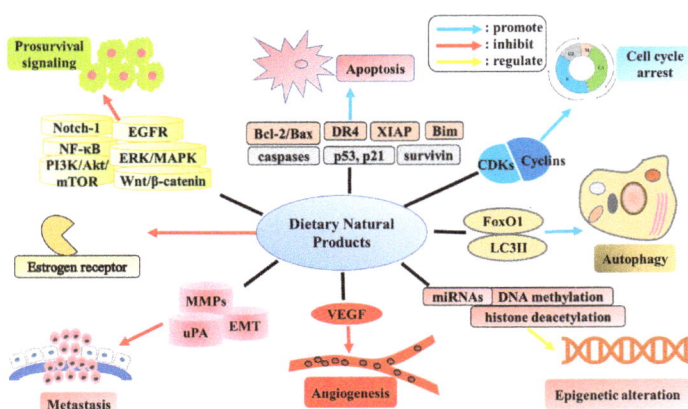

**Figure 4.** Mechanisms involved in the anti-breast cancer action of dietary natural products.

**Table 1.** Epidemiological studies on association between natural product intake and breast cancer.

| Natural Product | Study Type | Subject | Outcome | Association | Ref. |
|---|---|---|---|---|---|
| soy | cohort study | 70,578 Chinese women aged 40–70 years | BC risk | overall: HR = 0.78, 95% CI = 0.63–0.97, premenopausal women: HR = 0.46; 95% CI: 0.29–0.74), ER+/PR+ postmenopausal women: HR = 0.72; 95% CI = 0.53–0.96 ER-/PR- premenopausal women: HR = 0.46; 95% CI = 0.22–0.97 | [45] |
| soy | cohort study | 15,607 Japanese women aged 35 or above | BC risk | postmenopausal women: trend $p = 0.023$ for soy consumption; trend $p = 0.046$ for isoflavone consumption | [46] |
| soy | prospective study | 649 Chinese women with BC | BC death / BC prognosis | HR = 0.71, 95% CI = 0.52–0.98 ER+ patients: HR = 0.59, 95% CI = 0.40–0.93 | [47] |
| soy | cohort study | affected BC patients and unaffected high risk family members in Korea | BC risk | BRCA2 mutation carriers: HR = 0.39; 95% CI = 0.19– 0.79 | [48] |
| soy | cohort study | 9514 BC survivors | risk of recurrence | HR = 0.75; 95% CI = 0.61–0.92 | [30] |
| soy | cohort study | 3842 multiethnic women | all-cause mortality BC specific mortality | no significant association | [50] |
| soy | cohort study | 84,450 multiethnic women with BC | BC risk | no significant association | [51] |
| soy | cohort study | 339 Korean women with BC | risk of recurrence | no significant association | [52] |
| Citrus fruits | meta-analysis | 8393 participants: 3789 cases and 4,705 controls | BC risk | OR = 0.90; 95% CI = 0.85–0.96; $p < 0.001$ | [112] |
| cruciferous vegetables | meta-analysis | 18,673 BC cases | BC risk | RR = 0.85, 95% CI = 0.77–0.94 | [150] |
| garlic | case-control study | 285 Iranian women aged 25–65 years with BC | BC risk | ORs = 0.41, 95% CI = 0.20–0.83 | [211] |
| mushroom | case-control study | 362 women aged 30–65 years with BC | BC risk | postmenopausal women: for daily intake, OR=0.16, 95% CI = 0.04-0.54, $p$= 0.0058; for average frequency, OR = 0.17, 95% CI = 0.05–0.54, $p = 0.0037$ | [255] |
| mushroom | meta-analysis | 6890 BC cases | BC risk | premenopausal women: RR = 0.96, 95% CI = 0.91–1.00; postmenopausal women: RR = 0.94, 95% CI = 0.91–0.97 | [256] |

BC, stands for breast cancer.

**Table 2.** The in vitro and in vivo effects of dietary natural products against breast cancer.

| Natural Product | Constituents | Study Type | Main Effect and Possible Mechanism | Ref. |
|---|---|---|---|---|
| Soy | | | | |
| soy | genistein | in vitro | - inducing cell cycle arrest, - improving mitochondrial functionality, - regulating oxidative stress, uncoupling proteins, antioxidant enzymes and sirtuin, - enhancing effects of anticancer drugs | [58–60] |
| soy | genistein | in vivo | reducing breast cancer incidence in a high-oestrogen environment | [61] |
| fermented doenjang | NA | in vitro | inducing cell cycle arrest, proliferation inhibition, and apoptosis | [64] |
| soy | genistein | in vitro | inducing apoptosis through: - downregulation of the cancerous inhibitor of protein phosphatase 2A - the inactivation of the IGF-1R/p-Akt signaling pathway | [65,66] |
| soy | 6,7,4'-trihydroxyisoflavone | in vitro | inducing apoptosis and cell cycle arrest at S- and $G_2$/M phases | [67] |

Table 2. *Cont.*

| Natural Product | Constituents | Study Type | Main Effect and Possible Mechanism | Ref. |
|---|---|---|---|---|
| soybean | NA | in vitro | inducing cell death via activation of caspase-3 and upregulation of proapoptotic molecule expression | [68] |
| soy | genistein | in vitro | inhibiting DNA methylation and increasing expression of tumor suppressor genes | [69] |
| soy | genistein | in vitro | inhibiting cancer cell growth through modulating the DNA damage response and cell cycle | [70] |
| soy | genistein | in vitro | inhibiting cancer cell growth through inhibiting activity of NF-κB via the Nocth-1 signaling pathway | [71] |
| soy | genistein | in vitro and in vivo | decreasing breast cancer stem-like cell population through Hedgehog pathway | [72] |
| soy | daidzein, equol | in vitro | inhibiting the invasion through the down-regulation of MMP-2 expression | [63] |
| Fruits | | | | |
| pomegranate | NA | in vitro | inhibiting growth by inducing cell cycle arrest in $G_2/M$ and inducing apoptosis | [91] |
| pomegranate | NA | in vivo | preventing mammary tumorigenesis via concurrent disruption of ER and Wnt/-catenin signaling pathways | [92] |
| pomegranate | luteolin, ellagic acid, punicic acid | in vitro | inhibiting growth, increasing adhesion and decreasing migration of breast cancer cells | [94] |
| pomegranate | NA | in vitro and in vivo | showing cytotoxicities by targeting microRNAs155 and 27a, reducing cell proliferation and inducing apoptosis | [95,96] |
| pomegranate | ellagitannins, phenolic acids, conjugated octadecatrienoic acids | in vitro | inhibiting invasion and motility of cancer cells by inhibiting RhoC and RhoA protein expression | [97] |
| pomegranate | ellagitannin-derived compounds | in vitro | inhibiting aromatase activity and cell proliferation | [98] |
| pomegranate | NA | in vitro | inhibiting the cancerous lesion formation | [99,100] |
| mangosteen | NA | in vitro | inhibiting proliferation and inducing apoptosis | [101] |
| mangosteen | phenolics | in vitro | showing cytotoxicities | [102] |
| mangosteen | garcinone D, garcinone E, α-mangostin γ-mangostin | in vitro | dose-dependent anti-aromatase activity | [104] |
| mangosteen | α-mangostin | in vitro | inducing apoptosis through modulating HER2/PI3K/Akt and MAPK signaling pathways | [105] |
| mangosteen | α-mangostin | in vitro | inducing mitochondria-mediated apoptosis and cell cycle alterations | [106] |
| mangosteen | α-mangostin | in vitro | showing cytotoxicities | [107] |
| mangosteen | α-mangostin | in vitro | inhibiting FAS expression and activity, and inducing apoptosis | [108] |
| mangosteen | α-mangostin | in vitro | inducing apoptosis and decreasing the expression of ER alpha and pS2 | [109] |
| mangosteen | α-mangostin | in vivo | increasing survival rates and suppressing tumor volume and the multiplicity of lymph node metastases | [110] |
| | | in vitro | inducing apoptosis and cell cycle arrest | |
| mangosteen | panaxanthone | in vivo | suppressing tumor volumes and decreasing the multiplicity of lung metastasis and lymph node metastasis | [111] |
| | | in vitro | inducing apoptosis | |
| Citrus fruit | polysaccharides | in vitro | inhibiting angiogenesis and cell migration | [113] |

**Table 2.** *Cont.*

| Natural Product | Constituents | Study Type | Main Effect and Possible Mechanism | Ref. |
|---|---|---|---|---|
| Citrus fruit | NA | in vitro | inducing apoptosis | [114] |
| Citrus fruit | NA | in vitro | inducing apoptosis via upregulating the expression of bax and caspase-3 genes and downregulating the expression of bcl-2 gene | [115] |
| Citrus fruit | naringin | in vitro | inhibiting growth potential by targeting β-catenin pathway | [116] |
| | | in vivo | inhibiting cell proliferation and promoting cell apoptosis and G1 cycle arrest through modulating β-catenin pathway | |
| Citrus fruit | hesperidin | in vitro | anti-proliferative effect | [117] |
| apple | flavonoids | in vitro | inhibiting growth and inducing apoptosis | [118] |
| apple | polyphenol | in vitro | inhibiting tumorigenesis of pre-neoplastic cells by suppressing colony formation and ERK1/2 phosphorylation | [119] |
| apple | NA | in vitro | inhibiting proliferation and inducing cell cycle arrest at $G_1$ phase | [120] |
| apple | 2α-hydroxyursolic acid | in vitro | inhibit NF-κB activation through suppressing the proteasomal activities | [121, 122] |
| apple | 2α-hydroxyursolic acid | in vitro | antiproliferative and pro-apoptotic effect by regulating the p38/MAPK signal transduction pathway | [123] |
| apple | pectic acid | in vitro | inducing apoptosis and inhibiting cell growth preventing tumor metastasis mice via over-expression of P53 | [124] |
| | | in vivo | | |
| apple | NA | in vitro | enhancing the anti-proliferative effect of quercetin 3-beta-D-glucoside | [125] |
| grape | polyphenols | in vivo | inhibiting the lungs metastasis inhibiting migration by blocking the PI3k/Akt and MAPK pathways | [126] |
| | | in vitro | | |
| grape | NA | in vitro | suppressing migration and invasion | [127] |
| grape | polyphenols | in vitro | inducing membrane damage, disrupting mitochondrial function and inducing $G_2/M$ cell cycle arrest | [128] |
| grape | amurensin G | in vitro | inhibiting VEGF production | [129] |
| grape | anthocyanin | in vitro | decreasing invasion, migration and bone turnover, via inhibiting expression of Snail and phosphorylated STAT3 and abrogating Snail-mediated CatL activity | [130] |
| mango | polyphenolics | in vitro | showing cytotoxic effects reducing the tumor volume by regulating the PI3K/AKT pathway and miR-126 | [131] |
| | | in vivo | | |
| mango | polyphenols | in vitro | inhibiting cell viability | [132] |
| mango | NA | in vitro | inducing apoptosis via the activation of oxidative stress | [133, 134] |
| mango | pyrogallol | in vitro | inhibiting proliferation through mediating the AKT/mTOR signaling pathway | [135] |
| jujube | triterpenic acids | in vitro | inducing apoptotic cell death | [137] |
| jujube | betulinic acid | in vitro | inducing apoptosis through the mitochondria transduction pathway | [138] |
| jujube | NA | in vitro | inhibiting proliferation and inducing apoptosis | [139] |
| strawberry | NA | in vitro | showing cytotoxic effects inhibiting the proliferation of tumor cells by activating apoptosis | [140] |
| | | in vivo | | |
| bilberry | NA | in vitro | inhibiting proliferation and inducing apoptosis | [141] |
| jamun fruit | NA | in vitro | inhibiting proliferation and inducing apoptosis | [142] |
| cranberry | NA | in vitro | inducing apoptosis and G1 phase arrest | [143] |

Table 2. *Cont.*

| Natural Product | Constituents | Study Type | Main Effect and Possible Mechanism | Ref. |
|---|---|---|---|---|
| peach | polyphenolics | in vivo | suppressing tumor growth and lung metastasis by inhibition of metalloproteinases gene expression | [144] |
| plum | phenolics and condensed tannins | in vitro | inducing apoptosis | [145] |
| quince fruit | NA | in vitro | inhibiting proliferation and invasiveness | [146] |
| graviola fruit | NA | in vitro in vivo | inhibiting the growth of cancer cells inhibiting tumor growth by 32% ($p < 0.01$) through the EGFR/ERK signaling pathway | [147] |
| litchi fruit | NA | in vitro in vivo | inhibited cell growth reducing tumor mass volume | [148] |
| pineapple | bromelain | in vitro | inducing apoptosis | [149] |
| **Vegetables** | | | | |
| Cruciferous vegetables | benzyl isothiocyanate | in vitro | inducing apoptosis which was associated with: - inhibition of mitochondrial fusion - suppression of XIAP expression - generation of ROS | [155–157] |
| | | in vitro and in vivo | suppressing the invasion and migration involving: - suppression of uPA activity and of Akt signaling - suppression on EMT process | [158, 160] |
| | | in vitro and in vivo | - inducing FoxO1-mediated autophagic death, - acting against the oncogenic effects of leptin, - suppressing proliferation and neovascularization, - inhibiting breast cancer stem cells | [161–164] |
| Cruciferous vegetables | phenethyl isothiocyanate | in vitro and in vivo | - inducing apoptosis, - suppressing adhesion, aggregation, migration and invasion, - prolonging the tumor-free survival and reducing the tumor incidence, - causing alterations in some genes | [165–168] |
| Cruciferous vegetables | sulforaphane | in vitro and in vivo | - downregulating ER-α expression, - inducing apoptosis, - inhibiting metastasis, - activating tumor suppressor Egr1, - downregulating telomerase, - regulating p38 MAPK and caspase-7 activations | [169–175] |
| Cruciferous vegetables | indole-3-carbinol | in vitro and in vivo | suppressing metastasis through - up-regulation of BRCA1 and E-cadherin/catenin complexes - suppressing EMT process and downregulating FAK expression - inhibition on MMP-2 expression - inhibiting CXCR4 and MMP-9 expression by downregulation of the NF-κB signaling pathway | [176–179] |
| | | in vitro and in vivo | - regulating the cell cycle progression - downregulating expression of telomerase gene - inducing apoptotic cell death - suppressing the expression of IGF1R and IRS1 - inducing stress fibers and focal adhesion formation - stimulating expression of IFNγR1 | [180–186,188] |
| Cruciferous vegetables | 3,3′-diindolylmethane | in vitro | inducing apoptosis through: - inactivation of Akt and NF-κB activity - downregulating Bcl-2 and upregulating Bax - inducing cell cycle arrest | [189–191] |
| | | in vitro | - lowering the invasive and metastatic potential - stimulating the expression and secretion of IFNγ | [192–197] |
| red beetroot | betanin | in vitro | showing a dose-dependent cytotoxic effect | [198] |

**Table 2.** *Cont.*

| Natural Product | Constituents | Study Type | Main Effect and Possible Mechanism | Ref. |
|---|---|---|---|---|
| | | **Spices** | | |
| ginger | NA | in vitro | inhibiting the proliferation and colony formation | [200] |
| ginger | NA | in vitro | inducing apoptosis and inhibiting expression of c-Myc and hTERT | [201] |
| ginger | 10-gingerol | in vitro | inhibiting proliferation and metastasis, inducing cell cycle arrest | [202] |
| ginger | 6-gingerol | in vitro | inhibiting metastasis by suppressing MMP-2 and -9. | [203] |
| ginger | 6-shogaol | in vitro | inhibiting invasion by reducing MMP-9 expression via blockade of NF-κB activation | [204] |
| | | | inhibiting invasion by suppressing invadopodium formation and MMP activity | [205] |
| | | | inhibiting growth and sustainability of spheroid generated from adherent breast cancer cells | [206] |
| ginger | 6-dehydrogingerdione | in vitro | inducing apoptosis and cell cycle arrest in $G_2/M$ phase | [207] |
| garlic | diallyl disulfide | in vitro | inducing apoptosis though: - inhibition of histone deacetylation - inhibition of ERK and the activation of the SAPK/JNK and p38 pathways | [216, 217] |
| | | in vitro and in vivo | inhibit proliferation and metastasis via: - suppression of the SRC/Ras/ERK pathway - inactivation of the β-catenin signaling pathway | [218, 219] |
| garlic | diallyl trisulfide | in vitro and in vivo | inducing apoptosis though: - overproduction of ROS and subsequent activation of JNK and AP-1 - upregulating FAS, Bax and p53, and down-regulating Akt and Bcl-2 | [220, 221] |
| | | in vitro | - inhibiting migration and invasion; - inhibiting ER-α - decreasing protein level of FoxQ1 | [213,222, 223] |
| garlic | S-allyl mercaptocysteine | in vitro | inducing mitochondrial apoptosis and cell cycle arrest | [214] |
| garlic | allicin | in vitro | inhibiting invasion and metastasis | [215] |
| black cumin | extracts | in vitro | inducing apoptosis and inhibiting metastasis | [224, 225] |
| black cumin | thymoquinone | in vitro and in vivo | inducing apoptosis through: - inhibiting Akt phosphorylation - inducing p38 phosphorylation via ROS generation | [228– 230] |
| | | in vitro | inhibiting proliferation by modulation of the PPAR-γ activation pathway | [231] |
| | | in vitro | regulating COX-2 and E2 | [232] |
| red chili pepper | capsaicin | in vitro and in vivo | - inducing apoptosis - inhibiting growth and migration | [233– 235] |
| black pepper | piperine | in vitro and in vivo | - inhibiting growth, motility and metastasis - inducing apoptosis - suppressing the lung metastasis | [239– 241] |
| saffron | crocetin | in vitro | inhibiting proliferation and invasion, through decreasing MMP expression | [243] |
| clove | eugenol | in vitro and in vivo | inhibiting growth and proliferation, inducing apoptosis through targeting the E2F1/survivin pathway | [246, 247] |
| rosemary | extracts | in vitro | exerting antitumor activity through mediation of ER-α and HER2 signalings | [248] |

**Table 2.** *Cont.*

| Natural Product | Constituents | Study Type | Main Effect and Possible Mechanism | Ref. |
|---|---|---|---|---|
| wasabi | 6-(methylsulfinyl)hexyl isothiocyanate | in vivo | inducing apoptosis by inhibiting NF-κB and regulating the PI3K/AKT pathway | [249] |
| coriander | root extract | in vitro | affecting antioxidant enzymes, inducing $G_2/M$ phase arrest and apoptosis | [250] |
| **Edible Macro-Fungi** | | | | |
| *Antrodia camphorate* | methyl antcinate A | in vitro | suppressing the population of cancer stem-like cells | [257] |
| *Trametes robiniophila* Murr. | polysaccharides | in vitro | induced apoptosis through down-regulation of metadherin | [258] |
| *Pleurotus abalonus* | polysaccharides | in vitro | inhibiting antiproliferation and inducing apoptosis via ROS-mediated mitochondrial apoptotic pathway | [259] |
| *Ganoderma lucidum* | extracts | in vitro | inhibiting invasion via inhibiting the expression of uPA and uPA receptor | [260] |
| | | | causing both apoptosis and necrosis | [261] |
| *Agaricus bisporus* | extracts | in vitro | suppressing the aromatase activity dose-dependently | [262] |
| *Pleutorus eous* | polysaccharides | in vitro | inhibiting angiogenesis and inducing apoptosis | [263] |
| **Cereals** | | | | |
| Sorghum | extracts | in vivo | suppressing tumor growth, inducing cell cycle arrest, and inhibiting metastasis | [266] |
| | 3-deoxyanthocyanin | in vitro | inducing apoptosis by upregulating the p53 gene and downregulating the Bcl-2 gene | [267] |
| barley | extracts | in vitro and in vivo | exerting antiproliferative and pro-apoptotic activities | [268] |
| wheat | germinated wheat flour | in vitro | inhibiting growth and inducing apoptosis | [269] |

## 9. Conclusions

The intake of some dietary natural products, such as soy, citrus fruits, cruciferous vegetables and mushrooms, is suggested to be inversely correlated with the risk of breast cancer by epidemiological studies. Furthermore, experimental studies also indicated that many dietary natural products could be potential sources for prevention and treatment of breast cancer. The following natural products and the corresponding bioactive components are noteworthy, including soy (genistein and daidzein), pomegranate (ellagitannins), mangosteen (mangostin), citrus fruits (naringin), apple (2α-hydroxyursolic), grape, mango, cruciferous vegetables (isothiocyanates), ginger (gingerols and shogaols), garlic (organosulfur compounds), black cumin (thymoquinone), edible macro-fungi (polysaccharides), and cereals. The anti-breast cancer effects of these natural products involve various mechanisms of action, such as inhibiting proliferation, migration, metastasis and angiogenesis of tumor cells, inducing apoptosis and cell cycle arrest, and sensitizing tumor cells to radiotherapy and chemotherapy. In the future, more anti-breast cancer bioactive compounds should be isolated and identified from dietary natural products, and more efforts should be made to assess the underlying mechanisms, potential toxicity and adverse effects. Moreover, the clinical efficacy of dietary natural products and their bioactive components on breast cancer patients needs to be further studied.

**Acknowledgments:** This work was supported by the National Natural Science Foundation of China (No. 81372976), Key Project of Guangdong Provincial Science and Technology Program (No. 2014B020205002), and the Hundred-Talents Scheme of Sun Yat-Sen University.

**Author Contributions:** Y.L., S.L., R.Y.G. and H.B.L. conceived and designed the review. Y.L., X.M. and J.J.Z. wrote the review. S.L., R.Y.G. and H.B.L. revised the review. All authors discussed and approved the final version.

**Conflicts of Interest:** The authors declare no conflict of interest.

## Abbreviations

The following abbreviations are used in this manuscript: AP-1: active protein-1; ATF-2: activating transcription factor 2; Bax: Bcl-2-associated X protein; Bcl-2: B-cell lymphoma 2; Bcl-xL: B-cell lymphoma-xL; Bim: B-cell lymphoma 2 interacting mediator of cell death; BITC: benzyl isothiocyanate; CDKs: cyclin-dependent kinases; CXCR4: C-X-C chemokine receptor type 4; DADS: diallyl disulfide; DATS: diallyl trisulfide; DR4: death receptor 4; EGFR: epidermal growth factor receptor; EMT: epithelial-mesenchymal transition ER: estrogen receptor; ERK: extracellular regulated protein kinase; FAK: focal adhesion kinase; FAS: fatty acid synthase; FFQ: food frequency questionnaire; FoxQ1: Forkhead Box Q1; GSK-3β: glycogen synthase kinase 3β; HER2: human epidermal growth factor receptor 2; HIF: hypoxia-inducible factor; hTERT: human telomerase reserve transcriptase; I3C: indole-3-carbinol; IFNγ: interferon gamma; IGF1R: insulin-like growth factor-1 receptor; IL-2: interleukin 2; IRS1: insulin receptor substrate-1; Jak2: Janus kinase; JNK: c-Jun N-terminal kinase; MAA: methyl antcinate A; MAPK: mitogen-activated protein kinase; MMP: matrix metalloproteinase; mTOR: mechanistic target of rapamycin; NF-κB: nuclear factor kappa-light-chain-enhancer of activated B cells; NMU: N-methyl nitrosourea; PARP: poly-ADP-ribose polymerase; PCNA: proliferating cell nuclear antigen; PEITC: phenethyl isothiocyanate; PI3K: phosphatidylinositol 3-kinase; Pin1: Peptidyl-prolyl cis-trans isomerase; PR: progesterone receptor; PUMA: p53 upregulated modulator of apoptosis; RhoA: Ras homolog gene family, member A; RhoC: Ras homolog gene family, member C; ROS: reactive oxygen species; SAMC: S-allyl mercaptocysteine; SAPK: stress-activated protein kinase; SFN: sulforaphane; STAT3: signal transducers and activators of transcription 3; TNBC: triple-negative breast cancer; TNF-α: tumor necrosis factor α; TQ: thymoquinone; TRAIL: TNF related apoptosis inducing ligand; uPA: urokinase-type plasminogen activator; VCAM-1: vascular cell adhesion molecule 1; VEGF: vascular endothelial growth factor; XIAP: X-linked inhibitor of apoptosis.

## References

1. Torre, L.A.; Bray, F.; Siegel, R.L.; Ferlay, J.; Lortet-Tieulent, J.; Jemal, A. Global cancer statistics, 2012. *CA Cancer J. Clin.* **2015**, *65*, 87–108. [CrossRef] [PubMed]
2. Siegel, R.L.; Miller, K.D.; Jemal, A. Cancer statistics, 2017. *CA Cancer J. Clin.* **2017**, *67*, 7–30. [CrossRef] [PubMed]
3. Reis, J.S.; Pusztai, L. Breast Cancer 2 Gene expression profiling in breast cancer: Classification, prognostication, and prediction. *Lancet* **2011**, *378*, 1812–1823.
4. Perou, C.M.; Borresen-Dale, A.L. Systems biology and genomics of breast cancer. *Cold Spring Harb. Perspect. Biol.* **2011**, *3*. [CrossRef]
5. Hudis, C.A.; Gianni, L. Triple-negative breast cancer: An unmet medical need. *Oncologist* **2011**, *161*, 1–11. [CrossRef] [PubMed]
6. Moulder, S.; Hortobagyi, G.N. Advances in the treatment of breast cancer. *Clin. Pharmacol. Ther.* **2008**, *83*, 26–36. [PubMed]
7. DeSantis, C.; Ma, J.M.; Bryan, L.; Jemal, A. Breast cancer statistics, 2013. *CA Cancer J. Clin.* **2014**, *64*, 52–62. [CrossRef] [PubMed]
8. Cazzaniga, M.; Bonanni, B. Breast cancer chemoprevention: Old and new approaches. *J. Biomed. Biotechnol.* **2012**, *2012*, 985620. [PubMed]
9. Reddy, K.B. Triple-negative breast cancers: An updated review on treatment options. *Curr. Oncol.* **2011**, *18*, E173–E179. [CrossRef] [PubMed]
10. Bhadoria, A.S.; Kapil, U.; Sareen, N.; Singh, P. Reproductive factors and breast cancer: A case-control study in tertiary care hospital of North India. *Indian J. Cancer* **2013**, *50*, 316–321. [PubMed]
11. Rieder, V.; Salama, M.; Glockner, L.; Muhr, D.; Berger, A.; Tea, M.K.; Pfeiler, G.; Rappaport-Fuerhauser, C.; Gschwantler-Kaulich, D.; Weingartshofer, S. Effect of lifestyle and reproductive factors on the onset of breast cancer in female BRCA 1 and 2 mutation carriers. *Mol. Genet. Genom. Med.* **2016**, *4*, 172–177. [CrossRef] [PubMed]
12. Sisti, J.S.; Collins, L.C.; Beck, A.H.; Tamimi, R.M.; Rosner, B.A.; Eliassen, A.H. Reproductive risk factors in relation to molecular subtypes of breast cancer: Results from the nurses' health studies. *Int. J. Cancer* **2016**, *138*, 2346–2356. [CrossRef] [PubMed]
13. Ma, H.Y.; Ursin, G.; Xu, X.X.; Lee, E.; Togawa, K.; Duan, L.; Lu, Y.N.; Malone, K.E.; Marchbanks, P.A.; McDonald, J.A. Reproductive factors and the risk of triple-negative breast cancer in white women and African-American women: A pooled analysis. *Breast Cancer Res.* **2017**, *19*. [CrossRef] [PubMed]
14. Narod, S.A. Hormone replacement therapy and the risk of breast cancer. *Nat. Rev. Clin. Oncol.* **2011**, *8*, 669–676. [CrossRef] [PubMed]

15. Park, S.Y.; Kolonel, L.N.; Lim, U.; White, K.K.; Henderson, B.E.; Wilkens, L.R. Alcohol consumption and breast cancer risk among women from five ethnic groups with light to moderate intakes: The Multiethnic Cohort Study. *Int. J. Cancer* **2014**, *134*, 1504–1510. [CrossRef] [PubMed]

16. Park, Y.; O'Brien, K.M.; Zhao, S.S.; Weinberg, C.R.; Baird, D.D.; Sandler, D.P. Gestational diabetes mellitus may be associated with increased risk of breast cancer. *Br. J. Cancer* **2017**, *116*, 960–963. [CrossRef] [PubMed]

17. Charlot, M.; Castro-Webb, N.; Bethea, T.N.; Bertrand, K.; Boggs, D.A.; Denis, G.V.; Adams-Campbell, L.L.; Rosenberg, L.; Palmer, J.R. Diabetes and breast cancer mortality in Black women. *Cancer Cause Control* **2017**, *28*, 61–67. [CrossRef] [PubMed]

18. Pierobon, M.; Frankenfeld, C.L. Obesity as a risk factor for triple-negative breast cancers: A systematic review and meta-analysis. *Breast Cancer Res. Treat.* **2013**, *137*, 307–314. [CrossRef] [PubMed]

19. Jia, Y.J.; Lu, Y.S.; Wu, K.J.; Lin, Q.; Shen, W.; Zhu, M.J.; Huang, S.; Chen, J. Does night work increase the risk of breast cancer? A systematic review and meta-analysis of epidemiological studies. *Cancer Epidemiol.* **2013**, *37*, 197–206. [CrossRef] [PubMed]

20. Campeau, P.M.; Foulkes, W.D.; Tischkowitz, M.D. Hereditary breast cancer: New genetic developments, new therapeutic avenues. *Hum. Genet.* **2008**, *124*, 31–42. [CrossRef] [PubMed]

21. Zheng, J.; Zhou, Y.; Li, Y.; Xu, D.P.; Li, S.; Li, H.B. Spices for prevention and treatment of cancers. *Nutrients* **2016**, *8*, 495. [CrossRef] [PubMed]

22. Zhou, Y.; Zheng, J.; Li, Y.; Xu, D.P.; Li, S.; Chen, Y.M.; Li, H.B. Natural polyphenols for prevention and treatment of cancer. *Nutrients* **2016**, *8*, 515. [CrossRef] [PubMed]

23. Zhou, Y.; Li, Y.; Zhou, T.; Zheng, J.; Li, S.; Li, H.B. Dietary natural products for prevention and treatment of liver cancer. *Nutrients* **2016**, *8*, 156. [CrossRef] [PubMed]

24. Zhang, J.J.; Li, Y.; Zhou, T.; Xu, D.P.; Zhang, P.; Li, S.; Li, H.B. Bioactivities and health benefits of mushrooms mainly from China. *Molecules* **2016**, *21*, 938. [CrossRef] [PubMed]

25. Zhang, Y.J.; Gan, R.Y.; Li, S.; Zhou, Y.; Li, A.N.; Xu, D.P.; Li, H.B. Antioxidant Phytochemicals for the Prevention and Treatment of Chronic Diseases. *Molecules* **2015**, *20*, 21138–21156. [CrossRef] [PubMed]

26. Li, F.; Li, S.; Li, H.B.; Deng, G.F.; Ling, W.H.; Xu, X.R. Antiproliferative activities of tea and herbal infusions. *Food Funct.* **2013**, *4*, 530–538. [CrossRef] [PubMed]

27. Grosso, G.; Bella, F.; Godos, J.; Sciacca, S.; Del Rio, D.; Ray, S.; Galvano, F.; Giovannucci, E.L. Possible role of diet in cancer: Systematic review and multiple meta-analyses of dietary patterns, lifestyle factors, and cancer risk. *Nutr. Rev.* **2017**, *75*, 405–419. [CrossRef]

28. Farvid, M.S.; Chen, W.Y.; Michels, K.B.; Cho, E.; Willett, W.C.; Eliassen, A.H. Fruit and vegetable consumption in adolescence and early adulthood and risk of breast cancer: Population based cohort study. *BMJ Br. Med. J.* **2016**, *353*. [CrossRef] [PubMed]

29. Kim, M.K.; Kim, J.H.; Nam, S.J.; Ryu, S.; Kong, G. Dietary intake of soy protein and tofu in association with breast cancer risk based on a case-control study. *Nutr. Cancer* **2008**, *60*, 568–576. [CrossRef] [PubMed]

30. Nechuta, S.J.; Caan, B.J.; Chen, W.Y.; Lu, W.; Chen, Z.; Kwan, M.L.; Flatt, S.W.; Zheng, Y.; Zheng, W.; Pierce, J.P. Soy food intake after diagnosis of breast cancer and survival: An in-depth analysis of combined evidence from cohort studies of US and Chinese women. *Am. J. Clin. Nutr.* **2012**, *96*, 123–132. [CrossRef] [PubMed]

31. Thomson, C.A.; Rock, C.L.; Thompson, P.A.; Caan, B.J.; Cussler, E.; Flatt, S.W.; Pierce, J.P. Vegetable intake is associated with reduced breast cancer recurrence in tamoxifen users: A secondary analysis from the Women's Healthy Eating and Living Study. *Breast Cancer Res. Treat.* **2011**, *125*, 519–527. [CrossRef] [PubMed]

32. Lv, Z.D.; Liu, X.P.; Zhao, W.J.; Dong, Q.; Li, F.N.; Wang, H.B.; Kong, B. Curcumin induces apoptosis in breast cancer cells and inhibits tumor growth in vitro and in vivo. *Int. J. Clin. Exp. Pathol.* **2014**, *7*, 2818–2824. [PubMed]

33. Gallardo, M.; Calaf, G.M. Curcumin inhibits invasive capabilities through epithelial mesenchymal transition in breast cancer cell lines. *Int. J. Oncol.* **2016**, *49*, 1019–1027. [CrossRef] [PubMed]

34. Varinska, L.; Gal, P.; Mojzisova, G.; Mirossay, L.; Mojzis, J. Soy and breast cancer: Focus on angiogenesis. *Int. J. Mol. Sci.* **2015**, *16*, 11728–11749. [CrossRef] [PubMed]

35. Hu, X.J.; Xie, M.Y.; Kluxen, F.M.; Diel, P. Genistein modulates the anti-tumor activity of cisplatin in MCF-7 breast and HT-29 colon cancer cells. *Arch. Toxicol.* **2014**, *88*, 625–635. [CrossRef] [PubMed]

36. Bonofiglio, D.; Giordano, C.; de Amicis, F.; Lanzino, M.; Ando, S. Natural products as promising antitumoral agents in breast cancer: Mechanisms of action and molecular targets. *Mini Rev. Med. Chem.* **2016**, *16*, 596–604. [CrossRef] [PubMed]

37. Zhang, X.L.; Shu, X.O.; Gao, Y.T.; Yang, G.; Li, Q.; Li, H.L.; Jin, F.; Zheng, W. Soy food consumption is associated with lower risk of coronary heart disease in Chinese women. *J. Nutr.* **2003**, *133*, 2874–2878. [PubMed]

38. Mueller, N.T.; Odegaard, A.O.; Gross, M.D.; Koh, W.P.; Yu, M.C.; Yuan, J.M.; Pereira, M.A. Soy intake and risk of type 2 diabetes mellitus in Chinese Singaporeans. *Eur. J. Nutr.* **2012**, *51*, 1033–1040. [CrossRef] [PubMed]

39. Dong, J.Y.; Qin, L.Q. Soy isoflavones consumption and risk of breast cancer incidence or recurrence: A meta-analysis of prospective studies. *Breast Cancer Res. Treat.* **2011**, *125*, 315–323. [CrossRef] [PubMed]

40. Grosso, G.; Godos, J.; Lamuela-Raventos, R.; Ray, S.; Micek, A.; Pajak, A.; Sciacca, S.; D'Orazio, N.; Del Rio, D.; Galvano, F. A comprehensive meta-analysis on dietary flavonoid and lignan intake and cancer risk: Level of evidence and limitations. *Mol. Nutr. Food Res.* **2017**, *61*. [CrossRef] [PubMed]

41. Chi, F.; Wu, R.; Zeng, Y.C.; Xing, R.; Liu, Y.; Xu, Z.G. Post-diagnosis soy food intake and breast cancer survival: A meta-analysis of cohort studies. *Asian Pac. J. Cancer Prev.* **2013**, *14*, 2407–2412. [CrossRef] [PubMed]

42. Zhu, Y.Y.; Zhou, L.; Jiao, S.C.; Xu, L.Z. Relationship between soy food intake and breast cancer in China. *Asian Pac. J. Cancer Prev.* **2011**, *12*, 2837–2840. [PubMed]

43. Trock, B.J.; Hilakivi-Clarke, L.; Clarke, R. Meta-analysis of soy intake and breast cancer risk. *J. Natl. Cancer Inst.* **2006**, *98*, 459–471. [CrossRef] [PubMed]

44. Nagata, C. Factors to consider in the association between soy Iisoflavone intake and breast cancer risk. *J. Epidemiol.* **2010**, *20*, 83–89. [CrossRef] [PubMed]

45. Baglia, M.L.; Zheng, W.; Li, H.L.; Yang, G.; Gao, J.; Gao, Y.T.; Shu, X.O. The association of soy food consumption with the risk of subtype of breast cancers defined by hormone receptor and HER2 status. *Int. J. Cancer* **2016**, *139*, 742–748. [CrossRef] [PubMed]

46. Wada, K.; Nakamura, K.; Tamai, Y.; Tsuji, M.; Kawachi, T.; Hori, A.; Takeyama, N.; Tanabashi, S.; Matsushita, S.; Tokimitsu, N. Soy isoflavone intake and breast cancer risk in Japan: From the Takayama study. *Int. J. Cancer* **2013**, *133*, 952–960. [CrossRef] [PubMed]

47. Zhang, Y.F.; Kang, H.B.; Li, B.L.; Zhang, R.M. Positive effects of Ssoy isoflavone food on survival of breast cancer patients in China. *Asian Pac. J. Cancer Prev.* **2012**, *13*, 479–482. [CrossRef] [PubMed]

48. Ko, K.P.; Kim, S.W.; Ma, S.H.; Park, B.; Ahn, Y.; Lee, J.W.; Lee, M.H.; Kang, E.; Kim, L.S.; Jung, Y. Dietary intake and breast cancer among carriers and noncarriers of BRCA mutations in the Korean Hereditary Breast Cancer Study. *Am. J. Clin. Nutr.* **2013**, *98*, 1493–1501. [CrossRef] [PubMed]

49. Guo, X.Y.; Cai, Q.Y.; Bao, P.P.; Wu, J.; Wen, W.Q.; Ye, F.; Zheng, W.; Zheng, Y.; Shu, X.O. Long-term soy consumption and tumor tissue microRNA and gene expression in triple-negative breast cancer. *Cancer Am. Cancer Soc.* **2016**, *122*, 2544–2551. [CrossRef] [PubMed]

50. Conroy, S.M.; Maskarinec, G.; Park, S.Y.; Wilkens, L.R.; Henderson, B.E.; Kolonel, L.N. The effects of soy consumption before diagnosis on breast cancer survival: The multiethnic cohort study. *Nutr. Cancer* **2013**, *65*, 527–537. [CrossRef] [PubMed]

51. Morimoto, Y.; Maskarinec, G.; Park, S.Y.; Ettienne, R.; Matsuno, R.K.; Long, C.; Steffen, A.D.; Henderson, B.E.; Kolonel, L.N.; Le Marchand, L. Dietary isoflavone intake is not statistically significantly associated with breast cancer risk in the Multiethnic Cohort. *Br. J. Nutr.* **2014**, *112*, 976–983. [CrossRef] [PubMed]

52. Woo, H.D.; Park, K.S.; Ro, J.; Kim, J. Differential influence of dietary soy intake on the risk of breast cancer recurrence related to HER2 status. *Nutr. Cancer* **2012**, *64*, 198–205. [CrossRef] [PubMed]

53. Khan, S.A.; Chatterton, R.T.; Michel, N.; Bryk, M.; Lee, O.; Ivancic, D.; Heinz, R.; Zalles, C.M.; Helenowski, I.B.; Jovanovic, B.D. Soy isoflavone supplementation for breast cancer risk reduction: A randomized phase II trial. *Cancer Prev. Res.* **2012**, *5*, 309–319. [CrossRef] [PubMed]

54. Yamamoto, S.; Sobue, T.; Sasaki, S.; Kobayashi, M.; Arai, Y.; Uehara, M.; Adlercreutz, H.; Watanabe, S.; Takahashi, T.; Iitoi, Y. Validity and reproducibility of a self-administered food-frequency questionnaire to assess isoflavone intake in a Japanese population in comparison with dietary records and blood and urine isoflavones. *J. Nutr.* **2001**, *131*, 2741–2747. [PubMed]

55. Jemal, A.; Bray, F.; Center, M.M.; Ferlay, J.; Ward, E.; Forman, D. Global cancer statistics. *CA Cancer J. Clin.* **2011**, *61*, 69–90. [CrossRef] [PubMed]

56. Kuiper, G.G.; Lemmen, J.G.; Carlsson, B.; Corton, J.C.; Safe, S.H.; van der Saag, P.T.; van der Burg, B.; Gustafsson, J.A. Interaction of estrogenic chemicals and phytoestrogens with estrogen receptor beta. *Endocrinology* **1998**, *139*, 4252–4263. [CrossRef] [PubMed]

57. Kuiper, G.G.; Carlsson, B.; Grandien, K.; Enmark, E.; Häggblad, J.; Nilsson, S.; Gustafsson, J.A. Comparison of the ligand binding specificity and transcript tissue distribution of estrogen receptors alpha and beta. *Endocrinology* **1997**, *138*, 863–870. [CrossRef] [PubMed]

58. Pons, D.G.; Nadal-Serrano, M.; Blanquer-Rossello, M.M.; Sastre-Serra, J.; Oliver, J.; Roca, P. Genistein modulates proliferation and mitochondrial functionality in breast cancer cells depending on ERalpha/ERbeta ratio. *J. Cell. Biochem.* **2014**, *115*, 949–958. [CrossRef] [PubMed]

59. Nadal-Serrano, M.; Pons, D.G.; Sastre-Serra, J.; Blanquer-Rossello, M.D.; Roca, P.; Oliver, J. Genistein modulates oxidative stress in breast cancer cell lines according to ER alpha/ER beta ratio: Effects on mitochondrial functionality, sirtuins, uncoupling protein 2 and antioxidant enzymes. *Int. J. Biochem. Cell Biol.* **2013**, *45*, 2045–2051. [CrossRef] [PubMed]

60. Pons, D.G.; Nadal-Serrano, M.; Torrens-Mas, M.; Oliver, J.; Roca, P. The phytoestrogen genistein affects breast cancer cells treatment depending on the ER alpha/ER beta ratio. *J. Cell. Biochem.* **2016**, *117*, 218–229. [CrossRef] [PubMed]

61. Zhang, G.P.; Han, D.; Liu, G.; Gao, S.G.; Cai, X.Q.; Duan, R.H.; Feng, X.S. Effects of soy isoflavone and endogenous oestrogen on breast cancer in MMTV-erbB2 transgenic mice. *J. Int. Med. Res.* **2012**, *40*, 2073–2082. [CrossRef] [PubMed]

62. Li, Z.; Li, J.; Mo, B.Q.; Hu, C.Y.; Liu, H.Q.; Qi, H.; Wang, X.R.; Xu, J.D. Genistein induces cell apoptosis in MDA-MB-231 breast cancer cells via the mitogen-activated protein kinase pathway. *Toxicol. In Vitro* **2008**, *22*, 1749–1753. [CrossRef] [PubMed]

63. Magee, P.J.; Allsopp, P.; Samaletdin, A.; Rowland, I.R. Daidzein, *R*-(+)equol and *S*-(−)equol inhibit the invasion of MDA-MB-231 breast cancer cells potentially via the down-regulation of matrix metalloproteinase-2. *Eur. J. Nutr.* **2014**, *53*, 345–350. [CrossRef] [PubMed]

64. Seol, J.Y.; Youn, Y.N.; Koo, M.; Kim, H.J.; Choi, S.Y. Influence of water-soluble extracts of long-term fermented doenjang on bone metabolism bioactivity and breast cancer suppression. *Food Sci. Biotechnol.* **2016**, *25*, 517–524. [CrossRef]

65. Zhao, Q.X.; Zhao, M.; Parris, A.B.; Xing, Y.; Yang, X.H. Genistein targets the cancerous inhibitor of PP2A to induce growth inhibition and apoptosis in breast cancer cells. *Int. J. Oncol.* **2016**, *49*, 1203–1210. [CrossRef] [PubMed]

66. Chen, J.; Duan, Y.X.; Zhang, X.; Ye, Y.; Ge, B.; Chen, J. Genistein induces apoptosis by the inactivation of the IGF-1R/p-Akt signaling pathway in MCF-7 human breast cancer cells. *Food Funct.* **2015**, *6*, 995–1000. [CrossRef] [PubMed]

67. Lee, J.H.; Lee, H.J. A daidzein metabolite, 6,7,4′-trihydroxyisoflavone inhibits cellular proliferation through cell cycle arrest and apoptosis induction in MCF10CA1a human breast cancer cells. *J. Korean Soc. Appl. Biol. Chem.* **2013**, *56*, 695–700. [CrossRef]

68. Stocco, B.; Toledo, K.A.; Fumagalli, H.F.; Bianchini, F.J.; Fortes, V.S.; Fonseca, M.; Toloi, M. Biotransformed soybean extract induces cell death of estrogen-dependent breast cancer cells by modulation of apoptotic proteins. *Nutr. Cancer* **2015**, *67*, 612–619. [CrossRef] [PubMed]

69. Xie, Q.; Bai, Q.; Zou, L.Y.; Zhang, Q.Y.; Zhou, Y.; Chang, H.; Yi, L.; Zhu, J.D.; Mi, M.T. Genistein inhibits DNA methylation and increases expression of tumor suppressor genes in human breast cancer cells. *Genes Chromosomes Cancer* **2014**, *53*, 422–431. [CrossRef] [PubMed]

70. Fang, Y.; Zhang, Q.; Wang, X.; Yang, X.; Wang, X.Y.; Huang, Z.; Jiao, Y.C.; Wang, J. Quantitative phosphoproteomics reveals genistein as a modulator of cell cycle and DNA damage response pathways in triple-negative breast cancer cells. *Int. J. Oncol.* **2016**, *48*, 1016–1028. [CrossRef] [PubMed]

71. Pan, H.; Zhou, W.B.; He, W.; Liu, X.A.; Ding, Q.; Ling, L.J.; Zha, X.M.; Wang, S. Genistein inhibits MDA-MB-231 triple-negative breast cancer cell growth by inhibiting NF-kappa B activity via the Notch-1 pathway. *Int. J. Mol. Med.* **2012**, *30*, 337–343. [PubMed]

72. Fan, P.H.; Fan, S.J.; Wang, H.; Mao, J.; Shi, Y.; Ibrahim, M.M.; Ma, W.; Yu, X.T.; Hou, Z.H.; Wang, B. Genistein decreases the breast cancer stem-like cell population through Hedgehog pathway. *Stem Cell Res. Ther.* **2013**, *4*. [CrossRef] [PubMed]

73. Johnson, K.A.; Vemuri, S.; Alsahafi, S.; Castillo, R.; Cheriyath, V. Glycone-rich soy isoflavone extracts promote estrogen receptor positive breast cancer cell growth. *Nutr. Cancer* **2016**, *68*, 622–633. [CrossRef] [PubMed]

74. Wei, Y.; Gamra, I.; Davenport, A.; Lester, R.; Zhao, L.J.; Wei, Y.D. Genistein induces cytochrome P450 1B1 gene expression and cell proliferation in human breast cancer MCF-7 Ccells. *J. Environ. Pathol. Toxicol. Pathol.* **2015**, *34*, 153–159. [CrossRef]

75. Andrade, J.E.; Ju, Y.H.; Baker, C.; Doerge, D.R.; Helferich, W.G. Long-term exposure to dietary sources of genistein induces estrogen-independence in the human breast cancer (MCF-7) xenograft model. *Mol. Nutr. Food Res.* **2015**, *59*, 413–423. [CrossRef] [PubMed]

76. Yang, X.J.; Belosay, A.; Hartman, J.A.; Song, H.X.; Zhang, Y.K.; Wang, W.D.; Doerge, D.R.; Helferich, W.G. Dietary soy isoflavones increase metastasis to lungs in an experimental model of breast cancer with bone micro-tumors. *Clin. Exp. Metastasis* **2015**, *32*, 323–333. [CrossRef] [PubMed]

77. Gaete, L.; Tchernitchin, A.N.; Bustamante, R.; Villena, J.; Lemus, I.; Gidekel, M.; Cabrera, G.; Astorga, P. Daidzein-estrogen interaction in the rat uterus and its effect on human breast cancer cell growth. *J. Med. Food* **2012**, *15*, 1081–1090. [CrossRef] [PubMed]

78. Koo, J.; Cabarcas-Petroski, S.; Petrie, J.L.; Diette, N.; White, R.J.; Schramm, L. Induction of proto-oncogene BRF2 in breast cancer cells by the dietary soybean isoflavone daidzein. *BMC Cancer* **2015**, *15*. [CrossRef] [PubMed]

79. Rigalli, J.P.; Tocchetti, G.N.; Arana, M.R.; Villanueva, S.; Catania, V.A.; Theile, D.; Ruiz, M.L.; Weiss, J. The phytoestrogen genistein enhances multidrug resistance in breast cancer cell lines by translational regulation of ABC transporters. *Cancer Lett.* **2016**, *376*, 165–172. [CrossRef] [PubMed]

80. Xie, Q.; Chen, M.L.; Qin, Y.; Zhang, Q.Y.; Xu, H.X.; Zhou, Y.; Mi, M.T.; Zhu, J.D. Isoflavone consumption and risk of breast cancer: A dose-response meta-analysis of observational studies. *Asia Pac. J. Clin. Nutr.* **2013**, *22*, 118–127. [PubMed]

81. Li, Y.; Zhang, J.J.; Xu, D.P.; Zhou, T.; Zhou, Y.; Li, S.; Li, H.B. Bioactivities and health benefits of wild fruits. *Int. J. Mol. Sci.* **2016**, *17*, 1258. [CrossRef] [PubMed]

82. Li, F.; Li, S.; Li, H.B.; Deng, G.F.; Ling, W.H.; Wu, S.; Xu, X.R.; Chen, F. Antiproliferative activity of peels, pulps and seeds of 61 fruits. *J. Funct. Foods* **2013**, *5*, 1298–1309. [CrossRef]

83. Fu, L.; Xu, B.T.; Xu, X.R.; Gan, R.Y.; Zhang, Y.; Xia, E.Q.; Li, H.B. Antioxidant capacities and total phenolic contents of 62 fruits. *Food Chem.* **2011**, *129*, 345–350. [CrossRef]

84. Fu, L.; Xu, B.T.; Xu, X.R.; Qin, X.S.; Gan, R.Y.; Li, H.B. Antioxidant capacities and total phenolic contents of 56 wild fruits from South China. *Molecules* **2010**, *15*, 8602–8617. [CrossRef] [PubMed]

85. Xia, E.Q.; Deng, G.F.; Guo, Y.J.; Li, H.B. Biological activities of polyphenols from grapes. *Int. J. Mol. Sci.* **2010**, *11*, 622–646. [CrossRef] [PubMed]

86. Aune, D.; Chan, D.; Vieira, A.R.; Rosenblatt, D.; Vieira, R.; Greenwood, D.C.; Norat, T. Fruits, vegetables and breast cancer risk: A systematic review and meta-analysis of prospective studies. *Breast Cancer Res. Treat.* **2012**, *134*, 479–493. [CrossRef] [PubMed]

87. He, J.J.; Gu, Y.T.; Zhang, S.J. Consumption of vegetables and fruits and breast cancer survival: A systematic review and meta-analysis. *Sci. Rep.* **2017**, *7*. [CrossRef] [PubMed]

88. Wang, L.; Martins-Green, M. The potential of pomegranate and its components for prevention and treatment of breast cancer. *Agro Food Ind. Hi-Tech* **2013**, *24*, 58–61.

89. Adams, L.S.; Zhang, Y.; Navindra, P.; Seeram, N.P.; Heber, D; Chen, S. Pomegranate juice, total pomegranate ellagitannins, and punicalagin suppress inflammatory cell signaling in colon cancer cells. *J. Agric. Food Chem.* **2006**, *54*, 980–985. [CrossRef] [PubMed]

90. Legua, P.; Forner-Giner, M.A.; Nuncio-Jauregui, N.; Hernandez, F. Polyphenolic compounds, anthocyanins and antioxidant activity of nineteen pomegranate fruits: A rich source of bioactive compounds. *J. Funct. Foods* **2016**, *23*, 628–636. [CrossRef]

91. Shirode, A.B.; Kovvuru, P.; Chittur, S.V.; Henning, S.M.; Heber, D.; Reliene, R. Antiproliferative effects of pomegranate extract in MCF-7 breast cancer cells are associated with reduced DNA repair gene expression and induction of double strand breaks. *Mol. Carcinog.* **2014**, *53*, 458–470. [CrossRef] [PubMed]

92. Mandal, A.; Bishayee, A. Mechanism of breast cancer preventive action of pomegranate: Disruption of estrogen receptor and Wnt/beta-catenin signaling pathways. *Molecules* **2015**, *20*, 22315–22328. [CrossRef] [PubMed]

93. Costantini, S.; Rusolo, F.; De Vito, V.; Moccia, S.; Picariello, G.; Capone, F.; Guerriero, E.; Castello, G.; Volpe, M.G. Potential anti-inflammatory effects of the hydrophilic fraction of pomegranate (*Punica granatum* L.) seed oil on breast cancer cell lines. *Molecules* **2014**, *19*, 8644–8660. [CrossRef] [PubMed]

94.  Rocha, A.; Wang, L.; Penichet, M.; Martins-Green, M. Pomegranate juice and specific components inhibit cell and molecular processes critical for metastasis of breast cancer. *Breast Cancer Res. Treat.* **2012**, *136*, 647–658. [CrossRef] [PubMed]

95.  Banerjee, N.; Talcott, S.; Safe, S.; Mertens-Talcott, S.U. Cytotoxicity of pomegranate polyphenolics in breast cancer cells in vitro and vivo: Potential role of miRNA-27a and miRNA-155 in cell survival and inflammation. *Breast Cancer Res. Treat.* **2012**, *136*, 21–34. [CrossRef] [PubMed]

96.  Dikmen, M.; Ozturk, N.; Ozturk, Y. The antioxidant potency of *Punica granatum* L. fruit peel reduces cell proliferation and induces apoptosis on breast cancer. *J. Med. Food* **2011**, *14*, 1638–1646. [CrossRef] [PubMed]

97.  Khan, G.N.; Gorin, M.A.; Rosenthal, D.; Pan, Q.T.; Bao, L.W.; Wu, Z.F.; Newman, R.A.; Pawlus, A.D.; Yang, P.Y.; Lansky, E.P. Pomegranate fruit extract impairs invasion and motility in human breast cancer. *Integr. Cancer Ther.* **2009**, *8*, 242–253. [CrossRef] [PubMed]

98.  Adams, L.S.; Zhang, Y.J.; Seeram, N.P.; Heber, D.; Chen, S.A. Pomegranate ellagitannin-derived compounds exhibit antiproliferative and antiaromatase activity in breast cancer cells in vitro. *Cancer Prev. Res.* **2010**, *3*, 108–113. [CrossRef] [PubMed]

99.  Mehta, R.; Lansky, E.P. Breast cancer chemopreventive properties of pomegranate (*Punica granatum*) fruit extracts in a mouse mammary organ culture. *Eur. J. Cancer Prev.* **2004**, *13*, 345–348. [CrossRef] [PubMed]

100. Kim, N.D.; Mehta, R.; Yu, W.P.; Neeman, I.; Livney, T.; Amichay, A.; Poirier, D.; Nicholls, P.; Kirby, A.; Jiang, W.G. Chemopreventive and adjuvant therapeutic potential of pomegranate (*Punica granatum*) for human breast cancer. *Breast Cancer Res. Treat.* **2002**, *71*, 203–217. [CrossRef] [PubMed]

101. Moongkarndi, P.; Kosem, N.; Kaslungka, S.; Luanratana, O.; Pongpan, N.; Neungton, N. Antiproliferation, antioxidation and induction of apoptosis by *Garcinia mangostana* (mangosteen) on SKBR3 human breast cancer cell line. *J. Ethnopharmacol.* **2004**, *90*, 161–166. [CrossRef] [PubMed]

102. Yu, L.M.; Zhao, M.M.; Yang, B.; Bai, W.D. Immunomodulatory and anticancer activities of phenolics from *Garcinia mangostana* fruit pericarp. *Food Chem.* **2009**, *116*, 969–973. [CrossRef]

103. Gutierrez-Orozco, F.; Failla, M. Biological activities and bioavailability of mangosteen xanthones: A critical review of the current evidence. *Nutrients* **2013**, *5*, 3163–3183. [CrossRef] [PubMed]

104. Balunas, M.J.; Su, B.; Brueggemeier, R.W.; Kinghorn, A.D. Xanthones from the botanical dietary supplement mangosteen (*Garcinia mangostana*) with aromatase inhibitory activity. *J. Nat. Prod.* **2008**, *71*, 1161–1166. [CrossRef] [PubMed]

105. Kritsanawong, S.; Innajak, S.; Imoto, M.; Watanapokasin, R. Antiproliferative and apoptosis induction of alpha-mangostin in T47D breast cancer cells. *Int. J. Oncol.* **2016**, *48*, 2155–2165. [PubMed]

106. Kurose, H.; Shibata, M.A.; Iinuma, M.; Otsuki, Y. Alterations in cell cycle and induction of apoptotic cell death in breast cancer cells treated with alpha-mangostin extracted from mangosteen pericarp. *J. Biomed. Biotechnol.* **2012**, *2012*, 9p. [CrossRef] [PubMed]

107. Moongkarndi, P.; Jaisupa, N.; Samer, J.; Kosem, N.; Konlata, J.; Rodpai, E.; Pongpan, N. Comparison of the biological activity of two different isolates from mangosteen. *J. Pharm. Pharmacol.* **2014**, *66*, 1171–1179. [CrossRef] [PubMed]

108. Li, P.; Tian, W.X.; Ma, X.F. Alpha-mangostin inhibits intracellular fatty acid synthase and induces apoptosis in breast cancer cells. *Mol. Cancer* **2014**, *13*, 138. [CrossRef] [PubMed]

109. Won, Y.S.; Lee, J.H.; Kwon, S.J.; Kim, J.Y.; Park, K.H.; Lee, M.K.; Seo, K.I. Alpha-Mangostin-induced apoptosis is mediated by estrogen receptor alpha in human breast cancer cells. *Food Chem. Toxicol.* **2014**, *66*, 158–165. [CrossRef] [PubMed]

110. Shibata, M.A.; Iinuma, M.; Morimoto, J.; Kurose, H.; Akamatsu, K.; Okuno, Y.; Akao, Y.; Otsuki, Y. α-Mangostin extracted from the pericarp of the mangosteen (*Garcinia mangostana* Linn) reduces tumor growth and lymph node metastasis in an immunocompetent xenograft model of metastatic mammary cancer carrying a p53 mutation. *BMC Med.* **2011**, *9*, 69. [CrossRef] [PubMed]

111. Doi, H.; Shibata, M.A.; Shibata, E.; Morimoto, J.; Akao, Y.; Iinuma, M.; Tanigawa, N.; Otsuki, Y. Panaxanthone isolated from pericarp of *Garcinia mangostana* L. suppresses tumor growth and metastasis of a mouse model of mammary cancer. *Anticancer Res.* **2009**, *29*, 2485–2495. [PubMed]

112. Song, J.K.; Bae, J.M. Citrus fruit intake and breast cancer risk: A quantitative systematic review. *J. Breast Cancer* **2013**, *16*, 72–76. [CrossRef] [PubMed]

113. Park, J.Y.; Shin, M.S.; Kim, S.N.; Kim, H.Y.; Kim, K.H.; Shin, K.S.; Kang, K.S. Polysaccharides from Korean Citrus hallabong peels inhibit angiogenesis and breast cancer cell migration. *Int. J. Biol. Macromol.* **2016**, *85*, 522–529. [CrossRef] [PubMed]

114. Nguyen, L.T.T.; Song, Y.W.; Tran, T.A.; Kim, K.S.; Cho, S.K. Induction of apoptosis in anoikis-resistant breast cancer stem cells by supercritical $CO_2$ extracts from Citrus hassaku Hort ex Tanaka. *J. Korean Soc. Appl. Biol.* **2014**, *57*, 469–472. [CrossRef]

115. Alshatwi, A.A.; Shafi, G.; Hasan, T.N.; Al-Hazzani, A.A.; Alsaif, M.A.; Alfawaz, M.A.; Lei, K.Y.; Munshi, A. Apoptosis-mediated inhibition of human breast cancer cell proliferation by lemon citrus extract. *Asian Pac. J. Cancer Prev.* **2011**, *12*, 1555–1559. [PubMed]

116. Li, H.Z.; Yang, B.; Huang, J.; Xiang, T.X.; Yin, X.D.; Wan, J.Y.; Luo, F.; Zhang, L.; Li, H.Y.; Ren, G.S. Naringin inhibits growth potential of human triple-negative breast cancer cells by targeting beta-catenin signaling pathway. *Toxicol. Lett.* **2013**, *220*, 219–228. [CrossRef] [PubMed]

117. Lee, C.J.; Wilson, L.; Jordan, M.A.; Nguyen, V.; Tang, J.; Smiyun, G. Hesperidin suppressed proliferations of both human breast cancer and androgen-dependent prostate cancer cells. *Phytother. Res.* **2010**, *241*, S15–S19. [CrossRef] [PubMed]

118. Yang, S.F.; Zhang, H.S.; Yang, X.B.; Zhu, Y.L.; Zhang, M. Evaluation of antioxidative and antitumor activities of extracted flavonoids from Pink Lady apples in human colon and breast cancer cell lines. *Food Funct.* **2015**, *6*, 3789–3798. [CrossRef] [PubMed]

119. Schiavano, G.F.; De Santi, M.; Brandi, G.; Fanelli, M.; Bucchini, A.; Giamperi, L.; Giomaro, G. Inhibition of breast cancer cell proliferation and in vitro tumorigenesis by a new red apple cultivar. *PLoS ONE* **2015**, *10*, e135840. [CrossRef] [PubMed]

120. Sun, J.; Liu, R.H. Apple phytochemical extracts inhibit proliferation of estrogen-dependent and estrogen-independent human breast cancer cells through cell cycle modulation. *J. Agric. Food Chem.* **2008**, *56*, 11661–11667. [CrossRef] [PubMed]

121. Yoon, H.; Liu, R.H. Effect of selected phytochemicals and apple extracts on NF-kappa B activation in human breast cancer MCF-7 cells. *J. Agric. Food Chem.* **2007**, *55*, 3167–3173. [CrossRef] [PubMed]

122. Yoon, H.; Liu, R.H. Effect of 2 alpha-hydroxyursolic acid on NF-kappa B activation induced by TNF-alpha in human breast cancer MCF-7 cells. *J. Agric. Food Chem.* **2008**, *56*, 8412–8417. [CrossRef] [PubMed]

123. Jiang, X.; Li, T.; Liu, R.H. 2 alpha-Hydroxyursolic acid inhibited cell proliferation and induced apoptosis in MDA-MB-231 human breast cancer cells through the p38/MAPK signal transduction pathway. *J. Agric. Food Chem.* **2016**, *64*, 1806–1816. [CrossRef] [PubMed]

124. Delphi, L.; Sepehri, H. Apple pectin: A natural source for cancer suppression in 4T1 breast cancer cells in vitro and express p53 in mouse bearing 4T1 cancer tumors, in vivo. *Biomed. Pharmacother.* **2016**, *84*, 637–644. [CrossRef] [PubMed]

125. Yang, J.; Liu, R.H. Synergistic effect of apple extracts and quercetin 3-beta-D-glucoside combination on antiproliferative activity in MCF-7 human breast cancer cells in vitro. *J. Agric. Food Chem.* **2009**, *57*, 8581–8586. [CrossRef] [PubMed]

126. Sun, T.; Chen, Q.Y.; Wu, L.J.; Yao, X.M.; Sun, X.J. Antitumor and antimetastatic activities of grape skin polyphenols in a murine model of breast cancer. *Food Chem. Toxicol.* **2012**, *50*, 3462–3467. [CrossRef] [PubMed]

127. Dinicola, S.; Pasqualato, A.; Cucina, A.; Coluccia, P.; Ferranti, F.; Canipari, R.; Catizone, A.; Proietti, S.; D'Anselmi, F.; Ricci, G. Grape seed extract suppresses MDA-MB231 breast cancer cell migration and invasion. *Eur. J. Nutr.* **2014**, *53*, 421–431. [CrossRef] [PubMed]

128. Hakimuddin, F.; Paliyath, G.; Meckling, K. Treatment of MCF-7 breast cancer cells with a red grape wine polyphenol fraction results in disruption of calcium homeostasis and cell cycle arrest causing selective cytotoxicity. *J. Agric. Food Chem.* **2006**, *54*, 7912–7923. [CrossRef] [PubMed]

129. Kim, J.A.; Kim, M.R.; Kim, O.; Phuong, N.; Yoon, J.; Oh, W.K.; Bae, K.; Kang, K.W. Amurensin G inhibits angiogenesis and tumor growth of tamoxifen-resistant breast cancer via Pin1 inhibition. *Food Chem. Toxicol.* **2012**, *50*, 3625–3634. [CrossRef] [PubMed]

130. Burton, L.J.; Smith, B.A.; Smith, B.N.; Loyd, Q.; Nagappan, P.; McKeithen, D.; Wilder, C.L.; Platt, M.O.; Hudson, T.; Odero-Marah, V.A. Muscadine grape skin extract can antagonize Snail-cathepsin L-mediated invasion, migration and osteoclastogenesis in prostate and breast cancer cells. *Carcinogenesis* **2015**, *36*, 1019–1027. [CrossRef] [PubMed]

131. Banerjee, N.; Kim, H.; Krenek, K.; Talcott, S.T.; Mertens-Talcott, S.U. Mango polyphenolics suppressed tumor growth in breast cancer xenografts in mice: Role of the PI3K/AKT pathway and associated microRNAs. *Nutr. Res.* **2015**, *35*, 744–751. [CrossRef] [PubMed]

132. Hoang, V.; Pierson, J.T.; Curry, M.C.; Shaw, P.N.; Dietzgen, R.G.; Gidley, M.J.; Roberts-Thomson, S.J.; Monteith, G.R. Polyphenolic contents and the effects of methanol extracts from mango varieties on breast cancer cells. *Food Sci. Biotechnol.* **2015**, *24*, 265–271. [CrossRef]

133. Abdullah, A.H.; Mohammed, A.S.; Rasedee, A.; Mirghani, M. Oxidative stress-mediated apoptosis induced by ethanolic mango seed extract in cultured estrogen receptor positive breast cancer MCF-7 cells. *Int. J. Mol. Sci.* **2015**, *16*, 3528–3536. [CrossRef] [PubMed]

134. Abdullah, A.; Mohammed, A.S.; Rasedee, A.; Mirghani, M.; Al-Qubaisi, M.S. Induction of apoptosis and oxidative stress in estrogen receptor-negative breast cancer, MDA-MB231 cells, by ethanolic mango seed extract. *BMC Complement. Altern. Med.* **2015**, *15*, 1–7. [CrossRef] [PubMed]

135. Nemec, M.J.; Kim, H.; Marciante, A.B.; Barnes, R.C.; Talcott, S.T.; Mertens-Talcott, S.U. Pyrogallol, an absorbable microbial gallotannins-metabolite and mango polyphenols (*Mangifera Indica*, L.) suppress breast cancer ductal carcinoma in situ proliferation in vitro. *Food Funct.* **2016**, *7*, 3825–3833. [CrossRef] [PubMed]

136. Gao, Q.H.; Wu, C.S.; Wang, M. The jujube (*Ziziphus jujuba* Mill.) fruit: A review of current knowledge of fruit composition and health benefits. *J. Agric. Food Chem.* **2013**, *61*, 3351–3363. [CrossRef] [PubMed]

137. Plastina, P.; Bonofiglio, D.; Vizza, D.; Fazio, A.; Rovito, D.; Giordano, C.; Barone, I.; Catalano, S.; Gabriele, B. Identification of bioactive constituents of *Ziziphus jujube* fruit extracts exerting antiproliferative and apoptotic effects in human breast cancer cells. *J. Ethnopharmacol.* **2012**, *140*, 325–332. [CrossRef] [PubMed]

138. Sun, Y.F.; Song, C.K.; Viemstein, H.; Unger, F.; Liang, Z.S. Apoptosis of human breast cancer cells induced by microencapsulated betulinic acid from sour jujube fruits through the mitochondria transduction pathway. *Food Chem.* **2013**, *138*, 1998–2007. [CrossRef] [PubMed]

139. Abedini, M.R.; Erfanian, N.; Nazem, H.; Jamali, S.; Hoshyar, R. Anti-proliferative and apoptotic effects of *Ziziphus jujube* on cervical and breast cancer cells. *Avicenna J. Phytomed.* **2016**, *6*, 142–148. [PubMed]

140. Somasagara, R.R.; Hegde, M.; Chiruvella, K.K.; Musini, A.; Choudhary, B.; Raghavan, S.C. Extracts of strawberry fruits induce intrinsic pathway of apoptosis in breast cancer cells and inhibits tumor progression in mice. *PLoS ONE* **2012**, *7*, e47021. [CrossRef] [PubMed]

141. Nguyen, V.; Tang, J.; Oroudjev, E.; Lee, C.J.; Marasigan, C.; Wilson, L.; Ayoub, G. Cytotoxic effects of bilberry extract on MCF7-GFP-Tubulin breast cancer cells. *J. Med. Food* **2010**, *13*, 278–285. [CrossRef] [PubMed]

142. Li, L.Y.; Adams, L.S.; Chen, S.; Killian, C.; Ahmed, A.; Seeram, N.P. Eugenia Jambolana Lam. berry extract inhibits growth and induces apoptosis of human breast cancer but not non-tumorigenic breast cells. *J. Agric. Food Chem.* **2009**, *57*, 826–831. [CrossRef] [PubMed]

143. Sun, J.; Liu, R.H. Cranberry phytochemical extracts induce cell cycle arrest and apoptosis in human MCF-7 breast cancer cells. *Cancer Lett.* **2006**, *241*, 124–134. [CrossRef] [PubMed]

144. Noratto, G.; Porter, W.; Byrne, D.; Cisneros-Zevallos, L. Polyphenolics from peach (*Prunus persica* var. Rich Lady) inhibit tumor growth and metastasis of MDA-MB-435 breast cancer cells in vivo. *J. Nutr. Biochem.* **2014**, *25*, 796–800. [CrossRef] [PubMed]

145. Yu, M.H.; Im, H.G.; Lee, S.O.; Sung, C.; Park, D.C.; Lee, I.S. Induction of apoptosis by immature fruits of Prunus salicina Lindl. cv. Soldam in MDA-MB-231 human breast cancer cells. *Int. J. Food Sci. Nutr.* **2007**, *58*, 42–53. [CrossRef] [PubMed]

146. Lewandowska, U.; Szewczyk, K.; Owczarek, K.; Hrabec, Z.; Podsedek, A.; Koziolkiewicz, M.; Hrabec, E. Flavanols from Japanese quince (*Chaenomeles japonica*) fruit inhibit human prostate and breast cancer cell line invasiveness and cause favorable changes in Bax/Bcl-2 mRNA ratio. *Nutr. Cancer* **2013**, *65*, 273–285. [CrossRef] [PubMed]

147. Dai, Y.M.; Hogan, S.; Schmelz, E.M.; Ju, Y.H.; Canning, C.; Zhou, K.Q. Selective growth inhibition of human breast cancer cells by Graviola fruit extract in vitro and in vivo involving downregulation of EGFR expression. *Nutr. Cancer* **2011**, *63*, 795–801. [CrossRef] [PubMed]

148. Wang, X.J.; Yuan, S.L.; Wang, J.; Lin, P.; Liu, G.J.; Lu, Y.R.; Zhang, J.; Wang, W.D.; Wei, Y.Q. Anticancer activity of litchi fruit pericarp extract against human breast cancer in vitro and in vivo. *Toxicol. Appl. Pharm.* **2006**, *215*, 168–178. [CrossRef] [PubMed]

149. Dhandayuthapani, S.; Perez, H.D.; Paroulek, A.; Chinnakkannu, P.; Kandalam, U.; Jaffe, M.; Rathinavelu, A. Bromelain-induced apoptosis in GI-101A breast cancer cells. *J. Med. Food* **2012**, *15*, 344–349. [CrossRef] [PubMed]

150. Liu, X.J.; Lv, K.Z. Cruciferous vegetables intake is inversely associated with risk of breast cancer: A meta-analysis. *Breast J.* **2013**, *22*, 309–313. [CrossRef] [PubMed]

151. Kang, L.G.; Ding, L.; Wang, Z.Y. Isothiocyanates repress estrogen receptor a expression in breast cancer cells. *Oncol. Rep.* **2009**, *21*, 185–192. [PubMed]

152. Tseng, E.; Scott-Ramsay, E.A.; Morris, M.E. Dietary organic isothiocyanates are cytotoxic in human breast cancer MCF-7 and mammary epithelial MCF-12A cell lines. *Exp. Biol. Med.* **2004**, *229*, 835–842.

153. Bradlow, H.L. Indole-3-carbinol as a chemoprotective agent in breast and prostate cancer. *In Vivo* **2008**, *22*, 441–445. [PubMed]

154. Thomson, C.A.; Ho, E.; Strom, M.B. Chemopreventive properties of 3,3′-diindolylmethane in breast cancer: Evidence from experimental and human studies. *Nutr. Rev.* **2016**, *74*, 432–443. [CrossRef] [PubMed]

155. Sehrawat, A.; St Croix, C.; Baty, C.J.; Watkins, S.; Tailor, D.; Singh, R.P.; Singh, S.V. Inhibition of mitochondrial fusion is an early and critical event in breast cancer cell apoptosis by dietary chemopreventive benzyl isothiocyanate. *Mitochondrion* **2016**, *30*, 67–77. [CrossRef] [PubMed]

156. Kim, S.H.; Singh, S.V. p53-Independent apoptosis by benzyl isothiocyanate in human breast cancer cells is mediated by suppression of XIAP expression. *Cancer Prev. Res.* **2010**, *3*, 718–726. [CrossRef] [PubMed]

157. Xiao, D.; Vogel, V.; Singh, S.V. Benzyl isothiocyanate-induced apoptosis in human breast cancer cells is initiated by reactive oxygen species and regulated by Bax and Bak. *Mol. Cancer Ther.* **2006**, *5*, 2931–2945. [CrossRef] [PubMed]

158. Kim, E.J.; Eom, S.J.; Hong, J.E.; Lee, J.Y.; Choi, M.S.; Park, J. Benzyl isothiocyanate inhibits basal and hepatocyte growth factor-stimulated migration of breast cancer cells. *Mol. Cell. Biochem.* **2012**, *359*, 431–440. [CrossRef] [PubMed]

159. Hugo, H.; Ackland, M.L.; Blick, T.; Lawrence, M.G.; Clements, J.A.; Williams, E.D.; Thompson, E.W. Epithelial-mesenchymal and mesenchymal-Epithelial transitions in carcinoma progression. *J. Cell. Physiol.* **2007**, *213*, 374–383. [CrossRef] [PubMed]

160. Sehrawat, A.; Singh, S.V. Benzyl isothiocyanate inhibits epithelial-mesenchymal transition in cultured and vxenografted human breast cancer cells. *Cancer Prev. Res.* **2011**, *4*, 1107–1117. [CrossRef] [PubMed]

161. Xiao, D.; Bommareddy, A.; Kim, S.H.; Sehrawat, A.; Hahm, E.R.; Singh, S.V. Benzyl isothiocyanate causes FoxO1-mediated autophagic death in human breast cancer cells. *PLoS ONE* **2012**, *7*, e32597. [CrossRef] [PubMed]

162. Kim, S.H.; Nagalingam, A.; Saxena, N.K.; Singh, S.V.; Sharma, D. Benzyl isothiocyanate inhibits oncogenic actions of leptin in human breast cancer cells by suppressing activation of signal transducer and activator of transcription 3. *Carcinogenesis* **2011**, *32*, 359–367. [CrossRef] [PubMed]

163. Warin, R.; Xiao, D.; Arlotti, J.A.; Bommareddy, A.; Singh, S.V. Inhibition of human breast cancer xenograft growth by cruciferous vegetable constituent benzyl isothiocyanate. *Mol. Carcinogen.* **2010**, *49*, 500–507. [CrossRef] [PubMed]

164. Kim, S.H.; Sehrawat, A.; Singh, S.V. Dietary chemopreventative benzyl isothiocyanate inhibits breast cancer stem cells in vitro and in vivo. *Cancer Prev. Res.* **2013**, *6*, 782–790. [CrossRef] [PubMed]

165. Hahm, E.R.; Singh, S.V. Bim contributes to phenethyl isothiocyanate-induced apoptosis in breast cancer cells. *Mol. Carcinog.* **2012**, *51*, 465–474. [CrossRef] [PubMed]

166. Sarkar, R.; Mukherjee, S.; Biswas, J.; Roy, M. Phenethyl isothiocyanate, by virtue of its antioxidant activity, inhibits invasiveness and metastatic potential of breast cancer cells: HIF-1 alpha as a putative target. *Free Radic. Res.* **2016**, *50*, 84–100. [CrossRef] [PubMed]

167. Aras, U.; Gandhi, Y.A.; Masso-Welch, P.A.; Morris, M.E. Chemopreventive and anti-angiogenic effects of dietary phenethyl isothiocyanate in an *N*-methyl nitrosourea-induced breast cancer animal model. *Biopharm. Drug Dispos.* **2013**, *34*, 98–106. [CrossRef] [PubMed]

168. Moon, Y.J.; Brazeau, D.A.; Morris, M.E. Dietary phenethyl isothiocyanate alters gene expression in human breast cancer cells. *Evid.-Based Complement. Altern. Med.* **2011**, *2011*, 1–8. [CrossRef] [PubMed]

169. Ramirez, M.C.; Singletary, K. Regulation of estrogen receptor alpha expression in human breast cancer cells by sulforaphane. *J. Nutr. Biochem.* **2009**, *20*, 195–201. [CrossRef] [PubMed]

170. Pledgie-Tracy, A.; Sobolewski, M.D.; Davidson, N.E. Sulforaphane induces cell type-specific apoptosis in human breast cancer cell lines. *Mol. Cancer Ther.* **2007**, *6*, 1013–1021. [CrossRef] [PubMed]

171. Kanematsu, S.; Yoshizawa, K.; Uehara, N.; Miki, H.; Sasaki, T.; Kuro, M.; Lai, Y.C.; Kimura, A.; Yuri, T.; Tsubura, A. Sulforaphane inhibits the growth of KPL-1 human breast cancer cells in vitro and suppresses the growth and metastasis of orthotopically transplanted KPL-1 cells in female athymic mice. *Oncol. Rep.* **2011**, *26*, 603–608. [PubMed]

172. Lee, Y.R.; Noh, E.M.; Han, J.H.; Kim, J.M.; Hwang, B.M.; Kim, B.S.; Lee, S.H.; Jung, S.H.; Youn, H.J.; Chung, E.Y. Sulforaphane controls TPA-induced MMP-9 expression through the NF-kappa B signaling pathway, but not AP-1, in MCF-7 breast cancer cells. *BMB Rep.* **2013**, *46*, 201–206. [CrossRef] [PubMed]

173. Yang, M.; Teng, W.D.; Qu, Y.; Wang, H.Y.; Yuan, Q.P. Sulforaphane inhibits triple negative breast cancer through activating tumor suppressor Egr1. *Breast Cancer Res. Treat.* **2016**, *158*, 277–286. [CrossRef] [PubMed]

174. Meeran, S.M.; Patel, S.N.; Tollefsbol, T.O. Sulforaphane causes epigenetic repression of hTERT expression in human breast cancer cell lines. *PLoS ONE* **2010**, *5*, e11457. [CrossRef] [PubMed]

175. Jo, E.H.; Kim, S.H.; Ahn, N.S.; Park, J.S.; Hwang, J.W.; Lee, Y.S.; Kang, K.S. Efficacy of sulforaphane is mediated by p38 MAP kinase and caspase-7 activations in ER-positive and COX-2-expressed human breast cancer cells. *Eur. J. Cancer Prev.* **2007**, *16*, 505–510. [CrossRef] [PubMed]

176. Meng, Q.H.; Qi, M.; Chen, D.Z.; Yuan, R.Q.; Goldberg, I.D.; Rosen, E.M.; Auborn, K.; Fan, S.J. Suppression of breast cancer invasion and migration by indole-3-carbinol: Associated with up-regulation of BRCA1 and E-cadherin/catenin complexes. *J. Mol. Med.* **2000**, *78*, 155–165. [CrossRef] [PubMed]

177. Ho, J.N.; Jun, W.; Choue, R.; Lee, J. I3C and ICZ inhibit migration by suppressing the EMT process and FAK expression in breast cancer cells. *Mol. Med. Rep.* **2013**, *7*, 384–388. [PubMed]

178. Hung, W.C.; Chang, H.C. Indole-3-carbinol inhibits Sp1-induced matrix metalloproteinase-2 expression to attenuate migration and invasion of breast cancer cells. *J. Agric. Food Chem.* **2009**, *57*, 76–82. [CrossRef] [PubMed]

179. Rahman, K.; Sarkar, F.H.; Banerjee, S.; Wang, Z.W.; Liao, D.; Hong, X.; Sarkar, N.H. Therapeutic intervention of experimental breast cancer bone metastasis by indole-3-carbinol in SCID-human mouse model. *Mol. Cancer Ther.* **2006**, *5*, 2747–2756. [CrossRef] [PubMed]

180. Garcia, H.H.; Brar, G.A.; Nguyen, D.; Bjeldanes, L.F.; Firestone, G.L. Indole-3-carbinol (I3C) inhibits cyclin-dependent kinase-2 function in human breast cancer cells by regulating the size distribution, associated cyclin E forms, and subcellular localization of the CDK2 protein complex. *J. Biol. Chem.* **2005**, *280*, 8756–8764. [CrossRef] [PubMed]

181. Cram, E.J.; Liu, B.D.; Bjeldanes, L.F.; Firestone, G.L. Indole-3-carbinol inhibits CDK6 expression in human MCF-7 breast cancer cells by disrupting Sp1 transcription factor interactions with a composite element in the CDK6 gene promoter. *J. Biol. Chem.* **2001**, *276*, 22332–22340. [CrossRef] [PubMed]

182. Marconett, C.N.; Sundar, S.N.; Tseng, M.; Tin, A.S.; Tran, K.Q.; Mahuron, K.M.; Bjeldanes, L.F.; Firestone, G.L. Indole-3-carbinol downregulation of telomerase gene expression requires the inhibition of estrogen receptor-alpha and Sp1 transcription factor interactions within the hTERT promoter and mediates the G1 cell cycle arrest of human breast cancer cells. *Carcinogenesis* **2011**, *32*, 1315–1323. [CrossRef] [PubMed]

183. Rahman, K.; Aranha, O.; Glazyrin, A.; Chinni, S.R.; Sarkar, F.H. Translocation of Bax to mitochondria induces apoptotic cell death in Indole-3-carbinol (I3C) treated breast cancer cells. *Oncogene* **2000**, *19*, 5764–5771. [CrossRef] [PubMed]

184. Sarkar, F.H.; Rahman, K.; Li, Y.W. Bax translocation to mitochondria is an important event in inducing apoptotic cell death by indole-3-carbinol (I3C) treatment of breast cancer cells. *J. Nutr.* **2003**, *133S*, 2434S–2439S.

185. Marconett, C.N.; Singhal, A.K.; Sundar, S.N.; Firestone, G.L. Indole-3-carbinol disrupts estrogen receptor-alpha dependent expression of insulin-like growth factor-1 receptor and insulin receptor substrate-1 and proliferation of human breast cancer cells. *Mol. Cell. Endocrinol.* **2012**, *363*, 74–84. [CrossRef] [PubMed]

186. Brew, C.T.; Aronchik, I.; Kosco, K.; McCammon, J.; Bjeldanes, L.F.; Firestone, G.L. Indole-3-carbinol inhibits MDA-MB-231 breast cancer cell motility and induces stress fibers and focal adhesion formation by activation of Rho kinase activity. *Int. J. Cancer* **2009**, *124*, 2294–2302. [CrossRef] [PubMed]

187. Ikeda, H.; Old, L.J.; Schreiber, R.D. The roles of IFN gamma in protection against tumor development and cancer immunoediting. *Cytokine Growth Factor Rev.* **2002**, *13*, 95–109. [CrossRef]

188. Chatterji, U.; Riby, J.E.; Taniguchi, T.; Bjeldanes, E.L.; Bjeldanes, L.F.; Firestone, G.L. Indole-3-carbinol stimulates transcription of the interferon gamma receptor 1 gene and augments interferon responsiveness in human breast cancer cells. *Carcinogenesis* **2004**, *25*, 1119–1128. [CrossRef] [PubMed]

189. Hong, C.; Firestone, G.L.; Bjeldanes, L.F. Bcl-2 family-mediated apoptotic effects of 3,3′-diindolylmethane (DIM) in human breast cancer cells. *Biochem. Pharmacol.* **2002**, *63*, 1085–1097. [CrossRef]

190. Rahman, K.; Sarkar, F.H. Inhibition of nuclear translocation of nuclear factor-kappa B contributes to 3,3′-diindolylmethane-induced apoptosis in breast cancer cells. *Cancer Res.* **2005**, *65*, 364–371. [PubMed]

191. Nicastro, H.L.; Firestone, G.L.; Bjeldanes, L.F. 3,3′-Diindolylmethane rapidly and selectively inhibits hepatocyte growth factor/c-Met signaling in breast cancer cells. *J. Nutr. Biochem.* **2013**, *24*, 1882–1888. [CrossRef] [PubMed]

192. Jin, Y.C. 3,3′-Diindolylmethane inhibits breast cancer cell growth via miR-21-mediated Cdc25A degradation. *Mol. Cell. Biochem.* **2011**, *358*, 345–354. [CrossRef] [PubMed]

193. Hong, C.B.; Kim, H.A.; Firestone, G.L.; Bjeldanes, L.F. 3,3′-Diindolylmethane (DIM) induces a G1 cell cycle arrest in human breast cancer cells that is accompanied by Sp1-mediated activation of p21(WAF1/CIP1) expression. *Carcinogenesis* **2002**, *23*, 1297–1305. [CrossRef] [PubMed]

194. Gong, Y.X.; Sohn, H.; Xue, L.; Firestone, G.L.; Bjeldanes, L.F. 3,3′-diindolylmethane is a novel mitochondrial H+-ATP synthase inhibitor that can induce p21(Cip1/Waf1) expression by induction of oxidative stress in human breast cancer cells. *Cancer Res.* **2006**, *66*, 4880–4887. [CrossRef] [PubMed]

195. Hsu, E.L.; Chen, N.; Westbrook, A.; Wang, F.; Zhang, R.X.; Taylor, R.T.; Hankinson, O. CXCR4 and CXCL12 down-regulation: A novel mechanism for the chemoprotection of 3,3′-diindolylmethane for breast and ovarian cancers. *Cancer Lett.* **2008**, *265*, 113–123. [CrossRef] [PubMed]

196. Rahman, K.; Li, Y.W.; Wang, Z.W.; Sarkar, S.H.; Sarkar, F.H. Gene expression profiling revealed survivin as a target of 3,3′-diindolylmethane-induced cell growth inhibition and apoptosis in breast cancer cells. *Cancer Res.* **2006**, *66*, 4952–4960. [CrossRef] [PubMed]

197. Xue, L.; Firestone, G.L.; Bjeldanes, L.F. DIM stimulates IFN gamma gene expression in human breast cancer cells via the specific activation of JNK and p38 pathways. *Oncogene* **2005**, *24*, 2343–2353. [CrossRef] [PubMed]

198. Kapadia, G.J.; Azuine, M.A.; Rao, G.S.; Arai, T.; Iida, A.; Tokuda, H. Cytotoxic effect of the red beetroot (*Beta vulgaris* L.) extract compared to doxorubicin (Adriamycin) in the human prostate (PC-3) and breast (MCF-7) cancer cell lines. *Anti-Cancer Agents Med. Chem.* **2011**, *11*, 280–284. [CrossRef]

199. Butalla, A.C.; Crane, T.E.; Patil, B.; Wertheim, B.C.; Thompson, P.; Thomson, C.A. Effects of a carrot juice intervention on plasma carotenoids, oxidative stress, and inflammation in overweight breast cancer survivors. *Nutr. Cancer* **2012**, *64*, 331–341. [CrossRef] [PubMed]

200. Ansari, J.A.; Ahmad, M.K.; Khan, A.R.; Fatima, N.; Khan, H.J.; Rastogi, N.; Mishra, D.P.; Mahdi, A.A. Anticancer and antioxidant activity of Zingiber officinale Roscoe rhizome. *Indian J. Exp. Biol.* **2016**, *54*, 767–773.

201. Elkady, A.I.; Abuzinadah, O.A.; Baeshen, N.; Rahmy, T.R. Differential control of growth, apoptotic activity, and gene expression in human breast cancer cells by extracts derived from medicinal herbs *Zingiber officinale*. *J. Biomed. Biotechnol.* **2012**, *2012*, 614356. [CrossRef] [PubMed]

202. Joo, J.H.; Hong, S.S.; Cho, Y.R.; Seo, D.W. 10-Gingerol inhibits proliferation and invasion of MDA-MB-231 breast cancer cells through suppression of Akt and p38(MAPK) activity. *Oncol. Rep.* **2016**, *35*, 779–784. [PubMed]

203. Lee, H.S.; Seo, E.Y.; Kang, N.E.; Kim, W.K. (6)-Gingerol inhibits metastasis of MDA-MB-231 human breast cancer cells. *J. Nutr. Biochem.* **2008**, *19*, 313–319. [CrossRef] [PubMed]

204. Ling, H.; Yang, H.; Tan, S.H.; Chui, W.K.; Chew, E.H. 6-Shogaol, an active constituent of ginger, inhibits breast cancer cell invasion by reducing matrix metalloproteinase-9 expression via blockade of nuclear factor-kappa B activation. *Br. J. Pharmacol.* **2010**, *161*, 1763–1777. [CrossRef] [PubMed]

205. Hong, B.H.; Wu, C.H.; Yeh, C.T.; Yen, G.C. Invadopodia-associated proteins blockade as a novel mechanism for 6-shogaol and pterostilbene to reduce breast cancer cell motility and invasion. *Mol. Nutr. Food Res.* **2013**, *57*, 886–895. [CrossRef] [PubMed]

206. Ray, A.; Vasudevan, S.; Sengupta, S. 6-Shogaol inhibits breast cancer cells and stem cell-like spheroids by modulation of Notch signaling pathway and induction of autophagic cell death. *PLoS ONE* **2015**, *10*, e1376149. [CrossRef] [PubMed]

207. Hsu, Y.L.; Chen, C.Y.; Hou, M.F.; Tsai, E.M.; Jong, Y.J.; Hung, C.H.; Kuo, P.L. 6-Dehydrogingerdione, an active constituent of dietary ginger, induces cell cycle arrest and apoptosis through reactive oxygen species/c-Jun *N*-terminal kinase pathways in human breast cancer cells. *Mol. Nutr. Food Res.* **2010**, *54*, 1307–1317. [CrossRef] [PubMed]

208. Arslan, M.; Ozdemir, L. Oral intake of ginger for chemotherapy-induced nausea and vomiting among women with breast cancer. *Clin. J. Oncol. Nurs.* **2015**, *19*, E92–E97. [CrossRef] [PubMed]

209. Lua, P.L.; Salihah, N.; Mazlan, N. Effects of inhaled ginger aromatherapy on chemotherapy-induced nausea and vomiting and health-related quality of life in women with breast cancer. *Complement. Ther. Med.* **2015**, *23*, 396–404. [CrossRef] [PubMed]

210. Yun, H.M.; Ban, J.O.; Park, K.R.; Lee, C.K.; Jeong, H.S.; Han, S.B.; Hong, J.T. Potential therapeutic effects of functionally active compounds isolated from garlic. *Pharmacol. Ther.* **2014**, *142*, 183–195. [CrossRef] [PubMed]

211. Pourzand, A.; Tajaddini, A.; Pirouzpanah, S.; Asghari-Jafarabadi, M.; Samadi, N.; Ostadrahimi, A.R.; Sanaat, Z. Associations between dietary Allium vegetables and risk of breast cancer: A hospital-based matched case-control study. *J. Breast Cancer* **2016**, *19*, 292–300. [CrossRef] [PubMed]

212. Nakagawa, H.; Tsuta, K.; Kiuchi, K.; Senzaki, H.; Tanaka, K.; Hioki, K.; Tsubura, A. Growth inhibitory effects of diallyl disulfide on human breast cancer cell lines. *Carcinogenesis* **2001**, *22*, 891–897. [CrossRef] [PubMed]

213. Hahm, E.R.; Singh, S.V. Diallyl trisulfide inhibits estrogen receptor-alpha activity in human breast cancer cells. *Breast Cancer Res. Treat.* **2014**, *144*, 47–57. [CrossRef] [PubMed]

214. Zhang, H.; Wang, K.M.; Lin, G.M.; Zhao, Z.X. Antitumor mechanisms of *S*-allyl mercaptocysteine for breast cancer therapy. *BMC Complement. Altern. Med.* **2014**, *14*. [CrossRef] [PubMed]

215. Lee, C.G.; Lee, H.W.; Kim, B.O.; Rhee, D.K.; Pyo, S. Allicin inhibits invasion and migration of breast cancer cells through the suppression of VCAM-1: Regulation of association between p65 and ER-alpha. *J. Funct. Foods* **2015**, *15*, 172–185. [CrossRef]

216. Altonsy, M.O.; Habib, T.N.; Andrews, S.C. Diallyl disulfide-induced apoptosis in a breast-cancer cell line (MCF-7) may be caused by inhibition of histone deacetylation. *Nutr. Cancer* **2012**, *64*, 1251–1260. [CrossRef] [PubMed]

217. Lei, X.Y.; Yao, S.Q.; Zu, X.Y.; Huang, Z.X.; Liu, L.J.; Zhong, M.; Zhu, B.Y.; Tang, S.S.; Liao, D.F. Apoptosis induced by diallyl disulfide in human breast cancer cell line MCF-7. *Acta Pharmacol. Sin.* **2008**, *29*, 1233–1239. [CrossRef] [PubMed]

218. Xiao, X.S.; Chen, B.; Liu, X.P.; Liu, P.; Zheng, G.P.; Ye, F.; Tang, H.L.; Xie, X.M. Diallyl disulfide suppresses SRC/Ras/ERK signaling-mediated proliferation and metastasis in human breast cancer by up-regulating miR-34a. *PLoS ONE* **2014**, *9*, e11272011. [CrossRef] [PubMed]

219. Huang, J.; Yang, B.; Xiang, T.X.; Peng, W.Y.; Qiu, Z.; Wan, J.Y.; Zhang, L.; Li, H.Y.; Li, H.Z.; Ren, G.S. Diallyl disulfide inhibits growth and metastatic potential of human triple-negative breast cancer cells through inactivation of the β-catenin signaling pathway. *Mol. Nutr. Food Res.* **2015**, *59*, 1063–1075. [CrossRef] [PubMed]

220. Na, H.K.; Kim, E.H.; Choi, M.A.; Park, J.M.; Kim, D.H.; Surh, Y.J. Diallyl trisulfide induces apoptosis in human breast cancer cells through ROS-mediated activation of JNK and AP-1. *Biochem. Pharmacol.* **2012**, *84*, 1241–1250. [CrossRef] [PubMed]

221. Malki, A.; El-Saadani, M.; Sultan, A.S. Garlic constituent diallyl trisulfide induced apoptosis in MCF7 human breast cancer cells. *Cancer Biol. Ther.* **2009**, *8*, 2174–2184. [CrossRef]

222. Liu, Y.P.; Zhu, P.T.; Wang, Y.Y.; Wei, Z.H.; Tao, L.; Zhu, Z.J.; Sheng, X.B.; Wang, S.L.; Ruan, J.S.; Liu, Z.G. Antimetastatic therapies of the polysulfide diallyl Ttrisulfide against triple-negative breast cancer (TNBC) via suppressing MMP2/9 by blocking NF-kappa B and ERK/MAPK signaling pathways. *PLoS ONE* **2015**, *10*, e1237814.

223. Kim, S.H.; Kaschula, C.H.; Priedigkeit, N.; Lee, A.V.; Singh, S.V. Forkhead Box Q1 is a novel target of breast cancer stem cell inhibition by diallyl trisulfide. *J. Biol. Chem.* **2016**, *291*, 13495–13508. [CrossRef] [PubMed]

224. Baharetha, H.M.; Nassar, Z.D.; Aisha, A.F.; Ahamed, M.; Al-Suede, F.; Abd Kadir, M.O.; Ismail, Z.; Majid, A. Proapoptotic and antimetastatic properties of supercritical $CO_2$ extract of *Nigella sativa* Linn. against breast cancer cells. *J. Med. Food* **2013**, *16*, 1121–1130. [CrossRef] [PubMed]

225. Alhazmi, M.I.; Hasan, T.N.; Shafi, G.; Al-Assaf, A.H.; Alfawaz, M.A.; Alshatwi, A.A. Roles of p53 and caspases in induction of apoptosis in MCF-7 breast cancer cells treated with a methanolic extract of *Nigella sativa* seeds. *Asian Pac. J. Cancer Prev.* **2014**, *15*, 9655–9660. [CrossRef] [PubMed]

226. Schneider-Stock, R.; Fakhoury, I.H.; Zaki, A.M.; El-Baba, C.O.; Gali-Muhtasib, H.U. Thymoquinone: Fifty years of success in the battle against cancer models. *Drug Discov. Today* **2014**, *19*, 18–30. [CrossRef] [PubMed]

227. Franke, T.F.; Cantley, L.C. Apoptosis. A bad kinase makes good. *Nature* **1997**, *390*, 116–117. [CrossRef] [PubMed]

228. Arafa, E.; Zhu, Q.Z.; Shah, Z.I.; Wani, G.; Barakat, B.M.; Racoma, I.; El-Mandy, M.A.; Wani, A.A. Thymoquinone up-regulates PTEN expression and induces apoptosis in doxorubicin-resistant human breast cancer cells. *Mutat. Res.* **2011**, *706*, 28–35. [CrossRef] [PubMed]

229. Rajput, S.; Kumar, B.; Dey, K.K.; Pal, I.; Parekh, A.; Mandal, M. Molecular targeting of Akt by thymoquinone promotes G(1) arrest through translation inhibition of cyclin D1 and induces apoptosis in breast cancer cells. *Life Sci.* **2013**, *93*, 783–790. [CrossRef] [PubMed]

230. Woo, C.C.; Hsu, A.; Kumar, A.P.; Sethi, G.; Tan, K. Thymoquinone inhibits tumor growth and induces apoptosis in a breast cancer xenograft mouse model: The role of p38 MAPK and ROS. *PLoS ONE* **2013**, *8*, e75356. [CrossRef] [PubMed]

231. Woo, C.C.; Loo, S.Y.; Gee, V.; Yap, C.W.; Sethi, G.; Kumar, A.P.; Tan, K. Anticancer activity of thymoquinone in breast cancer cells: Possible involvement of PPAR-gamma pathway. *Biochem. Pharmacol.* **2011**, *82*, 464–475. [CrossRef] [PubMed]

232. Yu, S.M.; Kim, S.J. Thymoquinone (TQ) regulates cyclooxygenase-2 expression and prostaglandin E2 production through PI3kinase (PI3K)/p38 kinase pathway in human breast cancer cell line, MDA-MB-231. *Anim. Cells Syst.* **2012**, *16*, 274–279. [CrossRef]

233. Chou, C.C.; Wu, Y.C.; Wang, Y.F.; Chou, M.J.; Kuo, S.J.; Chen, D.R. Capsaicin-induced apoptosis in human breast cancer MCF-7 cells through caspase-independent pathway. *Oncol. Rep.* **2009**, *21*, 665–671. [PubMed]

234. Chang, H.C.; Chen, S.T.; Chien, S.Y.; Kuo, S.J.; Tsai, H.T.; Chen, D.R. Capsaicin may induce breast cancer cell death through apoptosis-inducing factor involving mitochondrial dysfunction. *Hum. Exp. Toxicol.* **2011**, *30*, 1657–1665. [CrossRef] [PubMed]

235. Thoennissen, N.H.; O'Kelly, J.; Lu, D.; Iwanski, G.B.; La, D.T.; Abbassi, S.; Leiter, A.; Karlan, B.; Mehta, R.; Koeffler, H.P. Capsaicin causes cell-cycle arrest and apoptosis in ER-positive and -negative breast cancer cells by modulating the EGFR/HER-2 pathway. *Oncogene* **2010**, *29*, 285–296. [CrossRef] [PubMed]

236. Liu, Z.G.; Zhu, P.T.; Tao, Y.; Shen, C.S.; Wang, S.L.; Zhao, L.G.; Wu, H.Y.; Fan, F.T.; Lin, C.; Chen, C. Cancer-promoting effect of capsaicin on DMBA/TPA-induced skin tumorigenesis by modulating inflammation, Erk and p38 in mice. *Food Chem. Toxicol.* **2015**, *81*, 1–8. [CrossRef] [PubMed]

237. Yang, J.; Li, T.Z.; Xu, G.H.; Luo, B.B.; Chen, Y.X.; Zhang, T. Low-concentration capsaicin promotes colorectal cancer metastasis by triggering ROS production and modulating Akt/mTOR and STAT-3 pathways. *Neoplasma* **2013**, *60*, 364–372. [CrossRef] [PubMed]

238. Caprodossi, S.; Amantini, C.; Nabissi, M.; Morelli, M.B.; Farfariello, V.; Santoni, M.; Gismondi, A.; Santoni, G. Capsaicin promotes a more aggressive gene expression phenotype and invasiveness in null-TRPV1 urothelial cancer cells. *Carcinogenesis* **2011**, *32*, 686–694. [CrossRef] [PubMed]

239. Greenshields, A.L.; Doucette, C.D.; Sutton, K.M.; Madera, L.; Annan, H.; Yaffe, P.B.; Knickle, A.F.; Dong, Z.M.; Hoskin, D.W. Piperine inhibits the growth and motility of triple-negative breast cancer cells. *Cancer Lett.* **2015**, *357*, 129–140. [CrossRef] [PubMed]

240. Do, M.T.; Kim, H.G.; Choi, J.H.; Khanal, T.; Park, B.H.; Tran, T.P.; Jeong, T.C.; Jeong, H.G. Antitumor efficacy of piperine in the treatment of human HER2-overexpressing breast cancer cells. *Food Chem.* **2013**, *141*, 2591–2599. [CrossRef] [PubMed]

241. Lai, L.H.; Fu, Q.H.; Liu, Y.; Jiang, K.; Guo, Q.M.; Chen, Q.Y.; Yan, B.; Wang, Q.Q.; Shen, J.G. Piperine suppresses tumor growth and metastasis in vitro and in vivo in a 4T1 murine breast cancer model. *Acta Pharmacol. Sin.* **2012**, *33*, 523–530. [CrossRef] [PubMed]

242. Chryssanthi, D.G.; Lamari, F.N.; Iatrou, G.; Pylara, A.; Karamanos, N.K.; Cordopatis, P. Inhibition of breast cancer cell proliferation by style constituents of different Crocus species. *Anticancer Res.* **2007**, *27*, 357–362. [PubMed]

243. Chryssanthi, D.G.; Dedes, P.G.; Karamanos, N.K.; Cordopatis, P.; Lamari, F.N. Crocetin inhibits invasiveness of MDA-MB-231 breast cancer cells via downregulation of matrix metalloproteinases. *Planta Med.* **2011**, *77*, 146–151. [CrossRef] [PubMed]

244. Sajjadi, M.; Bathaie, Z. Comparative study on the preventive effect of saffron carotenoids, crocin and crocetin, in NMU-induced breast cancer in rats. *Cell J.* **2017**, *19*, 94–101. [PubMed]

245. Lin, C.; Lin, S.H.; Lin, C.; Liu, Y.; Chen, C.; Chu, C.; Huang, H.; Lin, M. Inhibitory effect of clove methanolic extract and eugenol on dendritic cell functions. *J. Funct. Foods* **2016**, *27*, 439–447. [CrossRef]

246. Vidhya, N.; Devaraj, S.N. Induction of apoptosis by eugenol in human breast cancer cells. *Indian J. Exp. Biol.* **2011**, *49*, 871–878. [PubMed]

247. Al-Sharif, I.; Remmal, A.; Aboussekhra, A. Eugenol triggers apoptosis in breast cancer cells through E2F1/survivin down-regulation. *BMC Cancer* **2013**, *13*. [CrossRef] [PubMed]

248. Gonzalez-Vallinas, M.; Molina, S.; Vicente, G.; Sanchez-Martinez, R.; Vargas, T.; Garcia-Risco, M.R.; Fornari, T.; Reglero, G.; de Molina, A.R. Modulation of estrogen and epidermal growth factor receptors by rosemary extract in breast cancer cells. *Electrophoresis* **2014**, *35*, 1719–1727. [CrossRef] [PubMed]

249. Fuke, Y.; Hishinuma, M.; Namikawa, M.; Oishi, Y.; Matsuzaki, T. Wasabi-derived 6-(methylsulfinyl)hexyl isothiocyanate induces apoptosis in human breast cancer by possible involvement of the NF-kappa B pathways. *Nutr. Cancer* **2014**, *66*, 879–887. [CrossRef] [PubMed]

250. Tang, E.; Rajarajeswaran, J.; Fung, S.Y.; Kanthimathi, M.S. Antioxidant activity of *Coriandrum sativum* and protection against DNA damage and cancer cell migration. *BMC Complement. Altern. Med.* **2013**, *13*, 347. [CrossRef] [PubMed]

251. Deng, Y.; Verron, E.; Rohanizadeh, R. Molecular mechanisms of anti-metastatic activity of curcumin. *Anticancer Res.* **2016**, *36*, 5639–5647. [CrossRef] [PubMed]

252. Wang, Y.W.; Yu, J.Y.; Cui, R.; Lin, J.J.; Ding, X.T. Curcumin in treating breast cancer: A review. *JALA J. Lab. Autom.* **2016**, *21*, 723–731. [CrossRef] [PubMed]

253. Kumar, P.; Kadakol, A.; Shasthrula, P.K.; Mundhe, N.A.; Jamdade, V.S.; Barua, C.C.; Gaikwad, A.B. Curcumin as an adjuvant to breast cancer treatment. *Anti-Cancer Agents Med. Chem.* **2015**, *15*, 647–656. [CrossRef]

254. Liu, D.W.; Chen, Z.W. The effect of curcumin on breast cancer cells. *J. Breast Cancer* **2013**, *16*, 133–137. [CrossRef] [PubMed]

255. Hong, S.A.; Kim, K.; Nam, S.J.; Kong, G.; Kim, M.K. A case-control study on the dietary intake of mushrooms and breast cancer risk among Korean women. *Int. J. Cancer* **2008**, *122*, 919–923. [CrossRef] [PubMed]

256. Li, J.Y.; Zou, L.; Chen, W.; Zhu, B.B.; Shen, N.; Ke, J.T.; Lou, J.; Song, R.R.; Zhong, R.; Miao, X.P. Dietary mushroom intake may reduce the risk of breast cancer: Evidence from a meta-analysis of observational studies. *PLoS ONE* **2014**, *9*, e93437. [CrossRef] [PubMed]

257. Peng, C.Y.; Fong, P.C.; Yu, C.C.; Tsai, W.C.; Tzeng, Y.M.; Chang, W.W. Methyl antcinate A suppresses the population of cancer stem-like cells in MCF7 human breast cancer cell line. *Molecules* **2013**, *18*, 2539–2548. [CrossRef] [PubMed]

258. Luo, Z.Y.; Hu, X.P.; Xiong, H.; Qiu, H.; Yuan, X.L.; Zhu, F.; Wang, Y.H.; Zou, Y.M. A polysaccharide from Huaier induced apoptosis in MCF-7 breast cancer cells via down-regulation of MTDH protein. *Carbohydr. Polym.* **2016**, *151*, 1027–1033. [CrossRef] [PubMed]

259. Shi, X.L.; Zhao, Y.; Jiao, Y.D.; Shi, T.R.; Yang, X.B. ROS-dependent mitochondria molecular mechanisms underlying antitumor activity of *Pleurotus abalonus* acidic polysaccharides in human breast cancer MCF-7 cells. *PLoS ONE* **2013**, *8*, e64266. [CrossRef] [PubMed]

260. Sliva, D.; Labarrere, C.; Slivova, V.; Sedlak, M.; Lloyd, F.P.; Ho, N. *Ganoderma lucidum* suppresses motility of highly invasive breast and prostate cancer cells. *Biochem. Biophys. Res. Commun.* **2002**, *298*, 603–612. [CrossRef]

261. Choong, Y.K.; Noordin, M.M.; Mohamed, S.; Ali, A.M.; Umar, N.; Tong, C.C. The nature of apoptosis of human breast cancer cells induced by three species of genus *Ganoderma*, P. Karst. (aphyllophoromycetideae) crude extracts. *Int. J. Med. Mushrooms* **2008**, *10*, 115–125. [CrossRef]

262. Grube, S.J.; Eng, E.T.; Kao, Y.C.; Kwon, A.; Chen, S. White button mushroom phytochemicals inhibit aromatase activity and breast cancer cell proliferation. *J. Nutr.* **2001**, *131*, 3288–3293. [PubMed]

263. Xu, J.K.; Yuan, Q.G.; Luo, P.; Sun, X.L.; Ma, J.C. *Pleurotus eous* polysaccharides suppress angiogenesis and induce apoptosis via ROS-dependent JNK activation and mitochondrial mediated mechanisms in MCF-7 human breast cancer cells. *Bangladesh J. Pharmacol.* **2015**, *10*, 78–86. [CrossRef]

264. Aune, D.; Chan, D.; Greenwood, D.C.; Vieira, A.R.; Rosenblatt, D.; Vieira, R.; Norat, T. Dietary fiber and breast cancer risk: A systematic review and meta-analysis of prospective studies. *Ann. Oncol.* **2012**, *23*, 1394–1402. [CrossRef] [PubMed]

265. Awika, J.M.; Rooney, L.W. Sorghum phytochemicals and their potential impact on human health. *Phytochemistry* **2004**, *65*, 1199–1221. [CrossRef] [PubMed]

266. Park, J.H.; Darvin, P.; Lim, E.J.; Joung, Y.H.; Hong, D.Y.; Park, E.U.; Park, S.H.; Choi, S.K.; Moon, E.S.; Cho, B.W. Hwanggeumchal sorghum induces cell cycle arrest, and suppresses tumor growth and metastasis through Jak2/STAT pathways in breast cancer xenografts. *PLoS ONE* **2012**, *7*, e40531. [CrossRef] [PubMed]

267. Suganyadevi, P.; Saravanakumar, K.M.; Mohandas, S. The antiproliferative activity of 3-deoxyanthocyanins extracted from red sorghum (*Sorghum bicolor*) bran through P-53-dependent and Bcl-2 gene expression in breast cancer cell line. *Life Sci.* **2013**, *92*, 379–382. [CrossRef] [PubMed]

268. Kubatka, P.; Kello, M.; Kajo, K.; Kruzliak, P.; Vybohova, D.; Smejkal, K.; Marsik, P.; Zulli, A.; Gonciova, G.; Mojzis, J. Young barley indicates antitumor effects in experimental breast cancer in vivo and in vitro. *Nutr. Cancer* **2016**, *68*, 611–621. [CrossRef] [PubMed]

269. Cho, K.; Lee, C.W.; Ohm, J.B. In vitro study on effect of germinated wheat on human breast cancer cells. *Cereal Chem.* **2016**, *93*, 647–649. [CrossRef]

270. Xue, J.P.; Wang, G.; Zhao, Z.B.; Wang, Q.; Shi, Y. Synergistic cytotoxic effect of genistein and doxorubicin on drug-resistant human breast cancer MCF-7/Adr cells. *Oncol. Rep.* **2014**, *32*, 1647–1653. [CrossRef] [PubMed]

271. Kaushik, S.; Shyam, H.; Sharma, R.; Balapure, A.K. Genistein synergizes centchroman action in human breast cancer cells. *Indian J. Pharmacol.* **2016**, *48*, 637–642. [PubMed]

272. Charalambous, C.; Pitta, C.A.; Constantinou, A.I. Equol enhances tamoxifen's anti-tumor activity by induction of caspase-mediated apoptosis in MCF-7 breast cancer cells. *BMC Cancer* **2013**, *13*, 238. [CrossRef] [PubMed]

273. Taghizadeh, B.; Ghavami, L.; Nikoofar, A.; Goliaei, B. Equol as a potent radiosensitizer in estrogen receptor-positive and -negative human breast cancer cell lines. *Breast Cancer* **2015**, *22*, 382–390. [CrossRef] [PubMed]

274. Banerjee, S.; Kambhampati, S.; Banerjee, S.K.; Haque, I. Pomegranate sensitizes tamoxifen action in ER-alpha positive breast cancer cells. *J. Cell Commun. Signal.* **2011**, *5*, 317–324. [CrossRef] [PubMed]

275. McGuire, K.P.; Ngoubilly, N.; Neavyn, M.; Lanza-Jacoby, S. 3,3'-diindolylmethane and paclitaxel act synergistically to promote apoptosis in HER2/Neu human breast cancer cells. *J. Surg. Res.* **2006**, *132*, 208–213. [CrossRef] [PubMed]

276. Wang, W.J.; Lv, M.M.; Wang, Y.L.; Zhang, J.G. Development of novel application of 3,3'-diindolylmethane: Sensitizing multidrug resistance human breast cancer cells to gamma-irradiation. *Pharm. Biol.* **2016**, *54*, 3164–3168. [CrossRef] [PubMed]

277. Rahman, K.W.; Ali, S.; Aboukameel, A.; Sarkar, S.H.; Wang, Z.; Philip, P.A.; Sakr, W.A.; Raz, A. Inactivation of NF-κB by 3,3'-diindolylmethane contributes to increased apoptosis induced by chemotherapeutic agent in breast cancer cells. *Mol. Cancer Ther.* **2007**, *6*, 2757–2765. [CrossRef] [PubMed]

278. Ganji-Harsini, S.; Khazaei, M.; Rashidi, Z.; Ghanbari, A. Thymoquinone could increase the efficacy of tamoxifen induced apoptosis in human breast cancer cells: An in vitro study. *Cell J.* **2016**, *18*, 245–254. [PubMed]

279. Sakalar, C.; Izgi, K.; Iskender, B.; Sezen, S.; Aksu, H.; Cakir, M.; Kurt, B.; Turan, A.; Canatan, H. The combination of thymoquinone and paclitaxel shows anti-tumor activity through the interplay with apoptosis network in triple-negative breast cancer. *Tumor Biol.* **2016**, *37*, 4467–4477. [CrossRef] [PubMed]

280. Abdelhamed, S.; Yokoyama, S.; Refaat, A.; Ogura, K.; Yagita, H.; Awale, S.; Saiki, I. Piperine enhances the efficacy of TRAIL-based therapy for triple-negative breast cancer cells. *Anticancer Res.* **2014**, *34*, 1893–1899. [PubMed]

281. Gollapudi, S.; Ghoneum, M. MGN-3/Biobran, modified arabinoxylan from rice bran, sensitizes human breast cancer cells to chemotherapeutic agent, daunorubicin. *Cancer Detect. Prev.* **2008**, *32*, 1–6. [CrossRef] [PubMed]

282. Ghoneum, M.; El-Din, N.; Ali, D.A.; El-Dein, M.A. Modified arabinoxylan from rice bran, MGN-3/Biobran, sensitizes metastatic breast cancer cells to paclitaxel in vitro. *Anticancer Res.* **2014**, *34*, 81–87. [PubMed]

283. Bar-Sela, G.; Tsalic, M.; Fried, G.; Goldberg, H. Wheat grass juice may improve hematological toxicity related to chemotherapy in breast cancer patients: A pilot study. *Nutr. Cancer* **2007**, *58*, 43–48. [CrossRef] [PubMed]

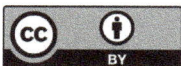

*nutrients*

MDPI

Review

# A Systematic Review and Meta-Analysis of the Effects of Flavanol-Containing Tea, Cocoa and Apple Products on Body Composition and Blood Lipids: Exploring the Factors Responsible for Variability in Their Efficacy

Antonio González-Sarrías [1,*], Emilie Combet [2], Paula Pinto [3], Pedro Mena [4],
Margherita Dall'Asta [4], Mar Garcia-Aloy [5,6], Ana Rodríguez-Mateos [7], Eileen R. Gibney [8],
Julie Dumont [9], Marika Massaro [10], Julio Sánchez-Meca [11], Christine Morand [12] and
María-Teresa García-Conesa [1,*]

1   Research Group on Quality, Safety and Bioactivity of Plant Foods, Campus de Espinardo,
    Centro de Edafologia y Biologia Aplicada del Segura-Consejo Superior de Investigaciones
    Científicas (CEBAS-CSIC), P.O. Box 164, 30100 Murcia, Spain
2   Human Nutrition, School of Medicine, Dentistry and Nursing, College of Medical, Veterinary and Life
    Sciences, University of Glasgow, Glasgow G31 2ER, UK; Emilie.CombetAspray@glasgow.ac.uk
3   Polytechnic Institute of Santarem, Escola Superior Agrária (ESA), Department of Food Technology,
    Biotechnology and Nutrition, 2001-904 Santarém, Portugal; paula.pinto@esa.ipsantarem.pt
4   Human Nutrition Unit, Department of Food & Drug, University of Parma, 43125 Parma, Italy;
    pedromiguel.menaparreno@unipr.it (P.M.); margherita.dallasta@unipr.it (M.D.)
5   Biomarkers and Nutrimetabolomic Laboratory, Department of Nutrition, Food Sciences and Gastronomy,
    University of Barcelona, 08028 Barcelona, Spain; margarcia@ub.edu
6   CIBER de Fragilidad y Envejecimiento Saludable (CIBERFES), Instituto de Salud Carlos III,
    08028 Barcelona, Spain
7   Division of Diabetes and Nutritional Sciences, King's College London, London SE1 9NH, UK;
    ana.rodriguez-mateos@kcl.ac.uk
8   Institute of Food and Health, School of Agriculture and Food Science, University College Dublin (UCD),
    Belfield, Dublin 4, Ireland; eileen.gibney@ucd.ie
9   U1167-RID-AGE-Facteurs de risque et Déterminants Moléculaires des Maladies Liées au Vieillissement,
    University Lille, Institut National de la Santé et de la Recherche Médicale (INSERM), Centre Hospitalier
    Universitaire (CHU) Lille, Institut Pasteur de Lille, F-59000 Lille, France; julie.dumont@pasteur-lille.fr
10  National Research Council (CNR), Institute of Clinical Physiology, 73100 Lecce, Italy; marika@ifc.cnr.it
11  Department of Basic Psychology & Methodology, Faculty of Psychology, University of Murcia, 30100 Murcia,
    Spain; jsmeca@um.es
12  Institut National de la Recherche Agronomique (INRA), Human Nutrition Unit,
    Université Clermont Auvergne (UCA), Centre de Recherches en Nutrition Humaine (CRNH) Auvergne,
    F-63000 Clermont-Ferrand, France; christine.morand@inra.fr
*   Correspondence: agsarrias@cebas.csic.es (A.G.-S.); mtconesa@cebas.csic.es (M.-T.G.-C.);
    Tel.: +34-968-396276 (A.G.-S. & M.-T.G.-C.); Fax: +34-968-396213(A.G.-S. & M.-T.G.-C.)

Received: 26 June 2017; Accepted: 10 July 2017; Published: 13 July 2017

**Abstract:** Several randomized controlled trials (RCTs) and meta-analyses support the benefits of flavanols on cardiometabolic health, but the factors affecting variability in the responses to these compounds have not been properly assessed. The objectives of this meta-analysis were to systematically collect the RCTs-based-evidence of the effects of flavanol-containing tea, cocoa and apple products on selected biomarkers of cardiometabolic risk and to explore the influence of various factors on the variability in the responses to the consumption of these products. A total of 120 RCTs were selected. Despite a high heterogeneity, the intake of the flavanol-containing products was associated using a random model with changes (reported as standardized difference in means (SDM)) in body mass index ($-0.15$, $p < 0.001$), waist circumference ($-0.29$, $p < 0.001$), total-cholesterol ($-0.21$,

$p < 0.001$), LDL-cholesterol ($-0.23$, $p < 0.001$), and triacylglycerides ($-0.11$, $p = 0.027$), and with an increase of HDL-cholesterol ($0.15$, $p = 0.005$). Through subgroup analyses, we showed the influence of baseline-BMI, sex, source/form of administration, medication and country of investigation on some of the outcome measures and suggest that flavanols may be more effective in specific subgroups such as those with a BMI $\geq 25.0$ kg/m$^2$, non-medicated individuals or by specifically using tea products. This meta-analysis provides the first robust evidence of the effects induced by the consumption of flavanol-containing tea, cocoa and apple products on weight and lipid biomarkers and shows the influence of various factors that can affect their bioefficacy in humans. Of note, some of these effects are quantitatively comparable to those produced by drugs, life-style changes or other natural products. Further, RCTs in well-characterized populations are required to fully comprehend the factors affecting inter-individual responses to flavanol and thereby improve flavanols efficacy in the prevention of cardiometabolic disorders.

**Keywords:** flavanols; tea; cocoa; apple; cardiometabolic disorders; meta-analysis; interindividual variability; blood lipids; body mass index; waist circumference

---

## 1. Introduction

Metabolic disorders, principally, abdominal obesity, dyslipidemia (high levels of triacylglycerides (TAGs) and low levels of high-density lipoprotein (HDL)), and insulin resistance have been associated to an increased risk of Type-2 diabetes mellitus (DM) and cardiovascular diseases (CVDs). CVDs remain the number one cause of death in developed countries and their prevalence is increasing rapidly in developing nations and in adolescents [1]. It is now well established from population studies that some aspects of CVDs risk can be modulated by various dietary interventions including an increased consumption of plant foods [2], as part of a healthy balanced diet. In addition to other protective compounds (i.e., fiber and vitamins), plant foods are an exclusive and abundant source of phytochemicals, a large and diverse group of compounds which exhibit an array of biological activities. The intake of these bioactive compounds are thought to contribute to the health benefits associated with the consumption of such foods [3]. Polyphenols are some of the most abundant phytochemicals in plant foods and increasing evidence from cohort studies indicate that the intake of some of these compounds such as diverse flavonoids and/or, importantly, some of their derived microbial metabolites (e.g., enterolactone) may help to reduce the development of CVDs and CVDs mortality risk [4–7]. This evidence is supported by animal and clinical studies reporting beneficial effects of the consumption of some polyphenol-rich foods or pure compounds on CVDs risk factors such as blood cholesterol, blood pressure, endothelial function and arterial stiffness [8].

Polyphenols encompass several families of compounds, the most represented in plant foods being phenolic acids and flavonoids [9]. A major group of flavonoids is constituted by flavanols that are abundant in green tea, red wine, cocoa and various fruits such as apples [10]. A summary of the major flavonoids present in tea (green and black), cocoa powder and apple is shown in Table S1. The assessment of daily intakes of flavanols across Europe revealed a large variation between countries (from 200 to 800 mg/day) depending on their dietary habits and the intake of tea [11]. The flavanol group is composed primarily of the epicatechin and catechin monomers, and of their oligomeric and polymeric forms, the procyanidins. Flavanol monomers and dimeric procyanidins are bioavailable. They undergo extensive phase II conjugation and are found in the blood circulation mostly as *O*-methylated, sulfated and glucuronidated conjugates (nM to µM range) [12,13]. In contrast, the procyanidins polymers are not absorbed and do not contribute to the systemic pool of flavanols in humans [14].

Human studies remain essential to understanding the effects of the plant bioactive compounds on health and thus, an increasing number of randomized controlled trials (RCTs) with flavanol-containing products have been carried out over the past two decades. Meta-analyses constitute a useful tool to integrate the accumulated RCTs and review the evidence in humans. Some of the main problems affecting the results of meta-analyses are the usually limited number of studies included as well as a range of factors that introduce heterogeneity in the findings. Identifying the factors underlying variability, as well as developing new and innovative methodologies to account for such variability constitute an overarching goal to ultimately optimize the beneficial health effects of plant food bioactives. Among the potential factors involved in such heterogeneity are: (i) factors inherent to the individuals: (epi) genetic factors, gut microbiota, baseline conditions (BMI, medication), sex, health status, ethnicity, and age; and (ii) factors intrinsic to the type of study (design, duration, dose, and type of product) [15].

The main goals of the present study were: (i) to systematically review and appraise, through meta-analysis, the impact of flavanol-containing tea, cocoa and apple products, three main sources of flavanols, on selected biomarkers of cardiometabolic risk, i.e., BMI, WC and blood lipid levels (total-, LDL-, HDL-cholesterol and TAGs); and (ii) to further explore some of the factors that may be implicated in the inter-individual variability in the response to the consumption of these flavanol-containing products.

## 2. Materials and Methods

This systematic review and meta-analysis followed the PRISMA (Preferred Reporting Items for Systematic Reviews and Meta-Analyses) statement guidelines [16], the Cochrane Handbook for Systematic Reviews of Interventions [17], and the Centre for Reviews and Dissemination's guidance for undertaking reviews in health care [18]. The protocol for this review was registered in the International Prospective Register of Systematic Reviews (PROSPERO, www.crd.york.ac.uk/prospero/index.asp) with the registration number CRD42016033878.

### 2.1. Search Strategy

A comprehensive search on PubMed and Web of Science databases was conducted in July 2015. Search terms included a combination of keywords referring to: (1) bioactive (polyphenols, flavonoids, flavanols, flavan-3-ol, (epi)catechin, (epi)gallocatechin gallate, theaflavins, thearubigin, and procyanidin); (2) food source (apple, tea, and cocoa); (3) type of study and participants (trial, experiment, study, intervention; human, subjects, men, women, patients, volunteers, and participants); and (4) cardiometabolic outcomes (BMI, WC, total cholesterol, LDL cholesterol, HDL cholesterol, and TAGs). No type of restriction was applied during the electronic searches.

### 2.2. Study Selection and Data Extraction

Two authors independently assessed all papers and in the case of disagreement, discussed findings to reach a consensus, or in the absence of resolution, a third author was contacted. Studies included in the meta-analysis were limited to human RCTs testing the effect of flavanol-containing tea, cocoa or apple products, which had a control group receiving a placebo and measured one or more of the defined outcomes (BMI, WC, total cholesterol, LDL cholesterol, HDL cholesterol, or TAGs). Manuscripts written in any European language were included, whereas other manuscripts were excluded. Additionally, the studies with the following characteristics were excluded: studies with flavanol-rich food sources other than tea, cocoa or apples; and studies with multifactorial interventions (i.e., flavanols given as a part of a multicomponent treatment; dietary or physical activity co-intervention). Data extraction was performed in duplicate by two authors, independently, and cross-checked by a third author using a standardized data extraction form. Extracted data included publication details (year of publication, contact details, clinical trial and registration number); participant characteristics (geographical origin, total number of participants included in the study and in the analysis, sex distribution, age, ethnicity, health status, menopausal status, smoking habits, and use of medication); study setting and design (cross-over or parallel design, duration of the intervention, number of arms and description, number of participants located in each arm and completing the study, composition of test and placebo, and dose and mode of administration); and outcomes (type of sample, changes in the outcome, values before and after intervention, and *p*-value).

### 2.3. Assessment of Quality and Data Analysis

The quality of the studies was assessed based on the Cochrane Collaboration measurement with some modifications [19]. The specific items used for the assessments are detailed in a previous meta-analysis following the same protocol [7].

Data for each outcome were analyzed using the Comprehensive Meta-Analysis Software, version 3.0 (Biostat, Englewood, NJ, USA) [20]. The free scale index standardized difference in means (SDM) was used to combine data from the highest number of collected valid studies, increasing the pool of studies and the power to detect significant differences. SDM, standard error (SE) and the corresponding 95% confidence intervals (CI) were calculated and pooled using random effects models to determine test/placebo differences across studies. Statistical heterogeneity between studies was assessed by using the Cochran $Q$ test, the between-studies variance ($T^2$) and $I^2$ (an estimate of the proportion of variance across studies caused by heterogeneity rather than by random errors) where $I^2$ values equal to 25%, 50% and 75% were considered as low, moderate and high heterogeneity, respectively. Publication bias was assessed visually with funnel plots and statistically by applying the Egger's regression test. Further assessment of the possible associations between the overall changes attributed to the supplementation with the flavanols and the duration of the intervention was examined using random-effects meta-regression analysis. Using the random model, we have additionally estimated the overall effect size as the difference in means (DM) and 95% CI.

Subgroup analyses were conducted to explore potential factors that may introduce heterogeneity into the studies and influence the inter-individual variability in the response to supplementation with the flavanol-containing products. We selected those factors that were more clearly described throughout articles (Table 1). We included factors that might be attributed to some of the individuals' characteristics, such as baseline BMI, sex, smoking habits and medication/health status. Age or ethnicity could not be assessed due to unclear reporting. We also included stratification by the country in which the study was carried out, the source and form of administration of the flavanols, as well as the type of diet reported to be followed during the intervention. For each subgroup, the pooled effects (SDM) and the significance of this value were estimated. Additionally, statistical comparisons between subgroups were performed by applying a random-effects analysis and calculation of the between-categories Q statistic, the *p*-value and the $R^2$ index (proportion of between-studies variance explained by each factor or covariate). Using some of the factors that partially explained some of the between-studies variance for a particular variable, we applied a multiple meta-regression analysis with a random-effects model to search for a potential combination of factors that best explained the between-study variance for this variable. Statistical significance of the findings was as follows: *p*-value < 0.05 was considered significant, while *p*-value $\geq$ 0.05 and < 0.1 was considered marginally significant.

**Table 1.** Potential factors influencing the heterogeneity in the responses to the supplementation with flavanols-containing products investigated in this meta-analysis.

| Factors | | | | | | |
|---|---|---|---|---|---|---|
| Baseline BMI | <25.0 [a] (normal and/or underweight) | | | ≥25.0 (overweight and/or obese) | | |
| Sex | Women | | | Men | | |
| Smoking | Non-smokers | | | Smokers | | |
| | East Asian | | | European countries | | |
| Country where the study was undertaken | countries (Japan, Korea, China, Thailand, Taiwan) | All other countries | North America (USA, Canada) | Non-Mediterranean countries (Denmark, Finland, The Netherlands, Germany, Poland, UK, Switzerland) | Mediterranean countries (Italy, Spain, Portugal, Greece) | |
| Medication | Yes | | | No | | |
| Healthy vs. non-healthy | Healthy individuals [b] | Individuals at a risk of disease [c] | Individuals with a reported disease [d] | Different disorders: overweight and/or obese, dyslipidemia, glucose disorders, blood pressure disorders, mixed [e] | | |
| Source of flavanols | Cocoa products | Apple products | Tea products | Tea drinks | Tea extracts (capsules, powder) | Tea purified EGCG |
| Diet during intervention | Controlled diet | | | Usual diet (includes usual with some restrictions and NR) | | |

[a]: BMI cut-off values as established by the WHO; [b]: Includes individuals specifically reported as healthy and not medicated (in some cases medication was not reported, NR); [c]: Includes individuals not medicated that were overweight and/or obese, or specifically indicated to be borderline, mild condition or at risk of a disease; [d]: Includes individuals with one or more than one of the following disorders: dyslipidemia, glucose disorders or type-2 diabetes, blood pressure disorders (hypertension), medicated obesity, metabolic syndrome (most cases were also medicated but in some cases medication was NR); [e]: Individuals reported to have only one of the specified disorders.

## 3. Results

### 3.1. Description of the Included Studies

A total of 1409 articles were initially identified through the search on the electronic databases. After removal of duplicates and screening, 188 trials were selected for data extraction. After detailed analysis of the full text, 71 articles were excluded, due to lack of relevant outcomes, aspects of study design or publication language. The final number of articles selected for meta-analysis was selected from a total of 117 articles published between 1997 and July 2015 (included) [21–137]. The detailed study selection flow diagram is shown in Figure 1.

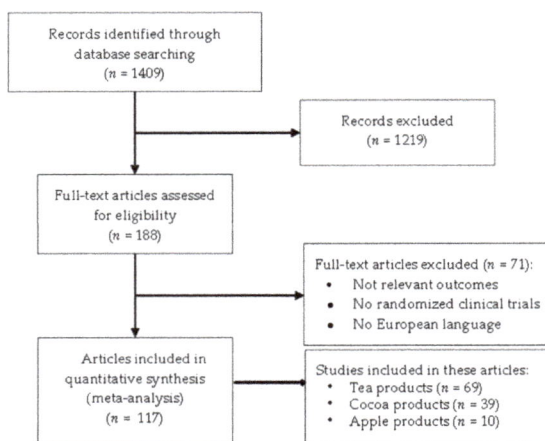

**Figure 1.** Flow diagram showing the study selection process.

## 3.2. Quality and Characteristics of the Selected Studies

Most of the studies (70%) were classified as studies with a moderate to low risk of bias (quality score ≥5.0 and <8.0 or ≥8.0 and ≤10.0, respectively) while 30% of the studies obtained a low quality score (<5.0) and were considered as a high risk of bias.

The studies were carried out in countries distributed over five continents: Asia (Japan, Korea, China, Taiwan, Thailand, Saudi Arabia, and Iran), North America (USA and Canada) and Latin America (Brazil and Mexico), Europe (Denmark, Finland, The Netherlands, Germany, Poland, UK, Switzerland, Italy, Spain, Portugal, and Greece), Africa (Mauritania, South Africa, and Republic of Mauritius), and Australia. Thus, they were considered representative of a global population. The participants in these studies also represent a mixed population of men and women ranging from young adults to elderly participants, and with a higher prevalence of individuals with a BMI ≥ 25.0 kg/m² (overweight and/or obese volunteers). The quality and depth of reporting of the factors potentially contributing toward inter-individual variability of the effect of flavanols varied among studies. The smoking habits were not reported in most studies but for those studies that did, the participants were typically non-smokers or a mixed sample population. Only two studies [34,57] were carried out specifically with smokers. The total sample population included healthy individuals, overweight and/or obese individuals as well as individuals with an incipient or with a reported chronic risk factor or metabolic disease, comprising principally hypertension, hyperlipidemias, type-2 diabetes, metabolic syndrome, atherosclerosis, coronary artery disease and heart failure. Among these, some participants were taking medication, others were not medicated or medication use was not reported. Studies were selected if the source of flavanols was tea, cocoa, or apple provided as liquid (tea drinks, cocoa beverages, and apple juice) or solid (powder or extracts in capsules, snacks, tablets, and foods) forms. Interventions ranged typically 1–6 months, during which participants followed either a controlled diet or their habitual diets.

## 3.3. Overall Impact of the Supplementation with Flavanol-Containing Tea, Cocoa or Apple Products on Blood Lipids, BMI and WC

The number of RCTs varied in function of the outcome measure studied, from 46 to 120 trials, recruiting a total high number of participants ranging from 2875 to 5931 individuals. Forest plots detailing weighted SDM, SE, 95% confidence intervals and relative weight for the impact of supplementation with flavanol-containing tea, cocoa or apple products on BMI, WC, and blood lipid levels are shown in Figures S1–S6. Visual inspection of the Funnel plots (Figures S7–S12) evidenced symmetrical shapes and absence of publication bias in the case of WC, total cholesterol, LDL, HDL and TAGs. Some asymmetry was however detected for BMI. These results were further confirmed by Egger's regression. A summary of the random overall effects for each lipid and obesity-related variable, heterogeneity and bias analyses is presented in Table 2.

**Table 2.** Overall changes (SDM), heterogeneity and publication bias analyses for the impact of flavanol-containing products on BMI, WC and blood lipids levels.

| | $n$ | $N_T$ | $N_S$ | $N_C$ | SDM | 95% CI | Z | $p$-Value | Tau² | Q | df ($p$-Value) | I² (%) | Egger's Regression Intercept | Egger's Regression $p$-Value (2-Tailed) |
|---|---|---|---|---|---|---|---|---|---|---|---|---|---|---|
| BMI | 74 | 4156 | 2127 | 2029 | −0.153 | −0.227, −0.078 | −4.009 | <0.001 | 0.027 | 99.6 | 73 (0.021) | 26.7 | 1.04 | 0.024 |
| WC | 46 | 2875 | 1478 | 1397 | −0.293 | −0.438, −0.147 | −3.932 | <0.001 | 0.168 | 156.7 | 45 (<0.001) | 71.3 | −1.47 | 0.101 |
| TC | 112 | 5812 | 2982 | 2830 | −0.214 | −0.328, −0.099 | −3.651 | <0.001 | 0.273 | 479.1 | 111 (<0.001) | 76.8 | −0.76 | 0.226 |
| LDL-C | 105 | 5726 | 2928 | 2798 | −0.235 | −0.345, −0.125 | −4.171 | <0.001 | 0.229 | 408.0 | 104 (<0.001) | 74.5 | −0.46 | 0.459 |
| HDL-C | 112 | 5928 | 3023 | 2905 | 0.152 | 0.047, 0.256 | 2.836 | 0.005 | 0.214 | 408.0 | 111 (<0.001) | 72.8 | 0.72 | 0.208 |
| TAGs | 120 | 5931 | 3023 | 2908 | −0.114 | −0.215, −0.013 | −2.213 | 0.027 | 0.209 | 407.7 | 119 (<0.001) | 70.8 | −0.33 | 0.570 |

BMI: Body Mass Index; WC: Waist Circumference; TC: Total Cholesterol; LDL-C: Low density Lipoprotein Cholesterol; HDL-C: High Density Lipoprotein Cholesterol; TAGs: Triglycerides; $n$: total number of studies included in the analysis; $N_T$: number of total participants; $N_S$: number of participants in the supplemented group; $N_C$: number of participants in the control group; SDM: standardized difference in means; 95% CI: lower and upper confidence limits for the average SDM: df: degrees of freedom; Z: statistic for testing the significance of the average SDM; Tau²: between-studies variance; Q: heterogeneity statistic; I²: heterogeneity index.

Despite a high heterogeneity across the studies ($I^2$ = 70–77% for most variables except for BMI which was more moderate, $I^2$ = 26.7%), the overall pooled analysis (shown as SDM) significantly confirmed a reduction of BMI (−0.153, *p*-value < 0.001), WC (−0.293, *p*-value < 0.001), blood total cholesterol (−0.214, *p*-value < 0.001), LDL (−0.235, *p*-value < 0.001), and TAGs (−0.114, *p*-value = 0.027). HDL levels were also significantly increased (0.152, *p*-value = 0.005). Sensitivity analyses were carried out using the leave-one-out approach where the meta-analysis was performed with each study removed in turn. The pooled estimates consistently showed a similar effect and significance emphasizing the robustness of these results and that the effect was not driven by any particular study (data not shown). Further support of these results was found by a significant relationship between the duration of the supplementation with the flavanol products and the reduction of WC; total-, LDL- and HDL-cholesterol; and TAGs using random-effects meta-regression analysis. Regression coefficients and *p*-values for each variable can be seen in Table S2.

### 3.4. Analysis of the Potential Factors Influencing Inter-Individual Responses to Flavanols Consumption

#### 3.4.1. Stratification by the Individuals' Baseline BMI, Sex, Smoking, and Country

Following stratification by the baseline BMI (Table 3), the effects of the flavanol-containing products on BMI, WC, total- and LDL-cholesterol remained significant only in those studies carried out in overweight/obese volunteers (BMI ≥ 25.0 kg/m$^2$). HDL-cholesterol levels were also increased in this subgroup (*p* = 0.063) whereas the reducing effects on TAGs levels were not significant in any of the two subgroups. Statistical comparison between ≥25.0 vs. <25.0 kg/m$^2$ subgroups did not reach significance for any of the variables investigated. Of note, 61% of the total between-study variance in BMI could be explained by the respective baseline BMI values (total between Q = 2.53, *p*-value = 0.112, R$^2$ index = 0.61).

Regarding stratification by sex, the reduction of WC was significant in both men and women after intervention with flavanol-containing products. However, total- and LDL-cholesterol were significantly reduced only in female whereas BMI was significantly lowered only in male. The effects on HDL and TAG levels were no longer significant after stratification by sex (Table 3). Between groups comparison indicated a difference between sexes (total between Q = 2.833, *p*-value = 0.092) and a considerable contribution of the sex to the between-study variance for BMI (R$^2$ index = 1.0).

The reduction of BMI, WC, and total- and LDL-cholesterol in response to the flavanol-containing products was significant in studies carried out in non-smoker volunteers. It was not possible, however, to establish a comparison with habitual smokers due to the very low number of studies carried out with this type of volunteers (*n* = 2 studies).

Comparison between studies carried out in East Asian countries (assuming Asian ethnicity) against those carried out elsewhere evidenced similar results for BMI, WC, total and LDL cholesterol in both subgroups although the results were slightly less significant in the East Asian subgroup. A small proportion (7%) of the BMI between-groups variance was explained by the study location (East Asian vs. others) (total between Q = 0.963, *p*-value = 0.327, R$^2$ index = 0.07). In addition, we found a significant difference in TAG levels in response to flavanol-containing products between the East Asian subgroup and the others with a more pronounced effect in the East Asian studies (total between Q = 7.419, *p*-value = 0.024, R$^2$ index < 0.01). When grouping in North America and European countries, we detected a significant reduction of BMI and WC in the Europe group but not in the American one, whereas the LDL-cholesterol reduction resulted significant in the American group only. Statistical comparison between North America and Europe groups showed a difference in the BMI response (total between Q = 3.143, *p*-value = 0.076) and a 28% of the between-group variance explained by this factor (R$^2$ index = 0.28). Within Europe, the studies carried out in countries of the Mediterranean area resulted in significant reductions of BMI, WC, total- and LDL-cholesterol and in an increase of HDL (*p* = 0.078). In the non-Mediterranean countries, we only detected a significant reduction of total-cholesterol. Comparison between the two subgroups indicated a significant difference in the WC reduction (Total between Q = 5.228, *p*-value = 0.022, R$^2$ index < 0.01).

**Table 3.** Stratification analysis of the influence of baseline BMI, sex, smoking and country where the study was carried out on the effects (SDM) on BMI, WC, and blood lipids levels following supplementation with flavanol-containing products.

| Factor | Baseline BMI | | Sex | | Smoking | | Country Where the Study Was Undertaken | | | | European Countries | |
|---|---|---|---|---|---|---|---|---|---|---|---|---|
| Subgroup | <25.0 | ≥25.0 | Women | Men | Non-Smokers | Smokers | East Asian Countries | All Other Countries | North America | All European Countries | Med Countries | Non-Med Countries |
| BMI | 0.003 [a] | −0.165 | −0.102 | −0.321 | −0.148 | NR | −0.204 | −0.126 | −0.042 | −0.235 | −0.306 | −0.176 |
| p-value | (NS) | (0.001) | (NS) | (0.003) | (0.018) | | (0.001) | (0.007) | (NS) | (0.001) | (0.024) | (0.091) |
| (n, N) | (11, 477) | (42, 2410) | (15, 831) | (8, 339) | (24, 1046) | | (23, 1511) | (51, 2645) | (15, 719) | (20, 1051) | (7, 392) | (13, 659) |
| WC | −0.102 | −0.362 | −0.643 | −0.932 | −0.252 | NR | −0.217 | −0.355 | −0.123 | −0.573 | −1.279 | −0.181 |
| p-value | (NS) | (0.000) | (0.037) | (0.024) | (0.008) | | (0.055) | (0.000) | (NS) | (0.006) | (0.001) | (NS) |
| (n, N) | (3, 253) | (36, 2002) | (9, 464) | (5, 266) | (16, 750) | | (19, 1458) | (27, 1471) | (6, 206) | (13, 757) | (5, 269) | (8, 488) |
| TC | −0.047 | −0.165 | −0.493 | −0.100 | −0.221 | 0.147 | −0.195 | −0.223 | −0.303 | −0.254 | −0.255 | −0.252 |
| p-value | (NS) | (0.011) | (0.012) | (NS) | (0.001) | (NS) | (0.054) | (0.002) | (0.027) | (0.032) | (0.003) | (0.003) |
| (n, N) | (19, 504) | (50, 2863) | (15, 873) | (14, 557) | (41, 1572) | (2, 88) | (37, 2297) | (75, 3515) | (23, 1097) | (30, 1296) | (15, 609) | (15, 639) |
| LDL-C | −0.062 | −0.195 | −0.545 | −0.131 | −0.156 | −0.341 | −0.236 | −0.234 | −0.379 | −0.185 | −0.246 | −0.140 |
| p-value | (NS) | (0.002) | (0.004) | (NS) | (0.039) | (NS) | (0.017) | (0.001) | (0.006) | (NS) | (0.042) | (NS) |
| (n, N) | (13, 396) | (48, 2698) | (15, 868) | (10, 416) | (42, 1764) | (2, 88) | (31, 2334) | (74, 3392) | (25, 1117) | (27, 1176) | (12, 537) | (15, 639) |
| HDL-C | 0.229 | 0.176 | 0.226 | 0.272 | 0.090 | 0.152 | 0.105 | 0.176 | 0.286 | 0.165 | 0.320 | 0.029 |
| p-value | (NS) | (0.063) | (NS) | (NS) | (NS) | (NS) | (NS) | (0.008) | (0.095) | (NS) | (0.078) | (NS) |
| (n, N) | (17, 455) | (52, 2872) | (15, 902) | (16, 634) | (45, 1945) | (2, 88) | (37, 2410) | (75, 3518) | (22, 978) | (34, 1495) | (15, 679) | (18, 816) |
| TAGs | −0.058 | −0.098 | −0.067 | 0.109 | −0.051 | 0.089 | −0.196 | −0.052 | −0.098 | −0.185 | −0.161 | −0.203 |
| p-value | (NS) | (NS) | (NS) | (NS) | (NS) | (NS) | (0.034) | (NS) | (NS) | (0.099) | (NS) | (NS) |
| (n, N) | (23, 596) | (53, 2599) | (16, 887) | (18, 781) | (55, 2243) | (2, 88) | (35, 1975) | (83, 3796) | (23, 921) | (41, 1969) | (18, 939) | (24, 1100) |

[a] Standardized difference in means (SDM); BMI: Body Mass Index; WC: Waist Circumference; TC: Total Cholesterol; LDL-C: Low density Lipoprotein Cholesterol; HDL-C: High Density Lipoprotein Cholesterol; TAGs: Triacylglycerides; Med: Mediterranean; p-value < 0.05 was considered significant; p-value < 0.1 and ≥ 0.05 was considered marginally significant.; NS: No significant change / effect; (n): Number of studies included; (N): Total number of participants; NR: Not reported.

### 3.4.2. Stratification by the Individuals' Medication and Health/Disease Status

The influence of medication on the response to the consumption of the flavanol-containing products was also explored (Table 4). The subgroup including participants without any reported medication showed significant reductions of BMI, WC, total- and LDL-cholesterol as well as a reduction of TAGs ($p = 0.063$). In contrast, in the subgroup of studies including participants under medication the effects did not reach statistical significance. Further comparison between the two subgroups (Yes vs. No medication) revealed no significant differences between them (total between Q = 2.59, $p$-value = 0.107) but 34% of the between-groups variance for the BMI response was explained by this factor ($R^2$ index = 0.34).

Regarding health/disease status, participants were stratified as healthy, at risk or with a reported disease. Both in healthy subjects and in participants with a disease, the total- and LDL-cholesterol levels were significantly reduced. Studies conducted with volunteers categorized as at a risk exhibited the most significant reduction of BMI and WC in response to the flavanols. Stratification of the studies by the type of disorder showed a significant reduction of BMI and WC in overweight and/or obese individuals, a significant increase of HDL-cholesterol levels in patients with a dyslipidemia and a significant reduction of LDL-cholesterol in patients with diabetes or hypertension (Table 4). Comparison between each of the subgroups against the healthy subgroup was not significant for any of the variables investigated.

### 3.4.3. Stratification by the Source/Administration Form of the Flavanols and the Diet during the Intervention

Among the sources of flavanols investigated, our meta-analysis confirmed that supplementation with tea derived products significantly impacts on all the investigated variables except for TAGs (Table 5). Studies carried out with cocoa as the source of flavanols exhibited a significant effect on total-, LDL-cholesterol and TAGs levels whereas intervention with the apple-derived products appears to only modulate total- and LDL-cholesterol levels. Statistical comparison between the sources of flavanols highlighted a significant difference in the effect on BMI between tea and cocoa products ($p$-value = 0.012) with a 29% of the between-groups variance explained by this factor ($R^2$ index = 0.29). The apple group resulted also significantly more efficient than the cocoa or tea groups in the reduction of total-cholesterol. In addition, the apple products showed a greater effect on LDL-cholesterol than the tea derived products.

Regarding the supplementation form, the results showed that the administration of tea as solid extracts caused a significant and efficient modulation of all the variables investigated except for HDL and TAGs, whereas the tea beverages were significant at reducing only BMI and LDL-cholesterol (Table 5). Statistical comparison between liquid and solid tea-flavanols administration pointed out at a difference between the two subgroups at reducing LDL cholesterol ($p$-value = 0.096) with 11% of the between-group variance explained by this factor ($R^2$ index = 0.11). A very limited number of studies have reported so far the effects of tea purified epigallocatechin gallate (EGCG), one of the main flavanols present in tea. Overall, these studies only support a significant reduction of BMI by this compound. Of note, and as opposed to tea products, the purified EGCG appears to reduce the levels of HDL (results not significant) and increase those of TAGs ($p = 0.077$) (Table 5). Comparison between the EGCG subgroup and the tea drink or the tea extract subgroups indicated that the form of administration (as a purified compound or as a mixture) partially contributed to explaining the between groups variances for HDL (total between Q = 5.211, $p$-value = 0.022, $R^2$ index = 0.10, EGCG vs. tea drink; total between Q = 3.835, $p$-value = 0.050, $R^2$ index = 0.12, EGCG vs. tea extract) and for TAGs (total between Q = 3.282, $p$-value = 0.070, $R^2$ index = 0.06, EGCG vs. tea drink; total between Q = 3.765, $p$-value = 0.052, $R^2$ index = 0.09, EGCG vs. tea extract).

**Table 4.** Analysis of the influence of medication and health status on the effects (SDM) of the supplementation with flavanols on BMI, WC, and blood lipids levels.

| Factor | Medication | | Health Status | | | | Type of Disorder | | |
|---|---|---|---|---|---|---|---|---|---|
| Subgroup | Yes | No | Healthy Individuals | Individuals at Risk | Individuals with a Disease | Overweight/Obese | Lipid Disorders | Glucose Disorders | Blood Pressure Disorders |
| BMI | −0.053[a] | −0.222 | −0.119 | −0.195 | −0.128 | −0.191 | −0.063 | −0.028 | −0.054 |
| $p$-value | (NS) | (0.001) | (NS) | (0.009) | (0.069) | (0.011) | (NS) | (NS) | (NS) |
| $(n, N)$ | (15, 744) | (28, 1312) | (18, 868) | (26, 1753) | (25, 1008) | (22, 1488) | (4, 179) | (5, 265) | (5, 225) |
| WC | −0.363 | −0.445 | −0.092 | −0.392 | −0.169 | −0.426 | NI | −0.057 | NI |
| $p$-value | (NS) | (0.003) | (NS) | (0.000) | (NS) | (0.000) | | (NS) | |
| $(n, N)$ | (5, 309) | (21, 1237) | (4, 250) | (26, 1485) | (9, 466) | (25, 1447) | | (4, 188) | |
| TC | −0.205 | −0.296 | −0.266 | −0.161 | −0.241 | −0.148 | −0.227 | −0.372 | −0.515 |
| $p$-value | (0.089) | (0.001) | (0.015) | (NS) | (0.014) | (NS) | (NS) | (NS) | (NS) |
| $(n, N)$ | (24, 1174) | (47, 2169) | (38, 1520) | (32, 2243) | (38, 1859) | (24, 1813) | (9, 491) | (8, 463) | (5, 275) |
| LDL-C | −0.200 | −0.289 | −0.210 | −0.192 | −0.311 | −0.187 | −0.336 | −0.579 | −0.754 |
| $p$-value | (NS) | (0.004) | (0.028) | (0.061) | (0.003) | (0.082) | (NS) | (0.042) | (0.041) |
| $(n, N)$ | (21, 1020) | (43, 2311) | (37, 1782) | (29, 2049) | (36, 1756) | (23, 1742) | (9, 491) | (6, 408) | (4, 146) |
| HDL-C | 0.162 | 0.128 | 0.163 | 0.229 | 0.091 | −0.062 | 0.476 | 0.032 | 0.115 |
| $p$-value | (NS) | (NS) | (NS) | (NS) | (NS) | (NS) | (NS) | (NS) | (NS) |
| $(n, N)$ | (25, 1212) | (48, 2042) | (37, 1670) | (32, 2187) | (39, 1881) | (20, 1541) | (12, 654) | (8, 488) | (6, 301) |
| TAGs | −0.165 | −0.063 | −0.144 | −0.08 | −0.103 | −0.008 | −0.258 | 0.065 | −0.251 |
| $p$-value | (NS) | (NS) | (NS) | (NS) | (NS) | (NS) | (NS) | (NS) | (NS) |
| $(n, N)$ | (23, 1132) | (63, 3019) | (45, 2669) | (31, 1205) | (39, 1931) | (24, 912) | (12, 585) | (7, 536) | (6, 250) |

[a] Standardized difference in means (SDM); BMI: Body Mass Index; WC: Waist Circumference; TC: Total Cholesterol; LDL-C: Low density Lipoprotein Cholesterol; HDL-C: High Density Lipoprotein Cholesterol; TAGs: Triacylglycerides; $p$-value < 0.05 was considered significant; $p$-value < 0.1 and $\geq$ 0.05 was considered marginally significant; NS: No significant change/effect; (n): Number of studies included; (N): Total number of participants.

**Table 5.** Analysis of the influence of the original source of flavanols and of the diet (during the intervention) on the effects (SDM) of the supplementation on BMI, WC, and blood lipids levels.

| Factor | Source of Flavanols | | | | | | Diet during Supplementation | |
|---|---|---|---|---|---|---|---|---|
| Subgroup | Cocoa Products | Apple Products | Tea Products | Tea Drinks | Tea Extracts | Tea Purified EGCG | Controlled | Usual |
| BMI | 0.001 [a] | −0.11 | −0.224 | −0.223 | −0.212 | −0.290 | −0.162 | −0.149 |
| *p*-value | (NS) | (NS) | (0.000) | −0.007 | (0.002) | (0.022) | (0.030) | (0.001) |
| (*n*, N) | (21, 1014) | (5, 319) | (46, 2704) | (20, 1167) | (26, 1537) | (7, 384) | (23, 1032) | (49, 2990) |
| WC | −0.106 | −0.206 | −0.354 | −0.22 | −0.506 | −0.465 | −0.500 | −0.164 |
| *p*-value | (NS) | (NS) | (0.000) | (NS) | (0.000) | (NS) | (0.000) | (0.084) |
| (*n*, N) | (8, 430) | (2, 155) | (34, 2228) | (16, 1074) | (17, 1110) | (2, 171) | (18, 903) | (27, 1868) |
| TC | −0.177 | −1.352 | −0.143 | −0.083 | −0.208 | −0.051 | −0.215 | −0.213 |
| *p*-value | −0.018 | −0.041 | (0.036) | (NS) | (0.008) | (NS) | (0.032) | (0.003) |
| (*n*, N) | (38, 1625) | (7, 402) | (65, 3666) | (36, 2051) | (26, 1615) | (7, 437) | (39, 1682) | (73, 4130) |
| LDL-C | −0.252 | −0.587 | −0.191 | −0.119 | −0.270 | −0.216 | −0.184 | −0.260 |
| *p*-value | −0.013 | −0.007 | (0.008) | −0.045 | (0.000) | (NS) | (0.062) | (0.000) |
| (*n*, N) | (35, 1577) | (8, 386) | (61, 3723) | (35, 2235) | (26, 1488) | (7, 206) | (38, 1540) | (67, 4186) |
| HDL-C | 0.16 | 0.197 | 0.150 | 0.17 | 0.13 | −0.291 | 0.245 | 0.104 |
| *p*-value | (NS) | (NS) | (0.031) | −0.071 | (NS) | (NS) | (0.008) | (NS) |
| (*n*, N) | (37, 1603) | (7, 386) | (66, 3820) | (38, 2292) | (27, 1484) | (7, 437) | (40, 1759) | (72, 4169) |
| TAGs | −0.183 | −0.173 | −0.050 | −0.047 | −0.053 | 0.314 | −0.139 | −0.105 |
| *p*-value | −0.047 | (NS) | (NS) | (NS) | (NS) | −0.077 | (NS) | (NS) |
| (*n*, N) | (39, 1691) | (10, 455) | (69, 3700) | (38, 2121) | (30, 1544) | (7, 437) | (46, 1939) | (73, 3922) |

[a] Standardized difference in means (SDM); BMI: Body Mass Index; WC: Waist Circumference; TC: Total Cholesterol; LDL-C: Low density Lipoprotein Cholesterol; HDL-C: High Density Lipoprotein Cholesterol; TAGs: Triacylglycerides; *p*-value < 0.05 was considered significant ; *p*-value < 0.1 and ≥ 0.05 was considered marginally significant ; NS: No significant change/effect; (*n*): Number of studies included; (N): Total number of participants; EGCG: Epigallocatechin gallate.

Regarding the type of diet (controlled vs. usual) during supplementation with the flavanol-containing products, the reducing effects on BMI, WC, total- and LDL-cholesterol remained significant or marginally significant in both subgroups. The levels of TAGs were also reduced although not significantly. We detected, however, a significant increase in the HDL-cholesterol levels only in the subgroup that followed a controlled diet (Table 5). Further, statistical comparison of the two subgroups highlighted a significant difference on the reduction of WC between them (total between Q = 4.761, *p*-value = 0.029) and a 7% explanation of the between-groups variance by this factor ($R^2$ index = 0.07).

### 3.4.4. Multiple Meta-Regression Analysis of BMI Modulators of the Response to Flavanol-Containing Products Consumption

Multiple meta-regression analysis was performed (Table 6) to derive the independent effect of some of the covariates previously found to partially explain some of the between-groups variance for BMI, i.e., baseline BMI (64%), country where the study was carried out (East-Asian vs. all other countries) (7%), medication use (34%) and source of flavanols (tea vs. cocoa products) (29%).

Although sex also appeared to contribute greatly to the BMI between-groups variance ($R^2$ = 1), it was not included in the multiple regression due to the limited number of studies clearly reporting sex and used in the analysis. The full model reached statistical significance, with a large proportion of variance (94%) accounted for and a considerable number of studies included (*n* = 40 studies). Both medication and source of flavanols were significantly correlated with the reducing effect on BMI, once controlled the influence of the other predictor. In particular, higher effects of the flavanols-products on BMI were found in the absence of the medication and with the consumption of tea products.

**Table 6.** Main results of the multiple random-effects meta-regression model for the contribution of the covariates, medication and source of flavanols, on BMI response (Standardized difference in means).

| Covariate | Coefficient | SE | 95% Lower | 95% Upper | Z | *p*-Value |
|---|---|---|---|---|---|---|
| Intercept | −0.0679 | 0.0899 | −0.2440 | 0.1082 | −0.76 | 0.4500 |
| Medication (No vs. Yes) | 0.2481 | 0.0995 | 0.0530 | 0.4431 | 2.49 | 0.0127 |
| Source of flavanols (Cocoa vs. Tea) | −0.3278 | 0.1022 | −0.5282 | −0.1274 | −3.21 | 0.0013 |
| **Test of the Model** | | | | | | |
| $Q_R$ | | | 15.64 | | | |
| *df* | | | 2 | | | |
| *p*-value | | | 0.0004 | | | |
| $R^2$ | | | 0.94 | | | |
| Number of studies included | | | 40 (54% of the total studies used in the meta-analysis) | | | |

SE: standard error for each regression coefficient; Z: statistic for testing the statistical significance of each predictor; P: probability level; $Q_R$: statistic for testing the statistical significance of the full meta-regression model; *df*: degrees of freedom; $R^2$: proportion of total between-studies variance explained by the model analog.

## 4. Discussion

The consumption of flavanols may contribute to improve cardiometabolic health via the moderation of a range of associated risk factors. Recent meta-analyses (Table S3) [138–151] suggest that the consumption of flavanol-containing tea and tea products could reduce total- and LDL-cholesterol as well as body mass index (BMI) and waist circumference (WC), while chocolate and cocoa flavanols also appear to regulate blood lipid levels. Nonetheless, the results of these analyses are inconsistent, partly due to the large heterogeneity of the clinical trials included. In addition, some of the anthropometric indicators of obesity such as BMI and WC have not yet been systematically investigated. We herein present the largest meta-analysis investigating the impact of flavanol-containing tea, cocoa and apple products, three major dietary sources of these bioactive compounds [152] on several biomarkers of lipid metabolism and anthropometric variables, such as BMI and WC. Our analysis confirms that the intake of these products is significantly associated with: (1) reduced BMI and WC; and (2) a more favorable lipid profile with a decrease in total- and LDL-cholesterol, and TAG plasma levels, and an increase in HDL-cholesterol levels. In addition, our analyses show that the changes in these biomarkers following consumption of the flavanol-containing products can be influenced by a number of factors and thus, the benefits of these products can significantly vary between specific population subgroups. It is of utmost interest to clarify the impact of these factors in order to discern which population subgroups could most benefit of the intake of these bioactive compounds.

### 4.1. Baseline BMI

There is evidence that baseline BMI may be a potential factor with an impact on the individuals' response to supplementation with different natural products. For instance, treatment with natural probiotics has been shown to significantly increase HDL only in patients with a baseline BMI $\geq$ 29 kg/m$^2$ [153] or significantly reduce BMI only in participants with a baseline BMI $\geq$ 25 kg/m$^2$ [154]. Regarding flavanol-containing products, a previous meta-analysis of the effects of black tea on blood cholesterol failed to detect differences in the modulation of cholesterol levels between individuals with normal weight or overweight and obese phenotype, but the results of this meta-analysis were estimated using a very small number of trials per subgroup (4 and 5, respectively) [141]. Our stratification approach by baseline BMI provides some evidence that the changes following consumption of flavanol-containing products on BMI, WC and cholesterol levels are more pronounced in individuals with a baseline BMI $\geq$ 25 kg/m$^2$ and supports the fact that supplementation with these products may have a better impact on these risk factors in overweight and/or obese people. Nevertheless, it is not yet clear whether there is a general better efficacy of natural treatments in overweight and/or obese people, or if the effects may vary depending on the biomarkers or the products investigated. More trials in individuals with a normal BMI < 25.0 kg/m$^2$ are still needed to further compare and demonstrate significant differences in the benefits of flavanol-containing products in relation to body weight, since most are conducted in populations of greater cardiometabolic risk, who are often obese in nature.

### 4.2. Sex

Understanding the differing responses by sex is becoming increasingly important. Previous work has shown that the reducing effects of green tea on total and LDL-cholesterol were significantly greater in men than in women, giving preliminary evidence of that supplementation with flavanol-containing green tea could have a different effect depending on the sex of the individuals [142]. Our results also support differences between women and men in their capacity to regulate the levels of total and LDL cholesterol in response to the consumption of flavanol-containing products with women exhibiting a more efficient reduction than men. A recent meta-analysis looking at the effects of flavonols (another flavonoids class) on lipids levels, failed to detect a difference between men and women, possibly due to the very low number of trials and participants in the two subgroups [7]. Comparing the regulation of cardiometabolic risk factors between women and men is complex because of the hormonal protection in premenopausal women [155]. We were not able to stratify our analyses based on the age or menopausal status of the women, as these factors were not sufficiently well characterized in the trials selected for the meta-analyses. Nevertheless, our results point out to a different response to flavanols consumption between sexes and reinforce the need to further investigate this factor in future trials specifically designed for this purpose.

### 4.3. Country Where the Study Was Carried Out

Ethno-cultural differences are associated with the risk of development of cardiometabolic disorders [156] and thus, it is important to explore and clarify whether different ethnic groups differ in their responses to consumption of plant bioactives as effective treatment against these diseases. Unfortunately, most of the clinical trials included in the present meta-analysis have not clearly identified the ethnicity of the participants. In the absence of this information, we have explored the potential influence of the country where the studies were carried out. A common comparison is that between studies undertaken in Asian countries vs. non-Asian ones. It has been reported that Asians showed a more marked decrease in the levels of TAGs in response to $\omega$-3 fatty acids supplementation as compared to subjects within a USA/European group but, no significant differences were found for total cholesterol or BMI [157]. Flavonols have also been shown to significantly reduce TAGs, total and LDL-cholesterol in studies conducted in Asian countries as compared to those in the EU/European subgroup [7]. Regarding flavanol-containing products, previous meta-analyses have suggested that tea and tea extracts reduce BMI and WC both in Asian and non-Asian trials [140] and that, cocoa products significantly reduce LDL-cholesterol in European countries as compared to USA [149]. Nevertheless, these analyses were all underpowered. Our stratification analysis by country included, in general, a big number of studies per subgroup and showed no apparent differences in the responses to the consumption of tea, cocoa and apple products between East Asian countries and all other countries except for TAGs which were significantly reduced only in the Asian subgroup. We also found some different responses between North American (USA/Canada) and European subgroups, as well as between European Mediterranean and non-Mediterranean ones. This may be partially related to features such as the ethnicity of the participants but also to other factors associated with the life-style of the country. More studies are needed in order to understand the influence of this factor in the response to interventions with plant natural compounds.

### 4.4. Health and Medication Status

Previous meta-analyses had suggested that the consumption of green tea [146,147], black tea [139], and cocoa products [149] had moderating effects on lipid levels both in healthy subjects and in patients with hyperlipidemia or at a higher cross-over or cross-over or s risk. Other bioactive compounds such as flavonols also had a more pronounced effect in the disease subgroup than in the healthy subgroup as significantly evidenced for LDL-cholesterol [7]. Our results show and corroborate a significant reduction of total- and LDL-cholesterol by the flavanol-containing tea, cocoa and apple products both in healthy participants and in individuals with a disease. On the other hand, BMI and WC were reduced and HDL increased in the three subgroups of healthy, "at risk" and individuals with a disease but the results reached statistical significance in the "at risk" group only. As a whole, these results support a metabolic benefit of the consumption of plant bioactive compounds, and in particular of flavanols, regardless of the health status of the individuals.

An important consideration regarding the use of plant bioactive compounds as modulators of cardiometabolic risk biomarkers is their potential use as treatment on their own or as coadjuvants in combination with pharmacological drugs [158]. Our results show that the use of flavanol-containing products in the absence of medication was significantly associated with the reduction of BMI, WC, total and LDL cholesterol, as well as TAGs giving some evidence of their efficacy as therapeutics. The number of clinical trials in which the flavanols were supplemented in combination with other drugs was in general smaller than studies carried out in the absence of medication (see Table 4) thus the pooled results did not reach significance. Nonetheless, these data point to a modulatory effect of the flavanol-containing products in medicated individuals. Whether the combined therapy is more efficient and safe than individual treatment with drugs or with natural plant bioactives warrants further investigation.

### 4.5. Source and Form of Administration of the Flavanols

Our results confirm that the flavanol-containing tea products are effective regulators of blood cholesterol (total, LDL and HDL) as well as of BMI and WC. The cocoa or apple products were effective at reducing total- and LDL-cholesterol and the cocoa products were also able to significantly decrease the levels of TAGs. These results might suggest that the metabolic regulatory efficacy of these three flavanol-containing products could be ranked as tea > cocoa > apple but caution should be taken with this interpretation due to the differences in the number of studies carried out with each source of flavanols as well as the differences in the doses and the composition of the products. Further studies are needed to corroborate this comparison. Our analysis also suggests that the administration of tea as a solid extract might be more efficient than tea beverages at reducing WC and total cholesterol. Earlier meta-analyses had suggested that the type of administration of green or black tea either in solid form (extracts and, capsules) or as a drink did not differ at reducing total- and LDL-cholesterol [139,146,147]. Unlike those previous analyses, where the number of studies per subgroup was very small, our stratification between tea drinks and tea extracts included a considerable number of studies per subgroup (>15) and gives preliminary evidence of a potentially higher efficacy of the tea when administered as a solid powder. We may hypothesize that this could be partially related to the presence of higher doses of the bioactive flavanols in such extracts.

### 4.6. Magnitude of the Changes

An interesting issue worth discussing here is the magnitude of the changes attributed to the intake of the flavanol-containing products and to the extent these changes can contribute to the regulation of the analyzed biomarkers in comparison with other approaches, i.e., drugs, lifestyle changes, or other natural compounds. Based on the Cohen guidelines [159], the effects of the flavanol-containing products (expressed as SDM) are, in general, small ($\leq$0.2) or medium (between 0.2 and 0.5) although changes in some specific risk markers in some specific subgroups can be considered high ($\geq$0.8). We used the same random effects model to generate the overall size effects by computing the difference in means (Table S4) and compare these values to some of the reported effects of pharmacological, behavioral or dietary interventions on BMI, WC and lipid levels. Some of the most potent reducing effects on BMI can be achieved with restricted energy diet ($-2.7$ kg/m$^2$) [160], pharmacological interventions ($-1.3$ kg/m$^2$) [161] or behavioral (diet, exercise) interventions ($-0.9$ to $-1.2$ kg/m$^2$) [162,163]. These reductions constitute between 5% and 10% of the WHO established limit values for overweight (BMI = 25.0–29.9 kg/m$^2$) and obesity (BMI $\geq$ 30.0 kg/m$^2$). Alternatively, intervention with probiotics [154] or nutraceuticals (e.g., lipoic acid) [164] shows a more modest but also significant reduction of BMI (approximately −0.5 kg/m$^2$, ~2% change of the WHO values). On average, the size effect of the flavanol-containing products on BMI was smaller (−0.15 kg/m$^2$, Table S3) but, notably, this effect may be enhanced in specific subpopulations (up to −0.91 kg/m$^2$ in studies conducted in European Mediterranean countries), more similar to other behavioral or dietary interventions. WC can also be significantly and efficiently reduced by brisk walking (−2.83 cm, ~3% of the established 102/88 cm risk values) [162] and, more modestly (−0.53 cm, ~0.5% of the established risk values) by intervention with supplements such as ω-3 polyunsaturated fatty acids [165]. Along these lines, intervention with the flavanol-containing products significantly reduces WC by 1.7 cm and can reach reducing values of −4.58 cm in studies conducted in European Mediterranean countries.

Regarding the cholesterol lowering effects, statins remain, at present, the first-choice agents. The pooled effects of various statins on total- and LDL-cholesterol were −0.89 mmol/L (~17% of the desirable 5.17 mmol/L limit level) and −0.92 mmol/L (~27% of the near optimal 3.36 mmol/L level), respectively [166]. Intervention with natural products such as red yeast rice or spirulina can be as effective as the statins, whereas other plant dietary bioactive compounds such as soluble fiber, sterols/stanols, probiotics and flavonols also significantly reduce total- and LDL-cholesterol by 0.5–0.1 mmol/L [7,167]. In this context, the flavanol-containing products show a similar efficiency at lowering total cholesterol (−0.13 mmol/L) and LDL cholesterol (−0.17 mmol/L). Again, in specific subgroups (e.g., supplementation with flavanol-containing apple products) the reduction of total cholesterol was much more efficient (−0.44 mmol/L). These results are very relevant considering that the reduction of LDL-cholesterol by 1 mmol/L has been associated with a 23% reduction of CVDs risk [168] and reinforce the interest in understanding the influence of different factors on the regulatory efficiency of plant bioactive compounds, in general, and of flavanols in particular.

### 4.7. Additional Recent Evidences

Since the completion of this meta-analysis, additional RCTs investigating the effects of tea or cocoa products containing flavanols on lipid and anthropometric variables have been added to the existing literature [111,169–183]. The heterogeneity of these trials remains high with population samples including mixed sexes and ages, obese, overweight, healthy, hyperlipidemic and/or diabetic subjects, etc. The products were administered in different forms, mostly as green tea extracts/capsules or cocoa drinks and at different doses and intervention periods. Some of these studies further support the reduction of total- and LDL-cholesterol by green tea or cocoa flavanols or the increase of HDL by dark chocolate or cocoa [111,169–171]. Others show no significant effects on these variables [175]. Noteworthy, some of these trials included stratification analyses by baseline conditions, medication, disease, age, sex, or even genotype and further point to specific responses in some subgroups [169,172,174,176,179]. Likewise, the intake of a cocoa product caused a greater increased of HDL in normocholesterolemic patients than in dyslipidemic patients [176], green tea capsules caused a significant reduction of total-cholesterol in women with a cholesterol baseline value above 5.17 mmol/L [169] or of LDL-cholesterol in patients not receiving anti-hyperlipidemic drugs [179]. Of note, the interactions between two factors: baseline BMI and catechol-O-methyltransferase (COMT) genotype, was also recently investigated although the COMT genotype did not modify the effect of green tea extract on any of the variables investigated including BMI [172]. In our study, we were able to identify several factors that may contribute to explaining the heterogeneity on the BMI changes in response to the flavanol-containing products. By multiple meta-regression analysis, we also found that supplementation with these products may be most effective at reducing BMI when specifically using tea products in non-medicated patients. These results highlight the importance of understanding not only the factors affecting the variability in the responses but also the interactions between these factors.

## 5. Conclusions

To the best of our knowledge, the meta-analysis conducted here is the largest one to date that compiles the evidence on the effects on various metabolic risk factors after supplementation with three sources of flavanols, tea, cocoa, and apple products. Our results show consistent and significant modulatory effects on BMI, WC and lipid levels. The size of these effects is modest but similar to that prompted by other natural products. We have also presented evidence of the influence of several factors on these beneficial effects that suggest that flavanols might be very effective in specific subpopulations such as overweight people or non-medicated individuals or when the source of these bioactive compounds is tea. Moreover, a combination of these factors may best explain interindividual variability in the response to the flavanols-containing products.

Although the total number of studies included in the meta-analysis was quite large, the number of studies (and of participants) remained small in some of the subgroup analyses. In addition, many of the studies reported limited or unclear information about the potential factors that may influence the treatment. These limitations affect the capability of the meta-analysis to unequivocally detect moderator variables and limit the significance of our findings. More randomized comparison studies with larger number of well-phenotyped volunteers and providing detailed descriptions of the participants and study characteristics are still needed. This research is crucial for a better understanding of the factors most relevantly involved in the variability of the responses to the consumption of these compounds and to achieve maximum efficacy so that flavanols may become an effective non-pharmacological alternative to battle hyperlipidemia, overweight/obesity and associated cardiometabolic disorders in humans.

**Supplementary Materials:** The following are available online at www.mdpi.com/2072-6643/9/7/746/s1. Figure S1: Forest plot of the meta-analysis evaluating the effects of supplementation with flavanols-containing tea, cocoa or apple products on human body mass index (BMI). A total of 74 studies (displayed in alphabetical order) were analysed. Pooled results are shown at the bottom using a random-effects model. SDM: Standardized difference in means, SE: standard error, 95% CI: lower and upper confidence limits for the average SDM, RW: relative weight; Figure S2: Forest plot of the meta-analysis evaluating the effects of supplementation with flavanols-containing tea, cocoa or apple products on human waist circumference (WC). A total of 46 studies (displayed in alphabetical order) were analysed. Pooled results are shown at the bottom using a random-effects model. SDM: standardized difference in means, SE: standard error, 95% CI: lower and upper confidence limits for the average SDM, RW: relative weight; Figure S3: Forest plot of the meta-analysis evaluating the effects of a prolonged supplementation with flavanols-containing tea, cocoa or apple products on human blood levels of total cholesterol. A total of 112 studies (displayed in alphabetical order) were analysed. Pooled results are shown at the bottom using a random-effects model. SDM: standardized difference in means, SE: standard error, 95% CI: lower and upper confidence limits for the average SDM, RW: relative weight; Figure S4: Forest plot of the meta-analysis evaluating the effects of a prolonged supplementation with flavanols-containing tea, cocoa or apple products on human blood levels of LDL cholesterol. A total of 105 studies (displayed in alphabetical order) were analysed. Pooled results are shown at the bottom using a random-effects model. SDM: standardized difference in means, SE: standard error, 95% CI: lower and upper confidence limits for the average SDM, RW: relative weight; Figure S5: Forest plot of the meta-analysis evaluating the effects of a prolonged supplementation with flavanols-containing tea, cocoa or apple products on human blood levels of HDL cholesterol. A total of 112 studies (displayed in alphabetical order) were analysed. Pooled results are shown at the bottom using a random-effects model. SDM: standardized difference in means, SE: standard error, 95% CI: lower and upper confidence limits for the average SDM, RW: relative weight; Figure S6: Forest plot of the meta-analysis evaluating the effects of a prolonged supplementation with flavanols-containing tea, cocoa or apple products on human blood levels of triglycerides (TAGs). A total of 120 studies (displayed in alphabetical order) were analysed. Pooled results are shown at the bottom using a random-effects model. SDM: standardized difference in means, SE: standard error, 95% CI: lower and upper confidence limits for the average SDM, RW: relative weight; Figure S7: Funnel plot and Eager statistics (intercept and 2-tailed *p*-value) of the meta-analysis evaluating the effects of a prolonged supplementation with flavanols-containing tea, cocoa or apple products on human BMI; Figure S8: Funnel plot and Eager statistics (intercept and 2-tailed *p*-value) of the meta-analysis evaluating the effects of a prolonged supplementation with flavanols-containing tea, cocoa or apple products on human WC; Figure S9: Funnel plot and Eager statistics (intercept and 2-tailed *p*-value) of the meta-analysis evaluating the effects of a prolonged supplementation with flavanols-containing tea, cocoa or apple products on human blood levels of total cholesterol; Figure S10: Funnel plot and Eager statistics (intercept and 2-tailed *p*-value) of the meta-analysis evaluating the effects of a prolonged supplementation with flavanols-containing tea, cocoa or apple products on human blood levels of LDL cholesterol; Figure S11: Funnel plot and Eager statistics (intercept and 2-tailed *p*-value) of the meta-analysis evaluating the effects of a prolonged supplementation with flavanols-containing tea, cocoa or apple products on human blood levels of HDL cholesterol; Figure S12: Funnel plot and Eager statistics (intercept and 2-tailed *p*-value) of the meta-analysis evaluating the effects of a prolonged supplementation with flavanols-containing tea, cocoa or apple products on human blood levels of triglycerides (TAGs); Table S1: Mean content (mg/100 fresh weight, FW) in flavonoids of green and black tea infusions, cocoa powder and whole apple illustrative of the composition of the three main sources of flavanols examined in this study: tea, cocoa and apple (data are based on the Phenol-Explorer database); Table S2: Results of the meta-regression of the changes in BMI, WC and blood lipids levels vs. duration of the supplementation with the flavanol-containing tea, cocoa or apple products; Table S3: Summary of most recent meta-analysis looking at the effects of flavanol-containing tea or cocoa products on anthropometric measurements and blood lipids associated with the development of metabolic disorders; Table S4: Overall effect size estimations (DM) for the impact of flavanols containing products on BMI, WC and blood lipids levels.

**Acknowledgments:** This article is based upon work from COST Action FA1403—POSITIVe "Interindividual variation in response to consumption of plant food bioactives and determinants involved" supported by COST (European Cooperation in Science and Technology, http://www.cost.eu/). The authors offer thanks for the financial support of the COST Action FA1403 "POSITIVe" to conduct two short-term scientific missions to A.G.-S. and P.P. at the University of Glasgow (E.C.) during which the data analysis was performed, and to M.G.-A. at the University College Dublin (E.G.) during which the protocol was developed. M.G.-A. also thanks to the Spanish Ministry of Economy and Competitiveness (MINECO) (PCIN-2014-133-MINECO, Spain), and CIBERFES (co-funded by the FEDER Program from EU).

**Author Contributions:** A.G.-S., A.R.-M., E.R.G., M.G.-A., E.C., P.P., C.M. and M.-T.G.-C. conceived and designed the study; A.G.-S., E.C., P.P., P.M., M.D'A., M.G.-A., A.R.-M., E.R.G., J.D., M.M., J.S.M., C.M., M.-T.G.-C. performed the data extraction; A.G.-S., J.S.M. and M.-T.G.-C. analyzed the data; A.G.-S., E.C., P.P., P.M., M.D'A., M.G.-A., A.R.-M., E.R.G., J.D., M.M., J.S.M., C.M., M.-T.G.-C. contributed to the discussions and preparation of the manuscript; and M.-T.G-C. wrote the article.

**Conflicts of Interest:** The authors declare no conflict of interest.

# References

1. Pucci, G.; Alcidi, R.; Tap, L.; Battista, F.; Mattace-Raso, F.; Schillaci, G. Sex- and gender-related prevalence, cardiovascular risk and therapeutic approach in metabolic syndrome: A review of the literature. *Pharmacol. Res.* **2017**, *120*, 34–42. [CrossRef] [PubMed]

2. Nothlings, U.; Schulze, M.B.; Weikert, C.; Boeing, H.; van der Schouw, Y.T.; Bamia, C.; Benetou, V.; Lagiou, P.; Krogh, V.; Beulens, J.W.; et al. Intake of vegetables, legumes, and fruit, and risk for all-cause, cardiovascular, and cancer mortality in a european diabetic population. *J. Nutr.* **2008**, *138*, 775–781. [PubMed]

3. Howes, M.J.; Simmonds, M.S. The role of phytochemicals as micronutrients in health and disease. *Curr. Opin. Clin. Nutr. Metab. Care* **2014**, *17*, 558–566. [CrossRef] [PubMed]

4. Wang, S.; Moustaid-Moussa, N.; Chen, L.; Mo, H.; Shastri, A.; Su, R.; Bapat, P.; Kwun, I.; Shen, C.L. Novel insights of dietary polyphenols and obesity. *J. Nutr. Biochem.* **2014**, *25*, 1–18. [CrossRef] [PubMed]

5. Grosso, G.; Micek, A.; Godos, J.; Pajak, A.; Sciacca, S.; Galvano, F.; Giovannucci, E.L. Dietary flavonoid and lignan intake and mortality in prospective cohort studies: Systematic review and dose-response meta-analysis. *Am. J. Epidemiol.* **2017**, 1–13. [CrossRef] [PubMed]

6. Rienks, J.; Barbaresko, J.; Nothlings, U. Association of polyphenol biomarkers with cardiovascular disease and mortality risk: A systematic review and meta-analysis of observational studies. *Nutrients* **2017**, *9*, 415. [CrossRef]

7. Menezes, R.; Rodriguez-Mateos, A.; Kaltsatou, A.; Gonzalez-Sarrias, A.; Greyling, A.; Giannaki, C.; Andres-Lacueva, C.; Milenkovic, D.; Gibney, E.R.; Dumont, J.; et al. Impact of flavonols on cardiometabolic biomarkers: A meta-analysis of randomized controlled human trials to explore the role of inter-individual variability. *Nutrients* **2017**, *9*, 117. [CrossRef] [PubMed]

8. Del Rio, D.; Rodriguez-Mateos, A.; Spencer, J.P.; Tognolini, M.; Borges, G.; Crozier, A. Dietary (poly)phenolics in human health: Structures, bioavailability, and evidence of protective effects against chronic diseases. *Antioxid. Redox Signal.* **2013**, *18*, 1818–1892. [CrossRef] [PubMed]

9. Rodriguez-Mateos, A.; Vauzour, D.; Krueger, C.G.; Shanmuganayagam, D.; Reed, J.; Calani, L.; Mena, P.; Del Rio, D.; Crozier, A. Bioavailability, bioactivity and impact on health of dietary flavonoids and related compounds: An update. *Arch. Toxicol.* **2014**, *88*, 1803–1853. [CrossRef] [PubMed]

10. Neveu, V.; Perez-Jiménez, J.; Vos, F.; Crespy, V.; du Chaffaut, L.; Mennen, L.; Knox, C.; Eisner, R.; Cruz, J.; Wishart, D.; et al. Phenol-explorer: An online comprehensive database on polyphenol contents in foods. *Database* **2010**. [CrossRef] [PubMed]

11. Vogiatzoglou, A.; Mulligan, A.A.; Luben, R.N.; Lentjes, M.A.; Heiss, C.; Kelm, M.; Merx, M.W.; Spencer, J.P.; Schroeter, H.; Kuhnle, G.G. Assessment of the dietary intake of total flavan-3-ols, monomeric flavan-3-ols, proanthocyanidins and theaflavins in the european union. *Br. J. Nutr.* **2014**, *111*, 1463–1473. [CrossRef] [PubMed]

12. Actis-Goretta, L.; Leveques, A.; Giuffrida, F.; Romanov-Michailidis, F.; Viton, F.; Barron, D.; Duenas-Paton, M.; Gonzalez-Manzano, S.; Santos-Buelga, C.; Williamson, G.; et al. Elucidation of (−)-epicatechin metabolites after ingestion of chocolate by healthy humans. *Free Radic. Biol. Med.* **2012**, *53*, 787–795. [CrossRef] [PubMed]

13. Manach, C.; Williamson, G.; Morand, C.; Scalbert, A.; Remesy, C. Bioavailability and bioefficacy of polyphenols in humans. I. Review of 97 bioavailability studies. *Am. J. Clin. Nutr.* **2005**, *81*, 230S–242S. [PubMed]

14. Ottaviani, J.I.; Kwik-Uribe, C.; Keen, C.L.; Schroeter, H. Intake of dietary procyanidins does not contribute to the pool of circulating flavanols in humans. *Am. J. Clin. Nutr.* **2012**, *95*, 851–858. [CrossRef] [PubMed]

15. Manach, C.; Milenkovic, D.; Van de Wiele, T.; Rodriguez-Mateos, A.; de Roos, B.; Garcia-Conesa, M.T.; Landberg, R.; Gibney, E.R.; Heinonen, M.; Tomas-Barberan, F.; et al. Addressing the inter-individual variation in response to consumption of plant food bioactives: Towards a better understanding of their role in healthy aging and cardiometabolic risk reduction. *Mol. Nutr. Food Res.* **2017**. [CrossRef] [PubMed]

16. Liberati, A.; Altman, D.G.; Tetzlaff, J.; Mulrow, C.; Gotzsche, P.C.; Ioannidis, J.P.; Clarke, M.; Devereaux, P.J.; Kleijnen, J.; Moher, D. The prisma statement for reporting systematic reviews and meta-analyses of studies that evaluate health care interventions: Explanation and elaboration. *PLoS Med.* **2009**, *6*, e1000100. [CrossRef] [PubMed]

17. Higgins, J.P.T.; Green, S. (Eds.) Cochrane Handbook for Systematic Reviews of Interventions Version 5.1.0 [Updated March 2011]. The Cochrane Collaboration, 2011. Available online: http://handbook-5-1.cochrane.org/ (accessed on 15 May 2015).

18. Centre for Reviews and Dissemination (CRD). *Systematic Reviews: CRD's Guidance for Undertaking Reviews in Health Care*; CRD, University of York: York, UK, 2009.

19. Higgins, J.P.T.; Altman, D.G.; Sterne, J.A.C. (Eds.) Assessing Risk of Bias in Included Studies. In Cochrane Handbook for Systematic Reviews of Interventions Version 5.1.0 [Updated March 2011]. The Cochrane Collaboration, 2011. Available online: http://handbook-5-1.cochrane.org/ (accessed on 15 October 2015).

20. Borenstein, M.J.; Hedges, L.V.; Higgins, J.; Rothstein, H. *Comprehensive Meta-Analysis Vers. 3.3 [Computer Program]*; Biostat, Inc.: Englewood, NJ, USA, 2014.

21. Akazome, Y.; Kametani, N.; Kanda, T.; Shimasaki, H.; Kobayashi, S. Evaluation of safety of excessive intake and efficacy of long-term intake of beverages containing apple polyphenols. *J. Oleo Sci.* **2010**, *59*, 321–338. [CrossRef] [PubMed]

22. Al-Faris, N.A. Short-term consumption of a dark chocolate containing flavanols is followed by a significant decrease in normotensive population. *Pak. J. Nutr.* **2008**, *7*, 773–781. [CrossRef]

23. Auvichayapat, P.; Prapochanung, M.; Tunkamnerdthai, O.; Sripanidkulchai, B.O.; Auvichayapat, N.; Thinkhamrop, B.; Kunhasura, S.; Wongpratoom, S.; Sinawat, S.; Hongprapas, P. Effectiveness of green tea on weight reduction in obese thais: A randomized, controlled trial. *Physiol. Behav.* **2008**, *93*, 486–491. [CrossRef] [PubMed]

24. Baba, S.; Natsume, M.; Yasuda, A.; Nakamura, Y.; Tamura, T.; Osakabe, N.; Kanegae, M.; Kondo, K. Plasma LDL and HDL cholesterol and oxidized LDL concentrations are altered in normo- and hypercholesterolemic humans after intake of different levels of cocoa powder. *J. Nutr.* **2007**, *137*, 1436–1441. [PubMed]

25. Baba, S.; Osakabe, N.; Kato, Y.; Natsume, M.; Yasuda, A.; Kido, T.; Fukuda, K.; Muto, Y.; Kondo, K. Continuous intake of polyphenolic compounds containing cocoa powder reduces LDL oxidative susceptibility and has beneficial effects on plasma HDL-cholesterol concentrations in humans. *Am. J. Clin. Nutr.* **2007**, *85*, 709–717. [PubMed]

26. Bahorun, T.; Luximon-Ramma, A.; Neergheen-Bhujun, V.S.; Gunness, T.K.; Googoolye, K.; Auger, C.; Crozier, A.; Aruoma, O.I. The effect of black tea on risk factors of cardiovascular disease in a normal population. *Prev. Med.* **2012**, *54*, S98–S102. [CrossRef] [PubMed]

27. Bajerska, J.; Mildner-Szkudlarz, S.; Walkowiak, J. Effects of rye bread enriched with green tea extract on weight maintenance and the characteristics of metabolic syndrome following weight loss: A pilot study. *J. Med. Food* **2015**, *18*, 698–705. [CrossRef] [PubMed]

28. Balzer, J.; Rassaf, T.; Heiss, C.; Kleinbongard, P.; Lauer, T.; Merx, M.; Heussen, N.; Gross, H.B.; Keen, C.L.; Schroeter, H.; et al. Sustained benefits in vascular function through flavanol-containing cocoa in medicated diabetic patients a double-masked, randomized, controlled trial. *J. Am. Coll. Cardiol.* **2008**, *51*, 2141–2149. [CrossRef] [PubMed]

29. Barth, S.W.; Koch, T.C.; Watzl, B.; Dietrich, H.; Will, F.; Bub, A. Moderate effects of apple juice consumption on obesity-related markers in obese men: Impact of diet-gene interaction on body fat content. *Eur. J. Nutr.* **2012**, *51*, 841–850. [CrossRef] [PubMed]

30. Basu, A.; Du, M.; Sanchez, K.; Leyva, M.J.; Betts, N.M.; Blevins, S.; Wu, M.; Aston, C.E.; Lyons, T.J. Green tea minimally affects biomarkers of inflammation in obese subjects with metabolic syndrome. *Nutrition* **2011**, *27*, 206–213. [CrossRef] [PubMed]

31. Basu, A.; Sanchez, K.; Leyva, M.J.; Wu, M.; Betts, N.M.; Aston, C.E.; Lyons, T.J. Green tea supplementation affects body weight, lipids, and lipid peroxidation in obese subjects with metabolic syndrome. *J. Am. Coll. Nutr.* **2010**, *29*, 31–40. [CrossRef] [PubMed]

32. Batista Gde, A.; Cunha, C.L.; Scartezini, M.; von der Heyde, R.; Bitencourt, M.G.; Melo, S.F. Prospective double-blind crossover study of camellia sinensis (green tea) in dyslipidemias. *Arq. Bras. Cardiol.* **2009**, *93*, 128–134. [PubMed]

33. Belcaro, G.; Ledda, A.; Hu, S.; Cesarone, M.R.; Feragalli, B.; Dugall, M. Greenselect phytosome for borderline metabolic syndrome. *Evid. Based Complement. Altern. Med.* **2013**, *2013*, 869061. [CrossRef] [PubMed]

34. Bingham, S.A.; Vorster, H.; Jerling, J.C.; Magee, E.; Mulligan, A.; Runswick, S.A.; Cummings, J.H. Effect of black tea drinking on blood lipids, blood pressure and aspects of bowel habit. *Br. J. Nutr.* **1997**, *78*, 41–55. [CrossRef] [PubMed]

35. Bogdanski, P.; Suliburska, J.; Szulinska, M.; Stepien, M.; Pupek-Musialik, D.; Jablecka, A. Green tea extract reduces blood pressure, inflammatory biomarkers, and oxidative stress and improves parameters associated with insulin resistance in obese, hypertensive patients. *Nutr. Res.* **2012**, *32*, 421–427. [CrossRef] [PubMed]

36. Bohn, S.K.; Croft, K.D.; Burrows, S.; Puddey, I.B.; Mulder, T.P.; Fuchs, D.; Woodman, R.J.; Hodgson, J.M. Effects of black tea on body composition and metabolic outcomes related to cardiovascular disease risk: A randomized controlled trial. *Food Funct.* **2014**, *5*, 1613–1620. [CrossRef] [PubMed]

37. Bondia-Pons, I.; Poho, P.; Bozzetto, L.; Vetrani, C.; Patti, L.; Aura, A.M.; Annuzzi, G.; Hyotylainen, T.; Rivellese, A.A.; Oresic, M. Isoenergetic diets differing in their *n*-3 fatty acid and polyphenol content reflect different plasma and HDL-fraction lipidomic profiles in subjects at high cardiovascular risk. *Mol. Nutr. Food Res.* **2014**, *58*, 1873–1882. [CrossRef] [PubMed]

38. Brown, A.L.; Lane, J.; Coverly, J.; Stocks, J.; Jackson, S.; Stephen, A.; Bluck, L.; Coward, A.; Hendrickx, H. Effects of dietary supplementation with the green tea polyphenol epigallocatechin-3-gallate on insulin resistance and associated metabolic risk factors: Randomized controlled trial. *Br. J. Nutr.* **2009**, *101*, 886–894. [CrossRef] [PubMed]

39. Brown, A.L.; Lane, J.; Holyoak, C.; Nicol, B.; Mayes, A.E.; Dadd, T. Health effects of green tea catechins in overweight and obese men: A randomised controlled cross-over trial. *Br. J. Nutr.* **2011**, *106*, 1880–1889. [CrossRef] [PubMed]

40. Cardoso, G.A.; Salgado, J.M.; Cesar, M.D.C.; Donado-Pestana, C.M. The effects of green tea consumption and resistance training on body composition and resting metabolic rate in overweight or obese women. *J. Med. Food.* **2013**, *16*, 120–127. [CrossRef] [PubMed]

41. Chai, S.C.; Hooshmand, S.; Saadat, R.L.; Payton, M.E.; Brummel-Smith, K.; Arjmandi, B.H. Daily apple versus dried plum: Impact on cardiovascular disease risk factors in postmenopausal women. *J. Acad. Nutr. Diet.* **2012**, *112*, 1158–1168. [CrossRef] [PubMed]

42. Chan, E.K.; Quach, J.; Mensah, F.K.; Sung, V.; Cheung, M.; Wake, M. Dark chocolate for children's blood pressure: Randomised trial. *Arch. Dis. Child.* **2012**, *97*, 637–640. [CrossRef] [PubMed]

43. Chen, I.J.; Liu, C.Y.; Chiu, J.P.; Hsu, C.H. Therapeutic effect of high-dose green tea extract on weight reduction: A randomized, double-blind, placebo-controlled clinical trial. *Clin. Nutr.* **2016**, *35*, 592–599. [CrossRef] [PubMed]

44. Coimbra, S.; Santos-Silva, A.; Rocha-Pereira, P.; Rocha, S.; Castro, E. Green tea consumption improves plasma lipid profiles in adults. *Nutr. Res.* **2006**, *26*, 604–607. [CrossRef]

45. Crew, K.D.; Ho, K.A.; Brown, P.; Greenlee, H.; Bevers, T.B.; Arun, B.; Sneige, N.; Hudis, C.; McArthur, H.L.; Chang, J.; et al. Effects of a green tea extract, polyphenon e, on systemic biomarkers of growth factor signalling in women with hormone receptor-negative breast cancer. *J. Hum. Nutr. Diet.* **2015**, *28*, 272–282. [CrossRef] [PubMed]

46. Crews, W.D., Jr.; Harrison, D.W.; Wright, J.W. A double-blind, placebo-controlled, randomized trial of the effects of dark chocolate and cocoa on variables associated with neuropsychological functioning and cardiovascular health: Clinical findings from a sample of healthy, cognitively intact older adults. *Am. J. Clin. Nutr.* **2008**, *87*, 872–880. [PubMed]

47. Davies, M.J.; Judd, J.T.; Baer, D.J.; Clevidence, B.A.; Paul, D.R.; Edwards, A.J.; Wiseman, S.A.; Muesing, R.A.; Chen, S.C. Black tea consumption reduces total and LDL cholesterol in mildly hypercholesterolemic adults. *J. Nutr.* **2003**, *133*, 3298S–3302S. [PubMed]

48. Davison, K.; Coates, A.M.; Buckley, J.D.; Howe, P.R. Effect of cocoa flavanols and exercise on cardiometabolic risk factors in overweight and obese subjects. *Int. J. Obes.* **2008**, *32*, 1289–1296. [CrossRef] [PubMed]

49. Romero-Prado, M.M.J.; Curiel-Beltran, J.A.; Miramontes-Espino, M.V.; Cardona-Munoz, E.G.; Rios-Arellano, A.; Balam-Salazar, L.B. Dietary flavonoids added to pharmacological antihypertensive therapy are effective in improving blood pressure. *Basic Clin. Pharmacol. Toxicol.* **2015**, *117*, 57–64. [CrossRef] [PubMed]

50. De la Torre, R.; De Sola, S.; Pons, M.; Duchon, A.; de Lagran, M.M.; Farre, M.; Fito, M.; Benejam, B.; Langohr, K.; Rodriguez, J.; et al. Epigallocatechin-3-gallate, a dyrk1a inhibitor, rescues cognitive deficits in down syndrome mouse models and in humans. *Mol. Nutr. Food Res.* **2014**, *58*, 278–288. [CrossRef] [PubMed]

51. Desideri, G.; Kwik-Uribe, C.; Grassi, D.; Necozione, S.; Ghiadoni, L.; Mastroiacovo, D.; Raffaele, A.; Ferri, L.; Bocale, R.; Lechiara, M.C.; et al. Benefits in cognitive function, blood pressure, and insulin resistance through cocoa flavanol consumption in elderly subjects with mild cognitive impairment: The cocoa, cognition, and aging (cocoa) study. *Hypertension* **2012**, *60*, 794–801. [CrossRef] [PubMed]

52. Diepvens, K.; Kovacs, E.M.; Vogels, N.; Westerterp-Plantenga, M.S. Metabolic effects of green tea and of phases of weight loss. *Physiol. Behav.* **2006**, *87*, 185–191. [CrossRef] [PubMed]

53. Dower, J.I.; Geleijnse, J.M.; Gijsbers, L.; Zock, P.L.; Kromhout, D.; Hollman, P.C. Effects of the pure flavonoids epicatechin and quercetin on vascular function and cardiometabolic health: A randomized, double-blind, placebo-controlled, crossover trial. *Am. J. Clin. Nutr.* **2015**, *101*, 914–921. [CrossRef] [PubMed]

54. Duffy, S.J.; Keaney, J.F., Jr.; Holbrook, M.; Gokce, N.; Swerdloff, P.L.; Frei, B.; Vita, J.A. Short- and long-term black tea consumption reverses endothelial dysfunction in patients with coronary artery disease. *Circulation* **2001**, *104*, 151–156. [CrossRef] [PubMed]

55. Erba, D.; Riso, P.; Bordoni, A.; Foti, P.; Biagi, P.L.; Testolin, G. Effectiveness of moderate green tea consumption on antioxidative status and plasma lipid profile in humans. *J. Nutr. Biochem.* **2005**, *16*, 144–149. [CrossRef] [PubMed]

56. Esser, D.; Mars, M.; Oosterink, E.; Stalmach, A.; Muller, M.; Afman, L.A. Dark chocolate consumption improves leukocyte adhesion factors and vascular function in overweight men. *FASEB J.* **2014**, *28*, 1464–1473. [CrossRef] [PubMed]

57. Farouque, H.M.; Leung, M.; Hope, S.A.; Baldi, M.; Schechter, C.; Cameron, J.D.; Meredith, I.T. Acute and chronic effects of flavanol-rich cocoa on vascular function in subjects with coronary artery disease: A randomized double-blind placebo-controlled study. *Clin. Sci.* **2006**, *111*, 71–80. [CrossRef] [PubMed]

58. Flammer, A.J.; Sudano, I.; Wolfrum, M.; Thomas, R.; Enseleit, F.; Periat, D.; Kaiser, P.; Hirt, A.; Hermann, M.; Serafini, M.; et al. Cardiovascular effects of flavanol-rich chocolate in patients with heart failure. *Eur. Heart J.* **2012**, *33*, 2172–2180. [CrossRef] [PubMed]

59. Frank, J.; George, T.W.; Lodge, J.K.; Rodriguez-Mateos, A.M.; Spencer, J.P.; Minihane, A.M.; Rimbach, G. Daily consumption of an aqueous green tea extract supplement does not impair liver function or alter cardiovascular disease risk biomarkers in healthy men. *J. Nutr.* **2009**, *139*, 58–62. [CrossRef] [PubMed]

60. Freese, R.; Basu, S.; Hietanen, E.; Nair, J.; Nakachi, K.; Bartsch, H.; Mutanen, M. Green tea extract decreases plasma malondialdehyde concentration but does not affect other indicators of oxidative stress, nitric oxide production, or hemostatic factors during a high-linoleic acid diet in healthy females. *Eur. J. Nutr.* **1999**, *38*, 149–157. [CrossRef] [PubMed]

61. Fu, D.; Ryan, E.P.; Huang, J.; Liu, Z.; Weir, T.L.; Snook, R.L.; Ryan, T.P. Fermented camellia sinensis, fu zhuan tea, regulates hyperlipidemia and transcription factors involved in lipid catabolism. *Food Res. Int.* **2011**, *44*, 2999–3005. [CrossRef]

62. Fujita, H.; Yamagami, T. Antihypercholesterolemic effect of Chinese black tea extract in human subjects with borderline hypercholesterolemia. *Nutr. Res.* **2008**, *28*, 450–456. [CrossRef] [PubMed]

63. Fukino, Y.; Ikeda, A.; Maruyama, K.; Aoki, N.; Okubo, T.; Iso, H. Randomized controlled trial for an effect of green tea-extract powder supplementation on glucose abnormalities. *Eur. J. Clin. Nutr.* **2008**, *62*, 953–960. [CrossRef] [PubMed]

64. Grassi, D.; Lippi, C.; Necozione, S.; Desideri, G.; Ferri, C. Short-term administration of dark chocolate is followed by a significant increase in insulin sensitivity and a decrease in blood pressure in healthy persons. *Am. J. Clin. Nutr.* **2005**, *81*, 611–614. [PubMed]

65. Grassi, D.; Necozione, S.; Lippi, C.; Croce, G.; Valeri, L.; Pasqualetti, P.; Desideri, G.; Blumberg, J.B.; Ferri, C. Cocoa reduces blood pressure and insulin resistance and improves endothelium-dependent vasodilation in hypertensives. *Hypertension* **2005**, *46*, 398–405. [CrossRef] [PubMed]

66. Hodgson, J.M.; Croft, K.D.; Woodman, R.J.; Puddey, I.B.; Fuchs, D.; Draijer, R.; Lukoshkova, E.; Head, G.A. Black tea lowers the rate of blood pressure variation: A randomized controlled trial. *Am. J. Clin. Nutr.* **2013**, *97*, 943–950. [CrossRef] [PubMed]

67. Hodgson, J.M.; Puddey, I.B.; Burke, V.; Watts, G.F.; Beilin, L.J. Regular ingestion of black tea improves brachial artery vasodilator function. *Clin. Sci.* **2002**, *102*, 195–201. [CrossRef] [PubMed]

68. Hsu, C.H.; Liao, Y.L.; Lin, S.C.; Tsai, T.H.; Huang, C.J.; Chou, P. Does supplementation with green tea extract improve insulin resistance in obese type 2 diabetics? A randomized, double-blind, and placebo-controlled clinical trial. *Altern. Med. Rev.* **2011**, *16*, 157–163. [CrossRef] [PubMed]

69. Hsu, C.H.; Tsai, T.H.; Kao, Y.H.; Hwang, K.C.; Tseng, T.Y.; Chou, P. Effect of green tea extract on obese women: A randomized, double-blind, placebo-controlled clinical trial. *Clin. Nutr.* **2008**, *27*, 363–370. [CrossRef] [PubMed]

70. Hsu, T.F.; Kusumoto, A.; Abe, K.; Hosoda, K.; Kiso, Y.; Wang, M.F.; Yamamoto, S. Polyphenol-enriched oolong tea increases fecal lipid excretion. *Eur. J. Clin. Nutr.* **2006**, *60*, 1330–1336. [CrossRef] [PubMed]

71. Hursel, R.; Westerterp-Plantenga, M.S. Green tea catechin plus caffeine supplementation to a high-protein diet has no additional effect on body weight maintenance after weight loss. *Am. J. Clin. Nutr.* **2009**, *89*, 822–830. [CrossRef] [PubMed]

72. Ibero-Baraibar, I.; Abete, I.; Navas-Carretero, S.; Massis-Zaid, A.; Martinez, J.A.; Zulet, M.A. Oxidised LDL levels decreases after the consumption of ready-to-eat meals supplemented with cocoa extract within a hypocaloric diet. *Nutr. Metab. Cardiovasc. Dis.* **2014**, *24*, 416–422. [CrossRef] [PubMed]

73. Ichinose, T.; Nomura, S.; Someya, Y.; Akimoto, S.; Tachiyashiki, K.; Imaizumi, K. Effect of endurance training supplemented with green tea extract on substrate metabolism during exercise in humans. *Scand. J. Med. Sci. Sports* **2011**, *21*, 598–605. [CrossRef] [PubMed]

74. Inami, S.; Takano, M.; Yamamoto, M.; Murakami, D.; Tajika, K.; Yodogawa, K.; Yokoyama, S.; Ohno, N.; Ohba, T.; Sano, J.; et al. Tea catechin consumption reduces circulating oxidized low-density lipoprotein. *Int. Heart J.* **2007**, *48*, 725–732. [CrossRef] [PubMed]

75. Ishikawa, T.; Suzukawa, M.; Ito, T.; Yoshida, H.; Ayaori, M.; Nishiwaki, M.; Yonemura, A.; Hara, Y.; Nakamura, H. Effect of tea flavonoid supplementation on the susceptibility of low-density lipoprotein to oxidative modification. *Am. J. Clin. Nutr.* **1997**, *66*, 261–266. [PubMed]

76. Kajimoto, O.; Kajimoto, Y.; Yabune, M.; Nakamura, T.; Kotani, K.; Suzuki, Y.; Nozawa, A.; Nagata, K.; Unno, T.; Sagesaka, Y.M.; et al. Tea catechins with a galloyl moiety reduce body weight and fat. *J. Health Sci.* **2005**, *51*, 161–171. [CrossRef]

77. Kajimoto, O.; Kajimoto, Y.; Yabune, M.; Nozawa, A.; Nagata, K.; Kakuda, T. Tea catechins reduce serum cholesterol levels in mild and borderline hypercholesterolemia patients. *J. Clin. Biochem. Nutr.* **2003**, *33*, 101–111. [CrossRef]

78. Koutelidakis, A.E.; Rallidis, L.; Koniari, K.; Panagiotakos, D.; Komaitis, M.; Zampelas, A.; Anastasiou-Nana, M.; Kapsokefalou, M. Effect of green tea on postprandial antioxidant capacity, serum lipids, c-reactive protein and glucose levels in patients with coronary artery disease. *Eur. J. Nutr.* **2014**, *53*, 479–486. [CrossRef] [PubMed]

79. Kovacs, E.M.; Lejeune, M.P.; Nijs, I.; Westerterp-Plantenga, M.S. Effects of green tea on weight maintenance after body-weight loss. *Br. J. Nutr.* **2004**, *91*, 431–437. [CrossRef] [PubMed]

80. Lettieri-Barbato, D.; Villaño, D.; Beheydt, B.; Guadagni, F.; Trogh, I.; Serafini, M. Effect of ingestion of dark chocolates with similar lipid composition and different cocoa content on antioxidant and lipid status in healthy humans. *Food Chem.* **2012**, *132*, 1305–1310. [CrossRef]

81. Liu, C.Y.; Huang, C.J.; Huang, L.H.; Chen, I.J.; Chiu, J.P.; Hsu, C.H. Effects of green tea extract on insulin resistance and glucagon-like peptide 1 in patients with type 2 diabetes and lipid abnormalities: A randomized, double-blinded, and placebo-controlled trial. *PLoS ONE* **2014**, *9*, e91163. [CrossRef] [PubMed]

82. Mahler, A.; Steiniger, J.; Bock, M.; Klug, L.; Parreidt, N.; Lorenz, M.; Zimmermann, B.F.; Krannich, A.; Paul, F.; Boschmann, M. Metabolic response to epigallocatechin-3-gallate in relapsing-remitting multiple sclerosis: A randomized clinical trial. *Am. J. Clin. Nutr.* **2015**, *101*, 487–495. [CrossRef] [PubMed]

83. Maki, K.C.; Reeves, M.S.; Farmer, M.; Yasunaga, K.; Matsuo, N.; Katsuragi, Y.; Komikado, M.; Tokimitsu, I.; Wilder, D.; Jones, F.; et al. Green tea catechin consumption enhances exercise-induced abdominal fat loss in overweight and obese adults. *J. Nutr.* **2009**, *139*, 264–270. [CrossRef] [PubMed]

84. Mastroiacovo, D.; Kwik-Uribe, C.; Grassi, D.; Necozione, S.; Raffaele, A.; Pistacchio, L.; Righetti, R.; Bocale, R.; Lechiara, M.C.; Marini, C.; et al. Cocoa flavanol consumption improves cognitive function, blood pressure control, and metabolic profile in elderly subjects: The cocoa, cognition, and aging (cocoa) study—A randomized controlled trial. *Am. J. Clin. Nutr.* **2015**, *101*, 538–548. [CrossRef] [PubMed]

85. Matsuyama, T.; Tanaka, Y.; Kamimaki, I.; Nagao, T.; Tokimitsu, I. Catechin safely improved higher levels of fatness, blood pressure, and cholesterol in children. *Obes. Silver Spring* **2008**, *16*, 1338–1348. [CrossRef] [PubMed]

86. Mellor, D.D.; Sathyapalan, T.; Kilpatrick, E.S.; Beckett, S.; Atkin, S.L. High-cocoa polyphenol-rich chocolate improves HDL cholesterol in type 2 diabetes patients. *Diabet. Med.* **2010**, *27*, 1318–1321. [CrossRef] [PubMed]

87. Mielgo-Ayuso, J.; Barrenechea, L.; Alcorta, P.; Larrarte, E.; Margareto, J.; Labayen, I. Effects of dietary supplementation with epigallocatechin-3-gallate on weight loss, energy homeostasis, cardiometabolic risk factors and liver function in obese women: Randomised, double-blind, placebo-controlled clinical trial. *Br. J. Nutr.* **2014**, *111*, 1263–1271. [CrossRef] [PubMed]

88. Mirzaei, K.; Hossein-Nezhad, A.; Karimi, M.; Hosseinzadeh-Attar, M.J.; Jafari, N.; Najmafshar, A.; Larijani, B. Effect of green tea extract on bone turnover markers in type 2 diabetic patients; a double-blind, placebo-controlled clinical trial study. *DARU J. Pharm. Sci.* **2009**, *17*, 38–44.

89. Miyazaki, R.; Kotani, K.; Ayabe, M.; Tsuzaki, K.; Shimada, J.; Sakane, N.; Takase, H.; Ichikawa, H.; Yonei, Y.; Ishii, K. Minor effects of green tea catechin supplementation on cardiovascular risk markers in active older people: A randomized controlled trial. *Geriatr. Gerontol. Int.* **2013**, *13*, 622–629. [CrossRef] [PubMed]

90. Mogollon, J.A.; Bujold, E.; Lemieux, S.; Bourdages, M.; Blanchet, C.; Bazinet, L.; Couillard, C.; Noel, M.; Dodin, S. Blood pressure and endothelial function in healthy, pregnant women after acute and daily consumption of flavanol-rich chocolate: A pilot, randomized controlled trial. *Nutr. J.* **2013**, *12*, 41. [CrossRef] [PubMed]

91. Monagas, M.; Khan, N.; Andres-Lacueva, C.; Casas, R.; Urpi-Sarda, M.; Llorach, R.; Lamuela-Raventos, R.M.; Estruch, R. Effect of cocoa powder on the modulation of inflammatory biomarkers in patients at high risk of cardiovascular disease. *Am. J. Clin. Nutr.* **2009**, *90*, 1144–1150. [CrossRef] [PubMed]

92. Monahan, K.D.; Feehan, R.P.; Kunselman, A.R.; Preston, A.G.; Miller, D.L.; Lott, M.E.J. Dose-dependent increases in flow-mediated dilation following acute cocoa ingestion in healthy older adults. *J. Appl. Physiol.* **2011**, *111*, 1568–1574. [CrossRef] [PubMed]

93. Mousavi, A.; Vafa, M.; Neyestani, T.; Khamseh, M.; Hoseini, F. The effects of green tea consumption on metabolic and anthropometric indices in patients with type 2 diabetes. *J. Res. Med. Sci.* **2013**, *18*, 1080–1086. [PubMed]

94. Mozaffari-Khosravi, H.; Jalali-Khanabadi, B.A.; Afkhami-Ardekani, M.; Fatehi, F. Effects of sour tea (hibiscus sabdariffa) on lipid profile and lipoproteins in patients with type ii diabetes. *J. Altern. Complement. Med.* **2009**, *15*, 899–903. [CrossRef] [PubMed]

95. Muniyappa, R.; Hall, G.; Kolodziej, T.L.; Karne, R.J.; Crandon, S.K.; Quon, M.J. Cocoa consumption for 2 wk enhances insulin-mediated vasodilatation without improving blood pressure or insulin resistance in essential hypertension. *Am. J. Clin. Nutr.* **2008**, *88*, 1685–1696. [CrossRef] [PubMed]

96. Murphy, K.J.; Chronopoulos, A.K.; Singh, I.; Francis, M.A.; Moriarty, H.; Pike, M.J.; Turner, A.H.; Mann, N.J.; Sinclair, A.J. Dietary flavanols and procyanidin oligomers from cocoa (theobroma cacao) inhibit platelet function. *Am. J. Clin. Nutr.* **2003**, *77*, 1466–1473. [PubMed]

97. Nagao, T.; Hase, T.; Tokimitsu, I. A green tea extract high in catechins reduces body fat and cardiovascular risks in humans. *Obes. Silver Spring* **2007**, *15*, 1473–1483. [CrossRef] [PubMed]

98. Nagao, T.; Komine, Y.; Soga, S.; Meguro, S.; Hase, T.; Tanaka, Y.; Tokimitsu, I. Ingestion of a tea rich in catechins leads to a reduction in body fat and malondialdehyde-modified LDL in men. *Am. J. Clin. Nutr.* **2005**, *81*, 122–129. [PubMed]

99. Nagao, T.; Meguro, S.; Hase, T.; Otsuka, K.; Komikado, M.; Tokimitsu, I.; Yamamoto, T.; Yamamoto, K. A catechin-rich beverage improves obesity and blood glucose control in patients with type 2 diabetes. *Obes. Silver Spring* **2009**, *17*, 310–317. [CrossRef] [PubMed]

100. Nagasako-Akazome, Y.; Kanda, T.; Ohtake, Y.; Shimasaki, H.; Kobayashi, T. Apple polyphenols influence cholesterol metabolism in healthy subjects with relatively high body mass index. *J. Oleo Sci.* **2007**, *56*, 417–428. [CrossRef] [PubMed]

101. Nantz, M.P.; Rowe, C.A.; Bukowski, J.F.; Percival, S.S. Standardized capsule of camellia sinensis lowers cardiovascular risk factors in a randomized, double-blind, placebo-controlled study. *Nutrition* **2009**, *25*, 147–154. [CrossRef]

102. Nickols-Richardson, S.M.; Piehowski, K.E.; Metzgar, C.J.; Miller, D.L.; Preston, A.G. Changes in body weight, blood pressure and selected metabolic biomarkers with an energy-restricted diet including twice daily sweet snacks and once daily sugar-free beverage. *Nutr. Res. Pract.* **2014**, *8*, 695–704. [CrossRef] [PubMed]

103. Njike, V.Y.; Faridi, Z.; Shuval, K.; Dutta, S.; Kay, C.D.; West, S.G.; Kris-Etherton, P.M.; Katz, D.L. Effects of sugar-sweetened and sugar-free cocoa on endothelial function in overweight adults. *Int. J. Cardiol.* **2011**, *149*, 83–88. [CrossRef] [PubMed]

104. Oi, Y.; Fujita, H. Body weight and body mass index (bmi) in preobese and overweight japanese adults treated with black chinese tea water extract (bte) using a more appropriate statistical analysis method. *Int. J. Food Prop.* **2015**, *18*, 1345–1349. [CrossRef]

105. Osakabe, N.; Baba, S.; Yasuda, A.; Iwamoto, T.; Kamiyama, M.; Tokunaga, T.; Kondo, K. Dose-response study of daily cocoa intake on the oxidative susceptibility of low-density lipoprotein in healthy human volunteers. *J. Health Sci.* **2004**, *50*, 679–684. [CrossRef]

106. Parsaeyan, N.; Mozaffari-Khosravi, H.; Absalan, A.; Mozayan, M.R. Beneficial effects of cocoa on lipid peroxidation and inflammatory markers in type 2 diabetic patients and investigation of probable interactions of cocoa active ingredients with prostaglandin synthase-2 (ptgs-2/cox-2) using virtual analysis. *J. Diabetes Metab. Disord.* **2014**, *13*, 30. [CrossRef] [PubMed]

107. Ravn-Haren, G.; Dragsted, L.O.; Buch-Andersen, T.; Jensen, E.N.; Jensen, R.I.; Nemeth-Balogh, M.; Paulovicsova, B.; Bergstrom, A.; Wilcks, A.; Licht, T.R.; et al. Intake of whole apples or clear apple juice has contrasting effects on plasma lipids in healthy volunteers. *Eur. J. Nutr.* **2013**, *52*, 1875–1889. [CrossRef] [PubMed]

108. Rostami, A.; Khalili, M.; Haghighat, N.; Eghtesadi, S.; Shidfar, F.; Heidari, I.; Ebrahimpour-Koujan, S.; Eghtesadi, M. High-cocoa polyphenol-rich chocolate improves blood pressure in patients with diabetes and hypertension. *ARYA Atheroscler.* **2015**, *11*, 21–29. [PubMed]

109. Rull, G.; Mohd-Zain, Z.N.; Shiel, J.; Lundberg, M.H.; Collier, D.J.; Johnston, A.; Warner, T.D.; Corder, R. Effects of high flavanol dark chocolate on cardiovascular function and platelet aggregation. *Vasc. Pharmacol.* **2015**, *71*, 70–78. [CrossRef] [PubMed]

110. Ryu, O.H.; Lee, J.; Lee, K.W.; Kim, H.Y.; Seo, J.A.; Kim, S.G.; Kim, N.H.; Baik, S.H.; Choi, D.S.; Choi, K.M. Effects of green tea consumption on inflammation, insulin resistance and pulse wave velocity in type 2 diabetes patients. *Diabetes Res. Clin. Pract.* **2006**, *71*, 356–358. [CrossRef] [PubMed]

111. Sansone, R.; Rodriguez-Mateos, A.; Heuel, J.; Falk, D.; Schuler, D.; Wagstaff, R.; Kuhnle, G.G.; Spencer, J.P.; Schroeter, H.; Merx, M.W.; et al. Cocoa flavanol intake improves endothelial function and framingham risk score in healthy men and women: A randomised, controlled, double-masked trial: The flaviola health study. *Br. J. Nutr.* **2015**, *114*, 1246–1255. [CrossRef] [PubMed]

112. Shiina, Y.; Funabashi, N.; Lee, K.; Murayama, T.; Nakamura, K.; Wakatsuki, Y.; Daimon, M.; Komuro, I. Acute effect of oral flavonoid-rich dark chocolate intake on coronary circulation, as compared with non-flavonoid white chocolate, by transthoracic doppler echocardiography in healthy adults. *Int. J. Cardiol.* **2009**, *131*, 424–429. [CrossRef] [PubMed]

113. Shimada, K.; Kawarabayashi, T.; Tanaka, A.; Fukuda, D.; Nakamura, Y.; Yoshiyama, M.; Takeuchi, K.; Sawaki, T.; Hosoda, K.; Yoshikawa, J. Oolong tea increases plasma adiponectin levels and low-density lipoprotein particle size in patients with coronary artery disease. *Diabetes Res. Clin. Pract.* **2004**, *65*, 227–234. [CrossRef] [PubMed]

114. Sone, T.; Kuriyama, S.; Nakaya, N.; Hozawa, A.; Shimazu, T.; Nomura, K.; Rikimaru, S.; Tsuji, I. Randomized controlled trial for an effect of catechin-enriched green tea consumption on adiponectin and cardiovascular disease risk factors. *Food Nutr. Res.* **2011**, *55*. [CrossRef] [PubMed]

115. Stendell-Hollis, N.R.; Thomson, C.A.; Thompson, P.A.; Bea, J.W.; Cussler, E.C.; Hakim, I.A. Green tea improves metabolic biomarkers, not weight or body composition: A pilot study in overweight breast cancer survivors. *J. Hum. Nutr. Diet.* **2010**, *23*, 590–600. [CrossRef] [PubMed]

116. Suliburska, J.; Bogdanski, P.; Szulinska, M.; Stepien, M.; Pupek-Musialik, D.; Jablecka, A. Effects of green tea supplementation on elements, total antioxidants, lipids, and glucose values in the serum of obese patients. *Biol. Trace Elem. Res.* **2012**, *149*, 315–322. [CrossRef] [PubMed]

117. Takahashi, M.; Miyashita, M.; Suzuki, K.; Bae, S.R.; Kim, H.K.; Wakisaka, T.; Matsui, Y.; Takeshita, M.; Yasunaga, K. Acute ingestion of catechin-rich green tea improves postprandial glucose status and increases serum thioredoxin concentrations in postmenopausal women. *Br. J. Nutr.* **2014**, *112*, 1542–1550. [CrossRef] [PubMed]

118. Taubert, D.; Roesen, R.; Lehmann, C.; Jung, N.; Schomig, E. Effects of low habitual cocoa intake on blood pressure and bioactive nitric oxide: A randomized controlled trial. *JAMA* **2007**, *298*, 49–60. [CrossRef] [PubMed]

119. Tinahones, F.J.; Rubio, M.A.; Garrido-Sanchez, L.; Ruiz, C.; Gordillo, E.; Cabrerizo, L.; Cardona, F. Green tea reduces LDL oxidability and improves vascular function. *J. Am. Coll. Nutr.* **2008**, *27*, 209–213. [CrossRef] [PubMed]

120. Toolsee, N.A.; Aruoma, O.I.; Gunness, T.K.; Kowlessur, S.; Dambala, V.; Murad, F.; Googoolye, K.; Daus, D.; Indelicato, J.; Rondeau, P.; et al. Effectiveness of green tea in a randomized human cohort: Relevance to diabetes and its complications. *Biomed. Res. Int.* **2013**, *2013*, 412379. [CrossRef] [PubMed]

121. Troup, R.; Hayes, J.H.; Raatz, S.K.; Thyagarajan, B.; Khaliq, W.; Jacobs, D.R.; Key, N.S.; Morawski, B.M.; Kaiser, D.; Bank, A.J.; et al. Effect of black tea intake on blood cholesterol concentrations in individuals with mild hypercholesterolemia: A diet-controlled randomized trial. *J. Acad. Nutr. Diet.* **2015**, *115*, 264–271. [CrossRef] [PubMed]

122. Tsai Ch, H.; Chiu, W.C.; Yang, N.C.; Ouyang, C.M.; Yen, Y.H. A novel green tea meal replacement formula for weight loss among obese individuals: A randomized controlled clinical trial. *Int. J. Food Sci. Nutr.* **2009**, *60* (Suppl. 6), 151–159. [CrossRef] [PubMed]

123. Tzounis, X.; Rodriguez-Mateos, A.; Vulevic, J.; Gibson, G.R.; Kwik-Uribe, C.; Spencer, J.P. Prebiotic evaluation of cocoa-derived flavanols in healthy humans by using a randomized, controlled, double-blind, crossover intervention study. *Am. J. Clin. Nutr.* **2011**, *93*, 62–72. [CrossRef] [PubMed]

124. Unno, T.; Tago, M.; Suzuki, Y.; Nozawa, A.; Sagesaka, Y.M.; Kakuda, T.; Egawa, K.; Kondo, K. Effect of tea catechins on postprandial plasma lipid responses in human subjects. *Br. J. Nutr.* **2005**, *93*, 543–547. [CrossRef] [PubMed]

125. Vafa, M.R.; Haghighatjoo, E.; Shidfar, F.; Afshari, S.; Gohari, M.R.; Ziaee, A. Effects of apple consumption on lipid profile of hyperlipidemic and overweight men. *Int. J. Prev. Med.* **2011**, *2*, 94–100. [PubMed]

126. Velliquette, R.A.; Grann, K.; Missler, S.R.; Patterson, J.; Hu, C.; Gellenbeck, K.W.; Scholten, J.D.; Randolph, R.K. Identification of a botanical inhibitor of intestinal diacylglyceride acyltransferase 1 activity via in vitro screening and a parallel, randomized, blinded, placebo-controlled clinical trial. *Nutr. Metab.* **2015**, *12*, 27. [CrossRef] [PubMed]

127. Vieira Senger, A.E.; Schwanke, C.H.; Gomes, I.; Valle Gottlieb, M.G. Effect of green tea (camellia sinensis) consumption on the components of metabolic syndrome in elderly. *J. Nutr. Health Aging* **2012**, *16*, 738–742. [CrossRef] [PubMed]

128. Villaño, D.; Pecorari, M.; Testa, M.F.; Raguzzini, A.; Stalmach, A.; Crozier, A.; Tubili, C.; Serafini, M. Unfermented and fermented rooibos teas (aspalathus linearis) increase plasma total antioxidant capacity in healthy humans. *Food Chem.* **2010**, *123*, 679–683. [CrossRef]

129. Vlachopoulos, C.; Aznaouridis, K.; Alexopoulos, N.; Economou, E.; Andreadou, I.; Stefanadis, C. Effect of dark chocolate on arterial function in healthy individuals. *Am. J. Hypertens.* **2005**, *18*, 785–791. [CrossRef] [PubMed]

130. Wang, H.; Wen, Y.; Du, Y.; Yan, X.; Guo, H.; Rycroft, J.A.; Boon, N.; Kovacs, E.M.; Mela, D.J. Effects of catechin enriched green tea on body composition. *Obes. Silver Spring* **2010**, *18*, 773–779. [CrossRef] [PubMed]

131. West, S.G.; McIntyre, M.D.; Piotrowski, M.J.; Poupin, N.; Miller, D.L.; Preston, A.G.; Wagner, P.; Groves, L.F.; Skulas-Ray, A.C. Effects of dark chocolate and cocoa consumption on endothelial function and arterial stiffness in overweight adults. *Br. J. Nutr.* **2014**, *111*, 653–661. [CrossRef] [PubMed]

132. Westphal, S.; Luley, C. Flavanol-rich cocoa ameliorates lipemia-induced endothelial dysfunction. *Heart Vessel.* **2011**, *26*, 511–515. [CrossRef] [PubMed]

133. Widlansky, M.E.; Hamburg, N.M.; Anter, E.; Holbrook, M.; Kahn, D.F.; Elliott, J.G.; Keaney, J.F., Jr.; Vita, J.A. Acute egcg supplementation reverses endothelial dysfunction in patients with coronary artery disease. *J. Am. Coll. Nutr.* **2007**, *26*, 95–102. [CrossRef] [PubMed]

134. Widmer, R.J.; Freund, M.A.; Flammer, A.J.; Sexton, J.; Lennon, R.; Romani, A.; Mulinacci, N.; Vinceri, F.F.; Lerman, L.O.; Lerman, A. Beneficial effects of polyphenol-rich olive oil in patients with early atherosclerosis. *Eur. J. Nutr.* **2013**, *52*, 1223–1231. [CrossRef] [PubMed]

135. Wu, A.H.; Spicer, D.; Stanczyk, F.Z.; Tseng, C.C.; Yang, C.S.; Pike, M.C. Effect of 2-month controlled green tea intervention on lipoprotein cholesterol, glucose, and hormone levels in healthy postmenopausal women. *Cancer Prev. Res.* **2012**, *5*, 393–402. [CrossRef] [PubMed]

136. Yang, H.Y.; Yang, S.C.; Chao, J.C.; Chen, J.R. Beneficial effects of catechin-rich green tea and inulin on the body composition of overweight adults. *Br. J. Nutr.* **2012**, *107*, 749–754. [CrossRef] [PubMed]

137. Yang, T.Y.; Chou, J.I.; Ueng, K.C.; Chou, M.Y.; Yang, J.J.; Lin-Shiau, S.Y.; Hu, M.E.; Lin, J.K. Weight reduction effect of puerh tea in male patients with metabolic syndrome. *Phytother. Res.* **2014**, *28*, 1096–1101. [CrossRef] [PubMed]

138. Li, Y.; Wang, C.; Huai, Q.; Guo, F.; Liu, L.; Feng, R.; Sun, C. Effects of tea or tea extract on metabolic profiles in patients with type 2 diabetes mellitus: A meta-analysis of ten randomized controlled trials. *Diabetes Metab. Res. Rev.* **2016**, *32*, 2–10. [CrossRef] [PubMed]

139. Zhao, Y.; Asimi, S.; Wu, K.; Zheng, J.; Li, D. Black tea consumption and serum cholesterol concentration: Systematic review and meta-analysis of randomized controlled trials. *Clin. Nutr.* **2015**, *34*, 612–619. [CrossRef] [PubMed]

140. Zhong, X.; Zhang, T.; Liu, Y.; Wei, X.; Zhang, X.; Qin, Y.; Jin, Z.; Chen, Q.; Ma, X.; Wang, R.; et al. Short-term weight-centric effects of tea or tea extract in patients with metabolic syndrome: A meta-analysis of randomized controlled trials. *Nutr. Diabetes* **2015**, *5*, e160. [CrossRef] [PubMed]

141. Wang, D.; Chen, C.; Wang, Y.; Liu, J.; Lin, R. Effect of black tea consumption on blood cholesterol: A meta-analysis of 15 randomized controlled trials. *PLoS ONE* **2014**, *9*, e107711. [CrossRef] [PubMed]

142. Onakpoya, I.; Spencer, E.; Heneghan, C.; Thompson, M. The effect of green tea on blood pressure and lipid profile: A systematic review and meta-analysis of randomized clinical trials. *Nutr. Metab. Cardiovasc. Dis.* **2014**, *24*, 823–836. [CrossRef] [PubMed]

143. Baladia, E.; Basulto, J.; Manera, M.; Martínez, R.; Calbet, D. Effect of green tea or green tea extract consumption on body weight and body composition; systematic review and meta-analysis. *Nutr. Hosp.* **2014**, *29*, 479–490. [PubMed]

144. Khalesi, S.; Sun, J.; Buys, N.; Jamshidi, A.; Nikbakht-Nasrabadi, E.; Khosravi-Boroujeni, H. Green tea catechins and blood pressure: A systematic review and meta-analysis of randomised controlled trials. *Eur. J. Nutr.* **2014**, *53*, 1299–1311. [CrossRef] [PubMed]

145. Hartley, L.; Flowers, N.; Holmes, J.; Clarke, A.; Stranges, S.; Hooper, L.; Rees, K. Green and black tea for the primary prevention of cardiovascular disease. *Cochrane Database Syst. Rev.* **2013**, CD009934. [CrossRef]

146. Kim, A.; Chiu, A.; Barone, M.K.; Avino, D.; Wang, F.; Coleman, C.I.; Phung, O.J. Green tea catechins decrease total and low-density lipoprotein cholesterol: A systematic review and meta-analysis. *J. Am. Diet. Assoc.* **2011**, *111*, 1720–1729. [CrossRef] [PubMed]

147. Zheng, X.X.; Xu, Y.L.; Li, S.H.; Liu, X.X.; Hui, R.; Huang, X.H. Green tea intake lowers fasting serum total and LDL cholesterol in adults: A meta-analysis of 14 randomized controlled trials. *Am. J. Clin. Nutr.* **2011**, *94*, 601–610. [CrossRef] [PubMed]

148. Phung, O.J.; Baker, W.L.; Matthews, L.J.; Lanosa, M.; Thorne, A.; Coleman, C.I. Effect of green tea catechins with or without caffeine on anthropometric measures: A systematic review and meta-analysis. *Am. J. Clin. Nutr.* **2010**, *91*, 73–81. [CrossRef] [PubMed]

149. Tokede, O.A.; Gaziano, J.M.; Djousse, L. Effects of cocoa products/dark chocolate on serum lipids: A meta-analysis. *Eur. J. Clin. Nutr.* **2011**, *65*, 879–886. [CrossRef] [PubMed]

150. Lin, X.; Zhang, I.; Li, A.; Manson, J.E.; Sesso, H.D.; Wang, L.; Liu, S. Cocoa Flavanol Intake and Biomarkers for Cardiometabolic Health: A Systematic Review and Meta-Analysis of Randomized Controlled Trials. *J. Nutr.* **2016**, *146*, 2325–2333. [CrossRef] [PubMed]

151. Hooper, L.; Kay, C.; Abdelhamid, A.; Kroon, P.A.; Cohn, J.S.; Rimm, E.B.; Cassidy, A. Effects of chocolate, cocoa, and flavan-3-ols on cardiovascular health: A systematic review and meta-analysis of randomized trials. *Am. J. Clin. Nutr.* **2012**, *95*, 740–751. [CrossRef] [PubMed]

152. De Pascual-Teresa, S.; Santos-Buelga, C.; Rivas-Gonzalo, J.C. Quantitative analysis of flavan-3-ols in Spanish foodstuffs and beverages. *J. Agric. Food. Chem.* **2000**, *48*, 5331–5337. [CrossRef] [PubMed]

153. Hendijani, F.; Akbari, V. Probiotic supplementation for management of cardiovascular risk factors in adults with type ii diabetes: A systematic review and meta-analysis. *Clin. Nutr.* **2017**. [CrossRef] [PubMed]

154. Zhang, Q.; Wu, Y.; Fei, X. Effect of probiotics on body weight and body-mass index: A systematic review and meta-analysis of randomized, controlled trials. *Int. J. Food. Sci. Nutr.* **2016**, *67*, 571–580. [CrossRef] [PubMed]

155. Sugiyama, M.G.; Agellon, L.B. Sex differences in lipid metabolism and metabolic disease risk. *Biochem. Cell Biol.* **2012**, *90*, 124–141. [CrossRef] [PubMed]

156. Wahi, G.; Anand, S.S. Race/ethnicity, obesity, and related cardio-metabolic risk factors: A life-course perspective. *Curr. Cardiovasc. Risk Rep.* **2013**, *7*, 326–335. [CrossRef] [PubMed]

157. Chen, C.; Yu, X.; Shao, S. Effects of omega-3 fatty acid supplementation on glucose control and lipid levels in type 2 diabetes: A meta-analysis. *PLoS ONE* **2015**, *10*, e0139565. [CrossRef] [PubMed]

158. Pereira, T.M.; Pimenta, F.S.; Porto, M.L.; Baldo, M.P.; Campagnaro, B.P.; Gava, A.L.; Meyrelles, S.S.; Vasquez, E.C. Coadjuvants in the diabetic complications: Nutraceuticals and drugs with pleiotropic effects. *Int. J. Mol. Sci.* **2016**, *17*, 1273. [CrossRef] [PubMed]

159. Cohen, J. *Statistical Power Analysis for the Behavioral Sciences*, 2nd ed.; Erlbaum: Hillsdale, NJ, USA, 1988.

160. Stelmach-Mardas, M.; Walkowiak, J. Dietary interventions and changes in cardio-metabolic parameters in metabolically healthy obese subjects: A systematic review with meta-analysis. *Nutrients* **2016**, *8*, 455. [CrossRef] [PubMed]

161. Mead, E.; Atkinson, G.; Richter, B.; Metzendorf, M.I.; Baur, L.; Finer, N.; Corpeleijn, E.; O'Malley, C.; Ells, L.J. Drug interventions for the treatment of obesity in children and adolescents. *Cochrane Database Syst. Rev.* **2016**, *11*, CD012436. [PubMed]

162. Mabire, L.; Mani, R.; Liu, L.; Mulligan, H.; Baxter, D. The influence of age, sex and body mass index on the effectiveness of brisk walking for obesity management in adults: A systematic review and meta-analysis. *J. Phys. Act. Health* **2017**, *14*, 389–407. [CrossRef] [PubMed]

163. Peirson, L.; Fitzpatrick-Lewis, D.; Morrison, K.; Warren, R.; Usman Ali, M.; Raina, P. Treatment of overweight and obesity in children and youth: A systematic review and meta-analysis. *CMAJ Open* **2015**, *3*, E35–E46. [CrossRef] [PubMed]

164. Kucukgoncu, S.; Zhou, E.; Lucas, K.B.; Tek, C. Alpha-lipoic acid (ala) as a supplementation for weight loss: Results from a meta-analysis of randomized controlled trials. *Obes. Rev.* **2017**, *18*, 594–601. [CrossRef] [PubMed]

165. Zhang, Y.Y.; Liu, W.; Zhao, T.Y.; Tian, H.M. Efficacy of omega-3 polyunsaturated fatty acids supplementation in managing overweight and obesity: A meta-analysis of randomized clinical trials. *J. Nutr. Health Aging* **2017**, *21*, 187–192. [CrossRef] [PubMed]

166. Taylor, F.; Huffman, M.D.; Macedo, A.F.; Moore, T.H.; Burke, M.; Davey Smith, G.; Ward, K.; Ebrahim, S. Statins for the primary prevention of cardiovascular disease. *Cochrane Database Syst. Rev.* **2013**, CD004816. [CrossRef]

167. Sahebkar, A.; Serban, M.C.; Gluba-Brzozka, A.; Mikhailidis, D.P.; Cicero, A.F.; Rysz, J.; Banach, M. Lipid-modifying effects of nutraceuticals: An evidence-based approach. *Nutrition* **2016**, *32*, 1179–1192. [CrossRef] [PubMed]

168. Silverman, M.G.; Ference, B.A.; Im, K.; Wiviott, S.D.; Giugliano, R.P.; Grundy, S.M.; Braunwald, E.; Sabatine, M.S. Association between lowering LDL-C and cardiovascular risk reduction among different therapeutic interventions: A systematic review and meta-analysis. *JAMA* **2016**, *316*, 1289–1297. [CrossRef] [PubMed]

169. Samavat, H.; Newman, A.R.; Wang, R.; Yuan, J.M.; Wu, A.H.; Kurzer, M.S. Effects of green tea catechin extract on serum lipids in postmenopausal women: A randomized, placebo-controlled clinical trial. *Am. J. Clin. Nutr.* **2016**, *104*, 1671–1682. [CrossRef] [PubMed]

170. Taub, P.R.; Ramirez-Sanchez, I.; Patel, M.; Higginbotham, E.; Moreno-Ulloa, A.; Roman-Pintos, L.M.; Phillips, P.; Perkins, G.; Ceballos, G.; Villarreal, F. Beneficial effects of dark chocolate on exercise capacity in sedentary subjects: Underlying mechanisms. A double blind, randomized, placebo controlled trial. *Food Funct.* **2016**, *7*, 3686–3693. [CrossRef] [PubMed]

171. Lu, P.H.; Hsu, C.H. Does supplementation with green tea extract improve acne in post-adolescent women? A randomized, double-blind, and placebo-controlled clinical trial. *Complement. Ther. Med.* **2016**, *25*, 159–163. [CrossRef] [PubMed]

172. Dostal, A.M.; Arikawa, A.; Espejo, L.; Kurzer, M.S. Long-term supplementation of green tea extract does not modify adiposity or bone mineral density in a randomized trial of overweight and obese postmenopausal women. *J. Nutr.* **2016**, *146*, 256–264. [CrossRef] [PubMed]

173. Most, J.; van Can, J.G.; van Dijk, J.W.; Goossens, G.H.; Jocken, J.; Hospers, J.J.; Bendik, I.; Blaak, E.E. A 3-day egcg-supplementation reduces interstitial lactate concentration in skeletal muscle of overweight subjects. *Sci. Rep.* **2015**, *5*, 17896. [CrossRef] [PubMed]

174. Dostal, A.M.; Samavat, H.; Espejo, L.; Arikawa, A.Y.; Stendell-Hollis, N.R.; Kurzer, M.S. Green tea extract and catechol-o-methyltransferase genotype modify fasting serum insulin and plasma adiponectin concentrations in a randomized controlled trial of overweight and obese postmenopausal women. *J. Nutr.* **2016**, *146*, 38–45. [CrossRef] [PubMed]

175. Basu, A.; Betts, N.M.; Leyva, M.J.; Fu, D.; Aston, C.E.; Lyons, T.J. Acute cocoa supplementation increases postprandial HDL cholesterol and insulin in obese adults with type 2 diabetes after consumption of a high-fat breakfast. *J. Nutr.* **2015**, *145*, 2325–2332. [CrossRef] [PubMed]

176. Sarria, B.; Martinez-Lopez, S.; Sierra-Cinos, J.L.; Garcia-Diz, L.; Goya, L.; Mateos, R.; Bravo, L. Effects of bioactive constituents in functional cocoa products on cardiovascular health in humans. *Food Chem.* **2015**, *174*, 214–218. [CrossRef] [PubMed]

177. Gutierrez-Salmean, G.; Meaney, E.; Lanaspa, M.A.; Cicerchi, C.; Johnson, R.J.; Dugar, S.; Taub, P.; Ramirez-Sanchez, I.; Villarreal, F.; Schreiner, G.; et al. A randomized, placebo-controlled, double-blind study on the effects of (−)-epicatechin on the triglyceride/HDLC ratio and cardiometabolic profile of subjects with hypertriglyceridemia: Unique in vitro effects. *Int. J. Cardiol.* **2016**, *223*, 500–506. [CrossRef] [PubMed]

178. Imbe, H.; Sano, H.; Miyawaki, M.; Fujisawa, R.; Miyasato, M.; Nakatsuji, F.; Haseda, F.; Tanimoto, K.; Terasaki, J.; Maeda-Yamamoto, M.; et al. "Benifuuki" green tea, containing o-methylated egcg, reduces serum low-density lipoprotein cholesterol and lectin-like oxidized low-density lipoprotein receptor-1 ligands containing apolipoprotein b: A double-blind, placebo-controlled randomized trial. *J. Funct. Foods* **2016**, *25*, 25–37. [CrossRef]

179. Lee, T.M.; Charng, M.J.; Tseng, C.D.; Lai, L.P. A double-blind, randomized, placebo-controlled study to evaluate the efficacy and safety of sta-2 (green tea polyphenols) in patients with chronic stable angina. *Acta Cardiol. Sin.* **2016**, *32*, 439–449. [PubMed]

180. Ide, K.; Yamada, H.; Takuma, N.; Kawasaki, Y.; Harada, S.; Nakase, J.; Ukawa, Y.; Sagesaka, Y.M. Effects of green tea consumption on cognitive dysfunction in an elderly population: A randomized placebo-controlled study. *Nutr. J.* **2016**, *15*, 49. [CrossRef] [PubMed]

181. Mahmoud, F.; Haines, D.; Al-Ozairi, E.; Dashti, A. Effect of black tea consumption on intracellular cytokines, regulatory t cells and metabolic biomarkers in type 2 diabetes patients. *Phytother. Res.* **2016**, *30*, 454–462. [CrossRef] [PubMed]

182. Ibero-Baraibar, I.; Suarez, M.; Arola-Arnal, A.; Zulet, M.A.; Martinez, J.A. Cocoa extract intake for 4 weeks reduces postprandial systolic blood pressure response of obese subjects, even after following an energy-restricted diet. *Food Nutr. Res.* **2016**, *60*, 30449. [CrossRef] [PubMed]

183. Kobayashi, M.; Kawano, T.; Ukawa, Y.; Sagesaka, Y.M.; Fukuhara, I. Green tea beverages enriched with catechins with a galloyl moiety reduce body fat in moderately obese adults: A randomized double-blind placebo-controlled trial. *Food Funct.* **2016**, *7*, 498–507. [CrossRef] [PubMed]

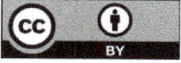

nutrients

MDPI

Article

# Dietary Phytochemicals Promote Health by Enhancing Antioxidant Defence in a Pig Model

Sophie N. B. Selby-Pham [1,2], Jeremy J. Cottrell [1], Frank R. Dunshea [1], Louise E. Bennett [2] and Kate S. Howell [1,*]

[1]   Faculty of Veterinary and Agricultural, The University of Melbourne, Parkville, VIC 3010, Australia;
      s.selbypham@gmail.com (S.N.B.S.-P.); jcottrell@unimelb.edu.au (J.J.C.);
      fdunshea@unimelb.edu.au (F.R.D.); ngkf@unimelb.edu.au (K.N.)
[2]   CSIRO Agriculture and Food, 671 Sneydes Road, Werribee, VIC 3010, Australia;
      louise.bennett1@monash.edu
*    Correspondence: khowell@unimelb.edu.au; Tel.: +61-3-9035-3119

Received: 8 June 2017; Accepted: 12 July 2017; Published: 14 July 2017

**Abstract:** Phytochemical-rich diets are protective against chronic diseases and mediate their protective effect by regulation of oxidative stress (OS). However, it is proposed that under some circumstances, phytochemicals can promote production of reactive oxygen species (ROS) in vitro, which might drive OS-mediated signalling. Here, we investigated the effects of administering single doses of extracts of red cabbage and grape skin to pigs. Blood samples taken at baseline and 30 min intervals for 4 hours following intake were analyzed by measures of antioxidant status in plasma, including Trolox equivalent antioxidant capacity (TEAC) and glutathione peroxidase (GPx) activity. In addition, dose-dependent production of hydrogen peroxide ($H_2O_2$) by the same extracts was measured in untreated commercial pig plasma in vitro. Plasma from treated pigs showed extract dose-dependent increases in non-enzymatic (plasma TEAC) and enzymatic (GPx) antioxidant capacities. Similarly, extract dose-dependent increases in $H_2O_2$ were observed in commercial pig plasma in vitro. The antioxidant responses to extracts by treated pigs were highly correlated with their respective yields of $H_2O_2$ production in vitro. These results support that dietary phytochemicals regulate OS via direct and indirect antioxidant mechanisms. The latter may be attributed to the ability to produce $H_2O_2$ and to thereby stimulate cellular antioxidant defence systems.

**Keywords:** hydrogen peroxide; reactive oxygen species; plant extracts; red cabbage; grape; glutathione peroxide; total antioxidant capacity; porcine; piglet; Landrace

## 1. Introduction

A phytochemical-rich diet is strongly associated with reducing the risk of chronic diseases including cancer [1], cardiovascular [2], and neurodegenerative diseases [3]. The health benefits of dietary phytochemicals have been attributed to their ability to mitigate oxidative stress and inflammation (OSI), which is associated with normal metabolism [4,5] but is also involved in the onset of chronic diseases [6]. Production of reactive oxygen species (ROS) occurs under normal conditions in cells, the main source from by-products of the electron transport chains [7]. Uncontrolled ROS can lead to OSI and unregulated OSI can result in molecular and cellular damage which in turn leads to an increased risk of chronic diseases [8]. However, OSI is an important defence mechanism of the body against infections and injuries [9]. Therefore, transient peaks or optimal steady state levels of ROS in the body are likely involved in maintaining good health and reducing the risk of disease [10].

It was believed that dietary phytochemicals exert protection via direct scavenging of ROS, as observed in many in vitro studies [11–13]. However, this concept has been challenged as the concentrations of phytochemicals in human plasma in vivo after consumption of phytochemicals are much lower (in the nM to low µM range) compared to concentrations used in the in vitro studies (in the low µM to mM range) [14,15]. There are clearly discrepancies between the studies of these mechanisms in the whole organism.

The health benefits of dietary phytochemicals are thought to be attributed to their ability to generate electrophilic or chemical stress signals, which trigger the cellular defence system to protect against molecular damage and subsequent chronic diseases [16–19]. The cellular antioxidant defence is made up of a non-enzymatic, inducible enzymatic defence and the DNA repair systems [20]. The non-enzymatic defence includes antioxidant molecules such as vitamin C, vitamin E, uric acid, glutathione, and thioredoxin that directly scavenge ROS and metal-chelating proteins such as transferrin, coeruloplasmin, and metallothionein that prevent ROS formation via controlling the level of pro-oxidative free metal ions [20]. The enzymatic antioxidant defence includes several pathways that remove ROS through enzymatic reactions. For example, superoxide dismutase converts superoxide anions into hydrogen peroxide ($H_2O_2$), which is subsequently transformed by catalase into oxygen and water or by glutathione peroxidase (GPx) into water [20]. The reduction of $H_2O_2$ by GPx consumes the reduced form of glutathione and generates the oxidised form, which can be recycled by glutathione reductase to restore the glutathione pool [20].

Dietary phytochemicals have been associated with increasing the levels of both non-enzymatic and enzymatic antioxidant defence in animal [21–26] and human dietary intervention studies [27–30]. Consumption of phytochemical-rich diets increased the expression of genes associated with DNA repair, immune, and inflammatory responses in humans [10,31–33]. The varied roles that dietary phytochemicals may play in the whole organism are complex, perhaps overlapping and have not been fully elucidated. The ability of dietary phytochemicals to generate stress signals can be related to their ability to produce ROS, in particular $H_2O_2$ [34]. Phytochemicals have been reported to produce $H_2O_2$ in cell culture media, which was potentially responsible for their cytotoxic effects in cell culture studies [35–38]. However, no research has been done on the ability of phytochemicals to produce $H_2O_2$ in plasma. Understanding this pro-oxidant action will provide information about how the phytochemicals can stimulate ROS-induced cellular antioxidant defence to provide protective effects against OSI.

Absorption of phytochemicals into circulation and uptake by target cells are essential for phytochemicals to exert biological effects [39]. As phytochemicals are recognised by the human body as xenobiotics, their presence in the human body is transient [40] and influenced by their physicochemical properties. Recently, we have developed the phytochemical absorption prediction (PCAP) model, allowing direct calculation of the time required for phytochemicals to reach their maximal plasma concentrations ($T_{max}$) after oral consumption, based on their molecular mass and lipophilicity descriptor log P [41]. Further, a liquid chromatography mass spectrometry (LC-MS) method has been developed to characterise $T_{max}$ ranges of phytochemical mixtures based on molecular mass and log P [42]. Here, we extend this modelling to dietary intervention in pigs, an animal model with physiological and anatomical similarities to the digestive tract of humans [43].

Phytochemicals across a broad range of chemical classes have been shown to impart positive health benefits [3,40]. Grape products and *Brassica* vegetables are among the most widely studied for their antioxidant capacity and protection against chronic diseases [44,45]. Grape skin contains predominately polyphenols including anthocyanidins, phenolic acids, and stilbenes [44], whilst red cabbage (a member of the *Brassica* vegetables) contains a wider variety of phytochemicals including polyphenols (anthocyanidins, phenolic acids), glucosinolates, and vitamins [46].

The aim of this study was to use a pig model to establish the absorption kinetics of phytochemical extracts from red cabbage and grape skin and to examine their effects on two measures of antioxidant status (plasma total antioxidant capacity and plasma GPx activity). Direct induction of the pro-oxidant effects of the plant extracts in pig plasma was measured by $H_2O_2$ production in pig plasma when exposed to the plant extracts in vitro. This study provides both in vitro and ex vivo evidence to support that one of the likely modes of action by phytochemicals is to induce $H_2O_2$ in plasma and to thereby initiate protective action by enzymatic and non-enzymatic cellular defences.

## 2. Materials and Methods

### 2.1. Materials

All chemicals including gallic acid, Folin-Ciocalteu reagent, sodium carbonate ($Na_2CO_3$), hydrogen peroxide ($H_2O_2$), sulfuric acid ($H_2SO_4$), xylenol orange, Iron(II) sulphate ($FeSO_4$), butylated hydroxytoluene (BHT), tris(hydroxymethyl)aminomethane (Tris), glycine, citrate, urea, hydrochloric acid (HCl), Trolox, bathocuproinedisulfonic acid sodium salt (BCS), copper(II) chloride ($CuCl_2$), methanol, formic acid, acetonitrile, L-histidine, (*S*)-dihydroorotate, shikimate, 4-pyridoxate, 3-hydroxybenzyl alcohol, 2,5-dihydroxybenzoate, 3-hydroxybenzaldehyde, trans-cinnamate, estradiol-17$\alpha$, deoxycholate, retinoate, oleic acid, and heptadecanoate were of analytical grade and from Sigma-Aldrich (St. Louis, MO, USA). 96 well plates were from Greiner UV-Star (Greiner Bio-One, Frickenhausen, Germany).

Tris-glycine-urea buffer pH 7 contained 0.086 M Tris, 0.09 M glycine, 4 mM citrate, and 8 M urea, adjusted to pH 7 using 2 M HCl. Ferrous ion oxidation-xylenol orange (FOX) reagent contained 25 mM $H_2SO_4$ containing 0.1 mM xylenol orange, 0.25 mM $FeSO_4$, and 4 mM BHT in 90% methanol.

### 2.2. Preparation of Plant Extracts

Grape skin extract was obtained from Tarac Technologies (Nuriootpa, South Australia, Australia). The extract was freeze-dried (Virtis Genesis 35EL, SP Scientific, Warmister, PA, USA) and stored with a small head space with desiccant at $-18$ °C.

Red cabbage extract was produced by the following process. Fresh red cabbage was purchased from a local retailer (Coles supermarket, Werribee, Victoria, Australia). Edible parts of the red cabbage were washed and blended in a food processor with water (1:2 ratio, *w/v*) before boiling by microwave heating at 800 W for 10 min. After cooling to ambient temperature, the mixture was ultrasonicated at 300 W for 11 min (Hielscher, Germany) before bag filtration (1 µm pore size, Sefar Filtration Inc., Depew, NY, USA). The filtrate was freeze-dried (Virtis Genesis 35EL, SP Scientific, Warmister, PA, USA) and stored with desiccant and low head space at $-18$ °C.

### 2.3. Total Phenolic Content of Plant Extracts

Total phenolic content of the plant extracts was quantified using the Folin-Ciocalteu assay [47]. In brief, 20 µL samples (blank, standard, or 2 mg/mL plant extract in 20% methanol) was added to 1 mL of 0.2 N Folin-Ciocalteu reagent and 180 µL of Milli-Q water and mixed for 15 s, and allowed to stand for 3 min before 800 µL of 7.5% $Na_2CO_3$ was added to the mixture. The mixture was shaken for 15 s followed by incubation at 37 °C for 1 h in the dark. The absorbance at 765 nm was measured using a Varioskan Flash microplate reader (Thermo Fisher Scientific, Waltham, MA, USA). The total phenolic content of plant extracts was reported as gallic acid equivalent (GAE) using a 7-point calibration curve of gallic acid standard with concentrations of 0–500 µg/mL in 20% methanol after blank subtraction. Total phenolic content of the plant extracts was 26.6 $\pm$ 1.5 mg GAE/g for red cabbage extract and 327.1 $\pm$ 13.9 mg GAE/g for grape skin extract. Analysis was performed in duplicate.

### 2.4. Prediction of Human Absorption Kinetics of Plant Extracts

Predicted human absorption kinetics, the "functional fingerprints" of plant extracts, were determined using untargeted liquid chromatography mass spectrometry (LC-MS) profiling method [42] in combination with the PCAP model [41]. Untargeted LC-MS profiling analysis was performed using an Agilent 6520 quadrupole time-of-flight (QTOF) MS system (Agilent, Santa Clara, CA, USA) with a dual sprayer electrospray ionisation (ESI) source attached to the Agilent 1200 series high performance liquid chromatography (HPLC) system (Santa Clara, CA, USA) comprised of a vacuum degasser and binary pump with a thermostated auto-sampler and column oven. The MS was operated in positive or negative mode using the following conditions (positive/negative, respectively): nebulizer pressure 30/45 psi, gas flow-rate 10 L/min, gas temperature 300 °C, capillary voltage 4000/−3500 V, fragmentor 150, and skimmer 65 V. The instrument was operated in the extended dynamic range mode with data collected in the mass to change ratio ($m/z$) range of 70–1700. Chromatography was carried out using an Agilent Zorbax Eclipse XDB-C18, 2.1 × 100 mm, 1.8 μm column maintained at 40 °C (±1 °C) at a flow rate of 400 μL/min with a 20-min run time. A gradient LC method was used with mobile phases comprised of (A) 0.1% formic acid in deionized water and (B) 0.1% formic acid in acetonitrile. Gradient: A 5-min linear gradient from 5% to 30% mobile phase B, followed by 5-min gradient to 100% mobile phase B and then a 5-min hold, followed by a 5-min re-equilibration at 5% mobile phase B. Molecular feature extraction (MFE) was conducted using Agilent MassHunter Qualitative analysis (version B.07.00, Agilent) and MassHunter Profinder (version B.06.00, Agilent). Binning and alignment tolerances were set to: retention time: ±0.1% + 0.15 min; mass window: ±20 ppm + 2 mDa. Allowed ion species: $H^+$, $Na^+$, $K^+$, $NH_4^+$, and neutral losses: $H_2O$, $H_3PO_4$, $CO_2$, $C_6H_{12}O_6$. MFE was restricted to the 1000 largest features and 1–2 charge states. After elimination of the molecular features which were common in the two plant extracts (i.e., primary metabolites), the remaining molecular features represented the phytochemicals (i.e., secondary metabolites) of the plant extracts.

The lipophilicity descriptor log P was determined using a calibration curve of retention time and log P of twelve standards including L-histidine, (*S*)-dihydroorotate, shikimate, 4-pyridoxate, 3-hydroxybenzyl alcohol, 2,5-dihydroxybenzoate, 3-hydroxybenzaldehyde, trans-cinnamate, estradiol-17α, deoxycholate, retinoate, oleic acid, and heptadecanoate. Log P values of standards were calculated using the Molinspiration Chemoinformatics calculator.

The combination of log P and molecular mass were used to calculate predicted time of maximal plasma absorption ($T_{max}$) in humans using the PCAP model [41]. The functional fingerprints of plant extracts were generated by plotting predicted human $T_{max}$ and peak area (relative ion count) of the phytochemicals detected by LC-MS [42].

## 2.5. Dietary Intervention Using an Animal Model

### 2.5.1. Animals and Background Diet

The study used six female pigs (Large White × Landrace, 2.5 months old, weight ~30 kg). The pigs weighed 23.2–25.4 kg (mean 24.4 kg, standard error (SE) 3 kg) at the start of the study and 42.8–45.4 kg (mean 44.5 kg, SE 0.3 kg) on study completion five week later. The pigs were housed in individual pens for the duration of the study (12 h light/dark cycle, temperature 18–24 °C). The animals were fed a commercial background diet (Ridley AgriProducts, Melbourne, VIC, Australia) at an energy intake of 0.5 MJ digestible energy/kg body weight (BW)/day representing about 80% of usual energy intake and consumed water ad libitum. The composition of the feed includes 18% protein, 40.37% starch, 2.73% sugar, 4.9% fat, 19.35% fibre, 4.95% ash, 0.9% calcium, and 0.65% phosphorus. The study was approved by the Animal Ethics Committee of the Faculty of Veterinary and Agricultural Sciences, The University of Melbourne, Australia (approval number 1513762.1).

### 2.5.2. Cephalic Vein Catheterisation Procedure

The cephalic veins of the animals were catheterised under general anaesthesia allowing 7-day post-surgery recovery. Pigs were injected intramuscularly with ketamine hydrochloride (10 mg/kg BW; Ketalar, Pfizer, NY, USA) mixed with xylazine (1 mg/kg BW; Rompun, Bayer, Leverkusen, Germany) to induce sedation and anesthesia. Pigs were then intubated and maintained on 1–4% isoflurane inhalation anaesthesia (Rhone Merieux, Footscray West, VIC, Australia). A silastic catheter was inserted into the external cephalic vein and advanced to the anterior vena cava via the cephalic vein; exteriorisation of the catheter in the interscapular space and storage of the catheter in a cloth pouch glued to the back of the animals was performed as described previously [48]. After catheterisation, the neck incision and exit site were irrigated with benzyl penicillin (BenPen, CSL, Parkville, VIC, Australia) and the animals were given 2 mL of 150 mg/mL of antibiotic amoxicillin (Moxylan, Jurox, Rutherford, NSW, Australia) and 2 mL of 100 mg/mL analgesic/anti-inflammatory ketoprofen (Troy Labs Pty. Ltd., Smithfield, NSW, Australia). After surgery, the animals were monitored for feeding behaviour, general disposition, and rectal temperature. Any animals with elevated temperatures (>39 °C) were given 2 mL of 150 mg/mL amoxicillin. Catheters were flushed daily with physiological saline containing 100 units/mL (U/mL) heparin.

### 2.5.3. Experimental Design and Procedure

The study was performed in a crossover $4 \times 2$ factorial design with the factors being two plant extracts at four doses (including placebo control) in triplicate. The wash-out period between treatments was for a minimum of two days. To account for differences in the total phenolic contents of the plant extracts, doses of red cabbage and grape skin extracts were standardised for their total phenolic content as gallic acid equivalents (GAE). On each experiment day, the pigs received a single dose of one of two treatments: red cabbage or grape skin extracts at one of four doses: 0, 2.22, 4.44, and 11.11 mg GAE/kg BW. Considering that the grape skin extract had a higher total phenolic content compared to the red cabbage extract, the doses were selected based on previous studies of grape skin extract administered safely to mice [49–51]. The maximal dose of 11.11 mg GAE/kg BW corresponding to 30 mg grape skin extract/kg BW was selected for our pig study, as this dose is equivalent to the proven safe dose of 200 mg grape skin extract/kg BW in mice [52].

At 8 am on each experiment day, pigs were weighed after an overnight fast. After a baseline (0 h) blood sample, pigs were gavaged with a single dose of plant extract solids reconstituted in water to 50 mL and blood samples collected every 0.5 h for 4 h. The catheter was washed before collecting each blood sample by withdrawing 10 mL of fresh blood. A 10-mL blood sample was then collected using a syringe and immediately placed into a heparinised collection tube (BD Vacutainer®, BD Australia, North Ryde, NSW, Australia) and immediately placed on ice. Lastly, the cannulas were refilled with 100 U/mL heparin in saline and secured in the interscapular pouch. Plasma was obtained by withdrawing supernatants of blood centrifuged at 2000× $g$ for 10 min at 4 °C, and aliquots were frozen at −20 °C until analysis. During 4 h of blood sampling period, no foods were given to pigs. After the last blood sampling, pigs were fed the background diet.

### 2.5.4. Plasma Total Antioxidant Capacity Assay

Plasma total antioxidant capacity ex vivo and in vitro was measured using the cupric reducing antioxidant capacity (CUPRAC) assay [53] and reported as Trolox equivalent antioxidant capacity (TEAC). Plasma TEAC ex vivo was performed on plasma samples collected from the pigs after oral intake of the plant extracts. Plasma TEAC in vitro was performed on reconstituted commercial pig plasma (3.8% trisodium citrate as anticoagulant, Sigma-Aldrich, St. Louis, MO, USA). Freeze-dried commercial pig plasma was reconstituted in Milli Q water to the indicated volume by the manufacture, and aliquots were frozen until analysis. On the day of plasma TEAC in vitro analysis, commercial pig plasma aliquots were thawed and spiked with either gallic acid standard, red cabbage, or grape skin extracts to final concentrations of 0.05, 0.1, 0.2, 0.4, and 0.5 mg GAE/mL. Plasma samples (collected from the pigs or spiked commercial plasma) were diluted 1:5 with Tris-glycine-urea buffer pH 7 before the CUPRAC assay.

The CUPRAC assay is based on the capacity of a sample to reduce a Cu(II) complex to a Cu(I) complex, which can be measured at 485 nm wavelength. Equal volumes (50 µL) of 7.5 mM BCS, 10 mM $CuCl_2$ and Tris-glycine-urea buffer were added to each well of a 96-well plate, followed by addition of 100 µL of samples (blank, standard, or diluted plasma). The plate was incubated at 22 °C for 1 h and absorbance at 485 nm was measured. Results were reported as TEAC based on a 6-point calibration curve using Trolox as the standard (0–100 µM) after blank subtraction. Analysis was performed in duplicate. Yields of increased plasma TEAC in vitro (nmol/µmol GAE) by the spiked phytochemicals were reported as the slope of linear regression of plasma TEAC as a function of phytochemical concentrations.

### 2.5.5. Plasma Glutathione Peroxidase Activity

Plasma GPx activity ex vivo was performed on plasma samples collected from the pigs after oral intake of the plant extracts using a commercial kit (Trevigen, Gaithersburg, MD, USA). Briefly, plasma samples (20 µL) were added to a reaction mixture containing premixed glutathione, reduced form of nicotiamide adenine dinucleotide phosphate (NADPH), glutathione reductase, and cumene hydroperoxide. Absorbance at 340 nm were monitored at 1 min intervals for 15 min, at 25 °C. The GPx activity was calculated from the rate of change in absorbance using GPx standard as a positive control. Results were reported as units/mL, where 1 unit of GPx activity was defined as the amount of enzyme that caused the oxidation of 1 nmol of NADPH to $NADP^+$ per minute at 25 °C. Analysis was performed in triplicate.

### 2.6. Hydrogen Peroxide Production of Plant Extracts in Pig Plasma In Vitro

The dose response production of $H_2O_2$ by phytochemicals in reconstituted commercial pig plasma (Sigma-Aldrich, St. Louis, MO, USA) was measured using the FOX assay [54]. Reconstituted commercial pig plasma was spiked with either gallic acid standard, red cabbage, or grape skin extracts to final concentrations of 0.05, 0.1, 0.2, 0.4, and 0.5 mg GAE/mL and was incubated at 37 °C for 1 h before the FOX assay of $H_2O_2$. The concentrations were selected to be in the equivalent range of the doses used in the animal study with pigs having 70 mL circulating blood/kg BW and plasma making up 55% of blood volume [55].

After incubation, the plasma sample was diluted 1:5 with Tris-glycine-urea buffer pH 7 and assays were conducted as follows. 90 µL of samples (blank, standard, or diluted plasma) were mixed with 10 µL of methanol and 900 µL of FOX reagent. The mixture was vortexed for 5 s followed by incubation at 22 °C for 30 min. After incubation, the mixture was centrifuged at 15,000 rpm for 10 min at 22 °C and absorbance of the supernatant was measured at 560 nm. Concentrations of plasma $H_2O_2$ were calculated based on a 6-point calibration curve using $H_2O_2$ as the standard (0–90 µM) after blank subtraction. Analysis was performed in duplicate. Yields of $H_2O_2$ production in vitro (nmol/µmol GAE) by the spiked phytochemicals were reported as the slope of the linear regression of $H_2O_2$ concentration as a function of phytochemical concentrations.

### 2.7. Data Analysis

All curve-fitting was performed using SigmaPlot for Windows Version 12.5 (Systat Software Inc., Chicago, IL, USA). The general linear model (GLM), analysis of covariance (ANCOVA), and Tukey's test 95% confidence grouping analyses were performed in Minitab 16 statistical software (Minitab Inc., State College, PA, USA). Pearson's correlation analysis was performed in Minitab 16 statistical software (Minitab Inc.).

## 3. Results

### 3.1. Predicted Human Absorption as Functional Fingerprints of Plant Extracts

Predicted absorption as 'functional fingerprints' of red cabbage and grape skin extracts were analysed by our LC-MS method with the application of the PCAP model. These functional fingerprints show the predicted ranges of time required for phytochemicals in the extracts to reach their maximal plasma concentrations in human ($T_{max}$) after oral consumption. Accordingly, red cabbage was predicted to have a long $T_{max}$ range of 0.4–11 h (Figure 1a) whilst grape skin was predicted to have shorter $T_{max}$ ranges of 0.4–3.7 h and 8.2–8.3 h (Figure 1b). The functional fingerprints of the plant extracts informed blood sampling time between 0–4 h at 0.5 h intervals in the current animal study.

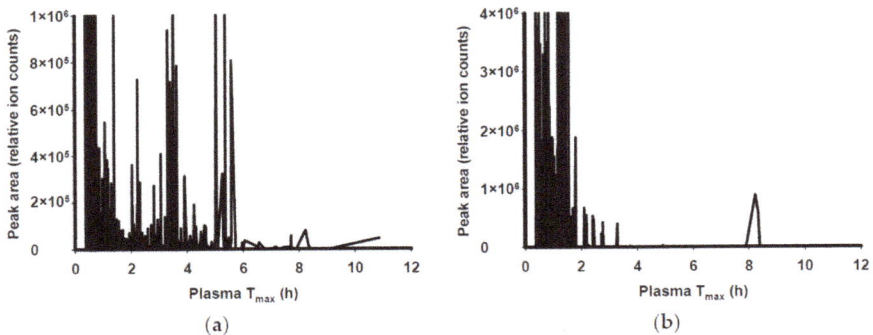

**Figure 1.** "Functional fingerprints" of plant extracts predicting absorption in humans based on the PCAP model [41] and the LC-MS method [42]. Functional fingerprints of (**a**) red cabbage; and (**b**) grape skin extracts. $T_{max}$, the time required for phytochemicals to reach their maximal plasma concentration.

### 3.2. Time Course Effects of Oral Consumption of Plant Extracts on Plasma Antioxidant Status Ex Vivo of Pigs

The animals consumed four doses of either red cabbage or grape skin extracts (0–11.11 mg GAE/kg BW) and plasma samples were taken every 0.5 h for 4 h. After oral consumption of red cabbage extract, in comparison to baseline at time 0, a significant increase in plasma TEAC was observed at 0.5 h in pigs consuming the maximal dose of 11.11 mg GAE/kg BW (Figure 2a) and a significant increase in plasma GPx activity was observed at 1.5 h in pigs consuming 2.22 mg GAE/kg BW (Figure 2b).

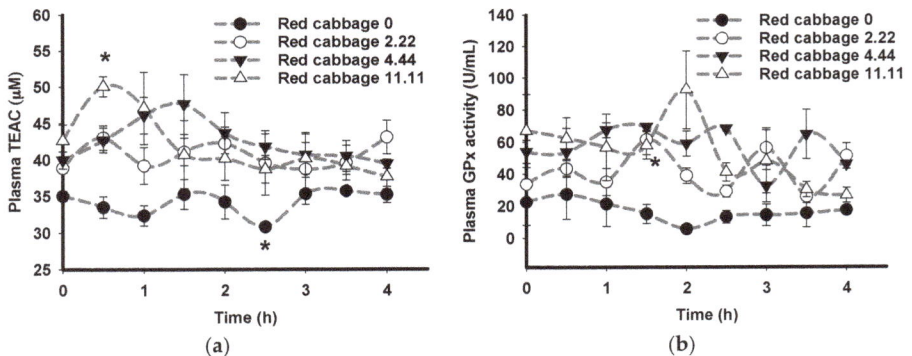

**Figure 2.** Effects of oral consumption of red cabbage extract on the plasma antioxidant status of pigs. Pigs consumed red cabbage extract at four doses in mg gallic acid equivalent/kg body weight: 0 (black circle), 2.22 (white circle), 4.44 (black triangle), and 11.11 (white triangle). Plasma antioxidant status was measured as: (**a**) plasma Trolox equivalent antioxidant capacity (TEAC); and (**b**) plasma glutathione peroxidase (GPx) activiy. Data points labelled "*" are significantly different from baseline at time 0 ($p \leq 0.05$, Tukey's test). Results represent the mean and error bars represent standard error of the mean ($N = 3$).

After consumption of grape skin extract, in comparison to baseline at time 0, a significant increase in plasma TEAC was observed after 1 h in pigs consuming 2.22 mg GAE/kg BW (Figure 3a) and significant increases of plasma GPx activity were observed at 2.5, 3.5, and 4 h in in pigs consuming

4.44 mg GAE/kg BW (Figure 3b). In contrast, a significant reduction in plasma GPx activity was observed at 1 h in pigs consuming 4.44 mg GAE/kg BW (Figure 3b).

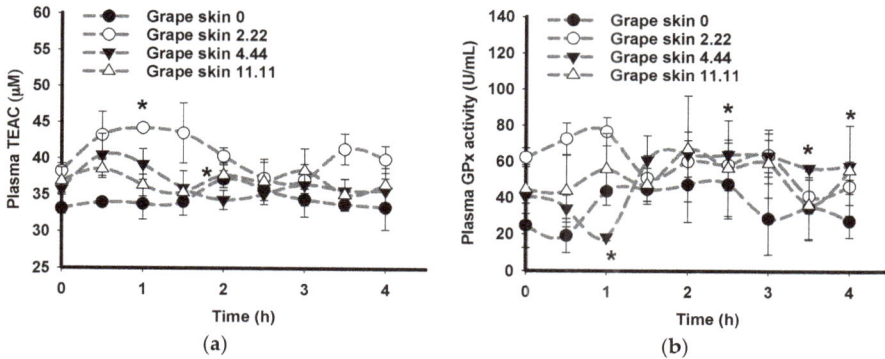

**Figure 3.** Effects of oral consumption of grape skin extract on the plasma antioxidant status of pigs. Pigs consumed grape skin extract at four doses in mg gallic acid equivalent/kg body weight: 0 (black circle), 2.22 (white circle), 4.44 (black triangle), and 11.11 (white triangle). Plasma antioxidant status was measured as: (**a**) plasma Trolox equivalent antioxidant capacity (TEAC); and (**b**) plasma glutathione peroxidase (GPx) activiy. Data points labelled "*" are significantly different from baseline at time 0 ($p \leq 0.05$, Tukey's test). Results represent the mean and error bars represent standard error of the mean ($N = 3$).

### 3.3. Effects of Plant Extracts on Plasma Total Antioxidant Capacity and Plasma Hydrogen Peroxide Concentration In Vitro

The dose response effects of the plant extracts on plasma TEAC and plasma $H_2O_2$ concentration in vitro were analysed after spiking plasma with either gallic acid standard, red cabbage, or grape skin extracts to final concentrations of 0.05, 0.1, 0.2, 0.4, and 0.5 mg GAE/mL. Proportional increase in plasma TEAC was observed with increased concentrations of all three phytochemical sources and followed linear regression relationships (Table 1). Yields of increased plasma TEAC in vitro by the phytochemicals were $1606.3 \pm 98.1$, $633.2 \pm 74.7$, and $1077.8 \pm 120.4$ nmol/µmol GAE for gallic acid standard, red cabbage, and grape skin extracts, respectively (Table 1).

**Table 1.** Effects of plant extracts on plasma Trolox equivalent antioxidant capacity (TEAC) and plasma levels of hydrogen peroxide ($H_2O_2$) in vitro.

| Phytochemical Sources | Plasma TEAC | | Plasma $H_2O_2$ | |
| --- | --- | --- | --- | --- |
| | Yield (nmol/µmol GAE) * | Linear Fit $R^2$ | Yield (nmol/µmol GAE) * | Linear Fit $R^2$ |
| Gallic acid standard | $1606.3 \pm 98.1$ | 0.99 | $68.7 \pm 4.5$ | 0.97 |
| Red cabbage extract | $633.2 \pm 74.7$ | 0.96 | $22.4 \pm 1.1$ | 0.99 |
| Grape skin extract | $1077.8 \pm 120.4$ | 0.96 | $44.2 \pm 2.1$ | 0.99 |

* Gallic acid standard and plant extracts were directly spiked into commercial pig plasma at concentrations of 0.05–0.5 mg gallic acid equivalent (GAE)/mL. Increased plasma TEAC and plasma $H_2O_2$ levels followed linear regressions with slopes representing yields of increase. Comparing three phytochemical sources, significant differences in yields of plasma TEAC and plasma $H_2O_2$ were observed ($p \leq 0.05$, analysis of covariance (ANCOVA)). Significantly high correlation between plasma TEAC and plasma $H_2O_2$ was observed ($r = 1$, $p \leq 0.05$, Pearson's correlation analysis). Results represent the mean ± standard error of the mean ($N = 2$).

Similar to plasma TEAC in vitro, proportional increase in plasma $H_2O_2$ concentrations was observed with increased concentrations of all three phytochemical sources and followed linear regression relationships (Table 1). Yields of $H_2O_2$ production in vitro by the phytochemicals in plasma were $68.7 \pm 4.5$, $22.4 \pm 1.1$, and $44.2 \pm 2.1$ nmol/µmol GAE for gallic acid standard, red cabbage, and grape skin extracts, respectively (Table 1).

Comparing the three phytochemical sources, significant differences in yields of plasma TEAC and plasma $H_2O_2$ were observed ($p \leq 0.05$, ANCOVA). Further, significantly high correlation between yields of plasma TEAC and plasma $H_2O_2$ were observed ($r = 1$, $p \leq 0.05$, Pearson's correlation analysis), with gallic acid having the strongest effect (highest yields) followed by grape skin and red cabbage extracts (Table 1).

### 3.4. Effects of Phytochemical Dose and Their $H_2O_2$ Production Capacity In Vitro on Plasma Antioxidant Status of Pigs Ex Vivo

Means across all pig plasma sampling points (0.5 h interval for 4 h, Figures 2 and 3) were combined to investigate the overall dose effects of the plant extracts on pig plasma antioxidant status (Figure 4). For both plant extracts, plasma TEAC ex vivo significantly increased at all three doses 2.22, 4.44, and 11.11 mg GAE/kg BW compared to dose 0 (Figure 4a). There was no significant difference in plasma TEAC among the three doses of red cabbage extract whilst plasma TEAC at grape skin extract dose of 4.44 and 11.11 mg GAE/kg BW was significantly reduced compared to the 2.22 mg GAE/kg BW dose (Figure 4a). The phytochemical dose (mg GAE/kg BW) of the two plant extracts was standardised to their in vitro $H_2O_2$ production yields (nmol/μmol GAE, Table 1) to estimate the $H_2O_2$ production (nmol/kg BW) by the plant extract dose used in the animal study. The in vitro $H_2O_2$ production yields of the two plant extracts had similar effects on the mean plasma TEAC of pigs compared to their phytochemical dose (Figure 4b).

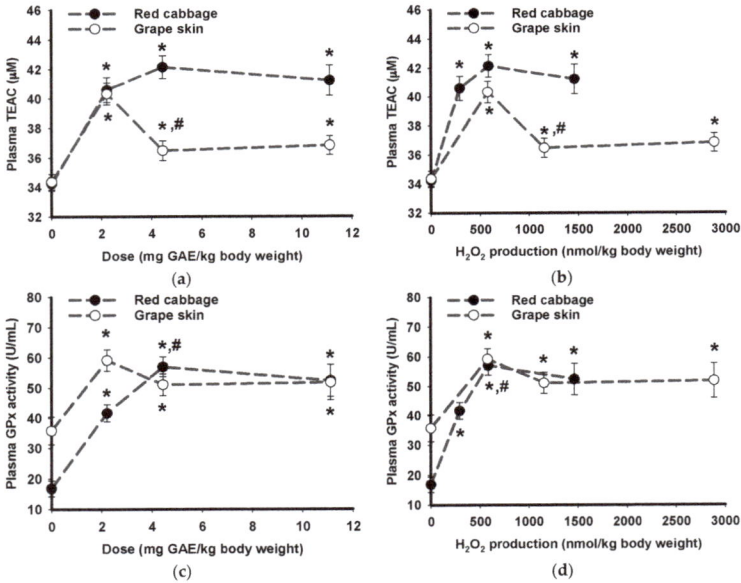

**Figure 4.** Total plasma antioxidant capacity and glutathione peroxidase activity of pig plasma as a function of phytochemical dose and $H_2O_2$ production efficacy. Means across all pig plasma sampling time points (0.5 h interval for 4 h) of plasma TEAC versus (a) phytochemical doses and (b) $H_2O_2$ production efficacy. Means across all pig plasma sampling time points of plasma GPx activity versus (c) phytochemical doses and (d) $H_2O_2$ production efficacy. The $H_2O_2$ production (nmol/kg body weight) was calculated based on the yield of $H_2O_2$ production (nmol/μmol GAE) of the plant extracts in vitro (Table 1). Data points labelled "*" are significantly different from dose 0 ($p \leq 0.05$, Tukey's test). Data points labelled "#" are significantly different from the previous dose ($p \leq 0.05$, Tukey's test). Results represent the mean and error bars represent standard error of the mean ($N = 27$).

Similarly, for both plant extracts, significant increases in pig plasma GPx activity were observed at all three doses (Figure 4c). There was no significant difference in GPx activity among the three doses of grape skin extract whilst GPx activity at a red cabbage extract dose of 4.44 mg GAE/kg BW was significantly increased compared to the 2.22 mg GAE/kg BW (Figure 4c). After standardisation of the phytochemical dose to their in vitro $H_2O_2$ production yields (Table 1), the plasma GPx activity in response to the two plant extracts was remarkably similar (Figure 4d).

## 4. Discussion

This study examines the consumption of dietary phytochemicals by pigs and shows that non-enzymatic and enzymatic antioxidant defences were increased. Absorption kinetics of red cabbage and grape skin extracts were characterised in pigs after oral consumption using plasma TEAC as a measure of the non-enzymatic antioxidant response [56] and plasma GPx (an antioxidant enzyme) activity [57]. The blood sampling time of the study (0.5 h interval for 4 hours) was chosen to capture the range of time expected for the phytochemicals to achieve their maximal plasma concentrations ($T_{max}$), predicted from their functional fingerprints (0.4–4 h). Consistent with the predicted functional fingerprints, a significant increase in plasma TEAC was observed at 0.5 h after consumption of red cabbage (11.11 mg GAE/kg BW) and at 1 h after consumption of grape skin (2.22 mg GAE/kg BW). Peaks of plasma TEAC have been observed to coincide with peaks of plasma phytochemicals in humans after consumption of tea [58] and chocolate [59]. Therefore, the identification of increased plasma TEAC within this selected time frame after plant extract ingestion validates the utility of the phytochemical absorption prediction (PCAP) model [41] and its application to the production of the functional fingerprints.

These results highlight the ability of the PCAP model to guide experimental design to ensure that the functional impact of the phytochemicals is captured during the sampling regime. For example, a previous study investigating the pharmacokinetics of three phytochemicals carvacrol, thymol, and eugenol in pigs reported the time of maximal absorption ($T_{max}$) at 1.39, 1.35, and 0.83 h, respectively [60]. Using our PCAP model [41], the $T_{max}$ of these phytochemicals for humans was predicted to be 1.76, 1.67, and 1.58 h, respectively. Comparing to the reported $T_{max}$ in pigs [60], the predicted $T_{max}$ of these phytochemicals in humans was very similar and followed the same sequence with $T_{max}$ of carvacrol > thymol > eugenol. This similarity of observed $T_{max}$ compared to predicted $T_{max}$ suggests that the PCAP model can be useful for predicting absorption of phytochemicals in pigs as well as in humans.

In the present study, the plant extract doses were standardised for their respective total phenolic contents as GAE analysed by the Folin-Ciocateu assay. Whilst ascorbic acid is known to interfere with this assay [61], based on analyses conducted by others [61–67], the contributions of ascorbic acid to the GAE results are estimated to be 0.3% and 4% for grape skin and red cabbage extracts, respectively. These minimal contributions of ascorbic acid to the GAE results reflected the naturally low ascorbic acid content of grape skin [62], and the effects of microwave cooking [66] and ultrasonication [67] which reduced the ascorbic acid content of red cabbage during plant processing. Accordingly, the GAE results presented herein are considered accurate indicators of the total phenolic content of the two plant extracts.

In comparison to plasma TEAC, a delayed increase in plasma GPx activity was observed at 1.5 h after consumption of red cabbage (2.22 mg GAE/kg BW) and at 2.5, 3.5, and 4 h after consumption of grape skin (4.44 mg GAE/kg BW). The observed time delay of plasma GPx activity after plasma TEAC is consistent with a previous study [68]. This delay may be explained by the induction of GPx activity occurring in response to the presence of phytochemicals in the plasma, as indicated by increased plasma TEAC [58,59]. Accordingly, increased plasma TEAC and increased plasma GPx activity after consumption of the plant extracts indicate that phytochemicals provide health benefits via both direct antioxidant activity and indirectly via the induction of enzymatic antioxidant defence mechanisms.

The dose response effects of red cabbage and grape skin extracts increased plasma TEAC in vitro after direct addition of the extracts to the pig plasma in the present study. As the phytochemical doses increased, there was a proportional increase in plasma TEAC in vitro (633.2–1606.3 nmol/µmol GAE), supporting the direct antioxidant activity of phytochemicals in vitro as observed in many studies [69–71]. In comparison to the in vitro experiments, same doses of red cabbage and grape skin extracts consumed by the pigs did not result in a proportional increase in plasma TEAC and plasma GPx activity ex vivo. When plant extracts were orally administered to pigs, increased plasma TEAC was observed at all doses compared to 0 but an increase in dose did not result in significant further increase of TEAC above the lowest dose. Further, an increase in dose of grape skin extract resulted in decreased plasma TEAC at doses of 4.44 and 11.11 mg GAE/kg BW compared to the dose at 2.22 mg/kg BW. The differences in plasma TEAC responses to the plant extracts may be attributed to their distinct phytochemical compositions [44,46]. Similarly, plasma GPx activity significantly increased for all doses compared to dose 0 but further increase of doses did not show a clear response relationship.

The observed differences between in vitro and ex vivo have also been observed in other studies [69,70]. Direct addition of tea [69] or apple phytochemicals [70] to human plasma in vitro increased plasma TEAC. However, consumption of the same or higher concentrations of tea [69] and apple phytochemicals [70] by humans did not reproduce the same effects as observed in vitro. The differences between in vitro and ex vivo results can be explained by the low bioavailability of phytochemicals in vivo as they are handled by the body as xenobiotics [40]. Further, these differences may be attributed to the increased complexity of the in vivo system wherein both direct and indirect antioxidant mechanisms may arise, as indicated by increased plasma GPx activity ex vivo.

Hypothetical pro-oxidant effects of phytochemicals in vitro via measurement of $H_2O_2$ levels in plasma were studied after direct addition of plant extracts. Similar to the results measuring plasma TEAC in vitro, incubation of red cabbage and grape skin extracts in pig plasma resulted in a proportional increase in plasma $H_2O_2$ levels (22.4–68.7 nmol/µmol GAE). Pro-oxidant effects of phytochemicals in vitro have been observed in the presence of oxygen and metal ions such as copper and iron [35–37,72–75]. Concentrations of iron and copper ions in human plasma are 2.13 and 0.81 µg/g, respectively [76], and iron levels of 0.1 µg/g [35] and copper levels of 3 µg/g [73] have been reported to initiate $H_2O_2$ production in vitro. The formation of $H_2O_2$ by phytochemicals in plasma observed here may be attributed to the electron transfer process between phytochemicals, oxygen, and metal ions present in plasma [73].

The ability of phytochemicals to produce $H_2O_2$ has been proposed to be responsible for the cytotoxic effects of phytochemicals in cell culture studies [35–37]. $H_2O_2$ has been widely used as an oxidative stress inducer in many studies investigating the protective effects of phytochemicals in response to oxidative stress [77–79]. However, the ability of phytochemicals to produce $H_2O_2$ may explain their indirect antioxidant protection mechanism. High concentrations of $H_2O_2$ ($\geq$100 µM) are harmful for cells but low concentrations of $H_2O_2$ ($\leq$50 µM) can be beneficial to initiate the antioxidant cellular defence [80,81]. Low concentrations of $H_2O_2$ have been observed to stimulate wound healing in keratinocytes [82] and in mice [83]. Similarly, the health benefits of regular exercise have been proposed to be associated with their production of low levels of ROS (such as $H_2O_2$) that induce adaptive responses to protect against molecular damage and, subsequently, aging [84,85]. Supporting this mechanism, $H_2O_2$ has been reported to activate the nuclear factor-erythroid-2-related factor 2 (Nrf2) de novo [86] which is a transcription factor involved in inducing the antioxidant response by regulating coordinated induction of stress response genes encoding antioxidant enzymes such as superoxide dismutase, catalase, and GPx [87]. Activation of Nrf2 has been proposed as a therapeutic potential for protection against chronic diseases [87,88]. Many phytochemicals are known as Nrf2 activators including curcumin (in turmeric) [89], epigallocatechin gallate (in green tea) [90], lycopene (in tomato) [91], resveratrol (in grape) [92], and sulforaphane (in broccoli) [93]. Accordingly, $H_2O_2$-mediated induction of Nrf2 in response to phytochemical supply may explain the correlation between $H_2O_2$ production and increased plasma GPx activity observed in our study.

## 5. Conclusions

The findings of the current study provide new insights in mechanisms by which dietary phytochemicals impact health, apart from direct ROS-scavenging pathways. An additional role is proposed whereby protection against oxidative tissue damage results from the promotion of cellular oxidative stress defence by dietary phytochemicals. This research demonstrates for the first time that $H_2O_2$ production analysis represents a useful predictive indicator of the in vivo efficacy of dietary phytochemicals.

**Acknowledgments:** This project has been funded by Horticulture Innovation Australia Limited using the Vegetable levy and funds from the Australian Government. We gratefully acknowledge the donation of the grape skin extract from Tarac Technologies and assistance during the animal trial by Maree Cox, Shannon Holbrook, Peter Cakebread, Ruslan Pustovit, Udanni Wijesiriwardana, Paula Andrea Giraldo Parra, and Caroline Storer.

**Author Contributions:** Conception and experimental design: S.N.B.S.-P., L.E.B., F.R.D. and J.J.C. Study execution: S.N.B.S.-P., J.J.C. and F.R.D. Data collection, analysis and interpretation: S.N.B.S.-P., L.E.B., F.R.D., J.J.C., K.N. and K.S.H. Manuscript writing and review: S. N.B.S.-P., L.E.B., K.S.H., J.J.C., K.N. and F.R.D. All authors read and approved the final manuscripts.

**Conflicts of Interest:** The authors declare no conflicts of interest.

## References

1.   Key, T.J. Fruit and vegetables and cancer risk. *Br. J. Cancer* **2011**, *104*, 6–11. [CrossRef] [PubMed]
2.   Dauchet, L.; Amouyel, P.; Dallongeville, J. Fruits, vegetables and coronary heart disease. *Nat. Rev. Cardiol.* **2009**, *6*, 599–608. [CrossRef] [PubMed]
3.   D'Onofrio, G.; Sancarlo, D.; Ruan, Q.; Yu, Z.; Panza, F.; Daniele, A.; Greco, A.; Seripa, D. Phytochemicals in the treatment of alzheimer's disease: A systematic review. *Curr. Drug Targets* **2016**, *17*. [CrossRef]
4.   Burton-Freeman, B. Postprandial metabolic events and fruit-derived phenolics: A review of the science. *Br. J. Nutr.* **2010**, *104*, S1–S14. [CrossRef] [PubMed]
5.   Van der Merwe, M.; Bloomer, R.J. The influence of methylsulfonylmethane on inflammation-associated cytokine release before and following strenuous exercise. *J. Sports Med.* **2016**, *2016*, 7498359. [CrossRef] [PubMed]
6.   Calder, P.C.; Albers, R.; Antoine, J.M.; Blum, S.; Bourdet-Sicard, R.; Ferns, G.A.; Folkerts, G.; Friedmann, P.S.; Frost, G.S.; Guarner, F.; et al. Inflammatory disease processes and interactions with nutrition. *Br. J. Nutr.* **2009**, *101*, S1–S45. [CrossRef] [PubMed]
7.   Halliwell, B. Reactive species and antioxidants. Redox biology is a fundamental theme of aerobic life. *Plant Physiol.* **2006**, *141*, 312–322. [CrossRef] [PubMed]
8.   Kryston, T.B.; Georgiev, A.B.; Pissis, P.; Georgakilas, A.G. Role of oxidative stress and DNA damage in human carcinogenesis. *Mutat. Res. Fund. Mol. Mech. Mut.* **2011**, *711*, 193–201. [CrossRef] [PubMed]
9.   Fang, F.C. Antimicrobial reactive oxygen and nitrogen species: Concepts and controversies. *Nat. Rev. Microbiol.* **2004**, *2*, 820–832. [CrossRef] [PubMed]
10.  Bøhn, S.K.; Myhrstad, M.C.; Thoresen, M.; Holden, M.; Karlsen, A.; Tunheim, S.H.; Erlund, I.; Svendsen, M.; Seljeflot, I.; Moskaug, J.Ø.; et al. Blood cell gene expression associated with cellular stress defense is modulated by antioxidant-rich food in a randomised controlled clinical trial of male smokers. *BMC Med.* **2010**, *8*, 54. [CrossRef] [PubMed]
11.  Krishnaiah, D.; Sarbatly, R.; Nithyanandam, R. A review of the antioxidant potential of medicinal plant species. *Food Bioprod. Process.* **2011**, *89*, 217–233. [CrossRef]
12.  Lee, J.; Koo, N.; Min, D.B. Reactive oxygen species, aging, and antioxidative nutraceuticals. *Compr. Rev. Food Sci. Food Saf.* **2004**, *3*, 21–33. [CrossRef]
13.  Seifried, H.E.; Anderson, D.E.; Fisher, E.I.; Milner, J.A. A review of the interaction among dietary antioxidants and reactive oxygen species. *J. Nutr. Biochem.* **2007**, *18*, 567–579. [CrossRef] [PubMed]
14.  Del Rio, D.; Rodriguez-Mateos, A.; Spencer, J.P.; Tognolini, M.; Borges, G.; Crozier, A. Dietary (poly)phenolics in human health: Structures, bioavailability, and evidence of protective effects against chronic diseases. *Antioxid. Redox. Signal.* **2013**, *18*, 1818–1892. [CrossRef] [PubMed]

15. Lotito, S.B.; Frei, B. Consumption of flavonoid-rich foods and increased plasma antioxidant capacity in humans: Cause, consequence, or epiphenomenon? *Free Radic. Biol. Med.* **2006**, *41*, 1727–1746. [CrossRef] [PubMed]

16. Kong, A.N.; Yu, R.; Lei, W.; Mandlekar, S.; Tan, T.H.; Ucker, D.S. Differential activation of MAPK and ICE/CED-3 protease in chemical-induced apoptosis. The role of oxidative stress in the regulation of mitogen-activated protein kinases (MAPKs) leading to gene expression and survival or activation of caspases leading to apoptosis. *Restor. Neurol. Neurosci.* **1998**, *12*, 63–70. [PubMed]

17. Kong, A.N.; Owuor, E.; Yu, R.; Hebbar, V.; Chen, C.; Hu, R.; Mandlekar, S. Induction of xenobiotic enzymes by the MAP kinase pathway and the antioxidant or electrophile response element (ARE/EpRE). *Drug Metab. Rev.* **2001**, *33*, 255–271. [CrossRef] [PubMed]

18. Finley, J.W.; Kong, A.N.; Hintze, K.J.; Jeffery, E.H.; Ji, L.L.; Lei, X.G. Antioxidants in foods: State of the science important to the food industry. *J. Agric. Food Chem.* **2011**, *59*, 6837–6846. [CrossRef] [PubMed]

19. Drew, J.E. Cellular defense system gene expression profiling of human whole blood: Opportunities to predict health benefits in response to diet. *Adv. Nutr.* **2012**, *3*, 499–505. [CrossRef] [PubMed]

20. Lee, W.L.; Huang, J.Y.; Shyur, L.F. Phytoagents for cancer management: Regulation of nucleic acid oxidation, ROS, and related mechanisms. *Oxid. Med. Cell. Longev.* **2013**, *2013*, 925804. [CrossRef] [PubMed]

21. Manjunatha, H.; Srinivasan, K. Protective effect of dietary curcumin and capsaicin on induced oxidation of low-density lipoprotein, iron-induced hepatotoxicity and carrageenan-induced inflammation in experimental rats. *FEBS J.* **2006**, *273*, 4528–4537. [CrossRef] [PubMed]

22. Srihari, T.; Sengottuvelan, M.; Nalini, N. Dose-dependent effect of oregano (*origanum vulgare* L.) on lipid peroxidation and antioxidant status in 1,2-dimethylhydrazine-induced rat colon carcinogenesis. *J. Pharm. Pharmacol.* **2008**, *60*, 787–794. [CrossRef] [PubMed]

23. Kim, B.; Ku, C.S.; Pham, T.X.; Park, Y.; Martin, D.A.; Xie, L.; Taheri, R.; Lee, J.; Bolling, B.W. *Aronia melanocarpa* (chokeberry) polyphenol-rich extract improves antioxidant function and reduces total plasma cholesterol in apolipoprotein E knockout mice. *Nutr. Res.* **2013**, *33*, 406–413. [CrossRef] [PubMed]

24. Ali, H.A.; Afifi, M.; Abdelazim, A.M.; Mosleh, Y.Y. Quercetin and omega 3 ameliorate oxidative stress induced by aluminium chloride in the brain. *J. Mol. Neurosci.* **2014**, *53*, 654–660. [CrossRef] [PubMed]

25. Gourineni, V.; Shay, N.F.; Chung, S.; Sandhu, A.K.; Gu, L. Muscadine grape (*vitis rotundifolia*) and wine phytochemicals prevented obesity-associated metabolic complications in C57BL/6J mice. *J. Agric. Food Chem.* **2012**, *60*, 7674–7681. [CrossRef] [PubMed]

26. Belviranli, M.; Gokbel, H.; Okudan, N.; Basarali, K. Effects of grape seed extract supplementation on exercise-induced oxidative stress in rats. *Br. J. Nutr.* **2012**, *108*, 249–256. [CrossRef] [PubMed]

27. Natella, F.; Belelli, F.; Gentili, V.; Ursini, F.; Scaccini, C. Grape seed proanthocyanidins prevent plasma postprandial oxidative stress in humans. *J. Agric. Food Chem.* **2002**, *50*, 7720–7725. [CrossRef] [PubMed]

28. Serafini, M.; Bugianesi, R.; Maiani, G.; Valtuena, S.; De Santis, S.; Crozier, A. Plasma antioxidants from chocolate. *Nature* **2003**, *424*, 1013. [CrossRef] [PubMed]

29. Pedersen, C.B.; Kyle, J.; Jenkinson, A.M.; Gardner, P.T.; McPhail, D.B.; Duthie, G.G. Effects of blueberry and cranberry juice consumption on the plasma antioxidant capacity of healthy female volunteers. *Eur. J. Clin. Nutr.* **2000**, *54*, 405–408. [CrossRef] [PubMed]

30. Sung, H.; Nah, J.; Chun, S.; Park, H.; Yang, S.E.; Min, W.K. In vivo antioxidant effect of green tea. *Eur. J. Clin. Nutr.* **2000**, *54*, 527–529. [CrossRef] [PubMed]

31. Guarrera, S.; Sacerdote, C.; Fiorini, L.; Marsala, R.; Polidoro, S.; Gamberini, S.; Saletta, F.; Malaveille, C.; Talaska, G.; Vineis, P.; et al. Expression of DNA repair and metabolic genes in response to a flavonoid-rich diet. *Br. J. Nutr.* **2007**, *98*, 525–533. [CrossRef] [PubMed]

32. Wang, J.; Siegmund, K.; Tseng, C.C.; Lee, A.S.; Wu, A.H. Soy food supplementation, dietary fat reduction and peripheral blood gene expression in postmenopausal women—A randomized, controlled trial. *Mol. Nutr. Food Res.* **2011**, *55*, S264–S277. [CrossRef] [PubMed]

33. Bakker, G.C.; van Erk, M.J.; Pellis, L.; Wopereis, S.; Rubingh, C.M.; Cnubben, N.H.; Kooistra, T.; van Ommen, B.; Hendriks, H.F. An antiinflammatory dietary mix modulates inflammation and oxidative and metabolic stress in overweight men: A nutrigenomics approach. *Am. J. Clin. Nutr.* **2010**, *91*, 1044–1059. [CrossRef] [PubMed]

34. Halliwell, B.; Whiteman, M. Measuring reactive species and oxidative damage in vivo and in cell culture: How should you do it and what do the results mean? *Br. J. Pharmacol.* **2004**, *142*, 231–255. [CrossRef] [PubMed]

35. Long, L.H.; Clement, M.V.; Halliwell, B. Artifacts in cell culture: Rapid generation of hydrogen peroxide on addition of (−)-epigallocatechin, (−)-epigallocatechin gallate, (+)-catechin, and quercetin to commonly used cell culture media. *Biochem. Biophys. Res. Commun.* **2000**, *273*, 50–53. [CrossRef] [PubMed]

36. Chai, P.C.; Long, L.H.; Halliwell, B. Contribution of hydrogen peroxide to the cytotoxicity of green tea and red wines. *Biochem. Biophys. Res. Commun.* **2003**, *304*, 650–654. [CrossRef]

37. Long, L.H.; Hoi, A.; Halliwell, B. Instability of, and generation of hydrogen peroxide by, phenolic compounds in cell culture media. *Arch. Biochem. Biophys.* **2010**, *501*, 162–169. [CrossRef] [PubMed]

38. Rodd, A.L.; Ververis, K.; Sayakkarage, D.; Khan, A.W.; Rafehi, H.; Ziemann, M.; Loveridge, S.J.; Lazarus, R.; Kerr, C.; Lockett, T.; et al. RNA sequencing supports distinct reactive oxygen species-mediated pathways of apoptosis by high and low size mass fractions of bay leaf (*Lauris nobilis*) in HT-29 cells. *Food Funct.* **2015**, *6*, 2507–2524. [CrossRef] [PubMed]

39. Lee, C.Y. Challenges in providing credible scientific evidence of health benefits of dietary polyphenols. *J. Funct. Foods* **2013**, *5*, 524–526. [CrossRef]

40. Holst, B.; Williamson, G. Nutrients and phytochemicals: From bioavailability to bioefficacy beyond antioxidants. *Curr. Opin. Biotechnol.* **2008**, *19*, 73–82. [CrossRef] [PubMed]

41. Selby-Pham, S.N.B.; Miller, R.B.; Howell, K.; Dunshea, F.; Bennett, L.E. Physicochemical properties of dietary phytochemicals can predict their passive absorption in the human small intestine. *Sci. Rep.* **2017**, *7*, 1931. [CrossRef] [PubMed]

42. Selby-Pham, S.N.B.; Howell, K.S.; Dunshea, F.R.; Ludbey, J.; Lutz, A.; Bennett, L.E. High throughput prediction of human absorption kinetics of plant extracts using LC-MS and statistical modelling. *Food Chem.* **2017**, in press.

43. Roura, E.; Koopmans, S.J.; Lalles, J.P.; Le Huerou-Luron, I.; de Jager, N.; Schuurman, T.; Val-Laillet, D. Critical review evaluating the pig as a model for human nutritional physiology. *Nutr. Res. Rev.* **2016**, *29*, 60–90. [CrossRef] [PubMed]

44. Flamini, R.; Mattivi, F.; De Rosso, M.; Arapitsas, P.; Bavaresco, L. Advanced knowledge of three important classes of grape phenolics: Anthocyanins, stilbenes and flavonols. *Int. J. Mol. Sci.* **2013**, *14*, 19651–19669. [CrossRef] [PubMed]

45. Wagner, A.E.; Terschluesen, A.M.; Rimbach, G. Health promoting effects of brassica-derived phytochemicals: From chemopreventive and anti-inflammatory activities to epigenetic regulation. *Oxid. Med. Cell. Longev.* **2013**, *2013*, 964539. [CrossRef] [PubMed]

46. Huang, H.; Jiang, X.; Xiao, Z.; Yu, L.; Pham, Q.; Sun, J.; Chen, P.; Yokoyama, W.; Yu, L.L.; Luo, Y.S.; et al. Red cabbage microgreens lower circulating low-density lipoprotein (LDL), liver cholesterol, and inflammatory cytokines in mice fed a high-fat diet. *J. Agric. Food Chem.* **2016**, *64*, 9161–9171. [CrossRef] [PubMed]

47. Ainsworth, E.A.; Gillespie, K.M. Estimation of total phenolic content and other oxidation substrates in plant tissues using folin-ciocalteu reagent. *Nat. Protoc.* **2007**, *2*, 875–877. [CrossRef] [PubMed]

48. Ostrowska, E.; Cross, R.F.; Muralitharan, M.; Bauman, D.E.; Dunshea, F.R. Effects of dietary fat and conjugated linoleic acid on plasma metabolite concentrations and metabolic responses to homeostatic signals in pigs. *Br. J. Nutr.* **2002**, *88*, 625–634. [CrossRef] [PubMed]

49. Asseburg, H.; Schafer, C.; Muller, M.; Hagl, S.; Pohland, M.; Berressem, D.; Borchiellini, M.; Plank, C.; Eckert, G.P. Effects of grape skin extract on age-related mitochondrial dysfunction, memory and life span in C57BL/6J mice. *Neuromol. Med.* **2016**, *18*, 378–395. [CrossRef] [PubMed]

50. Costa, M.R.; Pires, K.M.; Nalbones-Barbosa, M.N.; Dos Santos Valenca, S.; Resende, A.C.; de Moura, R.S. Grape skin extract-derived polyphenols modify programming-induced renal endowment in prenatal protein-restricted male mouse offspring. *Eur. J. Nutr.* **2016**, *55*, 1455–1464. [CrossRef] [PubMed]

51. Resende, A.C.; Emiliano, A.F.; Cordeiro, V.S.; de Bem, G.F.; de Cavalho, L.C.; de Oliveira, P.R.; Neto, M.L.; Costa, C.A.; Boaventura, G.T.; de Moura, R.S. Grape skin extract protects against programmed changes in the adult rat offspring caused by maternal high-fat diet during lactation. *J. Nutr. Biochem.* **2013**, *24*, 2119–2126. [CrossRef] [PubMed]

52. Nair, A.B.; Jacob, S. A simple practice guide for dose conversion between animals and human. *J. Basic Clin. Pharm.* **2016**, *7*, 27–31. [CrossRef] [PubMed]

53. Marques, S.; Magalhães, L.; Tóth, I.; Segundo, M. Insights on antioxidant assays for biological samples based on the reduction of copper complexes—The importance of analytical conditions. *Int. J. Mol. Sci.* **2014**, *15*, 11387–11402. [CrossRef] [PubMed]

54. Wolff, S.P. Ferrous ion oxidation in presence of ferric ion indicator xylenol orange for measurement of hydroperoxides. *Methods Enzymol.* **1994**, *233*, 182–189.

55. Wolfensohn, S.; Lloyd, M. The larger domestic species. In *Handbook of Laboratory Animal Management and Welfare*, 3rd ed.; Wolfensohn, S., Lloyd, M., Eds.; Blackwell Publishing: Ames, IA, USA, 2003; pp. 326–364.

56. Apak, R.; Guclu, K.; Ozyurek, M.; Karademir, S.E.; Altun, M. Total antioxidant capacity assay of human serum using copper(II)-neocuproine as chromogenic oxidant: The CUPRAC method. *Free Radic. Res.* **2005**, *39*, 949–961. [CrossRef] [PubMed]

57. Hayes, J.D.; McLellan, L.I. Glutathione and glutathione-dependent enzymes represent a co-ordinately regulated defence against oxidative stress. *Free Radic. Res.* **1999**, *31*, 273–300. [CrossRef] [PubMed]

58. Leenen, R.; Roodenburg, A.J.; Tijburg, L.B.; Wiseman, S.A. A single dose of tea with or without milk increases plasma antioxidant activity in humans. *Eur. J. Clin. Nutr.* **2000**, *54*, 87–92. [CrossRef] [PubMed]

59. Rein, D.; Lotito, S.; Holt, R.R.; Keen, C.L.; Schmitz, H.H.; Fraga, C.G. Epicatechin in human plasma: In vivo determination and effect of chocolate consumption on plasma oxidation status. *J. Nutr.* **2000**, *130*, 2109s–2114s. [PubMed]

60. Michiels, J.; Missotten, J.; Dierick, N.; Fremaut, D.; Maene, P.; De Smet, S. In vitro degradation and in vivo passage kinetics of carvacrol, thymol, eugenol and trans-cinnamaldehyde along the gastrointestinal tract of piglets. *J. Sci. Food Agric.* **2008**, *88*, 2371–2381. [CrossRef]

61. Everette, J.D.; Bryant, Q.M.; Green, A.M.; Abbey, Y.A.; Wangila, G.W.; Walker, R.B. Thorough study of reactivity of various compound classes toward the folin−ciocalteu reagent. *J. Agric. Food Chem.* **2010**, *58*, 8139–8144. [CrossRef] [PubMed]

62. Singha, I.; Das, S.K. Free radical scavenging properties of skin and pulp extracts of different grape cultivars in vitro and attentuation of $H_2O_2$-induced oxidative stress in liver tissue ex vivo. *Ind. J. Clin. Biochem.* **2015**, *30*, 305–312. [CrossRef] [PubMed]

63. Gabas, A.L.; Telis-Romero, J.; Menegalli, F.C. Thermodynamic models for water sorption by grape skin and pulp. *Drying Technol.* **1999**, *17*, 962–974. [CrossRef]

64. Singh, J.; Upadhyay, A.K.; Bahadur, A.; Singh, K.P.; Rai, M. Antioxidant phytochemicals in cabbage (*Brassica oleracea* L. Var. Capitata). *Sci. Hort.* **2006**, *108*, 233–237. [CrossRef]

65. Sivakumaran, S.; Huffman, L.; Sivakumaran, S. *The Concise New Zealand Food Composition Tables*, 12th ed.; The New Zealand Institute for Plant & Food Research Limited and Ministry of Health: Palmerston North, New Zealand, 2017.

66. Zeng, C. Effects of different cooking methods on the vitamin c content of selected vegetables. *Nutr. Food Sci.* **2013**, *43*, 438–443. [CrossRef]

67. Tiwari, B.K.; O'Donnell, C.P.O.; Patras, A.; Cullen, P.J. Anthocyanin and ascorbic acid degradation in sonicated strawberry juice. *J. Agric. Food Chem.* **2008**, *56*, 10071–10077. [CrossRef] [PubMed]

68. Alleva, R.; Di Donato, F.; Strafella, E.; Staffolani, S.; Nocchi, L.; Borghi, B.; Pignotti, E.; Santarelli, L.; Tomasetti, M. Effect of ascorbic acid-rich diet on in vivo-induced oxidative stress. *Br. J. Nutr.* **2012**, *107*, 1645–1654. [CrossRef] [PubMed]

69. Cherubini, A.; Beal, M.F.; Frei, B. Black tea increases the resistance of human plasma to lipid peroxidation in vitro, but not ex vivo. *Free Radic. Biol. Med.* **1999**, *27*, 381–387. [CrossRef]

70. Lotito, S.B.; Frei, B. Relevance of apple polyphenols as antioxidants in human plasma: Contrasting in vitro and in vivo effects. *Free Radic. Biol. Med.* **2004**, *36*, 201–211. [PubMed]

71. Kolodziejczyk-Czepas, J.; Nowak, P.; Moniuszko-Szajwaj, B.; Kowalska, I.; Stochmal, A. Free radical scavenging actions of three *trifolium* species in the protection of blood plasma antioxidant capacity in vitro. *Pharm. Biol.* **2015**, *53*, 1277–1284. [CrossRef] [PubMed]

72. Sahu, S.C.; Gray, G.C. Interactions of flavonoids, trace metals, and oxygen: Nuclear DNA damage and lipid peroxidation induced by myricetin. *Cancer Lett.* **1993**, *70*, 73–79. [CrossRef]

73. Zheng, L.F.; Wei, Q.Y.; Cai, Y.J.; Fang, J.G.; Zhou, B.; Yang, L.; Liu, Z.L. DNA damage induced by resveratrol and its synthetic analogues in the presence of Cu (II) ions: Mechanism and structure-activity relationship. *Free Radic. Biol. Med.* **2006**, *41*, 1807–1816. [CrossRef] [PubMed]

74. Fukumoto, L.R.; Mazza, G. Assessing antioxidant and prooxidant activities of phenolic compounds. *J. Agric. Food Chem.* **2000**, *48*, 3597–3604. [CrossRef] [PubMed]

75. Ahmad, M.S.; Fazal, F.; Rahman, A.; Hadi, S.M.; Parish, J.H. Activities of flavonoids for the cleavage of DNA in the presence of Cu(II): Correlation with generation of active oxygen species. *Carcinogenesis* **1992**, *13*, 605–608. [CrossRef]

76. Tautkus, S.; Irnius, A.; Speiciene, D.; Barkauskas, J.; Kareiva, A. Investigation of distribution of heavy metals between blood plasma and blood cells. *Ann. Chim.* **2007**, *97*, 1139–1142. [CrossRef]

77. Sandstrom, B.E.; Marklund, S.L. Effects of variation in glutathione peroxidase activity on DNA damage and cell survival in human cells exposed to hydrogen peroxide and t-butyl hydroperoxide. *Biochem. J.* **1990**, *271*, 17–23. [CrossRef] [PubMed]

78. Ajila, C.M.; Prasada Rao, U.J. Protection against hydrogen peroxide induced oxidative damage in rat erythrocytes by *Mangifera indica* L. Peel extract. *Food Chem. Toxicol.* **2008**, *46*, 303–309. [CrossRef] [PubMed]

79. Shui, G.; Bao, Y.M.; Bo, J.; An, L.J. Protective effect of protocatechuic acid from *alpinia oxyphylla* on hydrogen peroxide-induced oxidative PC12 cell death. *Eur. J. Pharmacol.* **2006**, *538*, 73–79. [CrossRef] [PubMed]

80. Halliwell, B.; Clement, M.V.; Long, L.H. Hydrogen peroxide in the human body. *FEBS Lett.* **2000**, *486*, 10–13. [CrossRef]

81. Ohguro, N.; Fukuda, M.; Sasabe, T.; Tano, Y. Concentration dependent effects of hydrogen peroxide on lens epithelial cells. *Br. J. Ophthalmol.* **1999**, *83*, 1064. [CrossRef] [PubMed]

82. Loo, A.E.; Halliwell, B. Effects of hydrogen peroxide in a keratinocyte-fibroblast co-culture model of wound healing. *Biochem. Biophys. Res. Commun.* **2012**, *423*, 253–258. [CrossRef] [PubMed]

83. Loo, A.E.; Wong, Y.T.; Ho, R.; Wasser, M.; Du, T.; Ng, W.T.; Halliwell, B. Effects of hydrogen peroxide on wound healing in mice in relation to oxidative damage. *PLoS ONE* **2012**, *7*, e49215. [CrossRef] [PubMed]

84. Radak, Z.; Chung, H.Y.; Goto, S. Exercise and hormesis: Oxidative stress-related adaptation for successful aging. *Biogerontology* **2005**, *6*, 71–75. [CrossRef] [PubMed]

85. Pallauf, K.; Giller, K.; Huebbe, P.; Rimbach, G. Nutrition and healthy ageing: Calorie restriction or polyphenol-rich "mediterrasian" diet? *Oxid. Med. Cell Longev.* **2013**, *2013*, 707421. [CrossRef] [PubMed]

86. Covas, G.; Marinho, H.S.; Cyrne, L.; Antunes, F. Activation of Nrf2 by $H_2O_2$: De novo synthesis versus nuclear translocation. *Methods Enzymol.* **2013**, *528*, 157–171. [PubMed]

87. Surh, Y.J.; Kundu, J.K.; Na, H.K. Nrf2 as a master redox switch in turning on the cellular signaling involved in the induction of cytoprotective genes by some chemopreventive phytochemicals. *Planta Med.* **2008**, *74*, 1526–1539. [CrossRef] [PubMed]

88. Hybertson, B.M.; Gao, B.; Bose, S.K.; McCord, J.M. Oxidative stress in health and disease: The therapeutic potential of Nrf2 activation. *Mol. Aspects Med.* **2011**, *32*, 234–246. [CrossRef] [PubMed]

89. Farombi, E.O.; Shrotriya, S.; Na, H.K.; Kim, S.H.; Surh, Y.J. Curcumin attenuates dimethylnitrosamine-induced liver injury in rats through Nrf2-mediated induction of heme oxygenase-1. *Food Chem. Toxicol.* **2008**, *46*, 1279–1287. [CrossRef] [PubMed]

90. Yuan, J.H.; Li, Y.Q.; Yang, X.Y. Inhibition of epigallocatechin gallate on orthotopic colon cancer by upregulating the Nrf2-ugt1a signal pathway in nude mice. *Pharmacology* **2007**, *80*, 269–278. [CrossRef] [PubMed]

91. Ben-Dor, A.; Steiner, M.; Gheber, L.; Danilenko, M.; Dubi, N.; Linnewiel, K.; Zick, A.; Sharoni, Y.; Levy, J. Carotenoids activate the antioxidant response element transcription system. *Mol. Cancer Ther.* **2005**, *4*, 177–186. [PubMed]

92. Kode, A.; Rajendrasozhan, S.; Caito, S.; Yang, S.R.; Megson, I.L.; Rahman, I. Resveratrol induces glutathione synthesis by activation of Nrf2 and protects against cigarette smoke-mediated oxidative stress in human lung epithelial cells. *Am. J. Physiol. Lung Cell. Mol. Physiol.* **2008**, *294*, L478–L488. [CrossRef] [PubMed]

93. Hong, F.; Freeman, M.L.; Liebler, D.C. Identification of sensor cysteines in human keap1 modified by the cancer chemopreventive agent sulforaphane. *Chem. Res. Toxicol.* **2005**, *18*, 1917–1926. [CrossRef] [PubMed]

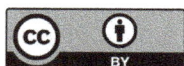

*nutrients*

MDPI

*Review*

# Whole Grain Intake and Glycaemic Control in Healthy Subjects: A Systematic Review and Meta-Analysis of Randomized Controlled Trials

Stefano Marventano [1], Claudia Vetrani [2], Marilena Vitale [2,*], Justyna Godos [3], Gabriele Riccardi [2] and Giuseppe Grosso [3]

[1]  Department of Medical and Surgical Sciences and Advanced Technologies "G.F. Ingrassia", University of Catania, 95123 Catania, Italy; stefano.marventano@studium.unict.it
[2]  Department of Clinical Medicine and Surgery, "Federico II" University, 80131 Naples, Italy; c.vetrani@libero.it (C.V.); riccardi@unina.it (G.R.)
[3]  Integrated Cancer Registry of Catania-Messina-Siracusa-Enna, Azienda Ospedaliero-Universitaria Policlinico Vittorio Emanuele, 95124 Catania, Italy; justyna.godos@student.uj.edu.pl (J.G.); giuseppe.grosso@studium.unict.it (G.G.)
*  Correspondence: marilena.vitale@unina.it; Tel.: +39-081-746-4736

Received: 18 May 2017; Accepted: 13 July 2017; Published: 19 July 2017

**Abstract:** Backgrounds: There is growing evidence from both observational and intervention studies that Whole Grain (WG) cereals exert beneficial effects on human health, especially on the metabolic profile. The aim of this study was to perform a meta-analysis of randomised controlled trials (RCT) to assess the acute and medium/long-term effect of WG foods on glycaemic control and insulin sensitivity in healthy individuals. Methods: A search for all the published RCT on the effect of WG food intake on glycaemic and insulin response was performed up to December 2016. Effect size consisted of mean difference (MD) and 95% CI between the outcomes of intervention and the control groups using the generic inverse-variance random effects model. Results: The meta-analysis of the 14 studies testing the acute effects of WG foods showed significant reductions of the post-prandial values of the glucose iAUC (0–120 min) by $-29.71$ mmol min/L (95% CI: $-43.57$, $-15.85$ mmol min/L), the insulin iAUC (0–120 min) by $-2.01$ nmol min/L (95% CI: $-2.88$, $-1.14$ nmol min/L), and the maximal glucose and insulin response. In 16 medium- and long-term RCTs, effects of WG foods on fasting glucose and insulin and homeostatic model assessment-insulin resistance values were not significant. Conclusions: The consumption of WG foods is able to improve acutely the postprandial glucose and insulin homeostasis compared to similar refined foods in healthy subjects. Further research is needed to better understand the long-term effects and the biological mechanisms.

**Keywords:** whole grain; glycemia; insulin; healthy subjects; meta-analysis; RTC

## 1. Introduction

Over the past decades, the burden of non-communicable chronic diseases, such as cardiovascular diseases (CVD), metabolic syndrome, diabetes and cancer, is rapidly increasing worldwide [1]. Non-communicable chronic diseases are generally preventable by managing modifiable risks factors, including dietary habits. Diet may play a key role in the promotion and maintenance of good health, but modern lifestyle is leading to a shifting away from traditional dietary patterns in favour of eating habits characterized by increased portion sizes, away-from-home foods, and unhealthy snacking. This process, known also as "Westernization" of the diet, is characterized by major consumption of refined sugars and fats, animal products and refined cereals, as well as decreased consumption of fruit, vegetable, and whole-grain (WG) cereals.

WG cereals contain all three parts of a natural grain kernel, including endosperm, germ, and bran and they are a rich source of dietary fibre, resistant starch, antioxidants, vitamins and minerals, such as folic acid, magnesium, and selenium [2]. The refinement process is performed by removing the bran and some of the germ, resulting in a loss of micronutrients and dietary fibre in favour of a softer texture and extended freshness. Thus, the endosperm alone, mainly composed of starchy carbohydrates, proteins, and small amounts of vitamins and minerals, is used to produce refined white flours.

There is growing evidence from both observational and intervention studies that WG cereals exert beneficial effects on human health [3]. WG food consumption has been associated with a modification of risk factors related to non-communicable chronic diseases, including post-prandial insulinaemic response, blood lipid profile, and intestinal microbiota [4–6]. A series of previous meta-analyses have shown a decreased risk of CVD [7], type-2 diabetes [8], metabolic syndrome [9], and cancer [10] associated with higher intake of WG foods. The mechanisms underlying the health benefits of WG foods may be explained, at least in part, by the high content of fibre that positively affects gut health (increasing transit time and faecal bulking). Moreover, other mechanisms, such as anti-inflammatory, antioxidant, hormonal (i.e., in hormone activation and synthesis of zinc, selenium, and nicotinic acid), anti-carcinogenic (i.e., content in phenolic compounds), and metabolic effects (i.e., vitamins and minerals), have to be considered [11].

A previous meta-analysis of 14 cohorts showed that WG food consumption was associated with lower fasting glucose and insulin concentrations independently from demographics and lifestyle factors, in non-diabetic European descents [12]. Although several clinical trials have been carried out to show the effects of WG consumption in healthy individuals, results are still conflicting. The aim of this study was to perform a meta-analysis of randomised controlled trials (RCT) to assess the acute and medium/long-term effect of WG foods on glycaemic control and insulin sensitivity in healthy individuals.

## 2. Methods

### 2.1. Search Strategy and Selection of the Studies

A search for all the published RCT on the effect of WG intake on glycaemic and insulin response was performed independently by three authors (J.G., C.V. and M.V.). Studies were identified from PubMed, Science Direct Online and The Cochrane Library up to December 2016. The search strategy included following key words: ("whole grain" or" whole meal" or "whole wheat" or "whole kernel") and ("blood glucose" or "HbA1c" or "glycated haemoglobin" or "fasting plasma glucose" or "glycolated haemoglobin" or "FBG" or "insulin" or "HOMA-IR"). The search was restricted to studies published in English. The reference list of the included studies was checked to identify relevant study not previously included. Inclusion criteria were: (i) studies conducted on healthy human subjects; (ii) parallel or crossover design; (iii) comparison of WG foods with foods with lower levels or no WG content; and (iv) presented means, standard deviations (SDs), or standards errors (SEs) at baseline and/or endpoint for the outcomes investigated. Exclusion criteria were the following: (i) studies with different design; (ii) studies evaluated only individual components of the grain; (iii) studies in which it was not possible to evaluate the WG foods effect because part of combined meals; and (iv) studies with fewer than 10 subjects in the intervention group.

### 2.2. Data Extraction and Study Quality

Data were independently extracted by three reviewers using a standard form. The information extracted included: first author and year of publication, country, study design, participant characteristics, number of subjects in comparison groups, type of WG foods, length of intervention, matching characteristics, and main results of the outcomes investigated. Primary outcomes consisted of changes from baseline in fasting glucose and insulin concentrations and in glucose and insulin incremental area under the curve (iAUC) values. Secondary outcomes included mean changes in HbA1c concentrations, peak and incremental glucose and insulin and homeostatic model assessment-insulin resistance (HOMA-IR) values. Changes from baseline were chosen as primary outcome as in many studies they were the only data presented, although this might not be the best approach (Bland and Altman).

The quality of each study was assessed following the principles of the Newcastle-Ottawa Quality Assessment Scale [13], consisting of 3 domains of quality as follows: selection (4 points), comparability (2 points), and outcome (3 points) for a total score of 9 points (9 representing the highest quality). Studies scoring 0–3 points, 3–6 points, and 7–9 points were identified as low, moderate, and high quality, respectively.

*2.3. Statistical Analysis*

In order to perform the comparison, all the values were converted to mmol/L for glucose concentrations and pmol/L for insulin concentrations. IAUC were converted to min x mmol/L for glucose iAUC values and min x nmol/L for insulin iAUC. When insulin was reported in μIU/mL (microunits of insulin per millilitre), a conversion factor of 6.945 was applied to convert to pmol/L (picomoles of insulin per litre) [14]. Change from baseline to endpoint was used for the analysis of fasting glucose, fasting insulin and HOMA-IR. When SD was not reported, it was derived from available data (95% confidence interval (CI), $p$-values, t or F statistics, and SE) using the method suggested by the Handbook for Systematic Review of Interventions [15]. When needed, the SD for changes from baseline was imputed using a pooled correlation coefficient according to a published procedure [15]. When it was not possible, a correlation coefficient of 0.5 was applied for imputing missing SDs, as it is a conservative value between 0 and 1. End-of-treatment values were used for glucose and insulin iAUC while data on HbA1 were insufficient to perform a meta-analysis. Results of trials containing multiple intervention or control arms were reported separately. Effect size consisted of mean difference (MD) and 95% CI between the outcomes of intervention and the control groups using the generic inverse-variance random effects model. A two-sided $p$-value 0.05 was considered statistically significant. Heterogeneity between trial results was tested using the $I^2$ statistic [16] and a value over 50% indicated a significant level of heterogeneity. Stability of results and possible source of heterogeneity between the studies was explored through sensitivity analyses by excluding results of one study at the time. In the analysis where SDs changes form baseline were imputed, a sensitivity analysis using also a 0.25 and a 0.75 correlation coefficients were performed to confirm the results. Moreover, subgroup analyses were used to evaluate the influence of some factors, including study design, geographical area, length of the study, and weight status. Publication bias was examined by visual inspection of the funnel plots. The analyses were carried out using Review Manager version 5.2 (RevMan 5.2, The Nordic Cochrane Centre, The Cochrane Collaboration, Copenhagen, Denmark).

## 3. Results

*3.1. Study Selection and Main Characteristics*

The flow chart of the search strategy is showed in Figure 1. From the initial 875 studies, a total of 51 articles were considered for the full-text examination. After the exclusion of 10 studies, 41 articles met the inclusion criteria for the qualitative analysis, while 30 were included in the quantitative meta-analysis.

Table 1 shows the characteristics of the 41 RCTs, which included 1033 healthy subjects (587 males and 682 females). Trials were conducted across 10 countries, including Sweden (eight trials) [17–24], Finland (five trial) [25–29], Canada (five trials) [30–34], UK (five trials) [4,35–38], Australia (three trial) [39–41], Denmark (three trials) [42–44], Italy (three trials) [5,45,46], USA (three trials) [47–49], Germany (one trial) [50], Japan (one trial) [51], Kuwait (one trial) [52], Singapore (one trial) [53], Spain (one trial) [54] and Switzerland (one trial) [55]. Five studies [35,37,42,45,47] had a parallel design and 36 [4,5,17–34,36,38–41,43,44,46,48–55] had a cross-over design. Twenty-five studies [17–22,24–34,40,41,43,44,46,49,52–54] evaluated the effects of the consumption of a single WG meal in an acute study, while 16 studies [4,5,23,32,35–42,45,47,48,50,51,55] evaluated the effects of a medium/long-term consumption in a RCT study with an intervention period ranging from two weeks to 16 weeks (median six weeks). The totality of the study included scored high quality. Even though studies were conducted on healthy individuals, 22 enrolled normal weight individuals [17–22,24–26,31,34,40,41,43,44,46,49,51–55], 11 overweight individuals [5,23,27–30,32,36–38,47], and seven obese individuals [33,35,39,42,45,48,50].

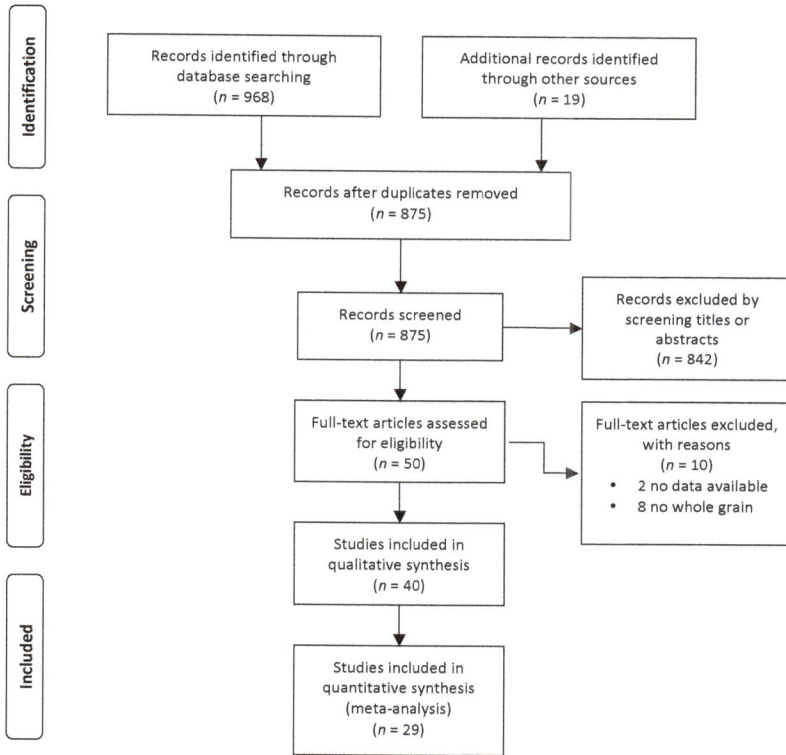

**Figure 1.** PRISMA flowchart indicating the results of the search strategy.

In the studies evaluating the acute effects of the consumption of a single WG meal, a wide variety of different meals were compared with control meals including mainly white wheat bread (Table 1). As regards medium/long-term RCT in 12 studies [5,23,35–41,48,50,51,55], participants consumed a diet in which food with refined cereals were substituted with WG foods, while in four studies the intervention groups were invited to consume WG sourdough bread [32], WG biscuits [45], WG breakfast cereals [4] or WG oats [47] during the normal diet.

**Table 1.** Characteristics and main findings of the clinical trials evaluating the effects of WG consumption in healthy subjects.

| Author, Year (Reference) | Country | Design (Washout or Arms) | Participants, Age, Year | BMI, kg/m² | Test Meals | Matching | Duration | Outcomes Evaluated | Main Results | Study Quality |
|---|---|---|---|---|---|---|---|---|---|---|
| **Acute Effect** | | | | | | | | | | |
| Stefoska-Needham, 2016 | Australia | C (3d) | 40 (20M/20F), 29.3 | 23.4 | I: Whole sorghum biscuits C: Wheat biscuits | none | - | Glucose and insulin iAUC | Greater insulin response (iAUC 4 h) after the red sorghum biscuit | No data |
| Gonzalez-Anton, 2015 | Spain | C (1w) | 23 (13M/10F), 25 ± 1 | 23.3 ± 0.5 | I: Wholemeal C: WWB | 50 g of available carbohydrates | - | Glucose and insulin iAUC | There were no differences in glucose and insulin iAUC | |
| Johansson, 2015 | Sweden | C (6d) | 23 (7M/16F), 60.1 ± 12.1 | 23.8 ± 3.4 | I: uRCB I2: RCB C: WCB | none | - | Glucose and insulin iAUC | Insulin response was lower for RCB (10%) and uRCB (21%) compared with WCB | TOTAL AUC |
| Mofidi, 2015 | Canada | C (1w) | 12M, 54.9 ± 2.0 | 29.1 ± 1.1 | I1: 11-grain I2: Sprouted-grain I3: 12-grain C: WBB | 50 g of available carbohydrates | - | Insulin iAUC | Only sprouted-grain improved postprandial glucose and insulin response | |
| Soong, 2015 | Singapore | C (na) | 12 (4M/8F), 26.2 ± 5.3 | 20.2 ± 1.7 | I1: WG barley flour I2: WG oat flour I3: WG yellow corn flour C: Refined wheat flour | 50 g of available carbohydrates | - | Glucose peak and iAUC | Improved postprandial glucose response for I1 and I2 but not for I3 | |
| Zafar, 2015 | Kuwait | C (na) | 13F, 21.4 ± 2.3 | 23.6 ± 2.4 | I: WGB C: WWB | 25 g available carbohydrate | - | Glucose peak and iAUC | Lower glucose peak and iAUC | |
| Luhovyy, 2014 | Canada | C (na) | 30M, 22.9 ± 0.6 | 22.6 ± 0.3 | I1: WG maize (high) I2: WG maize (low) C: Cookies | none | - | Glucose iAUC | Reduction in postprandial glucose response | |
| Moazzami, 2014 | Finland | C (1-2w) | 20F, 61.0 ± 4.8 | 26.0 ± 2.5 | I: WRB C: WWB | 50 g of available carbohydrates | - | Glucose and insulin iAUC | Improved postprandial insulin response but not glucose response | 15 |
| Poquette, 2014 | USA | C (1w) | 10M, 25.1 ± 4.0 | 24.2 ± 2.8 | I: Sorghum flour C: Wheat flour | 50 g of total starch | - | Glucose and insulin iAUC | Improved postprandial glucose and insulin response | 15 |
| Lappi, 2013 | Finland | C (3d) | 15 (6M/9F), 57 | 26 | I: WRB C: WWB | 50 g of available carbohydrates | - | Glucose and insulin iAUC | Improved postprandial insulin response but not glucose response | 15 |
| Keogh, 2011 | Australia | C (2d) | 10F, 29.4 | 21.8 | I: WGB C: WWB | none | - | Glucose and insulin iAUC | Improved postprandial glucose and insulin response | |
| Vuksan, 2010 | Canada | C (2d) | 11 (6M/5F), 30 ± 3.6 | 22.3 ± 2.8 | I1: WG low I2: WG intermediate I3: WG high C: WWB | 50 g of available carbohydrates | - | Glucose iAUC | Reduction in postprandial glucose response | |

**Table 1.** *Cont.*

| Author, Year (Reference) | Country | Design (Washout or Arms) | Participants, Age, Year | BMI, kg/m² | Test Meals | Matching | Duration | Outcomes Evaluated | Main Results | Study Quality |
|---|---|---|---|---|---|---|---|---|---|---|
| Rosén, 2011 | Sweden | C (1w) | 10 (5M/5F), 26.0 ± 1.1 | 22.6 ± 0.4 | I1: WGRB, I2: WGRB-lac, I3: RK, I4: WK, C: WWB | 50 g of available carbohydrates | - | Glucose and insulin total AUC, incremental glucose and insulin peak | Lower early glucose responses (0–60 min), insulin response and incremental glucose and insulin peak | 15 |
| Kristensen, 2010 | Denmark | C (na) | 16 (6M/10F), 24.1 ± 3.8 | 21.7 ± 2.2 | I1: WGB, I2: WGP, C: WWB and pasta | 50 g of available carbohydrates | - | Glucose iAUC | No differences between any WG product and R product | 15 |
| Hlebowicz, 2009 | Sweden | C (1w) | 10 (3M/7F), 26 ± 1 | 24.1 ± 0.8 | I: WRB, C: WWB | 50 g of available carbohydrates | - | Glucose iAUC | No differences between WG product and R product | 15 |
| Najjar, 2009 | Canada | C (>1w) | 10M, 59 ± 2.41 | 30.8 ± 0.95 | I1: WGB, I2: WG barley, C: WWB | 50 g of available carbohydrates | - | Glucose and insulin AUC | No differences between WG product and R product | 15 |
| Rosén, 2009 | Sweden | C (1w) | 12 (9M/3F), 25.3 ± 0.8 | 23.1 ± 0.6 | I1: WGRB, I2: WGRB-lac, I3: WGRP, C: WWB | 40 g of available carbohydrates | - | Glucose and insulin iAUC | Improved postprandial glucose and insulin response for WG products | 15 |
| Alminger, 2008 | Sweden | C (1w) | 13 (9F/4M), 56 ± 13.2 | 24.4 ± 2.6 | I1: Oat, I2: Barley, C: Glucose load | 25 g of available carbohydrates | - | Glucose and insulin iAUC | Improved postprandial glucose and insulin response for WG products | 15 |
| Nilsson, 2008 | Sweden | C (>3d) | 12 (7M/5F), 28.3 ± 5.1 | 22.1 ± 2.0 | I1: WK, I2: RK, I3: Oat kernels, I4: Barley kernels, I5: WG barley porridge, C: WWB | 50 g of available carbohydrates | - | Glucose iAUC | Improved postprandial glucose response for RK and barley kernels consumption | 15 |
| Hlebowicz, 2007 | Sweden | C (>1w) | 12 (6M/6F), 28 ± 4 | 22 ± 2 | I1: WG oat flakes, C: Cornflakes | None | - | Glucose iAUC | No differences between WG product and R product | 15 |
| Casiraghi, 2006 | Italy | C (2w) | 10 (5M/5F), 25.4 ± 0.5 | 22.6 ± 0.7 | I1: WWBCr, I2: WWBc, I3: BCr, I4: BC, C: WWB | 40 g of available carbohydrates | - | Glucose and insulin iAUC | Improved postprandial glucose and insulin response for WG products | 15 |
| Bakhøj, 2003 | Denmark | C (1w) | 11M, 25 ± 2 | 23 ± 4 | I1: Einkorn honey–salt, I2: Einkorn crushed, C: Wheat | 50 g of available carbohydrates | - | Glucose and insulin total AUC | No differences between WG product and R product | 15 |
| Juntunen, 2003 | Finland | C (1–2w) | 19F, 61 ± 4.8 | 26 ± 2.5 | I1: WRB, I2: High-fibre rye bread, C: WWB | 50 g of available carbohydrates | - | Glucose and insulin iAUC, maximal glucose and insulin response | Improved postprandial insulin response for WRB intake and maximal insulin response for both WRB and High-fibre rye bread. No differences for glucose iAUC and maximal response for any WG products | 15 |

**Table 1.** *Cont.*

| Author, Year (Reference) | Country | Design (Washout or Arms) | Participants, Age, Year | BMI, kg/m² | Test Meals | Matching | Duration | Outcomes Evaluated | Main Results | Study Quality |
|---|---|---|---|---|---|---|---|---|---|---|
| Juntunen, 2002 | Finland | C (1–2w) | 20 (10M/10F), 28.5 ± 1.8 | 22.9 ± 1 | I1: WKRB; I2: β-glucan rye bread; I3: WGP; C: WWB | 50 g of available carbohydrates | - | Maximal glucose and insulin response | Improved maximal glucose response for WGP and improved maximal insulin response for all the WG meals | 15 |
| Leinonnen, 1999 | Finland | C (na) | 20 (10M/10F), M 32 ± 3, F 27 ± 5 | M 24.5 ± 2.2; F 20.3 ± 1.1 | I1: WKRB; I2: WRB; I3: WRC; C: WWB | 50 g of available carbohydrates | - | Glucose and insulin iAUC, maximal glucose and insulin response | Improved insulin iAUC and maximal response for WKRB intake. No differences for glucose iAUC and maximal response for any WG products | 15 |
| Medium-long term effect | | | | | | | | | | |
| Ampatzoglou, 2015a | UK | C (4w) | 33 (12M/21F), 48.8 ± 1.1 | 27.9 ± 0.7 | I: WG pasta, rice, snacks, breakfast cereals; C: RG pasta, rice, snacks, breakfast cereals | isoenergetic (2000 kcal/day) | 6w | Fasting glucose | Fasting glucose did not differ between groups | 14 |
| Ampatzoglou, 2015b | UK | C (4w) | 33 (12M/21F), 48.8 ± 1.1 | 27.9 ± 0.7 | I: WG pasta, rice, snacks, breakfast cereals; C: RG pasta, rice, snacks, breakfast cereals | isoenergetic (2000 kcal/day) | 6w | Fasting insulin | Fasting insulin did not differ between groups | 14 |
| Vitaglione, 2015 | Italy | P (2 arms) | 68 (23M/45F), I: 40 ± 2, C: 37 ± 2 | I: 30.0 ± 0.5, C: 29.5 ± 0.4 | I: 3 WG biscuits; C: 1 package of crackers and 3 slices of toasted bread | isoenergetic (1500 kcal/day) | 8w | Fasting glucose and insulin | Fasting glucose and insulin did not differ between groups | 13 |
| Kristensen, 2012 | Denmark | P (2 arms) | 72F, I: 60.3 ± 5.3, C: 59.1 ± 5.6 | I: 30.4 ± 0.6, C: 30.0 ± 0.4 | I: WG pasta, bread and biscuits; C: RG pasta, bread and biscuits | hypocaloric (300–1200 kcal/day) | 12w | Fasting glucose and insulin, HOMA and HbA1c | HbA1c, fasting glucose and insulin, and HOMA did not differ between groups | 14 |
| MacKay, 2012 | Canada | C (4–5w) | 14 (10M/4F), 53 ± 6.0 | 26.5 ± 2.9 | I: WG sourdough bread; C: WWB | isoenergetic | 6w | Fasting glucose and insulin and HOMA | Fasting glucose and insulin and HOMA did not differ between groups | 13 |
| Ross, 2011 | Switzerland | C (5–7w) | 17 (6M/11F), M 36.5 ± 4.2, F 34.1 ± 3.0 | M 24.5 ± 0.6, F 23.1 ± 0.8 | I: WG pasta, rice, snacks and breakfast cereals; C: RG pasta, rice, snacks and breakfast cereals | isoenergetic (2000 kcal/day) | 2w | Fasting glucose | Fasting glucose did not differ between groups | 13 |
| Brownlee, 2010 | UK | P (3 arms) | 266 (132M/134F), 45.7 ± 10 | I: 30.0 ± 3.7, C: 30.3 ± 4.5 | I: WG pasta, rice, snacks and breakfast cereals; C: RG pasta, rice, snacks and breakfast cereals | none | 16w | Fasting glucose and insulin | Fasting glucose did not differ between groups | 14 |
| Giacco, 2010 | Italy | C (none) | 15 (12M/3F), 54.5 ± 7.6 | 27.4 ± 3.0 | I: WG bread, pasta, rusks and crackers; C: RG bread, pasta, rusks and crackers | isoenergetic (2000 kcal/day) | 3w | Fasting glucose and insulin and HOMA | Fasting glucose and insulin and HOMA did not differ between groups | 14 |

**Table 1.** *Cont.*

| Author, Year (Reference) | Country | Design (Washout or Arms) | Participants, Age, Year | BMI, kg/m² | Test Meals | Matching | Duration | Outcomes Evaluated | Main Results | Study Quality |
|---|---|---|---|---|---|---|---|---|---|---|
| Tighe, 2010 | UK | P (3 arms) | 206 (104M/102F), I1: 51.6 ± 0.8 I2: 52.1 ± 0.9 C: 51.8 ± 0.83 | I1: 28.0 ± 0.5; I2: 27.0 ± 0.4 C: 28.0 ± 0.5 | I1: WG bread and WG cereals I2: WG wheat food plus oat C: RG bread and cereals | isoenergetic (2100 kcal/day) | 16w | Fasting glucose and insulin and HOMA | Fasting glucose and insulin and HOMA did not differ between groups | 13 |
| Costabile, 2008 | UK | C (2w) | 31 (15M/16F), 25 | 20–30 range | I: WG cereals C: Wheat bran cereals | 48 g/day portion | 3w | Fasting glucose and insulin | No significant differences were observed | |
| Anderson, 2007 | Sweden | C (6–8w) | 30 (8M/22F), 59 ± 5 | 28.3 ± 2.0 30.0 ± 4.0 C; | I1: WG bread, crispbread, muesli, pasta, pancakes, scones, pie, pizza C: RG bread, crispbread, muesli, pasta, pancakes, scones, pie, pizza | isoenergetic (2100 kcal/day) | 6w | Fasting glucose and insulin | Fasting glucose and insulin did not differ between groups | 12 |
| Rave, 2007 | Germany | C (2w) | 31 (13M/18F), 51 ± 13 | 33.9 ± 2.3 | I: WG C: MR | isoenergetic (1700 kcal/day) | 4w | Fasting glucose and insulin, HOMA | HOMA, fasting glucose and insulin did not differ between groups | |
| Li, 2003 | Japan | C (4w) | 10F, 20.4 ± 1.3 | 19.2 ± 2.0 | I: Barley diet C: standard diet | isoenergetic (1900 kcal/day) | 4w | Fasting glucose and HbA1 | Fasting glucose and HbA1 did not differ between group | 15 |
| McIntosh, 2003 | Australia | C (none) | 28M, range 40–65 | 30 ± 0.9 | I1: WG bread, crispbread and breakfast cereal I2: WG rye bread, rye crispbread and rye breakfast cereal C: WWB, RG crispbread and rice cereal | isoenergetic (2300 kcal/day) | 4w | Fasting glucose and insulin | Fasting glucose and insulin were lower in the WG groups | 13 |
| Pereira, 2002 | USA | C (6–9w) | 11 (5M-6f), 41.6 ± 2.67 | 30.2 ± 1.01 | I: WG pasta, rice, snacks, breakfast cereals C: RG pasta, rice, snacks, breakfast cereals | isoenergetic (2000 kcal/day) | 6w | Fasting glucose and insulin and HOMA | Fasting insulin and HOMA were significantly lower in the WG group | 13 |
| Saltzman, 2001 | USA | P (2 arms) | 43 (20M/23F), I: 45.1 ± 22.7 C: 44.1 ± 21.3 | I: 26.1 ± 3.4 C: 26.7 ± 3.2 | I: Standard diet plus WG oat C: Standard diet | hypocaloric (1900 kcal/day) | 6w | Fasting glucose and insulin and HOMA | Fasting glucose and insulin and HOMA did not differ between groups | 15 |

BC, barley crackers; BCr, barley crackers; C, control; HOMA, homeostatic model assessment; I, intervention; iAUC: incremental area under the curve; na, not available; RCB, fermented whole grain rye crisp bread; RG, refined grain; RK, rye kernels; uRCB, Unfermented whole grain rye crisp bread; WCB, refined wheat crisp bread; WG, Whole grain; WGB, whole grain bread; WGRB, whole grain rye bread; WGRB-lac, whole grain rye bread with lactic acid; WGRP, whole grain rye porridge; WGP, whole grain pasta; WK, wholegrain wheat kernels; WKRB, whole kernel rye bread; WRB, Whole rye bread; WRC, Whole rye Crispbread; WWB: white wheat bread; WWBc, whole-wheat cookies; WWBCr, whole-wheat crackers.

## 3.2. Acute Studies

### 3.2.1. Glucose iAUC

Fourteen studies reported data on glucose iAUC, two of which relative to the time period 0–90 min [24,52], 10 to the time period 0–120 min (145 subjects) [18–21,31,34,40,46,53,54], four to the time period 0–180 min (61 subjects) [25,27,43,49], and two to the time period 0–240 [28,41]. Four studies were not reported because there was no information on the AUC calculation or because of different type of AUC was used [17,29,33,44]. Six studies [24,28,34,41,44] did not present relevant data for the meta-analysis.

Plasma glucose concentrations after the WG meal for the time periods 0–120 min were lower compared with the control meal (MD = −29.71 mmol min/L, 95% CI: −43.57, −15.85 mmol min/L; Figure 2). Significant heterogeneity was found between studies ($I^2$ = 80%; $p$ <0.001).

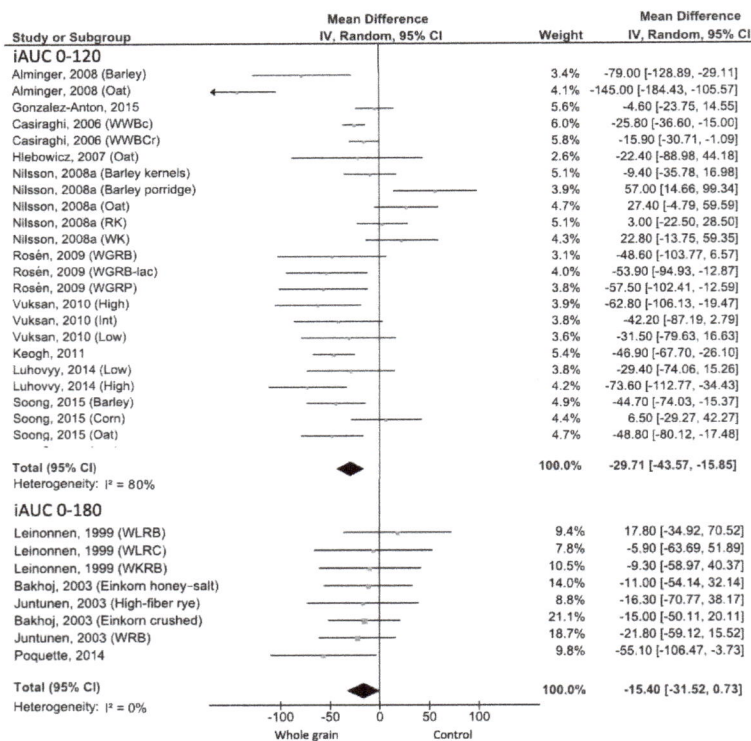

**Figure 2.** Forest plot of the meta-analysis carried out to investigate the effect of whole grain consumption on glucose iAUC. iAUC: incremental area under the curve; WWBc, whole-wheat cookies; WWBCr, whole-wheat crackers RK, rye kernels; WK, wholegrain wheat kernels; WGRB, whole grain rye bread; WGRB-lac, whole grain rye bread with lactic acid; WGRP, whole grain rye porridge; WLRB, wholemeal rye bread; WLRC, wholemeal rye crispbread; WKRB, whole kernel rye bread; WRB, Whole rye bread.

The visual inspection of the funnel plot showed asymmetry due to the study of Alminger et al. [18] (Supplementary Materials, Figure S1). Heterogeneity was reduced to 40% ($p$ = 0.06) when three studies were excluded [18,20,54], with no change in the results (MD = −36.46 mmol min/L, 95% CI: −46.80, −26.12 mmol min/L), despite no substantial differences between these three studies and the others have been observed. These results did not achieve statistical significance in the 0–180 min analysis (MD = −15.40 mmol min/L, 95% CI: −31.52, 0.73 mmol min/L; Figure 2) with no evidence of heterogeneity ($I^2$ = 0%, $p$ = 0.76).

Among the excluded studies, glucose response after consumption of the WG meal did not significantly differ from the refined grain meal across all the studies (Table 1).

### 3.2.2. Insulin iAUC

Insulin iAUC 0–120 min was evaluated in 5 studies [17,18,21,40,54] (58 subjects), while 8 studies [25,27,29,30,33,43,46,49] evaluated the iAUC 0–180 min (83 subjects). Two studies reported data on insulin iAUC relative to the time period 0–240 min [28,41] and were excluded from the analysis. Three studies were excluded because there was no information on the AUC calculation or because of different type of AUC was used [17,29,33].

The WG products induced significantly lower 0–120 min incremental areas than foods with lower amount or no WG foods (MD = −2.01 nmol min/L, 95% CI: −2.88, −1.14 nmol min/L; Figure 3), with no evidence of heterogeneity ($I^2$ = 0%; $p$ = 0.49). In the studies evaluating the iAUC 0–180 min, a significant insulin iAUC reduction with no evidence of heterogeneity was found (MD = −3.64 nmol min/L, 95% CI: −5.00, −2.28 nmol min/L; $I^2$ = 1%, $p$ = 0.44; Figure 3). Four [17,28,29,41] out of the five excluded trials showed a significantly smaller iAUC for the WG consumption in comparison with the WWB, while one study [33] found no difference between the WG and refined grain meals.

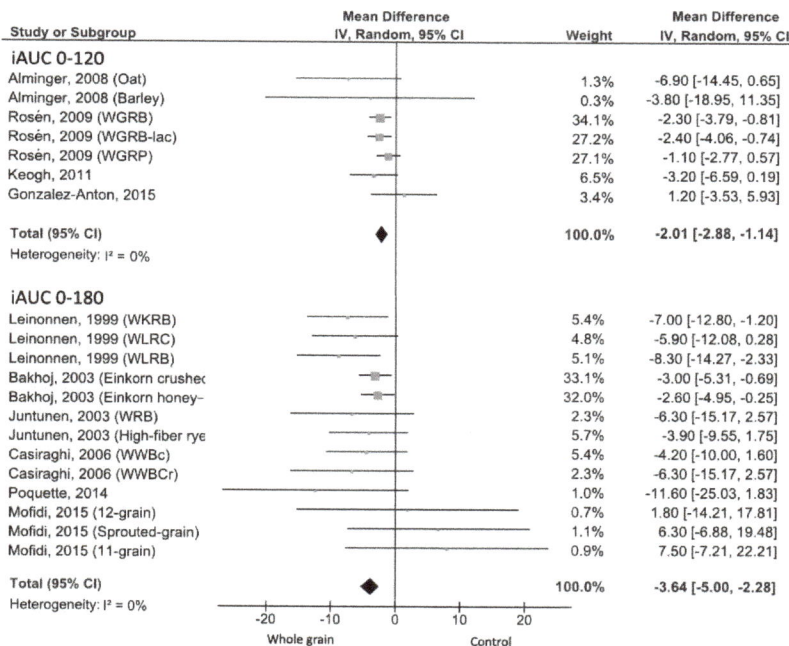

| Study or Subgroup | Mean Difference IV, Random, 95% CI | Weight | Mean Difference IV, Random, 95% CI |
|---|---|---|---|
| **iAUC 0-120** | | | |
| Alminger, 2008 (Oat) | | 1.3% | -6.90 [-14.45, 0.65] |
| Alminger, 2008 (Barley) | | 0.3% | -3.80 [-18.95, 11.35] |
| Rosén, 2009 (WGRB) | | 34.1% | -2.30 [-3.79, -0.81] |
| Rosén, 2009 (WGRB-lac) | | 27.2% | -2.40 [-4.06, -0.74] |
| Rosén, 2009 (WGRP) | | 27.1% | -1.10 [-2.77, 0.57] |
| Keogh, 2011 | | 6.5% | -3.20 [-6.59, 0.19] |
| Gonzalez-Anton, 2015 | | 3.4% | 1.20 [-3.53, 5.93] |
| **Total (95% CI)** | | **100.0%** | **-2.01 [-2.88, -1.14]** |
| Heterogeneity: $I^2$ = 0% | | | |
| | | | |
| **iAUC 0-180** | | | |
| Leinonnen, 1999 (WKRB) | | 5.4% | -7.00 [-12.80, -1.20] |
| Leinonnen, 1999 (WLRC) | | 4.8% | -5.90 [-12.08, 0.28] |
| Leinonnen, 1999 (WLRB) | | 5.1% | -8.30 [-14.27, -2.33] |
| Bakhoj, 2003 (Einkorn crushed) | | 33.1% | -3.00 [-5.31, -0.69] |
| Bakhoj, 2003 (Einkorn honey-) | | 32.0% | -2.60 [-4.95, -0.25] |
| Juntunen, 2003 (WRB) | | 2.3% | -6.30 [-15.17, 2.57] |
| Juntunen, 2003 (High-fiber rye) | | 5.7% | -3.90 [-9.55, 1.75] |
| Casiraghi, 2006 (WWBc) | | 5.4% | -4.20 [-10.00, 1.60] |
| Casiraghi, 2006 (WWBCr) | | 2.3% | -6.30 [-15.17, 2.57] |
| Poquette, 2014 | | 1.0% | -11.60 [-25.03, 1.83] |
| Mofidi, 2015 (12-grain) | | 0.7% | 1.80 [-14.21, 17.81] |
| Mofidi, 2015 (Sprouted-grain) | | 1.1% | 6.30 [-6.88, 19.48] |
| Mofidi, 2015 (11-grain) | | 0.9% | 7.50 [-7.21, 22.21] |
| **Total (95% CI)** | | **100.0%** | **-3.64 [-5.00, -2.28]** |
| Heterogeneity: $I^2$ = 0% | | | |

**Figure 3.** Forest plot of the meta-analysis carried out to investigate the effect of whole grain consumption on insulin iAUC. iAUC: incremental area under the curve; WGRB, whole grain rye bread; WGRB-lac, whole grain rye bread with lactic acid; WGRP, whole grain rye porridge; WKRB, whole kernel rye bread; WLRB, wholemeal rye bread; WLRC, wholemeal rye crispbread; WRB, Whole rye bread; WWBc, whole-wheat cookies; WWBCr, whole-wheat crackers.

### 3.2.3. Maximal Glucose and Insulin Response

Four studies [25–27,53] for a total of 71 subjects and 11 different test meals considered maximal glucose and insulin response incremental as outcome. The meta-analysis showed a significantly lower maximal glucose response (MD = −0.25 mmol/L, 95% CI: −0.43, −0.06 mmol/L) with low evidence of heterogeneity ($I^2$ = 40%; $p$ = 0.08) for the experimental compared with control groups (Figure 4). Concerning the study of Zafar et al. [52], blood glucose concentrations were significantly lower after WG products compared to refined food, however it was excluded from the analysis due to the lack of data. As regards maximal insulin responses, all test meals products induced a lower maximal insulin response with a MD of −73.78 pmol/L (95% CI: −108.56, −38.99 pmol/L) and moderate evidence of heterogeneity ($I^2$ = 49%; $p$ = 0.05; Figure 4).

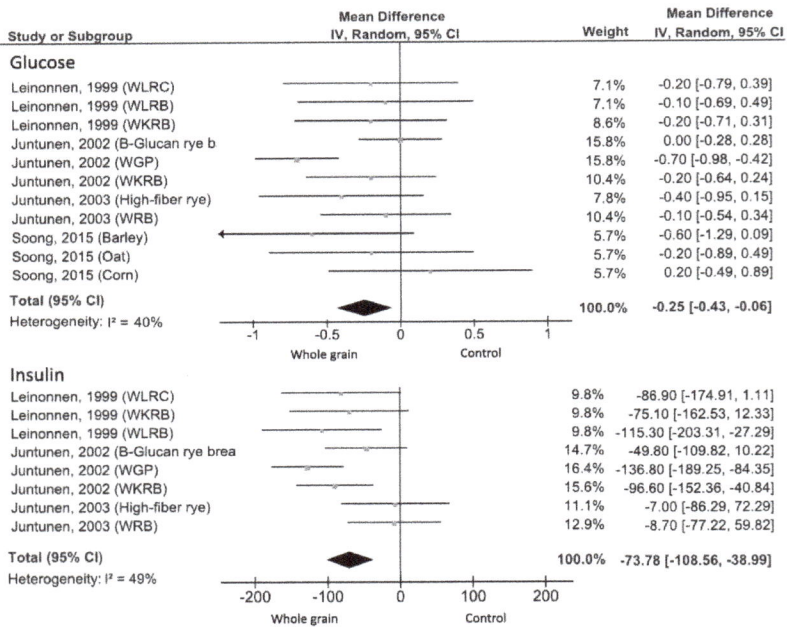

**Figure 4.** Forest plot of the meta-analysis carried out to investigate the effect of whole grain consumption on maximal glucose and insulin response. WLRC, wholemeal rye crispbread; WLRB, wholemeal rye bread; WKRB, whole kernel rye bread; WGP, whole grain pasta; WKRB, whole kernel rye bread; WRB, Whole rye bread.

### 3.3. Medium- and Long-Term Studies

### 3.3.1. Fasting Glucose

In total, 10 crossover studies [4,5,23,32,36,39,48,50,51,55] and five parallel studies [35,37,42,45,47] accounting for 773 subjects (325 males and 448 females) reported fasting glucose outcomes for medium- and long-term WG meals intake. Two studies [4,39] were excluded because baseline fasting glucose values were not reported. When the results from all of the studies were grouped in a meta-analysis, there was no summary effect on fasting glucose in the WG group compared to the control group (MD = −0.04 mmol/L, 95% CI: −0.13, 0.04 mmol/L) with no significant evidence of heterogeneity ($I^2$ = 33%; $p$ = 0.11; Figure 5). The visual inspection of the funnel plot showed asymmetry due to the study of Li et al. (Supplementary Material, Figure S2) [51]. Sensitivity analyses showed that, after excluding results of Vitaglione et al. [45], where subjects were selected specifically with unhealthy dietary and lifestyle behaviours, and Rave et al. [50], where participants were obese subjects with elevated fasting blood glucose, summary effect size resulted in a low significant reduction of fasting glucose in favour of the intervention group with no evidence of heterogeneity (MD = $-0.08$ mmol/L, 95% CI: $-0.16$, $-0.01$ mmol/L; $I^2 = 0\%$, $p = 0.72$).

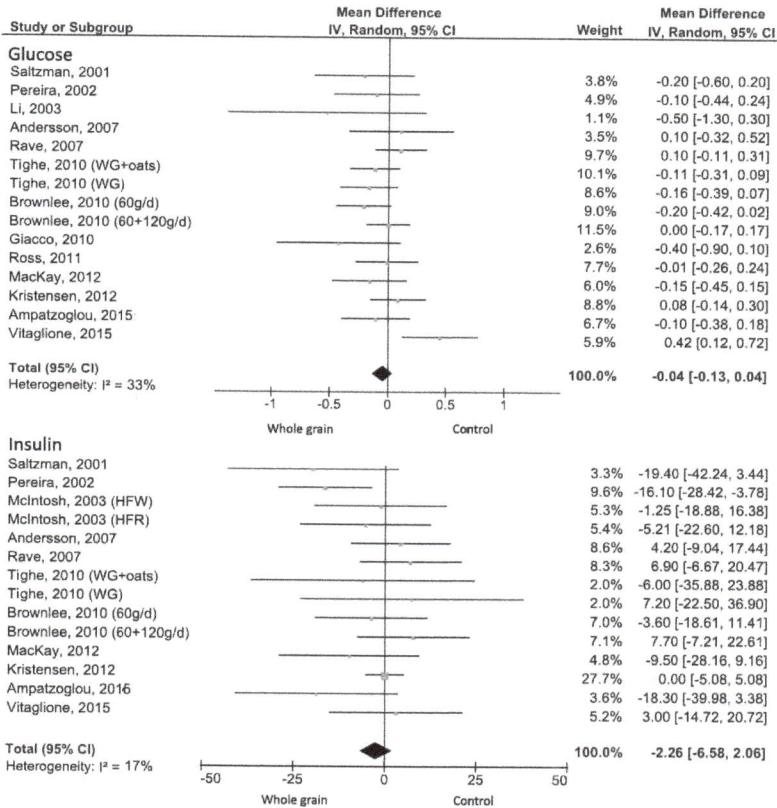

**Figure 5.** Forest plot of the meta-analysis carried out to investigate the effect of whole grain consumption on fasting glucose and insulin. WG, whole grain; HFW, high-fibre wheat; HFR, high-fibre rye.

### 3.3.2. Fasting Insulin

Plasma insulin was evaluated in 13 studies [4,5,23,32,35,37–39,42,45,47,48,50] with a total of 730 subjects (355 males and 375 females) and the meta-analysis was not significantly different in the WG group compared to the controls (MD= $-2.26$ pmol/L, 95% CI: $-6.58$, 2.06 pmol/L; $I^2 = 17\%$, $p = 0.27$; Figure 5). Two studies [4,5] were excluded for the lack of baseline values.

### 3.3.3. HOMA-IR

Data on HOMA-IR were reported in seven studies [5,32,37,42,47,48,50] accounting for 377 healthy subjects (152 males and 225 females). The study of Giacco et al. [5] was excluded because of the lack of baseline values. The results of the meta-analysis showed no evidence of an effect on HOMA-IR for the medium- and long-term WG consumption compared to the control group (MD = $-0.18$, 95% CI:

−0.48, 0.13) with no significant evidence of heterogeneity ($I^2 = 35\%$; $p = 0.16$; Figure 6). Sensitivity analyses showed that the exclusion of two studies [42,50] changed the summary effect size from non-significant to significant (MD = −0.39, 95% CI: −0.69, −0.08; $I^2 = 0\%$, $p = 0.52$). A possible reason for heterogeneity relied on the fact that the intervention, in both studies, was conducted in the context of a strict hypocaloric diet.

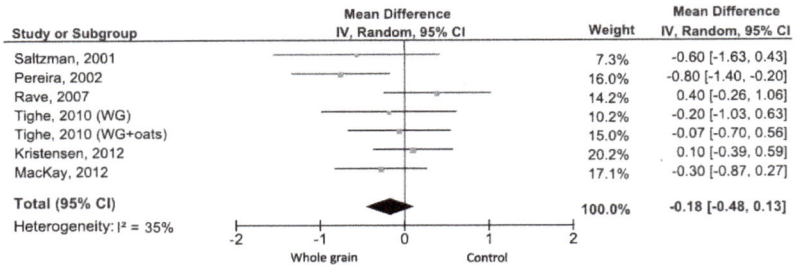

| Study or Subgroup | Mean Difference IV, Random, 95% CI | Weight | Mean Difference IV, Random, 95% CI |
|---|---|---|---|
| Saltzman, 2001 | | 7.3% | -0.60 [-1.63, 0.43] |
| Pereira, 2002 | | 16.0% | -0.80 [-1.40, -0.20] |
| Rave, 2007 | | 14.2% | 0.40 [-0.26, 1.06] |
| Tighe, 2010 (WG) | | 10.2% | -0.20 [-1.03, 0.63] |
| Tighe, 2010 (WG+oats) | | 15.0% | -0.07 [-0.70, 0.56] |
| Kristensen, 2012 | | 20.2% | 0.10 [-0.39, 0.59] |
| MacKay, 2012 | | 17.1% | -0.30 [-0.87, 0.27] |
| Total (95% CI) | | 100.0% | -0.18 [-0.48, 0.13] |
| Heterogeneity: I² = 35% | | | |

**Figure 6.** Forest plot of the meta-analysis carried out to investigate the effect of whole grain consumption on HOMA-IR. WG, whole grain.

### 3.3.4. Subgroup Analyses

Table 2 shows the results of categorical subgroup analyses for the effect of medium- and long-term consumption of wholegrain meals on fasting glucose and insulin. The subgroup analyses of fasting glucose concentrations indicated that the overall outcome of fasting glucose did not differ between subgroups. Instead, a significant reduction in fasting insulin concentrations were observed for studies not conducted in the European region (MD = −10.71 pmol/L, 95% CI: −18.19, −3.24 pmol/L). No significant heterogeneity was observed across the studies ($I^2 = 0\%$). The sensitivity analysis of the duration subgroups resulted in a significant lower fasting insulin (MD = −8.17 pmol/L, 95% CI: −15.24, −1.10 pmol/L; $I^2 = 19\%$, $p = 0.28$) after the removing of the study of Rave et al. [50], which was conducted on obese subjects with elevated fasting blood glucose.

**Table 2.** Subgroup analyses of medium- and long-term wholegrain intake effect on fasting glucose and insulin.

| | Glucose | | | | Insulin | | | |
|---|---|---|---|---|---|---|---|---|
| | No. of Datasets | OR (95% CI) | Heterogeneity $I^2$ (%) | $p$ | No. of Datasets | OR (95% CI) | Heterogeneity $I^2$ (%) | $p$ |
| **Study design** | | | | | | | | |
| Parallel | 8 | −0.03 (−0.17, 0.11) | 58 | 0.03 | 7 | −0.14 (−4.40, 4.12) | 0 | 0.61 |
| Crossover | 8 | −0.04 (−0.15, 0.07) | 0 | 0.49 | 6 | −4.76 (−12.37, 2.86) | 38 | 0.14 |
| **Geographical area** | | | | | | | | |
| Europe | 11 | −0.02 (−0.12, 0.08) | 44 | 0.06 | 8 | 0.78 (−3.09, 4.66) | 0 | 0.80 |
| Other | 4 | −0.17 (−0.36, 0.02) | 0 | 0.84 | 5 | −10.71 (−18.19, −3.24) | 0 | 0.59 |
| **BMI category** | | | | | | | | |
| Normal/overweight | 9 | −0.12 (−0.22, −0.02) | 0 | 0.83 | 5 | −3.15 (−12.14, 5.84) | 2 | 0.40 |
| Obese | 5 | 0.04 (−0.11, 0.19) | 58 | 0.04 | 8 | −1.17 (−6.21, 3.86) | 23 | 0.25 |
| **Duration** | | | | | | | | |
| ≤6 weeks | 10 | −0.05 (−0.16, 0.05) | 0 | 0.54 | 8 | −5.93 (−13.31, 1.44) | 13 | 0.38 |
| >6 weeks | 5 | −0.01 (−0.16, 0.13) | 64 | 0.02 | 6 | 0.56 (−3.78, 5.89) | 0 | 0.89 |

## 4. Discussion

The present study showed significant advantages in iAUC peak and incremental, both for post-prandial glucose and insulin in favour of the WG compared to control meals in acute studies.

In some studies, benefits on glycaemic excursions [20,56], feeling of fullness, lower feeling of hunger and lower desire to eat [22] were found after the consumption of a WG meal. Overall, these results contribute to explain, from a mechanistic point of view, the association between WG food consumption and lower risk of type-2 diabetes [57], metabolic syndrome [58], and CVD [59] in epidemiological studies. Diets rich in refined carbohydrates induce a rapid increase in blood glucose concentrations with a high demand for insulin from the pancreatic β-cells [60], which in turn may increase the risk of insulin resistance [61]. In contrast, WG cereals are able to acutely lower blood glucose levels, which may improve insulin sensitivity and beta-cell function.

In relation to the postprandial blood glucose response, the difference between WG and refined grain meals was more relevant and statistically significant when the two hours' response was evaluated. This is in line with other studies on the impact of different carbohydrates foods on postprandial blood glucose [62–64]. In fact, meal carbohydrates influence directly the early postprandial blood glucose response, whereas the late blood glucose levels are linked mainly to the hormonal (mainly insulin and glucagon) and metabolic (free fatty acids) response.

Results from medium and long-term trials showed no statistically significant difference in HOMA-IR, fasting plasma glucose and insulin levels after WG compared to refined grain meals. This is not in line with evidence reported in some cross-sectional studies [62,64]. However, after a sensitivity analysis with exclusion of studies including obese individuals with unhealthy dietary habits at baseline, both fasting plasma glucose and HOMA-IR showed a significant difference between WG and the control meal. This suggests that the evidence available from intervention trials on the long-term effects of WG is still inadequate to drawn definitive conclusions and the analysis on a more homogenous group of individuals might lead to more consistent results.

The possible mechanisms for the beneficial effects of WG foods include the slow rate of digestion and the fermentation of fibre and resistant starch by microbiota in the large intestine with the production of short-chain fatty acids (SCFA). SCFA in the liver increase glucose oxidation, decrease fatty acid release, and increase insulin clearance, thus improving glucose homeostasis and insulin sensitivity [65]. Moreover, the pancreatic beta cells are extremely sensible to oxidative damage [66] and could be protected by some antioxidants present in WG cereals, such as polyphenols (ferulic acid, lignans, and anthocyanins) and alkylresorcinols, demonstrated to be direct radical scavengers in animal models [67]. Nevertheless, the ability of WG cereals to improve glycaemic control may be related to the synergistic action of multiple compounds more than a single component [68].

The results of this meta-analysis should be considered in light of some limitations. First, the lack of a clear universal definition of the concept of WG food as well as the different properties of the source of dietary WG could lead to some bias. Separate investigations across the various whole grain foods produced from different crops may be useful to reduce heterogeneity and to obtain a more robust scientific evidence of the impact of WG from specific sources on glycaemic responses. Second, the sample sizes of some RCTs were relatively small and some of the variables analysed were not primary outcomes of the studies. Third, the imputation of SD could lead to a bias of the results. However, the sensitivity analyses imputing different values of correlation confirmed that the general results were robust. Fourth, several studies were not included due to the lack of available information necessary for the quantitative analysis; as some of these studies reported not significant results, the possibility of selection bias should be considered. Finally, only few studies reported HbA1c and no conclusions about the effect of WG foods on blood glucose levels over a period of time can be made.

In conclusion, the results of the present meta-analysis suggest that consumption of WG foods may improve acutely the postprandial glucose and insulin homeostasis compared to similar refined foods in healthy subjects. These effects, in addition to a better appetite regulation, need to be confirmed by future long-term studies designed ad hoc to test whether WG foods may contribute to reduce the risk of type 2 diabetes and other chronic diseases. Moreover, the results of the acute studies included in this meta-analysis relied mostly on studies evaluating the effects of oat, rye and barley; these cereals provide a relatively lower contribution to the overall cereal intake worldwide [69] than wheat. In fact,

*Nutrients* **2017**, *9*, 769

WG wheat products have a larger diffusion at the population level, at least in Western countries. Therefore, further research is needed to better understand the long-term effects and the biological mechanisms that underline the health benefits of WG food consumption.

**Supplementary Materials:** The following are available online at www.mdpi.com/2072-6643/9/7/769/s1.

**Acknowledgments:** No grants received in support of the present study.

**Conflicts of Interest:** The authors declare no conflict of interest.

## References

1.   World Health Organization. *World Health Statistics*; World Health Organization: Geneva, Switzerland, 2009.
2.   Slavin, J.L. Why wholegrains are protective: Biological mechanisms. *Proc. Nutr. Soc.* **2003**, *62*, 129–134. [CrossRef] [PubMed]
3.   Seal, C.J.; Brownlee, I.A. Whole-grain foods and chronic disease: Evidence from epidemiological and intervention studies. *Proc. Nutr. Soc.* **2015**, *74*, 313–319. [CrossRef] [PubMed]
4.   Costabile, A.; Klinder, A.; Fava, F.; Napolitano, A.; Fogliano, V.; Leonard, C.; Gibson, G.R.; Tuohy, K.M. Whole-grain wheat breakfast cereal has a prebiotic effect on the human gut microbiota: A double-blind, placebo-controlled, crossover study. *Br. J. Nutr.* **2008**, *99*, 110–120. [CrossRef] [PubMed]
5.   Giacco, R.; Clemente, G.; Cipriano, D.; Luongo, D.; Viscovo, D.; Patti, L.; Di Marino, L.; Giacco, A.; Naviglio, D.; Bianchi, M.A.; et al. Effects of the regular consumption of wholemeal wheat foods on cardiovascular risk factors in healthy people. *Nutr. Metab. Cardiovasc. Dis. NMCD* **2010**, *20*, 186–194. [CrossRef] [PubMed]
6.   Juntunen, K.S.; Laaksonen, D.E.; Poutanen, K.S.; Niskanen, L.K.; Mykkanen, H.M. High-fiber rye bread and insulin secretion and sensitivity in healthy postmenopausal women. *Am. J. Clin. Nutr.* **2003**, *77*, 385–391. [PubMed]
7.   Kelly, S.A.; Summerbell, C.D.; Brynes, A.; Whittaker, V.; Frost, G. Wholegrain cereals for coronary heart disease. *Cochrane Database Syst. Rev.* **2007**, *18*, CD005051.
8.   Aune, D.; Norat, T.; Romundstad, P.; Vatten, L.J. Whole grain and refined grain consumption and the risk of type 2 diabetes: A systematic review and dose-response meta-analysis of cohort studies. *Eur. J. Epidemiol.* **2013**, *28*, 845–858. [CrossRef] [PubMed]
9.   Ye, E.Q.; Chacko, S.A.; Chou, E.L.; Kugizaki, M.; Liu, S. Greater whole-grain intake is associated with lower risk of type 2 diabetes, cardiovascular disease, and weight gain. *J. Nutr.* **2012**, *142*, 1304–1313. [CrossRef] [PubMed]
10.  Aune, D.; Chan, D.S.; Lau, R.; Vieira, R.; Greenwood, D.C.; Kampman, E.; Norat, T. Dietary fibre, whole grains, and risk of colorectal cancer: Systematic review and dose-response meta-analysis of prospective studies. *BMJ* **2011**, *343*, d6617. [CrossRef] [PubMed]
11.  Fardet, A. New hypotheses for the health-protective mechanisms of whole-grain cereals: What is beyond fibre? *Nutr. Res. Rev.* **2010**, *23*, 65–134. [CrossRef] [PubMed]
12.  Nettleton, J.A.; McKeown, N.M.; Kanoni, S.; Lemaitre, R.N.; Hivert, M.F.; Ngwa, J.; van Rooij, F.J.; Sonestedt, E.; Wojczynski, M.K.; Ye, Z.; et al. Interactions of dietary whole-grain intake with fasting glucose- and insulin-related genetic loci in individuals of european descent: A meta-analysis of 14 cohort studies. *Diabetes Care* **2010**, *33*, 2684–2691. [CrossRef] [PubMed]
13.  Wells, G.A.; Shea, B.; O'Connell, D.; Peterson, J.; Welch, V.; Losos, M.; Tugwell, P. *The Newcastle-Ottawa Scale (nos) for Assessing the Quality of Nonrandomised Studies in Meta-Analyses*; Ottawa Health Research Institute: Ottawa, ON, Canada, 1999.
14.  The Journal of the American Medical Association. *Author Instructions: Systeme International (si) Conversion Factors for Selected Laboratory Components*; The Journal of the American Medical Association: Berlin, Germany, 2001.
15.  Higgins, J.P.T.; Green, S. *Cochrane Handbook for Systematic Reviews of Interventions Version 5.1.0 (Updated March 2011)*; The Cochrane Collaboration: London, UK, 2011.
16.  Higgins, J.P.; Thompson, S.G.; Deeks, J.J.; Altman, D.G. Measuring inconsistency in meta-analyses. *BMJ* **2003**, *327*, 557–560. [CrossRef] [PubMed]
17.  Johansson, D.P.; Lee, I.; Riserus, U.; Langton, M.; Landberg, R. Effects of unfermented and fermented whole grain rye crisp breads served as part of a standardized breakfast, on appetite and postprandial glucose and insulin responses: A randomized cross-over trial. *PLoS ONE* **2015**, *10*, e0122241. [CrossRef] [PubMed]

18. Alminger, M.; Eklund-Jonsson, C. Whole-grain cereal products based on a high-fibre barley or oat genotype lower post-prandial glucose and insulin responses in healthy humans. *Eur. J. Nutr.* **2008**, *47*, 294–300. [CrossRef] [PubMed]

19. Hlebowicz, J.; Wickenberg, J.; Fahlstrom, R.; Bjorgell, O.; Almer, L.O.; Darwiche, G. Effect of commercial breakfast fibre cereals compared with corn flakes on postprandial blood glucose, gastric emptying and satiety in healthy subjects: A randomized blinded crossover trial. *Nutr. J.* **2007**, *6*, 22. [CrossRef] [PubMed]

20. Nilsson, A.C.; Ostman, E.M.; Granfeldt, Y.; Bjorck, I.M. Effect of cereal test breakfasts differing in glycemic index and content of indigestible carbohydrates on daylong glucose tolerance in healthy subjects. *Am. J. Clin. Nutr.* **2008**, *87*, 645–654. [PubMed]

21. Rosen, L.A.; Silva, L.O.; Andersson, U.K.; Holm, C.; Ostman, E.M.; Bjorck, I.M. Endosperm and whole grain rye breads are characterized by low post-prandial insulin response and a beneficial blood glucose profile. *Nutr. J.* **2009**, *8*, 42. [CrossRef] [PubMed]

22. Rosen, L.A.; Ostman, E.M.; Bjorck, I.M. Effects of cereal breakfasts on postprandial glucose, appetite regulation and voluntary energy intake at a subsequent standardized lunch; focusing on rye products. *Nutr. J.* **2011**, *10*, 7. [CrossRef] [PubMed]

23. Andersson, A.; Tengblad, S.; Karlstrom, B.; Kamal-Eldin, A.; Landberg, R.; Basu, S.; Aman, P.; Vessby, B. Whole-grain foods do not affect insulin sensitivity or markers of lipid peroxidation and inflammation in healthy, moderately overweight subjects. *J. Nutr.* **2007**, *137*, 1401–1407. [PubMed]

24. Hlebowicz, J.; Jonsson, J.M.; Lindstedt, S.; Bjorgell, O.; Darwich, G.; Almer, L.O. Effect of commercial rye whole-meal bread on postprandial blood glucose and gastric emptying in healthy subjects. *Nutr. J.* **2009**, *8*, 26. [CrossRef] [PubMed]

25. Leinonen, K.; Liukkonen, K.; Poutanen, K.; Uusitupa, M.; Mykkanen, H. Rye bread decreases postprandial insulin response but does not alter glucose response in healthy finnish subjects. *Eur. J. Clin. Nutr.* **1999**, *53*, 262–267. [CrossRef] [PubMed]

26. Juntunen, K.S.; Niskanen, L.K.; Liukkonen, K.H.; Poutanen, K.S.; Holst, J.J.; Mykkanen, H.M. Postprandial glucose, insulin, and incretin responses to grain products in healthy subjects. *Am. J. Clin. Nutr.* **2002**, *75*, 254–262. [PubMed]

27. Juntunen, K.S.; Laaksonen, D.E.; Autio, K.; Niskanen, L.K.; Holst, J.J.; Savolainen, K.E.; Liukkonen, K.H.; Poutanen, K.S.; Mykkanen, H.M. Structural differences between rye and wheat breads but not total fiber content may explain the lower postprandial insulin response to rye bread. *Am. J. Clin. Nutr.* **2003**, *78*, 957–964. [PubMed]

28. Lappi, J.; Aura, A.M.; Katina, K.; Nordlund, E.; Kolehmainen, M.; Mykkanen, H.; Poutanen, K. Comparison of postprandial phenolic acid excretions and glucose responses after ingestion of breads with bioprocessed or native rye bran. *Food Funct.* **2013**, *4*, 972–981. [CrossRef] [PubMed]

29. Moazzami, A.A.; Shrestha, A.; Morrison, D.A.; Poutanen, K.; Mykkanen, H. Metabolomics reveals differences in postprandial responses to breads and fasting metabolic characteristics associated with postprandial insulin demand in postmenopausal women. *J. Nutr.* **2014**, *144*, 807–814. [CrossRef] [PubMed]

30. Mofidi, A.; Ferraro, Z.M.; Stewart, K.A.; Tulk, H.M.; Robinson, L.E.; Duncan, A.M.; Graham, T.E. The acute impact of ingestion of sourdough and whole-grain breads on blood glucose, insulin, and incretins in overweight and obese men. *J. Nutr. Metab.* **2012**, *2012*, 184710. [CrossRef] [PubMed]

31. Luhovyy, B.L.; Mollard, R.C.; Yurchenko, S.; Nunez, M.F.; Berengut, S.; Liu, T.T.; Smith, C.E.; Pelkman, C.L.; Anderson, G.H. The effects of whole grain high-amylose maize flour as a source of resistant starch on blood glucose, satiety, and food intake in young men. *J. Food Sci.* **2014**, *79*, H2550–H2556. [CrossRef] [PubMed]

32. MacKay, K.A.; Tucker, A.J.; Duncan, A.M.; Graham, T.E.; Robinson, L.E. Whole grain wheat sourdough bread does not affect plasminogen activator inhibitor-1 in adults with normal or impaired carbohydrate metabolism. *Nutr. Metab. Cardiovasc. Dis. NMCD* **2012**, *22*, 704–711. [CrossRef] [PubMed]

33. Najjar, A.M.; Parsons, P.M.; Duncan, A.M.; Robinson, L.E.; Yada, R.Y.; Graham, T.E. The acute impact of ingestion of breads of varying composition on blood glucose, insulin and incretins following first and second meals. *Br. J. Nutr.* **2009**, *101*, 391–398. [CrossRef] [PubMed]

34. Vuksan, V.; Jenkins, A.L.; Dias, A.G.; Lee, A.S.; Jovanovski, E.; Rogovik, A.L.; Hanna, A. Reduction in postprandial glucose excursion and prolongation of satiety: Possible explanation of the long-term effects of whole grain Salba (Salvia Hispanica L.). *Eur. J. Clin. Nutr.* **2010**, *64*, 436–438. [CrossRef] [PubMed]

35. Brownlee, I.A.; Moore, C.; Chatfield, M.; Richardson, D.P.; Ashby, P.; Kuznesof, S.A.; Jebb, S.A.; Seal, C.J. Markers of cardiovascular risk are not changed by increased whole-grain intake: The wholeheart study, a randomised, controlled dietary intervention. *Br. J. Nutr.* **2010**, *104*, 125–134. [CrossRef] [PubMed]

36. Ampatzoglou, A.; Atwal, K.K.; Maidens, C.M.; Williams, C.L.; Ross, A.B.; Thielecke, F.; Jonnalagadda, S.S.; Kennedy, O.B.; Yaqoob, P. Increased whole grain consumption does not affect blood biochemistry, body composition, or gut microbiology in healthy, low-habitual whole grain consumers. *J. Nutr.* **2015**, *145*, 215–221. [CrossRef] [PubMed]

37. Tighe, P.; Duthie, G.; Vaughan, N.; Brittenden, J.; Simpson, W.G.; Duthie, S.; Mutch, W.; Wahle, K.; Horgan, G.; Thies, F. Effect of increased consumption of whole-grain foods on blood pressure and other cardiovascular risk markers in healthy middle-aged persons: A randomized controlled trial. *Am. J. Clin. Nutr.* **2010**, *92*, 733–740. [CrossRef] [PubMed]

38. Ampatzoglou, A.; Williams, C.L.; Atwal, K.K.; Maidens, C.M.; Ross, A.B.; Thielecke, F.; Jonnalagadda, S.S.; Kennedy, O.B.; Yaqoob, P. Effects of increased wholegrain consumption on immune and inflammatory markers in healthy low habitual wholegrain consumers. *Eur. J. Nutr.* **2016**, *55*, 183–195. [CrossRef] [PubMed]

39. McIntosh, G.H.; Noakes, M.; Royle, P.J.; Foster, P.R. Whole-grain rye and wheat foods and markers of bowel health in overweight middle-aged men. *Am. J. Clin. Nutr.* **2003**, *77*, 967–974. [PubMed]

40. Keogh, J.; Atkinson, F.; Eisenhauer, B.; Inamdar, A.; Brand-Miller, J. Food intake, postprandial glucose, insulin and subjective satiety responses to three different bread-based test meals. *Appetite* **2011**, *57*, 707–710. [CrossRef] [PubMed]

41. Stefoska-Needham, A.; Beck, E.J.; Johnson, S.K.; Chu, J.; Tapsell, L.C. Flaked sorghum biscuits increase postprandial glp-1 and gip levels and extend subjective satiety in healthy subjects. *Mol. Nutr. Food Res.* **2016**, *60*, 1118–1128. [CrossRef] [PubMed]

42. Kristensen, M.; Toubro, S.; Jensen, M.G.; Ross, A.B.; Riboldi, G.; Petronio, M.; Bugel, S.; Tetens, I.; Astrup, A. Whole grain compared with refined wheat decreases the percentage of body fat following a 12-week, energy-restricted dietary intervention in postmenopausal women. *J. Nutr.* **2012**, *142*, 710–716. [CrossRef] [PubMed]

43. Bakhoj, S.; Flint, A.; Holst, J.J.; Tetens, I. Lower glucose-dependent insulinotropic polypeptide (gip) response but similar glucagon-like peptide 1 (glp-1), glycaemic, and insulinaemic response to ancient wheat compared to modern wheat depends on processing. *Eur. J. Clin. Nutr.* **2003**, *57*, 1254–1261. [CrossRef] [PubMed]

44. Kristensen, M.; Jensen, M.G.; Riboldi, G.; Petronio, M.; Bugel, S.; Toubro, S.; Tetens, I.; Astrup, A. Wholegrain vs. Refined wheat bread and pasta. Effect on postprandial glycemia, appetite, and subsequent ad libitum energy intake in young healthy adults. *Appetite* **2010**, *54*, 163–169. [CrossRef] [PubMed]

45. Vitaglione, P.; Mennella, I.; Ferracane, R.; Rivellese, A.A.; Giacco, R.; Ercolini, D.; Gibbons, S.M.; La Storia, A.; Gilbert, J.A.; Jonnalagadda, S.; et al. Whole-grain wheat consumption reduces inflammation in a randomized controlled trial on overweight and obese subjects with unhealthy dietary and lifestyle behaviors: Role of polyphenols bound to cereal dietary fiber. *Am. J. Clin. Nutr.* **2015**, *101*, 251–261. [CrossRef] [PubMed]

46. Casiraghi, M.C.; Garsetti, M.; Testolin, G.; Brighenti, F. Post-prandial responses to cereal products enriched with barley beta-glucan. *J. Am. Coll. Nutr.* **2006**, *25*, 313–320. [CrossRef] [PubMed]

47. Saltzman, E.; Das, S.K.; Lichtenstein, A.H.; Dallal, G.E.; Corrales, A.; Schaefer, E.J.; Greenberg, A.S.; Roberts, S.B. An oat-containing hypocaloric diet reduces systolic blood pressure and improves lipid profile beyond effects of weight loss in men and women. *J. Nutr.* **2001**, *131*, 1465–1470. [PubMed]

48. Pereira, M.A.; Jacobs, D.R., Jr.; Pins, J.J.; Raatz, S.K.; Gross, M.D.; Slavin, J.L.; Seaquist, E.R. Effect of whole grains on insulin sensitivity in overweight hyperinsulinemic adults. *Am. J. Clin. Nutr.* **2002**, *75*, 848–855. [PubMed]

49. Poquette, N.M.; Gu, X.; Lee, S.O. Grain sorghum muffin reduces glucose and insulin responses in men. *Food Funct.* **2014**, *5*, 894–899. [CrossRef] [PubMed]

50. Rave, K.; Roggen, K.; Dellweg, S.; Heise, T.; Tom Dieck, H. Improvement of insulin resistance after diet with a whole-grain based dietary product: Results of a randomized, controlled cross-over study in obese subjects with elevated fasting blood glucose. *Br. J. Nutr.* **2007**, *98*, 929–936. [CrossRef] [PubMed]

51. Li, J.; Kaneko, T.; Qin, L.Q.; Wang, J.; Wang, Y. Effects of barley intake on glucose tolerance, lipid metabolism, and bowel function in women. *Nutrition* **2003**, *19*, 926–929. [CrossRef]

52. Zafar, T.A.; Al-Hassawi, F.; Al-Khulaifi, F.; Al-Rayyes, G.; Waslien, C.; Huffman, F.G. Organoleptic and glycemic properties of chickpea-wheat composite breads. *J. Food Sci. Technol.* **2015**, *52*, 2256–2263. [CrossRef] [PubMed]

53. Soong, Y.Y.; Quek, R.Y.; Henry, C.J. Glycemic potency of muffins made with wheat, rice, corn, oat and barley flours: A comparative study between in vivo and in vitro. *Eur. J. Nutr.* **2015**, *54*, 1281–1285. [CrossRef] [PubMed]

54. Gonzalez-Anton, C.; Rico, M.C.; Sanchez-Rodriguez, E.; Ruiz-Lopez, M.D.; Gil, A.; Mesa, M.D. Glycemic responses, appetite ratings and gastrointestinal hormone responses of most common breads consumed in spain. A randomized control trial in healthy humans. *Nutrients* **2015**, *7*, 4033–4053. [CrossRef] [PubMed]

55. Ross, A.B.; Bruce, S.J.; Blondel-Lubrano, A.; Oguey-Araymon, S.; Beaumont, M.; Bourgeois, A.; Nielsen-Moennoz, C.; Vigo, M.; Fay, L.B.; Kochhar, S.; et al. A whole-grain cereal-rich diet increases plasma betaine, and tends to decrease total and ldl-cholesterol compared with a refined-grain diet in healthy subjects. *Br. J. Nutr.* **2011**, *105*, 1492–1502. [CrossRef] [PubMed]

56. Granfeldt, Y.; Wu, X.; Bjorck, I. Determination of glycaemic index; some methodological aspects related to the analysis of carbohydrate load and characteristics of the previous evening meal. *Eur. J. Clin. Nutr.* **2006**, *60*, 104–112. [CrossRef] [PubMed]

57. Ardisson Korat, A.V.; Willett, W.C.; Hu, F.B. Diet, lifestyle, and genetic risk factors for type 2 diabetes: A review from the nurses' health study, nurses' health study 2, and health professionals' follow-up study. *Curr. Nutr. Rep.* **2014**, *3*, 345–354. [CrossRef] [PubMed]

58. Sahyoun, N.R.; Jacques, P.F.; Zhang, X.L.; Juan, W.; McKeown, N.N. Whole-grain intake is inversely associated with the metabolic syndrome and mortality in older adults. *Am. J. Clin. Nutr.* **2006**, *83*, 124–131. [PubMed]

59. Aune, D.; Keum, N.; Giovannucci, E.; Fadnes, L.T.; Boffetta, P.; Greenwood, D.C.; Tonstad, S.; Vatten, L.J.; Riboli, E.; Norat, T. Whole grain consumption and risk of cardiovascular disease, cancer, and all cause and cause specific mortality: Systematic review and dose-response meta-analysis of prospective studies. *BMJ* **2016**, *353*, i2716. [CrossRef] [PubMed]

60. Willett, W.; Manson, J.; Liu, S. Glycemic index, glycemic load, and risk of type 2 diabetes. *Am. J. Clin. Nutr.* **2002**, *76*, 274S–280S. [PubMed]

61. Lopez-Alarcon, M.; Perichart-Perera, O.; Flores-Huerta, S.; Inda-Icaza, P.; Rodriguez-Cruz, M.; Armenta-Alvarez, A.; Bram-Falcon, M.T.; Mayorga-Ochoa, M. Excessive refined carbohydrates and scarce micronutrients intakes increase inflammatory mediators and insulin resistance in prepubertal and pubertal obese children independently of obesity. *Mediat. Inflamm.* **2014**, *2014*, 849031. [CrossRef] [PubMed]

62. Liese, A.D.; Roach, A.K.; Sparks, K.C.; Marquart, L.; D'Agostino, R.B., Jr.; Mayer-Davis, E.J. Whole-grain intake and insulin sensitivity: The insulin resistance atherosclerosis study. *Am. J. Clin. Nutr.* **2003**, *78*, 965–971. [PubMed]

63. Meynier, A.; Goux, A.; Atkinson, F.; Brack, O.; Vinoy, S. Postprandial glycaemic response: How is it influenced by characteristics of cereal products? *Br. J. Nutr.* **2015**, *113*, 1931–1939. [CrossRef] [PubMed]

64. Steffen, L.M.; Jacobs, D.R., Jr.; Murtaugh, M.A.; Moran, A.; Steinberger, J.; Hong, C.P.; Sinaiko, A.R. Whole grain intake is associated with lower body mass and greater insulin sensitivity among adolescents. *Am. J. Epidemiol.* **2003**, *158*, 243–250. [CrossRef] [PubMed]

65. Canfora, E.E.; Jocken, J.W.; Blaak, E.E. Short-chain fatty acids in control of body weight and insulin sensitivity. *Nat. Rev. Endocrinol.* **2015**, *11*, 577–591. [CrossRef] [PubMed]

66. Robertson, R.P. Chronic oxidative stress as a central mechanism for glucose toxicity in pancreatic islet beta cells in diabetes. *J. Biol. Chem.* **2004**, *8*, 42351–42354. [CrossRef] [PubMed]

67. Ohnishi, M.; Matuo, T.; Tsuno, T.; Hosoda, A.; Nomura, E.; Taniguchi, H.; Sasaki, H.; Morishita, H. Antioxidant activity and hypoglycemic effect of ferulic acid in stz-induced diabetic mice and kk-ay mice. *BioFactors* **2004**, *21*, 315–319. [CrossRef] [PubMed]

68. Marventano, S.; Kolacz, P.; Castellano, S.; Galvano, F.; Buscemi, S.; Mistretta, A.; Grosso, G. A review of recent evidence in human studies of n-3 and n-6 pufa intake on cardiovascular disease, cancer, and depressive disorders: Does the ratio really matter? *Int. J. Food Sci. Nutr.* **2015**, *66*, 611–622. [CrossRef] [PubMed]

69. Food and Agriculture Organization of the United Nations (FAOSTAT). *Cereal Production*; Food and Agriculture Organization of the United Nations: Rome, Italy, 2016.

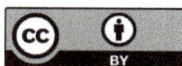

MDPI

St. Alban-Anlage 66

4052 Basel

Switzerland

Tel. +41 61 683 77 34

Fax +41 61 302 89 18

www.mdpi.com

*Nutrients* Editorial Office

E-mail: nutrients@mdpi.com

www.mdpi.com/journal/nutrients

www.ingramcontent.com/pod-product-compliance
Lightning Source LLC
Chambersburg PA
CBHW051704210326
41597CB00032B/5367